ircebook, 2nd Edition
ehold Safety Sourcebook
ine System Disorders Sourcebook
& Toddler Health Sourcebook
ious Diseases Sourcebook
y & Trauma Sourcebook
Kidney & Urinary Tract Diseases & Disorders Sourcebook
Learning Disabilities Sourcebook, 2nd Edition
Leukemia Sourcebook
Liver Disorders Sourcebook
Lung Disorders Sourcebook
Medical Tests Sourcebook, 2nd Edition
Men's Health Concerns Sourcebook, 2nd Edition
Mental Health Disorders Sourcebook, 2nd Edition
Mental Retardation Sourcebook
Movement Disorders Sourcebook
Obesity Sourcebook
Osteoporosis Sourcebook
Pain Sourcebook, 2nd Edition
Pediatric Cancer Sourcebook
Physical & Mental Issues in Aging Sourcebook
Podiatry Sourcebook
Pregnancy & Birth Sourcebook, 2nd Edition
Prostate Cancer
Public Health Sourcebook
Reconstructive & Cosmetic Surgery Sourcebook
Rehabilitation Sourcebook
Respiratory Diseases & Disorders Sourcebook
Sexually Transmitted Diseases Sourcebook, 2nd Edition
Skin
Sleep D
Sports I
Stress-Related Disorders Sourcebook
Stroke Sourcebook
Substance Abuse Sourcebook
Surgery Sourcebook
Transplantation Sourcebook
Traveler's Health Sourcebook
Vegetarian Sourcebook
Women's Health Concerns Sourcebook, 2nd Edition
Workplace Health & Safety Sourcebook
Worldwide Health Sourcebook

Teen Health Series

Cancer Information for Teens
Diet Information for Teens
Drug Information for Teens
Fitness Information for Teens
Mental Health Information for Teens
Sexual Health Information for Teens
Skin Health Information for Teens
Sports Injuries Information for Teens

Contagious Diseases
SOURCEBOOK

Health Reference Series

First Edition

Contagious Diseases SOURCEBOOK

Basic Consumer Health Information about Infectious Diseases Spread by Person-to-Person Contact through Direct Touch, Airborne Transmission, Sexual Contact, or Contact with Blood or Other Body Fluids, Including Hepatitis, Herpes, Influenza, Lice, Measles, Mumps, Pinworm, Ringworm, Severe Acute Respiratory Syndrome (SARS), Streptococcal Infections, Tuberculosis, and Others

Along with Facts about Disease Transmission, Antimicrobial Resistance, and Vaccines, with a Glossary and Directories of Resources for More Information

Edited by
Karen Bellenir

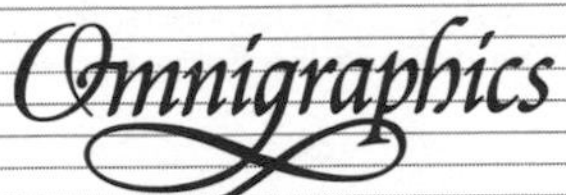

615 Griswold Street • Detroit, MI 48226

Bibliographic Note

Because this page cannot legibly accommodate all the copyright notices, the Bibliographic Note portion of the Preface constitutes an extension of the copyright notice.

Edited by Karen Bellenir

Health Reference Series

Karen Bellenir, *Managing Editor*
David A. Cooke, M.D., *Medical Consultant*
Elizabeth Barbour, *Permissions Associate*
Dawn Matthews, *Verification Assistant*
Laura Pleva Nielsen, *Index Editor*
EdIndex, Services for Publishers, *Indexers*

* * *

Omnigraphics, Inc.

Matthew P. Barbour, *Senior Vice President*
Kay Gill, *Vice President—Directories*
Kevin Hayes, *Operations Manager*
Leif Gruenberg, *Development Manager*
David P. Bianco, *Marketing Director*

* * *

Peter E. Ruffner, *Publisher*

Frederick G. Ruffner, Jr., *Chairman*

ISBN 0-7808-0736-7

Library of Congress Cataloging-in-Publication Data

Contagious diseases sourcebook : basic consumer health information about infectious diseases spread by person-to-person contact through direct touch, airborne transmission, sexual contact, or contact with blood or other body fluids, including hepatitis, herpes, influenza, lice, measles, mumps, pinworm, ringworm, severe acute respiratory syndrome (SARS), streptococcal infections, tuberculosis, and others; along with facts about disease transmission, antimicrobial resistance, and vaccines, with a glossary and directories of resources for more information / edited by Karen Bellenir.-- 1st ed.
p. cm. -- (Health reference series)
Includes index.
ISBN 0-7808-0736-7 (hardcover : alk. paper)
1. Communicable diseases--Popular works. I. Bellenir, Karen. II. Series.
RC113.C664 2004
616.9--dc22

2004010210

This book is printed on acid-free paper meeting the ANSI Z39.48 Standard. The infinity symbol that appears above indicates that the paper in this book meets that standard.

Printed in the United States

Table of Contents

Part III: Viral Diseases

Part IV: Parasitic, Fungal, and Other Diseases

Part V: Vaccination Information

Part VI: Additional Help and Information

Preface

About This Book

From early in human history—perhaps from the very beginning—and continuing to the present day, contagious diseases have caused human suffering and death. Ancient Egyptian writings describe smallpox and polio. European records document a syphilis outbreak in the late fifteenth century. An influenza virus killed more than 20 million people worldwide in 1918–1919, and the human immunodeficiency virus (HIV), which was identified in 1984, resulted in 36.1 million deaths during the years that led to the close of the 20th century, and the epidemic is far from over. As of the end of 2003, an estimated 40 million people around the world were living with HIV.

Disease-causing microbes, such as bacteria, viruses, fungi, and parasites, lead to a wide variety of illnesses. Some may produce mild symptoms or even no symptoms; others can lead to chronic disorders or be life threatening. As recently as a generation ago, people believed that vaccinations, antibiotics, and improved sanitation would triumph over contagious diseases. The fight against afflictions such as smallpox, pertussis, polio, tuberculosis, pneumonia, and streptococcal infections seemed like it could be won. Despite the successes, however, contagious diseases still pose a significant threat. For example,

- Chlamydia, one of the most widespread bacterial diseases transmitted by sexual contact, infects more than four million people in the United States every year. Related health care costs exceed $2 billion.

- Tuberculosis (TB), an airborne disease that is spread when people cough, sneeze, speak, sing, or laugh, infects two billion people worldwide—approximately one-third of the global population. Most infections are latent (without symptoms), but every year eight million people develop active TB and three million die. In the United States, TB is re-emerging as a public health concern, and some newly identified strains are resistant to traditional medications.
- Influenza viruses cause disease epidemics almost every winter. In the United States, the peak of flu season can occur anywhere from late December through March, and annual flu outbreaks result in 114,000 hospitalizations and 36,000 deaths.

Contagious Diseases Sourcebook provides information about bacterial, viral, fungal, parasitic, and other diseases spread by person-to-person contact. It explains what microbes are, how they cause disease, how they are spread and treated, and how the risk of contracting contagious illnesses can be reduced through techniques like handwashing, using a condom, or vaccination. The problem of antimicrobial resistance is described, and steps that need to be taken to lessen its potential impact on future disease control efforts are explained. A section on vaccination tells how immunity is acquired through vaccines, discusses vaccine safety, provides facts about research related to vaccines, and gives current immunization schedules for children, adolescents, and adults. A glossary of terms related to contagious diseases and directories of additional resources are also included.

Readers seeking information about infectious diseases spread by means other than person-to-person contact, including through contaminated food and drinking water, by insects and animals, or by contact with microorganisms in the environment, may wish to consult *Infectious Diseases Sourcebook,* a separate volume in the *Health Reference Series*.

How to Use This Book

This book is divided into parts and chapters. Parts focus on broad areas of interest. Chapters are devoted to single topics within a part.

Part I: What You Need to Know about Germs provides basic information about various types of microbes, including bacteria, viruses, and parasites. It explains the diseases they cause and outlines steps that can be taken to minimize exposure risks. The use of antibiotics to combat infectious diseases, the resulting problem of antimicrobial resistance, and steps being taken to preserve the effectiveness of current antibiotics are also explained.

Part II: Bacterial Diseases describes contagious diseases caused by bacteria, including chlamydia, diphtheria, gonorrhea, streptococcal disease, tuberculosis, and many others. Individual chapters describe the organism responsible for the disease, how it is spread, symptoms, and current treatment options.

Part III: Viral Diseases describes contagious diseases caused by viruses, including chickenpox, hepatitis, herpes, influenza, measles, polio, and smallpox. Individual chapters explain the different disease-causing viruses, their modes of transmission, symptoms, and treatments.

Part IV: Parasitic, Fungal, and Other Diseases explains the causes, symptoms, and treatments of some of the most commonly occurring diseases associated with parasites, prions, and fungal infections. These include tinea infections (which are responsible for ringworm, athlete's foot, jock itch, and nail fungus), cryptosporidiosis, lice, pinworm, and scabies.

Part V: Vaccination Information provides facts about the use of immunizations to combat contagious diseases. It includes recommended vaccination schedules for children, adolescents, and adults and explains issues related to vaccine safety.

Part VI: Additional Help and Information includes a glossary of terms and directories of resources for more information about contagious diseases, antimicrobial resistance, vaccines, and vaccine safety.

Bibliographic Note

This volume contains documents and excerpts from publications issued by the National Institutes of Health (NIH) and its subagencies, including the National Institute of Allergy and Infectious Diseases (NIAID) and its Division of Microbiology and Infectious Diseases; the National Institute on Drug Abuse (NIDA), and the National Institute of Neurological Disorders and Stroke (NINDS). Also included are documents and excerpts from publications issued by the Centers for Disease Control and Prevention (CDC) and its subagencies, including: *Morbidity and Mortality Weekly Report*; the National Center for Infectious Diseases (NCID) and its Division of Bacterial and Mycotic Diseases and

Division of Parasitic Diseases; the National Immunization Program (NIP); and Public Health Emergency Preparedness and Response. Additional information is included from other U.S. government agencies, including: Health Resources and Services Administration (HRSA); National Hansen's Disease Programs; President's Council on Physical Fitness and Sports, *Research Digest*; U.S. Department of Health and Human Services (HHS); and the U.S. Food and Drug Administration (FDA).

In addition, this volume contains copyrighted documents from the following organizations and individuals: A.D.A.M., Inc.; Alliance for the Prudent Use of Antibiotics; American Academy of Dermatology; American Association of Blood Banks; American Lung Association; American Osteopathic College of Dermatology; Association for Professionals in Infection Control and Epidemiology; Hepatitis Foundation; Jere Mammino, DO; March of Dimes Birth Defects Foundation; National Foundation for Infectious Disease; Nemours Center for Children's Health Media, a division of The Nemours Foundation; New York State Department of Health; University of Iowa's Virtual Children's Hospital; Wisconsin Department of Health and Family Services; and the World Health Organization.

Full citation information is provided on the first page of each chapter. Every effort has been made to secure all necessary rights to reprint the copyrighted material. If any omissions have been made, please contact Omnigraphics to make corrections for future editions.

Acknowledgements

In addition to the organizations, agencies, and individuals listed above, special thanks go to many others who have worked hard to help bring this book to fruition. They include editorial assistant Michael Bellenir, permissions associate Liz Barbour, and indexer Edward J. Prucha.

Note from the Editor

This book is part of Omnigraphics' *Health Reference Series*. The *Series* provides basic information about a broad range of medical concerns. It is not intended to serve as a tool for diagnosing illness, in prescribing treatments, or as a substitute for the physician/patient relationship. All persons concerned about medical symptoms or the possibility of disease are encouraged to seek professional care from an appropriate health care provider.

Our Advisory Board

The *Health Reference Series* is reviewed by an Advisory Board comprised of librarians from public, academic, and medical libraries. We would like to thank the following board members for providing guidance to the development of this series:

Dr. Lynda Baker,
Associate Professor of Library and Information Science,
Wayne State University, Detroit, MI

Nancy Bulgarelli,
William Beaumont Hospital Library, Royal Oak, MI

Karen Imarisio,
Bloomfield Township Public Library, Bloomfield Township, MI

Karen Morgan,
Mardigian Library, University of Michigan-Dearborn,
Dearborn, MI

Rosemary Orlando,
St. Clair Shores Public Library, St. Clair Shores, MI

Medical Consultant

Medical consultation services are provided to the *Health Reference Series* editors by David A. Cooke, M.D. Dr. Cooke is a graduate of Brandeis University, and he received his M.D. degree from the University of Michigan. He completed residency training at the University of Wisconsin Hospital and Clinics. He is board-certified in Internal Medicine. Dr. Cooke currently works as part of the University of Michigan Health System and practices in Brighton, MI. In his free time, he enjoys writing, science fiction, and spending time with his family.

Health Reference Series *Update Policy*

The inaugural book in the *Health Reference Series* was the first edition of *Cancer Sourcebook* published in 1989. Since then, the *Series* has been enthusiastically received by librarians and in the medical community. In order to maintain the standard of providing high-quality health information for the layperson the editorial staff at Omnigraphics felt it was necessary to implement a policy of updating volumes when warranted.

Medical researchers have been making tremendous strides, and it is the purpose of the *Health Reference Series* to stay current with the most recent advances. Each decision to update a volume will be made on an individual basis. Some of the considerations will include how much new information is available and the feedback we receive from people who use the books. If there is a topic you would like to see added to the update list, or an area of medical concern you feel has not been adequately addressed, please write to:

Editor
Health Reference Series
Omnigraphics, Inc.
615 Griswold Street
Detroit, MI 48226
E-mail: editorial@omnigraphics.com

Part One

What You Need to Know about Germs

Chapter 1

How Microbes Make Us Sick

What Are Microbes?

Microbes are tiny organisms—too tiny to see without a microscope, yet they are abundant on Earth. They live everywhere—in air, soil, rock, and water. Some of them live happily in searing heat, and others in freezing cold. Like humans, some microbes need oxygen to live, but others cannot exist with it. These microscopic organisms are in plants, animals, and in the human body.

Some microbes cause disease in humans, plants, and animals. Others are essential for a healthy life, and we could not exist without them. Indeed, the relationship between microbes and humans is very delicate and complex. In this chapter, we will learn that some microbes keep us healthy while others can make us sick.

Most microbes belong to one of four major groups: bacteria, viruses, fungi, or protozoa. A familiar, often-used word for microbes that cause disease is "germs." Some people refer to disease-causing microbes as "bugs." "I've got the flu bug," for example, is a phrase you may hear during the wintertime to describe an influenza virus infection.

Since the 19th century, we have known microbes cause infectious diseases. Near the end of the 20th century, researchers began to learn that microbes also contribute to many chronic diseases and conditions. Mounting scientific evidence strongly links them to some forms of

---

"Microbes in Sickness and in Health," National Institute of Allergy and Infectious Diseases (NIAID), National Institutes of Health (NIH), September 2001.

cancer, coronary artery disease, diabetes, multiple sclerosis, autism, and chronic lung diseases.

Bacteria

Microbes belonging to the bacteria group are made up of only one cell. Under a microscope, bacteria look like balls, rods, or spirals. Bacteria are so small that a line of 1,000 could fit across the eraser of a pencil. Life in any form on Earth could not exist without these tiny cells.

Scientists have discovered fossilized remains of bacteria that date back more than 3.5 billion years, placing them among the oldest living things on Earth. Bacteria inhabit a variety of environments. Psychrophiles, or cold-loving bacteria, can live in the subfreezing temperature of the Arctic. Thermophiles are heat-loving bacteria that can live in extreme heat, such as in the hot springs in Yellowstone National Park. Extreme thermophiles, or hyperthermophiles, thrive at 235 degrees Fahrenheit near volcanic vents on the ocean floor. Many bacteria prefer the milder temperature of the healthy human body.

Like humans, some bacteria (aerobic bacteria) need oxygen to survive, but others (anaerobic bacteria) do not. Amazingly, some can adapt to new environments by learning to survive with or without oxygen.

Like all living cells, each bacterium requires food for energy and building materials. There are countless numbers of bacteria on Earth—most are harmless and many are even beneficial to humans. In fact, less than 1 percent of them cause diseases in humans. For example, harmless anaerobic bacteria, such as *Lactobacilli acidophilus*, live in human intestines, where they help to digest food, destroy disease-causing microbes, fight cancer cells, and give the body needed vitamins. Healthy food products, such as yogurt, sauerkraut, and cheese, are made using bacteria.

Some bacteria produce poisons called toxins, which also can make us sick.

Are Toxins Always Harmful?

Certain bacteria give off toxins that can seriously affect your health. Botulism, a severe form of food poisoning, affects the nerves and is caused by toxins from *Clostridium botulinum* bacteria. Under certain circumstances, however, bacterial toxins can be helpful. Several vaccines that protect us from getting sick are made from bacterial toxins. One type of pertussis vaccine, which protects infants and children from whooping cough, contains toxins from *Bordetella pertussis* bacteria. This vaccine is safe and effective and causes fewer reactions than other types of pertussis vaccine.

Viruses

Viruses are among the smallest microbes, much smaller even than bacteria. Viruses are not cells. They consist of one or more molecules of DNA or RNA, which contain the virus's genes surrounded by a protein coat. Viruses can be rod-shaped, sphere-shaped, or multisided. Some look like tadpoles.

Unlike most bacteria, most viruses do cause disease because they invade living, normal cells, such as those in the human body. They then multiply and produce other viruses like themselves. Each virus is very particular about which cell it attacks. Various human viruses specifically attack particular cells in the body's organs, systems, or tissues, such as the liver, respiratory system, or blood cells.

Although types of viruses behave differently, most survive by taking over the machinery that makes a cell work. Briefly, when a single virus particle, a "virion", comes in contact with a cell it likes, it may attach to special landing sites on the surface of that cell. From there, the virus may inject molecules into the cell, or the cell may swallow up the virion. Once inside the cell, viral molecules such as DNA or RNA direct the cell to make new virus offspring. That's how a virus "infects" a cell.

Viruses can even "infect" bacteria. These viruses, called bacteriophages, may help researchers develop alternatives to antibiotic medicines for wiping out bacterial infections.

Many viral infections do not result in disease. For example, by the time most people in the United States become adults, they have been infected by cytomegalovirus (CMV). Most of these people, however, do not develop CMV disease symptoms. Other viral infections can result in deadly diseases, such as HIV infection, which causes acquired immunodeficiency syndrome (AIDS).

Fungi

A fungus is actually a primitive vegetable. Fungi can be found in air, in soil, on plants, and in water. Thousands, perhaps millions, of different types of fungi exist on Earth. The most familiar ones to us are mushrooms, yeast, mold, and mildew. Some live in the human body, usually without causing illness. In fact, only about half of all types of fungi cause disease in humans. Those conditions are called mycoses.

Mycoses can affect your skin, nails, body hair, internal organs such as the lungs, and body systems such as the nervous system. *Aspergillus fumigatus*, for example, can cause aspergillosis, a fungal infection in the respiratory system.

Some fungi have made our lives easier. Penicillin and other antibiotics, which kill harmful bacteria in our bodies, are made from fungi. Other fungi, like certain yeasts, also can be beneficial. For example, when a warm liquid like water and a food source are added to certain yeasts, the fungus ferments. The process of fermentation is essential for making healthy foods like some breads and cheeses.

Protozoa

Protozoa are a group of microscopic one-celled animals. Protozoa can be parasites or predators. In humans, protozoa usually cause disease. Some protozoa, like plankton, live in water environments and serve as food for marine animals, such as some species of whales. Protozoa also can be found on land in decaying matter and in soil, but they must have a moist environment to survive. Termites wouldn't be able to do such a good job of digesting wood without these microorganisms in their guts.

Table 1.1. Microbes in the healthy human body*

Microbe found in:	
Ear (outer)	*Aspergillus* (fungus)
Skin	*Candida* (fungus)
Small intestine	*Clostridium*
Intestines	*Escherichia coli*
Vagina	*Gardnerella vaginalis*
Stomach	*Lactobacillus*
Urethra	*Mycobacterium*
Nose	*Staphylococcus aureus*
Eye	*Staphylococcus epidermis*
Mouth	*Streptococcus salivarius*
Large intestine	*Trichomonas hominis* (protozoa)

*A selection of usually harmless microbes, some of which help keep our bodies functioning normally. If their numbers become unbalanced, however, these microbes may make us sick. All are bacteria, unless otherwise noted.

Malaria is caused by a protozoan parasite. Another protozoan parasite, *Toxoplasma gondii*, causes toxoplasmosis in humans. This is an especially troublesome infection in pregnant women because of its effects on the fetus and in people with HIV infection or other immune deficiency.

Microbes Have Bothered Us for Millennia

Microbes have probably always caused diseases in humans. Since ancient times, historians have documented some of those diseases, and present-day archeologists and microbiologists are discovering evidence of infectious disease in prehistoric human skeletons.

In a fascinating find in the late 20th century, researchers uncovered evidence in the mountains of northern Italy that prehistoric humans were troubled by microbial parasites and used natural remedies against them. Along with the frozen mummy of the "Ice Man", who lived between 3300 and 3100 B.C., scientists found a type of tree fungus containing oils that are toxic to intestinal parasites. Later in the laboratory, researchers found the eggs of a microscopic parasitic intestinal roundworm, *Trichuris trichiura* (whipworm), in his intestines.

Smallpox, which is caused by a variola virus, was described in ancient Egyptian and Chinese writings. According to some researchers, over the centuries smallpox was responsible for more deaths than all other infectious diseases combined. It killed millions of people over thousands of years before being eradicated late in the 20th century by worldwide vaccination. The last case of smallpox was recorded in 1977.

The protozoan parasite *Plasmodium* causes malaria, a tropical disease that usually is transmitted to humans during the bite of the *Anopheles* mosquito. In ancient times, this disease was mentioned in Egyptian writings called hieroglyphics and was described in detail by the Greek physician Hippocrates. Malaria ravaged invaders from the Roman Empire. Though rare in the United States, malaria remains a serious public health threat worldwide. It kills 3 million people each year, most of whom are children.

Evidence on a 1300 B.C. Egyptian stone engraving shows that poliomyelitis (polio) has been around since ancient times. In the 1990s, public health officials launched a massive international vaccination campaign to eradicate the polio virus, which causes paralysis and can be deadly. Polio has been virtually eliminated in the United States and in much of the rest of the world.

Table 1.2. Here are some other significant scientific events and advances.

Date	Event
Approximately 300 B.C.	Aristotle, Greek philosopher and scientist, studied and wrote about living organisms.
1675	Antony van Leeuwenhoek discovered bacteria.
1796	Edward Jenner laid the foundation for developing vaccines.
1848	Ignác Fülöp Semmelweis discovered simple handwashing could prevent passage of infection from one patient to another.
1857	Louis Pasteur introduced the germ theory of disease.
1867	Joseph Lister showed evidence that microbes caused disease and pioneered the use of antiseptics during surgery to kill germs.
1876	Robert Koch, by studying anthrax, showed the role of bacteria in disease.
1928	Alexander Fleming is credited with discovering penicillin.

In the 14th century, a bacterium scientists later identified as *Yersinia pestis* caused the bubonic plague, or Black Death. Bubonic plague entered Europe and Africa through infected rodents and fleas that accompanied travelers along trade routes from Mongolia. The plague epidemic spread through Europe, Africa, and the Middle East, killing about 20 million people in Europe alone. Plague is spread to humans through the bites of fleas, which pick up the bacteria while sucking blood from rodents, especially rats. In the United States, health care workers report cases of plague even today, most of which are found in the Southwest.

Viruses caused two major pandemics during the 20th century. From 1918 to 1919, the influenza virus ravaged worldwide populations. Estimates of the number of people killed during the so-called "Spanish flu" pandemic range from 20 million to 40 million. HIV, which was identified in 1984, had killed 36.1 million people worldwide by the end of 2000.

Microbes Can Make Us Sick

According to health care experts, infectious diseases caused by microbes are responsible for more deaths worldwide than any other single cause. They estimate the annual cost of medical care for treating infectious diseases in the United States alone is about $120 billion.

The science of microbiology explores how microbes work and how to control them, and it seeks ways to use that knowledge to prevent and treat the diseases microbes cause. The 20th century saw an extraordinary increase in knowledge about microbes. Microbiologists (scientists who study microbes) and other researchers scored many successes in learning how microbes cause certain infectious diseases and how to combat those microbes.

Common Microbial Causes of Diseases and Infections

Bacteria

- Diarrheal disease
- Meningitis
- Pneumonia
- Sinusitis
- Skin diseases
- Strep throat
- Tuberculosis
- Urinary tract infection
- Vaginal infections

Fungus

- Athlete's foot
- Pneumonia
- Sinusitis
- Skin diseases
- Vaginal infections

Protozoa

- Diarrheal disease
- Malaria
- Skin diseases

Virus

- Chickenpox
- Common cold
- Diarrheal disease
- Flu
- Genital herpes
- Meningitis
- Pneumonia
- Skin diseases
- Viral hepatitis

Unfortunately, microbes are much better at adapting to new environments than people are. On Earth for billions of years, microbes are constantly challenging human newcomers with ingenious new survival tactics.

- Many microbes are developing new properties to resist drug treatments that once effectively combated them. Drug resistance has become a serious problem worldwide.
- Changes in the environment have put certain human populations in contact with newly identified microbes that cause diseases never seen before or that previously occurred only in isolated populations.
- Newly emerging diseases are a growing global health concern. Since 1976, scientists have identified approximately 30 new pathogens.

Microbes Can Infect Us

Some Microbes Can Travel Through the Air

Microbes can be transmitted from person to person through the air, as in coughing or sneezing. These are common ways to get viruses that cause colds or flu or the bacterium that causes tuberculosis (TB). Interestingly, international airplane travel can expose passengers to germs not common in their own countries.

Germs Can Be Passed Directly from Person to Person

Scientists have identified more than 500 types of bacteria that live in the human mouth. Some keep the oral environment healthy, while others cause gum disease, for example. One way to transmit oral bacteria from person to person is by kissing. Microbes such as HIV, herpes simplex virus 1, and gonorrhea bacteria are examples of germs that can be transmitted directly during sexual intercourse.

You Can Pick up and Spread Germs by Touching Infectious Material

A common way for some microbes to enter the body, especially when caring for young children, is to unintentionally pass feces on your hand to your mouth or the mouths of young children. Infant diarrhea is often spread in this way. Day care workers, for example, can pass diarrhea-causing rotavirus or *Giardia lamblia* (protozoa) from one baby to the next between diaper changes and other childcare practices.

It also is possible to pick up cold viruses from shaking someone's hand or from touching surfaces such as a handrail or telephone.

A Healthy Person Can Be a Germ Carrier and Pass It on to Others

The story of "Typhoid Mary" is a famous example from medical history about how a person can pass germs on to others, yet not be affected by them. The germs in this case were *Salmonella typhi* bacteria, which cause typhoid fever and are usually spread through food or water.

Mary Mallon, an Irish immigrant who lived at the turn of the 20th century, worked as a cook for several New York City families. More than half of the first family she worked for came down with typhoid fever. Through a clever deduction, a researcher determined that the disease was caused by the family cook. He concluded that although Mary had no symptoms of the disease, she probably had had a mild typhoid infection sometime in the past. Though not sick, she still carried the bacteria and was able to spread them to others through the food she prepared.

Germs from Your Household Pet Can Make You Sick

You can catch a variety of germs from animals, especially household pets. The rabies virus, which can infect cats and dogs, is one of the most serious and deadly of these microbes. Fortunately, the rabies vaccine prevents animals from getting rabies. Vaccines also protect people from accidentally getting the virus from an animal and prevent people who have been exposed to the virus, such as through an animal bite, from getting sick.

Dog and cat saliva can contain any of more than 100 different germs that can make you sick. Pasteurella bacteria, the most common, can be transmitted through bites that break the skin causing serious, and sometimes fatal, diseases such as blood infections and meningitis.

Warm-blooded animals are not the only ones that can cause you harm. Pet reptiles such as turtles, snakes, and iguanas can transmit Salmonella bacteria to their unsuspecting owners.

Selected Diseases We Can Get Directly or Indirectly from Animals

- Anthrax
- Babesiosis
- Brucellosis
- Cat scratch disease
- Cryptosporidiosis
- Fascioliasis
- Giardiasis
- Hantavirus pulmonary syndrome

- Histoplasmosis
- Listeriosis
- Psittacosis
- Q fever
- Rabies
- Salmonellosis
- Toxocariasis
- Toxoplasmosis
- Trichinosis

You Can Get Microbes from Tiny Critters

Mosquitoes may be the most common insect carriers (vectors) of pathogens. *Anopheles* mosquitoes can pick up *Plasmodium*, which causes malaria, from the blood of an infected person and transmit the protozoan to an uninfected person.

Fleas that pick up *Yersinia pestis* bacteria from rodents can then transmit plague to humans.

Ticks, which are more closely related to crabs than to insects, are another common vector. The tiny deer tick can infect humans with *Borrelia burgdorferi*, the bacterium that causes Lyme disease, which it picks up from deer.

Microbes in the Food You Eat or Water You Drink Could Make You Sick

Every year, millions of people worldwide become ill from eating contaminated foods. Although many cases of foodborne illness or "food poisoning" are not reported, the U.S. Centers for Disease Control and Prevention (CDC) estimates there are 76 million illnesses, 325,000 hospitalizations, and 5,200 deaths in the United States each year that are caused by foodborne bacteria. Bacteria, viruses, and protozoa can cause these illnesses, some of which can be fatal if not treated properly.

Poor manufacturing processes or poor food preparation can allow microbes to grow in food and subsequently infect you. *Escherichia coli* (*E. coli*) bacteria sometimes persist in food products such as undercooked hamburger meat and unpasteurized fruit juice. These bacteria can have deadly consequences in vulnerable people, especially children and the elderly.

Cryptosporidia are bacteria found in fecal matter and can get into lake, river, and ocean water from sewage spills, animal waste, and water runoff. They can be released in the millions from infectious fecal matter. People who drink, swim, or play in infected water can get sick.

People, including babies, with diarrhea caused by *Cryptosporidia* or other diarrhea-causing microbes, such as *Giardia* and *Salmonella*, can infect others while using swimming pools, waterparks, hot tubs, and spas.

Transplanted Animal Organs May Harbor Germs

As researchers investigate the possibility of transplanting animal organs, such as pig hearts, into people, they must guard against the risk that organs also may transmit microbes that were harmless to the animal into humans, where they indeed may cause disease.

Some People Are Immune to Certain Diseases

As long ago as the 5th century B.C., Greek physicians noticed that people who had recovered from the plague would never get it again—they seemed to have become immune or resistant to the germ. People can become immune, or develop immunity, to a microbe in several ways. The first time T cells and B cells in a person's immune system meet up with an antigen, such as a virus or bacterium, they prepare the immune system to destroy the antigen. Because the immune system often can remember its enemies, those cells become active if they meet that particular antigen again. This is called naturally acquired immunity.

Another example of naturally acquired immunity occurs when a pregnant woman passes antibodies to her unborn baby. Babies are born with weak immune responses, but they are protected from some diseases for their first few months of life by antibodies received from their mothers before birth. Babies who are nursed also receive antibodies from breast milk that help protect their digestive tracts.

Immunization with vaccines is a safe way to get protection from germs. Some vaccines contain microorganisms or parts of microorganisms that have been weakened or killed. If you get this type of vaccine, those microorganisms (or their parts) will start your body's immune response, which will demolish the foreign invader but not make you sick. This is a type of artificially acquired immunity.

Immunity can be strong or weak and short- or long-lived, depending on the type of antigen, the amount of antigen, and the route by which it enters your body. When faced with the same antigen, some people's immune systems will respond forcefully, others feebly, and some not at all.

The genes you inherit also can influence your likelihood of getting a disease. In simple terms, the genes you get from your parents can influence how your body reacts to certain microbes.

Microbes Cause Different Kinds of Infections

Some disease-causing microbes can make you very sick very quickly and then not bother you again. Some can last for a long time and continue to damage tissues. Others can last forever, but you won't feel sick any more, or you will only feel sick once in a while. Most infections caused by microbes fall into three major groups:

- Acute infections
- Chronic infections
- Latent infections

Acute Infections

Acute infections usually last a short time, but they can make you feel very uncomfortable, with signs and symptoms such as tiredness, achiness, coughing, and sneezing. The common cold is such an infection. The signs and symptoms of a cold can last for 2 to 24 days (but usually a week), though it may seem like a lot longer. Once your body's immune system has successfully fought off one of the many different types of rhinoviruses that caused your cold, the cold doesn't come back. If you get another cold, it's probably because you have been infected with someone else's rhinoviruses.

Chronic Infections

Chronic infections usually develop from acute infections and can last for days to months to a lifetime. Sometimes, people are totally unaware they are infected but still may be able to transmit the germ to others. For example, hepatitis C, which affects the liver, is a chronic viral infection. In fact, most people who have been infected with the hepatitis C virus don't know it until they have a blood test that shows antibodies to the virus. Recovery from this infection is rare—about 85 percent of infected persons become chronic carriers of the virus. In addition, serious signs of liver damage, like cirrhosis or cancer, may not appear until as long as 20 years after the infection began.

Latent Infections

Latent infections are "hidden" or "silent" and may or may not cause symptoms again after the initial acute episode. Some infectious microbes, usually viruses, can "wake up" and become active again, sometimes off and on for months or years, and cause symptoms. When active, these microbes can be transmitted to other people. *Herpes simplex* viruses, which cause genital herpes and common cold sores, can remain latent in nerve cells for short or long periods of time, or forever.

Chickenpox is another example of a latent infection. Before the chickenpox vaccine became available in the 1990s, most children in the United States got chickenpox. After the first acute episode, usually when children are very young, the *Varicella zoster* virus goes into hiding in the body. In many people, it emerges many years later when they are older adults and causes a painful disease of the nerves called herpes zoster, or shingles.

Researchers are studying what turns these microbial antics off and on and are looking for ways to finally stop the process.

Difference between Infection and Disease

A disease occurs when cells or molecules in a person's body stop working properly, causing symptoms of illness. Many things can cause a disease, including altered genes, chemicals, aging, and infections. An infection occurs when another organism—such as a virus, bacterium, or parasite—enters a person's body and begins to reproduce. The invading microbe can directly damage cells, or the immune system can cause disease symptoms, such as fever, as it tries to rid the body of the invader. Some infections do not cause disease because the microbe is quickly killed or it hides out where it cannot be detected.

You Can Prevent Catching or Passing on Germs

Handwashing

Handwashing is one of the simplest, easiest, and most effective ways to prevent getting or passing on many germs. Amazingly, it is also one of the most overlooked. Health care experts recommend scrubbing your hands vigorously for at least 15 seconds with soap and water, about as long as it takes to recite the English alphabet. This will wash away cold viruses and staph and strep bacteria as well as many other disease-causing microbes. This also will help prevent accidentally passing those germs on to others.

It is especially important to wash your hands:

- Before preparing or eating food
- After coughing or sneezing
- After changing a diaper

- After using the bathroom

Health care providers should be especially conscientious about washing their hands before and after examining any patient. Day care workers, too, should be vigilant about handwashing around their young children.

Medicines

There are medicines on the market that help prevent people from getting infected by germs. For example, you can prevent getting the flu by taking a medicine such as Tamiflu, Flumadine, or Symmetrel. Vaccines, however, are the best defense against influenza viruses. Under specific circumstances, doctors may prescribe antibiotics to protect patients from getting certain bacteria such as *Mycobacterium tuberculosis*, which causes TB. Health care experts usually advise people traveling to areas where malaria is present to take antiparasitic medicines to prevent possible infection.

Vaccines

Edward Jenner laid the foundation for modern vaccines by discovering one of the basic principles of immunization. He had used a relatively harmless microbe, cowpox virus, to bring about an immune response that would help protect people from getting infected by the related but deadly smallpox virus.

Dr. Jenner's discovery helped researchers find ways to ease human disease suffering worldwide. By the beginning of the 20th century, doctors were immunizing patients with vaccines for diphtheria, typhoid fever, and smallpox.

Today, safe and effective vaccines prevent childhood diseases, including measles, whooping cough, chickenpox, and meningitis caused by *Haemophilus influenzae* type B (Hib).

Vaccines are not only for young children. Adolescents and adults should get vaccinated regularly for tetanus and diphtheria. In addition, adults who never had diseases such as measles or chickenpox during childhood or who never received vaccines to prevent them should consider being immunized. Childhood diseases can be far more serious in adults.

More people travel all over the world today. So, finding out which immunizations are recommended for travel to your destination(s) is even more important than ever. Vaccines also can prevent yellow fever, polio, typhoid fever, hepatitis A, cholera, rabies, and other bacterial and viral diseases that are more prevalent abroad than in the United States.

In the fall of the year, many adults and children may benefit from getting the flu vaccine. A doctor also may recommend immunizations for pneumococcal pneumonia and hepatitis B for people at risk of getting these diseases.

Some Vaccine-Preventable Infectious Diseases

- Anthrax
- Bacterial meningitis
- Chickenpox
- Cholera
- Diphtheria
- *Haemophilus influenzae* type B
- Hepatitis A
- Hepatitis B
- Influenza (Flu)
- Measles
- Mumps
- Pertussis
- Pneumococcal pneumonia
- Polio
- Rabies
- Rubella
- Tetanus
- Yellow fever

When You Should Go to the Doctor

Call a doctor immediately when:

- You have been bitten by an animal
- You are having difficulty breathing
- You have a cough that has lasted for more than a week
- You have a fever of 100 degrees Fahrenheit or higher
- You have episodes of rapid heartbeat
- You have a rash (especially if you have a fever at the same time)
- You have swelling
- You suddenly start having difficulty with seeing (for example, your vision is blurry)
- You have been vomiting

Generally, you should consult a doctor or other health care professional if you have or think you may have contracted an infectious disease.

These trained professionals can determine whether you have been infected, determine the seriousness of your infection, and give you the best advice for treating or preventing disease. Sometimes, however, a visit to the doctor may not be necessary.

Some infectious diseases, such as the common cold, usually do not require a visit to the doctor. They often last a short time and are not life-threatening, or there is no specific treatment. We've all heard the advice to rest and drink plenty of liquids to treat colds. Unless there are complications, most victims of colds find their immune systems successfully ward off the viral culprits. In fact, the coughing, sneezing, and fever that make you feel miserable are part of your immune system's way of fighting them off.

If, however, you have other conditions in which your immune system doesn't function properly, you should be in contact with your doctor whenever you suspect you have any infectious disease, even the common cold. Such conditions can include asthma and immunodeficiency diseases like HIV infection and AIDS.

In addition, some common, usually mild infectious diseases, such as chickenpox or flu, can cause serious harm in very young children or the elderly.

Infectious Diseases Are Diagnosed in Many Ways

Sometimes a doctor or other health care professional can diagnose an infectious disease by listening to your medical history and doing a physical exam. For example, listening to a patient describe what happened and any symptoms they have noticed plays an important part in helping a doctor find out what's wrong.

Blood and urine tests are other ways to diagnose an infection. A laboratory expert can sometimes see the offending microbe in a sample of blood or urine viewed under a microscope. One or both of these tests may be the only way to determine what caused the infection, or they may be used to confirm a diagnosis that was made based on taking a history and doing a physical exam.

In another type of test, a doctor will take a sample of blood or other body fluid, such as vaginal secretion, and then put it into a special container called a Petri dish to see if any microbe "grows." This test is called a culture. Certain bacteria, such as chlamydia and strep, and viruses, such as herpes simplex, usually can be identified using this method.

X-rays, scans, and biopsies (taking a tiny sample of tissue from the infected area and inspecting it under a microscope) are among other tools the doctor can use to make an accurate diagnosis.

All of the above procedures are relatively safe, and some can be done in a doctor's office or a clinic. Others pose a higher risk to patients because they involve procedures that go inside the body. One such invasive procedure is taking a biopsy from an internal organ. For example, one way a doctor can diagnose *Pneumocystis carinii* pneumonia, a lung disease caused by a fungus, is by doing a biopsy on lung tissue and then examining the sample under a microscope.

Infectious Diseases Are Treated in Many Ways

How an infectious disease is treated depends on the microbe that caused it and sometimes on the age and medical condition of the person affected. Certain diseases are not treated at all, but are allowed to run their course, with the immune system doing its job alone. Some diseases, such as the common cold, are treated only to relieve the symptoms. Others, such as strep throat, are treated to destroy the offending microbe as well as to relieve symptoms.

By Your Immune System

Your immune system has an arsenal of ways to fight off invading microbes. Most begin with B and T cells and antibodies whose sole purpose it is to keep your body healthy. Some of these cells sacrifice their lives to rid you of disease and restore your body to a healthy state. Some microbes normally present in your body also help destroy microbial invaders. For example, normal bacteria in your digestive system help destroy disease-causing microbes, such as listeria in that hot dog you had at lunch.

Other important ways your body reacts to an infection include fever and coughing and sneezing.

Fever

Fever is one of your body's special ways of fighting an infection. Many microbes are very sensitive to temperature changes and cannot survive in temperatures higher than normal body heat, which is usually around 98.6 degrees Fahrenheit. Your body uses fever to destroy flu viruses, for example.

Coughing and Sneezing

Another piece in your immune system's reaction to invading infection-causing microbes is mucus production. Coughing and sneezing help mucus move those germs out of your body efficiently and quickly.

Other methods your body may use to fight off an infection include:

- Inflammation
- Diarrhea
- Cramping
- Vomiting
- Fatigue

By Your Doctor

For Bacteria

The last century saw an explosion in our knowledge about how microbes work and in our methods of treating infectious diseases. For example, the discovery of antibiotics to treat and cure many bacterial diseases was a major breakthrough in medical history.

Doctors, however, sometimes prescribe antibiotics unnecessarily for a variety of reasons, including pressure from patients with viral infections. Patients may insist on being prescribed an antibiotic without knowing that it won't work on viruses. Colds and flu are two notable viral infections for which some doctors send their patients to the drugstore with a prescription for an antibiotic.

Because antibiotics have been over-prescribed or inappropriately prescribed over the years, bacteria have become resistant to the killing effects of these drugs. This resistance, called antimicrobial or drug resistance, has become a very serious problem, especially in hospital settings.

Bacteria that are not killed by the antibiotic become strong enough to resist the same medicine the next time it's given. Because bacteria multiply so rapidly, changed or mutated bacteria that resist antibiotics will quickly outnumber those that can be destroyed by those same drugs.

For Viruses

Viral diseases can be very difficult to treat because viruses live inside the body's cells where they are protected from medicines in the blood stream. Researchers developed the first antiviral drug in the late 20th century. The drug, acyclovir, was first approved by the U.S. Food and Drug Administration to treat herpes simplex virus infections. Only a few other antiviral medicines are available to prevent and treat viral infections and diseases.

Health care professionals treat HIV infection with a group of powerful medicines which can keep the virus in check. Known as highly active antiretroviral therapy, or HAART, the new treatment has improved the lives of many suffering from this deadly infection.

Viral diseases should never be treated with antibiotics. Sometimes a person with a viral disease will develop a bacterial disease as a complication of the initial viral disease. For example, children with chickenpox often scratch the skin sores caused by the viral infection. Bacteria such as staph can enter those lesions and cause a bacterial infection. The doctor may then prescribe an antibiotic to destroy the bacteria. The antibiotic, however, will not work on the chickenpox virus. It will work only against staph.

Unfortunately, safe and effective treatments and cures for most viral diseases have eluded researchers, but there are safe vaccines to protect you from viral infections and diseases.

For Fungi

Medicines applied directly to the infected area are available by prescription and over the counter for treating skin and nail fungal infections. Unfortunately, many people have had limited success with them. During the 1990s, oral prescription medicines became available for treating fungal infections of the skin and nails.

For many years, very powerful oral antifungal medicines were used only to treat systemic (within the body) fungal infections, such as histoplasmosis. Doctors usually prescribe oral antifungal medications cautiously because all of them, even the milder ones for skin and nail fungi, can have very serious side effects.

For Protozoa

Diseases caused by protozoan parasites are among the leading causes of death and disease in tropical and subtropical regions of the world. Developing countries within these areas contain three-quarters of the world's population, and their populations suffer the most from these diseases. Controlling parasitic diseases is a problem because there are no vaccines for any of them.

In many cases, controlling the insects that transmit these diseases is difficult because of pesticide resistance, concerns regarding environmental damage, and lack of adequate public health systems to apply existing insect-control methods. Thus, control of these diseases relies heavily on the availability of medicines. Doctors usually use antiparasitic medicines to treat protozoal infections. Unfortunately, there are very few medicines that fight protozoal infections, and some of those are either harmful to humans or are becoming ineffective.

The fight against the protozoan *Plasmodium falciparum*, the cause of the most deadly form of malaria, is a good example. This protozoan has become resistant to most of the medicines currently available to destroy it. A major focus of malaria research is on developing a vaccine to prevent people from getting the disease. In the meantime, many worldwide programs hope to eventually control malaria by keeping people from contact with infected mosquitoes or from getting infected if contact can't be avoided.

"New" and "Old" Microbes Emerge on the Scene

Although at odds with the belief that medicine had mastered infectious diseases, the emergence of new microbes and the re-emergence of old ones are nothing new. The factors involved in this process also go back centuries. For example, microbes have always traveled, like the bacteria that emerged in the 14th century to spread bubonic plague through Mongolia, Europe, and finally North Africa.

Emerging Microbes

From time to time, strange new disease-causing microbes seem to come out of nowhere. Scientists usually define newly emerging infectious diseases as those that have only recently appeared in a population or have existed but are rapidly increasing in incidence or geographic range. Recent examples include West Nile fever, *E. coli* infection, chronic hepatitis C, flu, hantavirus infection, and Lyme disease. Re-emerging infectious diseases, like TB, are those that were once under control.

In addition, pathogens previously not seen in the United States, like West Nile virus, may become more common here because of the increased speed of international travel and because more people are traveling.

In the early summer of 1999, cases of encephalitis (inflammation of the brain) and death began to appear in New York City. Researchers later identified West Nile virus as the cause. Prior to that time, health care experts had never seen cases of illness caused by this virus in the United States. The virus is common in Africa, West Asia, and the Middle East. Mosquitoes become infected when they feed on infected birds, which may circulate the virus in their blood for a few days. Infected mosquitoes can then transmit West Nile virus to humans and animals while biting to take blood. Every summer since it first appeared, West Nile virus has been found in a continuously increasing number of states.

Identified in 1989, the hepatitis C virus causes approximately 20 percent of all cases of acute viral liver disease each year in the United

States. CDC estimates that nearly 4 million Americans are infected with hepatitis C, many of whom are not aware of their infection. Chronic liver disease due to hepatitis C causes between 8,000 and 10,000 deaths and leads to about 1,000 liver transplants each year in the United States. Over the next two decades, the number of annual deaths from hepatitis C is expected to triple if there continues to be no effective treatment.

Some Newly Recognized Pathogens

- Babesia protozoa
- *Bartonella henselae* bacteria
- *Borrelia burgdorferi* bacteria
- Ebola virus
- Ehrlichiosis bacteria
- Hantaviruses
- *Helicobacter pylori* bacteria
- Hepatitis C virus
- Hepatitis E virus
- Human herpesvirus 6
- Human herpesvirus 8
- Human immunodeficiency virus
- Nipah virus
- Parvovirus B19

Within the past few years, many outbreaks of intestinal disease with bloody diarrhea have been reported in the United States and abroad. These outbreaks are often due to the newly pathogenic O157:H7 strain of *E. coli*, which was first recognized in 1982. Other strains of *E. coli* are common in other countries but less frequent in the United States. Approximately 10 to 15 percent of people infected with these organisms develop hemolytic uremic syndrome (HUS), a serious complication that can lead to kidney failure and death. Children and the elderly are particularly at risk for developing HUS.

Environmental changes can cause a microbe to become a health threat to humans. Lyme disease and hantavirus pulmonary syndrome are two examples.

Lyme disease emerged in 1975 in the northeastern United States as people expanded their communities into wooded areas occupied by infected deer ticks. It is the most common tick-borne infection in this country, affecting people in almost every state. Although not deadly, Lyme disease can cause serious illness. In 1982, scientists at the National Institute of Allergy and Infectious Diseases identified *B. burgdorferi* bacteria as the cause of Lyme disease. From then until 1999, health care workers reported more than 128,000 cases of the disease to CDC.

In 1993, an outbreak of a mysterious, often fatal lung disease occurred in the southwestern United States. That outbreak occurred in part from weather changes like those brought about by El Niño, which fosters increases in the rodent populations that carry diseases. Scientists quickly determined the illness was caused by a previously unknown strain of hantavirus, a family of disease-causing viruses that occurs naturally in mice and other rodents. By April 2001, health care workers had reported that 283 people had developed the condition known as hantavirus pulmonary syndrome. More than a third have died from the disease.

Re-Emerging Microbes

The reappearance of microbes that had been successfully conquered or controlled by medicines is distressing to the scientific and medical communities as well as to the public. A major cause of this re-emergence is that microbes, which cause these diseases, are becoming resistant to the drugs used to treat them.

According to the World Health Organization (WHO), nearly 2 billion people, one-third of the world's population, have TB. This includes between 10 and 15 million people in the United States. TB is the world's leading cause of death from a single infectious organism, killing 2 million people each year. The TB crisis has intensified because multidrug-resistant (MDR) microbes have emerged. An incurable form of the disease may develop from infections caused by these organisms. WHO estimates more than 50 million people worldwide may be infected with MDR strains of TB.

Malaria, the most deadly of all tropical parasitic diseases, has been resurging dramatically. Increasing resistance of *Plasmodium* protozoa to inexpensive and effective medicines presents problems for treating active infections. WHO estimates between 300 million and 500 million new cases of malaria occur worldwide each year. At least 2.7 million people die annually. In the United States, approximately 1,000 cases are reported annually, which researchers estimate represent only 25 to 50 percent of actual cases. Although most of these cases occurred in people who had been infected while traveling abroad, others occurred in people bitten by infected mosquitoes in states such as New York.

In the United States, approximately 25 percent of the population has flu-associated illness annually, leading to an average of 20,000 to 40,000 deaths per year. Influenza viruses change from year to year and powerful strains have re-emerged throughout history to cause worldwide, catastrophic pandemics. Many scientists believe the next pandemic is long overdue. In addition, in the 1990s, people in Hong Kong became infected with avian influenza—the first known case of an influenza virus jumping directly from birds to people.

Re-Emerging Pathogens

- Cholera bacteria
- *Coccidioides immitis* fungus
- *E. coli* bacteria
- Enterovirus
- Dengue virus
- Group A Streptococcus bacteria
- Influenza virus
- West Nile virus

[Source: NIAID Division of Microbiology and Infectious Diseases, February 2001.]

Research

The National Institute of Allergy and Infectious Diseases (NIAID), a component of the National Institutes of Health (NIH), is the Federal Government's lead agency for conducting and funding research on many infectious diseases, including their causes, diagnoses, treatments, and prevention methods. Biomedical research supported by NIAID provides the tools necessary to develop diagnostic tests, new and improved treatments, vaccines, and other means to combat the microbial threats of today and tomorrow.

NIAID's research activities include:

- Projects to sequence the whole or partial genomes of a variety of pathogenic microbes. These projects should help scientists understand how the organisms cause disease and identify new drug and vaccine targets.
- A broad malaria research program. This program is conducted by scientists at institutions throughout the United States and in several countries where malaria is endemic, and by scientists working in NIAID's laboratories in Bethesda, Maryland, and Hamilton, Montana. NIAID and other NIH components also participate in the Multilateral Initiative on Malaria, a global group that boosts international collaboration among malaria scientists and identifies resources to enhance malaria research.

- Research on the basic biology of influenza viruses and on efforts to find more effective vaccines and treatments for flu.
- Clinical trials involving several experimental HIV vaccines. NIAID scientists and grantees have been conducting these trials since 1987. In 1999, NIAID began the first HIV vaccine trial in Africa, an important step for developing global vaccines.
- The HIV Vaccine Trials Network (HVTN). HVTN is a network of domestic and international clinical research institutions. Established in 2000, HVTN conducts all phases of vaccine clinical trials.
- Emerging Virus Research Groups. NIAID supports three groups to learn more about emerging viruses. By learning how these viruses work, researchers hope to develop better ways to diagnose and treat the diseases they cause.

Institute researchers work closely with other agencies, institutions, and individuals from across the United States and around the world to achieve the common goal of controlling and eliminating infectious diseases. Information on current NIAID research activities is available at the institute website http://www.niaid.nih.gov.

Chapter 2

Contagious Diseases: A Statistical Summary

Introduction

The statistics in this chapter were collected and compiled from reports sent by state health departments to the National Notifiable Diseases Surveillance System (NNDSS), which is operated by Centers for Disease Control and Prevention (CDC) in collaboration with the Council of State and Territorial Epidemiologists (CSTE).

The infectious diseases designated as notifiable at the national level during 2001 are listed in Table 2.1. A notifiable disease is one for which regular, frequent, and timely information regarding individual cases is considered necessary for the prevention and control of the disease.

Highlights

AIDS

Since the use of highly active antiretroviral therapy (HAART) in the United States became widespread in 1996, the number of persons diagnosed with acquired immunodeficiency syndrome (AIDS) has declined. The number of deaths among persons with AIDS has also

---

Excerpted from "Summary of Notifiable Diseases—United States, 2001," *Morbidity and Mortality Weekly Report (MMWR),* Centers for Disease Control and Prevention (CDC), Vol. 50, No. 53, May 2, 2003. The full text including tables and references is available online at www.cdc.gov/mmwr/summary .html.

declined substantially; as a result, the number of persons living with AIDS has increased. By December 2001, a total of 807,075 adults and 9,074 children had been reported with AIDS.

In 1996, sharp declines in AIDS incidence occurred for the first time; during 1998–1999, declines in AIDS incidence began to level, and essentially no change occurred from 1999 through 2000. Through December 2001, 462,653 adult and 5,257 pediatric AIDS cases resulted in death. Since 1996, the number of deaths among persons with AIDS declined sharply and continued to decline each year through 2000. The number of persons living with AIDS, approximately 362,827, was the highest ever reported; of these persons, 78% were men and 61% were black or Hispanic. Of the 282,250 adult and adolescent men with AIDS, 57% were men who have sex with men, 24%

Table 2.1. Infectious Diseases Designated as Notifiable at the National Level During 2001 (*continued on next page*)

Acquired immunodeficiency syndrome (AIDS)
Anthrax
Botulism
Brucellosis
Chancroid
Chlamydia trachomatis, genital infection
Cholera
Coccidioidomycosis
Cryptosporidiosis
Cyclosporiasis
Diphtheria
Ehrlichiosis, human granulocytic
Ehrlichiosis, human monocytic
Ehrlichiosis, human, other or unspecified agent
Encephalitis, California serogroup viral
Encephalitis, eastern equine
Encephalitis, St. Louis
Encephalitis, western equine
Escherichia coli, enterohemorrhagic (EHEC), O157:H7
EHEC, serogroup non-O157
EHEC, not serogrouped
Gonorrhea
Haemophilus influenzae, invasive disease
Hansen disease (leprosy)
Hantavirus pulmonary syndrome
Hemolytic uremic syndrome, postdiarrheal
Hepatitis A, acute
Hepatitis B, acute
Hepatitis B, perinatal
Hepatitis C; non-A, non-B
Human immunodeficiency virus (HIV) infection, adult
HIV infection, pediatric (<13 yrs)
Legionellosis
Listeriosis
Lyme disease

were injecting drug users, 9% were exposed through heterosexual contact, and 8% were both men who have sex with men and injecting drug users. Of the 76,696 adult and adolescent women with AIDS, 59% were exposed through heterosexual contact and 38% through injecting drug use.

To provide better data for prevention of human immunodeficiency virus (HIV) infection (the virus that causes AIDS), CDC and CSTE recommend that national surveillance include the monitoring of both HIV infection and AIDS. CDC supports several supplemental surveillance projects that collect data on barriers to preventing AIDS cases and deaths of persons with AIDS, including access to HIV testing and treatment in accordance with current public health service guidelines.

Table 2.1. Infectious Diseases Designated as Notifiable at the National Level During 2001 (*continued from previous page*)

Malaria
Measles
Meningococcal disease
Mumps
Pertussis
Plague
Poliomyelitis, paralytic
Psittacosis
Q fever
Rabies, animal
Rabies, human
Rocky Mountain spotted fever
Rubella
Rubella, congenital syndrome
Salmonellosis
Shigellosis
Streptococcal disease, invasive, group A
Streptococcal toxic-shock syndrome
Streptococcus pneumoniae, invasive, drug-resistant
Streptococcus pneumoniae, invasive, <5 yrs
Syphilis
Syphilis, congenital
Tetanus
Toxic-shock syndrome
Trichinosis
Tuberculosis
Tularemia
Typhoid fever
Varicella (chickenpox)*
Varicella deaths
Yellow fever

* Although varicella (chickenpox) is not a nationally notifiable disease, the Council of State and Territorial Epidemiologists recommends reporting cases of this disease to CDC.

Chancroid

During 2001, a total of 38 cases of chancroid were reported (rate: 0.01 cases/100,000 population), representing a 51% decline from 2000 and a continuing decline since 1987. However, chancroid is difficult to culture and could be substantially underdiagnosed. Several studies that used DNA amplification tests (which are not commercially available) have identified this infection in cities where it was previously undetected.

Chlamydia Trachomatis, *Genital Infection*

During 2001, a total of 783,242 cases of genital chlamydial infection were reported (rate: 278.32/100,000). This rate was the highest since voluntary case reporting began in the mid-1980s and the highest since genital chlamydial infection became a nationally notifiable disease in 1995. This increase could be caused in part by the continued expansion of chlamydia screening programs and increased use of more sensitive diagnostic tests for this condition.

Diphtheria

During 2001, two probable diphtheria cases were reported to CDC. Both patients had membranous pharyngitis. The first was a man aged 59 years from Montana. A specimen for culture was not obtained from this patient. The second patient was a woman aged 19 years from Michigan. Although a throat swab culture from this patient did not yield *Corynebacterium diphtheriae*, a weakly positive TaqMan polymerase chain reaction test result was obtained from the membranous tissue. Neither patient had a history of recent travel or had contact with international or local visitors. Both patients survived.

Gonorrhea

During 2001, a total of 361,705 cases of gonorrhea were reported (rate: 128.53/ 100,000). The 2001 rate was similar to rates for 2000 (129.04/100,000), 1999 (132.32/ 100,000), and 1998 (131.89/100,000) and has remained stable among men and women. Nevertheless, increases have been observed in some areas among men who have sex with men. Decreased susceptibility to the fluoroquinolone antibiotics and azithromycin has been reported from some regions. In 2001, the prevalence of fluoroquinolone-resistant *Neisseria gonorrhoeae* infections increased in California. As a result, fluoroquinolones are no longer advised for treatment of gonorrhea in Hawaii or California or for infections that may have been acquired in those states.

Haemophilus Influenzae, *Invasive Disease*

Since 1990, when *Haemophilus influenzae* type b (Hib) conjugate vaccines were licensed for use in infants beginning at age 2 months, Hib has become a rare cause of invasive disease (for example, meningitis) among children aged less than 5 years in the United States. Surveillance information is used to monitor the effectiveness of immunization programs and vaccines and to assess progress toward disease elimination. To continue to assess progress toward the elimination of Hib invasive disease, accurate laboratory information is essential to correctly identify the serotype of the causative *H. influenzae* (Hi) isolate. Serotyping Hi by slide agglutination can sometimes be inaccurate, especially since it is not performed frequently in most laboratories. Recently, CDC reported discrepancies in Hi slide agglutination serotyping results obtained by state health department laboratories participating in active surveillance and those obtained by CDC. In this study, 28 (70%) of 40 Hi isolates that had been reported as Hib to CDC were actually identified at CDC as nontypeable Hi. Because of these discrepancies, CDC requests state health department laboratories to send all Hi invasive disease isolates from children aged less than 5 years to CDC for testing to reconfirm serotype.

Hansen Disease

A total of 81 Hansen disease cases were reported to CDC through the NNDSS database from 20 states, Puerto Rico and American Samoa in 2001; three states (California, Hawaii and New York) accounted for 74% of the total number of cases reported. In contrast, 110 Hansen disease cases were reported to the National Hansen Disease Program from 27 states and Puerto Rico in 2001; six states (Texas, New York, Louisiana, Washington, Florida and California) accounted for 71% of the total number of cases reported. These data suggest that the annual number of cases in the United States may not be declining and underscore the need for coordination between the multiple surveillance systems as well as the need to continue to identify and treat patients with Hansen disease.

Hepatitis A

Hepatitis A vaccine is recommended for persons at increased risk of acquiring hepatitis A (for example, illegal drug users, men who have sex with men [MSM]) and also for children in states and counties that have historically had consistently elevated rates of hepatitis A. After routine childhood vaccination was recommended, the overall hepatitis A rate has declined steadily, and in 2001 it was the lowest yet recorded (4.0/100,000). Because hepatitis A rates tend to vary from year to year and from region to region, continued monitoring of hepatitis A incidence is needed to determine whether this low rate is due to routine immunization or natural variability in infection rates. However, declines in rates have been greater among children and in the states where routine childhood vaccination is recommended, suggesting an impact of childhood vaccination. Despite declining overall rates, some states reported increasing rates in 2000–2001. In several states, these increases were related to outbreaks occurring among high-risk adults, including MSM, and cases among adults in high-risk groups represent an increasing proportion of reported cases nationwide. For example, cases among MSM increased from 4% (1990) to 8% (1995) to 12% (2000).

Hepatitis B

During 2001, a total of 7,843 acute hepatitis B cases were reported, representing a decrease of more than 60% decrease since 1990 (21,102 cases). Surveillance data are being used to monitor the impact of the national strategy for eliminating hepatitis B virus (HBV) infection. *Healthy People 2010* objectives call for a 75%–90% reduction in the national incidence of hepatitis B among adults (baseline: 15–24 cases/100,000), a 99% reduction among children aged 2–18 years (baseline: 945 cases/year), and a 75% reduction in the number of perinatal HBV infections (baseline: 1,682 infections/year). The effect of routine infant and adolescent vaccination can already be seen in the declining rate of disease among persons aged less than 19 years. In contrast, the continued high incidence among persons in other risk groups for which vaccination is recommended (for example, injection drug users and persons engaging in high-risk sexual behaviors) indicates that programs for reaching these populations need to be developed or strengthened.

Hepatitis C; Non-A, Non-B

Cases of hepatitis C reported to CDC are considered unreliable because 1) no serologic marker for acute infection exists, and 2) most health departments do not have the resources to determine if a positive laboratory report for hepatitis C virus (HCV) infection represents acute infection, chronic infection, repeated testing of a person previously reported, or a false-positive result. Historically, the most reliable national estimates of acute disease incidence have come from sentinel surveillance. After adjusting for underreporting and asymptomatic infections, the annual number of new infections has decreased more than 80% since 1989 to 25,000 cases in 2001 (CDC, unpublished data, 2002). Because surveillance for acute hepatitis C can be used to evaluate the effectiveness of prevention efforts and identify missed opportunities for prevention, efforts are under way to help states establish and improve surveillance.

HIV Infection, Adult

Persons with HIV infection are living longer without progressing to AIDS. As a result, AIDS incidence is decreasing and no longer provides the most accurate information on the HIV epidemic. Recommendations for implementing national HIV case surveillance were published in December 1999, and the revised surveillance case definition became effective January 1, 2000.

By December 31, 2001, 37 areas had laws or regulations requiring confidential reporting by name of adults/adolescents with confirmed HIV infection. Nine areas (Washington, DC, Hawaii, Illinois, Kentucky, Maryland, Massachusetts, Puerto Rico, Rhode Island, and Vermont) had implemented a code-based system to conduct case surveillance for HIV infection. Other areas (Delaware, Maine, Montana, Oregon, and Washington) had implemented a name-to-code system to conduct HIV infection surveillance: names are collected initially and later are converted to codes. Data on cases of HIV infection from those areas conducting code-based or name-to code systems are not included in this report pending evaluations demonstrating acceptable performance under CDC guidelines and the development of methods to report such data to CDC.

Trend analysis is possible by examining data from the 25 states that have continually conducted HIV surveillance since 1994. These 25 states represent 24% of all AIDS cases diagnosed in the United States. During 1994–2000, HIV infection was diagnosed in 128,813 persons from the 25 states. The number of persons newly diagnosed each year with HIV infection declined steadily during 1994–1997. From 1997 through 2000, case counts have been stable in all age, race/ethnicity and HIV exposure categories. The largest declines were observed in the following groups: persons aged 25–44 years, men who have sex with men, and injection-drug users. The majority (55%) of persons with newly diagnosed HIV in these 25 states were black non-Hispanic, and 36% were white non-Hispanic. Because persons with newly diagnosed HIV infections include those who may have had previously unrecognized infections for a long time, these data do not represent incident infections. However, the stability in the number of infections diagnosed each year during the latter part of the 1990s and the small declines in the proportion of persons presenting with AIDS indicate that improvements in the targeting of HIV counseling and testing are needed to facilitate earlier diagnoses. Early diagnosis is a critical factor in ensuring that infected persons are linked to effective treatment and prevention services to reduce further transmission and improve quality of life.

HIV Infection, Pediatric

As of December 2001, 39 areas conducted name-based surveillance for HIV infection among children aged less than 13 years. In 2001, 543 children whose infection had not progressed to AIDS and 175 children who had AIDS were reported. These states also received reports of perinatally exposed children who required follow-up with health-care providers to determine their HIV infection status.

In 2000, an estimated 6,075–6,422 infants were born to HIV-positive mothers in the United States. Of these infants, an estimated 280–370 were infected with HIV, representing a decline of more than 80% from the 1991 peak of 1,760 estimated HIV-positive U.S. births. Declines in perinatal HIV infections have been attributed to the use of zidovudine to reduce perinatal HIV transmission and to nationwide efforts to implement routine, voluntary prenatal HIV testing for all pregnant women. Continued declines in perinatal HIV infections may be difficult to sustain unless new HIV infections in women of child-bearing age are reduced.

Measles

A total of 116 confirmed measles cases were reported in 2001; cases occurred in 22 states. Fifty-four of the cases were internationally imported, and exposure to these cases resulted in 25 additional cases. Twelve other cases had virologic evidence of importation (genotypic analysis of measles viruses indicated an imported source). The remaining 25 cases were classified as unknown source cases because no link to importation was detected. The majority of confirmed measles cases

(61 cases) occurred in persons aged more than 20 years; 29 cases occurred in persons 5–19 years, and 26 occurred in children aged less than 5 years. Ten outbreaks, ranging in size from 3 to 14 cases, accounted for 49% of cases (n = 57). All 10 outbreaks were linked to international importation; nine had an epidemiologic link to imported cases and one had virologic evidence of importation.

Meningococcal Disease

Rates of meningococcal disease have been relatively stable in the United States. A total of 2,333 cases were reported in 2001, of which 1,931 were confirmed, 77 probable, seven suspected, and 318 of unknown case status. Serogroup information was reported for 33% of cases, and serogroup Y accounted for 33% of those reported. Most other cases were caused by serogroup B (32%) or serogroup C (27%). Although rates of meningococcal disease are usually highest among children aged less than 1 year, 55% of cases in 2001 occurred among persons aged greater than 18 years.

Using the technology applied to the development of *Haemophilus influenzae* type b (Hib) conjugate vaccines, several companies are in the final stages of developing and testing meningococcal conjugate vaccines with various serogroup-specific formulas and in combination with other antigens for licensure in the United States. Three serogroup C meningococcal conjugate vaccines were licensed and integrated into routine childhood immunization in the United Kingdom in 2000; early results confirm 85%–95% efficacy in infants, toddlers and teenagers and suggest herd immunity.

Mumps

Because of the recommendation of two doses of measles/mumps/rubella vaccine and its high coverage rate in the United States, mumps is at record low levels. During the 1990s, mumps cases declined substantially, from 5,292 reported cases in 1990 to 266 reported cases in 2001, meeting the *Healthy People 2000* objective of less than 500 cases per year.

Pertussis

During 2001, a total of 7,580 cases of pertussis were reported. Of these, 22% occurred among infants aged less than 6 months, who were too young to have received the recommended three doses of diphtheria and tetanus toxoids and acellular pertussis (DTaP) vaccine; 3% occurred among children aged 6–11 months; 13% among preschool-aged children (those aged 1–4 years); 10% among children aged 5–9 years; 30% among persons aged 10–19 years; and 22% among persons aged greater than 20 years.

Since 1995, the coverage rate with more than 3 doses of a pertussis-containing vaccine has been greater than 94% among U.S. children aged 19–35 months. Since 1980, the number of reported cases of pertussis in infants aged less than 7 months and in adolescents and adults has increased markedly in some states. The reasons for this rise are unknown but could include increased awareness of pertussis among health-care providers, increased use of more sensitive diagnostic tests, better reporting of cases to health departments, and possibly an increase in circulating pertussis. In contrast, the incidence of reported pertussis among children aged 7 months to 9 years has not increased markedly and suggests protection against pertussis. Adolescents and adults can become susceptible to disease because vaccine-induced immunity is believed to wane approximately 5–10 years after pertussis vaccination.

Rubella

Because of the success of the U.S. rubella vaccination program, rubella is at a record low level, with 23 reported cases in 2001. Rubella now mostly occurs among adults born in countries that do not have routine rubella vaccination programs or that have only recently implemented such programs. In 2000 and 2001, 10 mothers of the 11 children with reported congenital rubella syndrome were foreign-born Hispanics.

Shigellosis

Shigella sonnei infections continue to account for approximately 75% of shigellosis in the United States. Prolonged, community-wide outbreaks of *S. sonnei* infections that are transmitted in child care centers and other settings where maintenance of good hygienic conditions requires special care account for much of the problem. In 2001, one such outbreak in Ohio and Kentucky accounted for several hundred laboratory-confirmed infections. *S. sonnei* can also be transmitted through contaminated foods and through water used for drinking or recreational purposes. Recent evidence suggests that *S. sonnei* infections are increasing among men who have sex with men.

Streptococcal Disease, Invasive, Group A

During 2001, 1,147 cases of invasive group A streptococcal (GAS) disease were reported from nine states (California, Colorado, Connecticut, Georgia, Maryland, Minnesota, New York, Oregon, and Tennessee) through the Active Bacterial Core Surveillance (ABCs) project under CDC's Emerging Infections Program. Based on these 1,147 cases, CDC estimates that approximately 9,930 cases of invasive GAS disease (rate: 3.5/100,000) and 1,350 deaths occurred nationally during 2001. Disease incidence was highest among children aged less than 1 year (5.5/100,000) and adults aged more than 65 years (9.9/ 100,000). Streptococcal toxic-shock syndrome and necrotizing fasciitis accounted for approximately 5.9% and 6.7% of invasive cases, respectively. The overall case-fatality rate among persons with invasive GAS disease was 13.2%.

In 2002, CDC published recommendations for the control of invasive group A streptococcal disease among household contacts of persons with invasive GAS infections and for responding to postpartum and postsurgical infections. These recommendations are based on routine surveillance data, studies of the epidemiology of subsequent invasive GAS infections among household contacts of case-patients and postpartum and postsurgical GAS clusters, and studies of the effectiveness of chemoprophylactic regimens for eradicating carriage.

Streptococcus Pneumoniae, *Invasive, Drug-Resistant*

In 2001, the ABCs project of CDC's Emerging Infections Program collected information on invasive pneumococcal disease, including drug-resistant *Streptococcus pneumoniae*, in nine states (California, Colorado, Connecticut, Georgia, Maryland, Minnesota, New York, Oregon, and Tennessee). For the first time, the proportion of pneumococcal isolates that were drug resistant was lower in the current year than reported in the previous year. Of the 3,418 *S. pneumoniae* isolates collected in 2001, 9.7% exhibited intermediate resistance to penicillin (minimum inhibitory concentration [MIC] 0.1–1 µg/mL), and 15.6% were fully resistant (MIC >2 µg/mL); in 2000, 9.8% were intermediate and 17.1% were fully resistant. For cefotaxime, 10.5% of all isolates had intermediate resistance and 5.7% were fully resistant in 2001, compared with 9.8% of all isolates with intermediate resistance and 7.5% fully resistant in 2000. For erythromycin, 19.4% were resistant in 2001 versus 21.3% in 2000. Approximately one in six (16.9%) isolates had reduced susceptibility to at least three classes of drugs commonly used to treat pneumococcal infections, a decline from approximately one fifth (18.9%) of isolates in 2000.

In February 2000, the Food and Drug Administration licensed a pneumococcal conjugate vaccine for use in infants and young children. In October 2000, the Advisory Committee on Immunization Practices issued recommendations for use of the vaccine in children aged less than 5 years. Among isolates from children aged less than 5 years reported to ABCs during 2001, 63.9% of all strains (n = 587) and 75.9% of strains not susceptible to penicillin (n = 199) were serotypes included in this 7-valent vaccine.

Streptococcus Pneumoniae, *Invasive, Less Than 5 Years*

Invasive *Streptococcus pneumoniae* infection in children aged less than 5 years was reportable in 28 states and the District of Columbia in 2001. Of these 29 jurisdictions with mandated reporting, only 11 states and the District of Columbia reported cases. The incidence rate in these reporting areas was 13.3/100,000, which is lower than the rate of 39.7 cases/100,000 population estimated from data collected through the Active Bacterial Core Surveillance (CDC, unpublished data).

Syphilis, Congenital

During 2001, a total of 441 cases of congenital syphilis were reported (rate: 11.1/ 100,000 live births). Like primary and secondary syphilis, the rate of congenital syphilis has declined sharply in recent years, from a peak of 107.3/100,000 in 1991. The continuing decrease in the rate of congenital syphilis likely reflects the substantial reduction in the rate of primary and secondary syphilis among women that has occurred in the last decade. Congenital syphilis persists in the United States because a substantial number of women do not receive syphilis serologic testing until late in their pregnancy or not at all. This lack of screening is often related to absent or late prenatal care.

Syphilis, Primary and Secondary

During 2001, a total of 6,103 primary and secondary syphilis cases were reported. From 1990 to 2000, the primary and secondary syphilis rate declined 90%, from 20.34/ 100,000 to 2.12/100,000. The overall 2001 rate (2.17/100,000) is a 2% increase from the 2000 rate, which was the lowest since reporting began in 1941 and the first annual increase since 1990. The 2001 primary and secondary syphilis rate reflects a 15.4% increase among men but a 17.7% decrease among women. This disparity between men and women, observed across all racial and ethnic groups, along with reported outbreaks of syphilis among men who have sex with men (MSM) in large urban areas, suggests that increases in syphilis are occurring among MSM. Rates also remain disproportionately high in the South and among non-Hispanic blacks.

Tuberculosis

During 2001, a total of 15,989 cases (rate: 5.6/100,000 population) of tuberculosis (TB) were reported to CDC from the 50 states and the District of Columbia, representing a 2% decrease from 2000 and a 40% decrease from 1992, when the number of cases and the case rate most recently peaked in the United States. In 1991, 73% of reported cases were among U.S.-born persons (rate: 8.2/100,000), and 27% were among foreign-born persons (33.9/100,000). In comparison in 2001, there was an equal distribution (50%) in the number of TB cases among these two groups (case rates: 3.1/100,000 for U.S.-born persons and 26.6/100,000 for foreign-born persons).

Despite the decrease in case rate among foreign-born persons during the past decade, half of the TB cases in the United States in 2001 occurred in this population, and the case rate was eight times greater in this population than among U.S.-born persons. To address the high rate, CDC is collaborating with public health partners to implement TB control initiatives among recent international arrivals and residents along the border between the United States and Mexico and to strengthen TB programs in countries with a high incidence of TB disease. CDC has recently updated its comprehensive national action plan to reflect the alignment of its priorities with the Institute of Medicine report and to ensure that priority prevention activities are undertaken with optimal collaboration and coordination among national and international public health partners.

Typhoid Fever

In 2001, typhoid fever was diagnosed in 368 persons in the United States. Despite the availability of two effective vaccines, NNDSS reports 350–450 cases each year. Approximately 80% of these cases occur among persons who report international travel during the 6 weeks before illness. Persons visiting friends and relatives in their country of origin appear to be at high risk. In many areas of the world, *Salmonella typhi* strains have acquired resistance to multiple antimicrobial agents, including ampicillin, chloramphenicol, and trimethoprim-sulfamethoxazole. *S. typhi* outbreaks in the United States are generally small in size, but they can cause significant morbidity and are often foodborne, warranting thorough investigation.

Chapter 3

How to Keep the Germs Away

Being Sick Costs You a Lot

- **It costs you a lot of time.** Each year Americans are sick more than 4 billion days.
- **It costs you a lot of money.** They spend almost $950 billion on direct medical costs.
- **But the biggest cost of all is the cost of a life.** Over 160,000 die due to infectious diseases as the underlying cause of death.

Being sick does cost too much. Especially since there are some steps you can take to prevent getting sick in the first place.

Scientists at the Centers for Disease Control and Prevention (CDC) have identified some simple things you and your family can do to prevent getting infectious diseases. But first, you may be wondering, what are infectious diseases?

Well, they are diseases caused by various types of microscopic germs such as:

- Viruses
- Bacteria
- Parasites
- Fungi

"An Ounce of Prevention: Keeps the Germs Away," National Center for Infectious Diseases, Centers for Disease Control and Prevention (CDC), reviewed April 5, 2000.

These germs cause illnesses that range from common ailments like a cold and the flu; to disabling conditions such as Lyme disease and polio; to deadly diseases like hantavirus and AIDS. The bad news is that some of these diseases can be quite serious.

The good news is that many of those diseases can be prevented through amazingly simple and extremely inexpensive methods. Many of these methods are not new. And many were taught to us by our parents. But we get in a hurry and get out of the habit of practicing these simple but important prevention steps.

Wash Your Hands Often

The most important thing that you can do to keep from getting sick is to wash your hands.

By frequently washing your hands you wash away germs that you have picked up from other people, or from contaminated surfaces, or from animals and animal waste.

What happens if you do not wash your hands frequently?

You pick up germs from other sources and then you infect yourself when you:

- Touch your eyes
- Touch your nose
- Touch your mouth

One of the most common ways people catch colds is by rubbing their nose or their eyes after their hands have been contaminated with the cold virus.

You can also spread germs directly to others or onto surfaces that other people touch. And before you know it, everybody around you is getting sick.

The important thing to remember is that, in addition to colds, some pretty serious diseases—like hepatitis A, meningitis, and infectious diarrhea—can easily be prevented if people make a habit of washing their hands.

When should you wash your hands?

You should wash your hands often. Probably more often than you do now because you can't see germs with the naked eye or smell them, so you do not really know where they are hiding.

It is especially important to wash your hands:

- Before, during, and after you prepare food
- Before you eat, and after you use the bathroom
- After handling animals or animal waste
- When your hands are dirty, and
- More frequently when someone in your home is sick

What is the correct way to wash your hands?

- First wet your hands and apply liquid or clean bar soap. Place the bar soap on a rack and allow it to drain.
- Next rub your hands vigorously together and scrub all surfaces.
- Continue for 10–15 seconds or about the length of a little tune. It is the soap combined with the scrubbing action that helps dislodge and remove germs.
- Rinse well and dry your hands.

It is estimated that one out of three people do not wash their hands after using the restroom. So these tips are also important when you are out in public.

Washing your hands regularly can certainly save a lot on medical bills. Because it costs less than a penny, you could say that this penny's worth of prevention can save you a $50 visit to the doctor.

Routinely Clean and Disinfect Surfaces

Another way to help you keep the germs away is to routinely clean and disinfect surfaces.

What is the difference between cleaning and disinfecting?

Cleaning and disinfecting are not the same thing. In most cases, cleaning with soap and water is adequate. It removes dirt and most of the germs. However, in other situations disinfecting provides an extra margin of safety.

You should disinfect areas where there are both high concentrations of dangerous germs and a possibility that they will be spread to others. That is because disinfectants, including solutions of household bleach, have ingredients that destroy bacteria and other germs. While surfaces may look clean, many infectious germs may be lurking around. Given the right conditions some germs can live on surfaces for hours and even for days.

Do you know where the "hot zones", or the contaminated areas, are in your home?

The kitchen is one of the most dangerous places in the house because of the infectious bacteria that are sometimes found in raw food such as chicken. Also, there is a potential for germs to be spread to other people because that is where food is prepared. You cannot always tell where or when germs are hiding. When you touch a contaminated object you can contaminate other surfaces that you touch afterwards and spread the germs to others.

Another potential hot zone is the bathroom. Routinely cleaning and disinfecting the bathroom reduces odors and may help prevent the spread of germs when someone in the house has a diarrheal illness. And do not forget your child's changing table and diaper pail.

What is the best way to routinely clean and disinfect surfaces?

- You should follow the directions on the cleaning product labels. And be sure to read safety precautions as well.
- If you are cleaning up body fluids such as blood, vomit, or feces, you should wear rubber gloves, particularly if you have cuts or scratches on your hands or if a family member has AIDS, hepatitis B, or another bloodborne disease. And it is also a good idea to clean and disinfect surfaces when someone in the home is sick.
- To begin, clean the surface thoroughly with soap and water or another cleaner.
- After cleaning, if you need to use a disinfectant, apply it to the area, and let it stand for a few minutes or longer, depending on the manufacturers recommendations. This keeps the germs in contact with the disinfectant longer.
- Wipe the surface with paper towels that can be thrown away or cloth towels that can be washed afterwards.
- Store cleaners and disinfectants out of the reach of children.
- And remember, even if you use gloves, wash your hands after cleaning or disinfecting surfaces.

Handle and Prepare Food Safely

- Buy perishable foods at the end of your shopping trip.
- Store food properly.
- Use care when preparing meals and cook foods well.
- Cool and promptly store leftovers.

Almost everyone has experienced a foodborne illness at some point in time. But do we only get sick from restaurant food? No, in fact many cases of foodborne illnesses occur when food is prepared at home. If food is handled and prepared safely, most of those can be avoided. All food may contain some natural bacteria, and improper handling gives the bacteria a chance to grow. Also, food can be contaminated with bacteria from other sources that can make you ill. Contaminated or unclean food can be very dangerous, especially to young children, older adults, pregnant women, and people with weakened immune systems. Each year in the United States, approximately 76 million people get sick, more than 300,000 are hospitalized, and 5,000 Americans die each from foodborne illness.

There are four major tips you can use to prevent contaminating food:

Use Caution When You Buy Your Food

- Buy perishable food such as meat, eggs, and milk last.
- Avoid raw or unpasteurized milk.
- Because eggs, meat, seafood, and poultry are most likely to contain bacteria, do not allow their juices to drip on other food.
- Shop for groceries when you can take food home right away so that it does not spoil in a hot car.

Store Your Food Properly

- Store eggs, raw meat, poultry, and seafood in the refrigerator.
- Use containers to prevent contaminating other foods or kitchen surfaces.
- Your refrigerator should be set at 40° F.
- Your freezer should be set at 0° F.
- Regularly clean and disinfect the refrigerator and freezer.

Use Special Precautions when Preparing and Cooking Food

- Wash your hands and clean and disinfect kitchen surfaces before, during and after handling, cooking, and serving food.
- Wash raw fruits and vegetables before eating them.
- Defrost frozen food on a plate either in the refrigerator or in a microwave, but not on the counter.
- Cook food immediately after defrosting.
- Use different dishes and utensils for raw foods than you use for cooked foods.

Cooking Guidelines

Eggs

- Cook eggs until they are firm and not runny.
- Do not eat raw or partially cooked eggs.
- Avoid eating other foods that include raw or partially cooked eggs.

Poultry

- Cook poultry until it has an internal temperature of 180° F.
- It is done when the juices run clear and it is white in the middle.
- Never eat rare poultry.

Fish

- Cook fish until it is opaque or white and flaky.
- Cook ground meat to 160° F.

Meat

- It is done when it is brown inside. This is especially critical with hamburger meat.

Cool and Promptly Store Leftovers after Food Has Been Served

- Because harmful bacteria grow at room temperature keep hot food hot at 140° F or higher, and keep cold food cold at 40° F or cooler. This is especially important during picnics and buffets.

- Do not leave perishable foods out for more than two hours.
- Promptly refrigerate or freeze leftovers in shallow containers or wrapped tightly in bags.

Basically use common sense and when in doubt, throw it out. It is much cheaper to throw out bad food than it is to pay expensive medical bills or miss work.

Get Immunized

Getting immunizations is easy, inexpensive, and can save lives. Make sure you and your children get immunizations as recommended by your health care provider.

Did you know that in the United States measles and diphtheria used to kill thousands of people a year? Or that in 1952, 20,000 people were crippled from polio? We might think we do not have to worry about these diseases today because, thanks to vaccines, we do not see them nearly as often as we used to. But they're still around and they're still dangerous.

Why are immunizations important?

Getting you and your family immunized is a very easy way to prevent getting some very serious diseases. About 128,000 people still get infected with hepatitis B virus each year. There's no cure but a simple immunization can prevent it. By getting immunized your family fights disease in two ways. First, you protect yourselves, but also you protect others, because if you don't have a disease you can't spread it to someone else.

What is an immunization?

Sometimes immunizations are called vaccinations or just shots. And they help our body fight diseases.

What diseases can immunizations prevent?

The following ten dangerous diseases are prevented by routine shots given to children.

- Polio
- Measles
- Mumps
- Rubella (or German measles)
- Diphtheria
- Tetanus

- Whooping cough
- Chicken pox
- Meningitis
- Hepatitis B

There are other shots for diseases given to both adults and children if they are at risk of getting those diseases or they are likely to have serious complications if they get them. Examples of these include:

- Hepatitis A
- Pneumonia
- Flu

Without shots your children could get these diseases. And these diseases can also lead to pneumonia, brain damage, severe eye problems, paralysis, or other serious problems.

When should you or your family be immunized?

Immunizations for Children

Many "baby shots" protect your children for the rest of their lives. The following schedule is recommended:

- Children should get their first shots no later than 2 months of age, and
- Return for shots 4 or more times before they're two years old.
- Some diseases need booster shots when your child is older.

Ask your doctor when you and your family need vaccines. And be sure to keep your immunization records in a safe place.

Immunizations for Adults

Adults need immunizations too, because each year thousands of adults die unnecessarily from flu, pneumonia and hepatitis B.

- You need tetanus and diphtheria shots repeated every 10 years.
- You may need shots when traveling to other countries.

How much do immunizations cost?

Shots are inexpensive but the diseases they prevent can be very expensive. While public health clinics may charge a small service fee, they may provide free vaccines. And ask your doctor about special programs that provide free shots to your children.

Most people are getting their families immunized so many serious diseases are at an all time low in the United States. But some of them are still common in other countries. If we stop vaccinating, they could easily return to the United States. Thanks to vaccinations smallpox, a deadly disease, has been wiped out and polio will soon be gone, too. With immunizations we not only can prevent some very serious diseases, but actually eliminate them from the world. It is easy, inexpensive, and it saves lives.

Use Antibiotics Appropriately

Antibiotics don't work against viruses such as colds and flu. Unnecessary antibiotics can be harmful. Antibiotics should be taken exactly as prescribed by your health care provider.

Getting you and your family immunized is an important way to prevent getting sick. But if you do get sick it is important to use antibiotics appropriately. Antibiotics are powerful drugs used to treat certain illnesses. But antibiotics do not cure everything, and unnecessary antibiotics can even be harmful.

Viruses Versus Bacteria

Basically, there are two main types of germs that cause most infections. These are viruses and bacteria.

Viruses cause:

- All colds and flu
- Most coughs
- Most sore throats

Antibiotics cannot kill viruses.

Bacteria cause:

- Most ear infections
- Some sinus infections
- Strep throat
- Urinary tract infections

Antibiotics do kill specific bacteria.

Drug-Resistant Bacteria

Each time you take an antibiotic, bacteria are killed. Sometimes bacteria may be resistant or become resistant. Resistant bacteria do not respond to the antibiotics and continue to cause infection.

Each time you take an antibiotic unnecessarily or improperly, you increase your chance of developing drug-resistant bacteria. So it is really important to take antibiotics only when necessary. Because of these resistant bacteria, some diseases that used to be easy to treat are now becoming nearly impossible to treat.

What do you need to know about antibiotics?

- Remember that antibiotics don't work against colds and flu, and that unnecessary antibiotics can be harmful.
- Talk to your health care provider about antibiotics and find out about the differences between viruses and bacteria—and when antibiotics should and shouldn't be used.
- If you do get an antibiotic, be sure to take it exactly as prescribed—that may help decrease the development of resistant bacteria.
- Antibiotic resistance is particularly dangerous for children, but it can occur in adults as well.

One final note is that taking antibiotics appropriately and getting immunized will help prevent having to take more dangerous and more costly medications. If we use antibiotics appropriately we can avoid developing drug resistance. We just need to take our medicine exactly as it is prescribed and not expect to take antibiotics every time we're sick.

Keep Pets Healthy

Pets should be adopted from an animal shelter or purchased from a reputable pet store or breeder. Pets should be routinely cared for by a veterinarian.

Owning a pet can be a rewarding experience for children and adults. And you can make sure it's a healthy experience by following a few simple tips. It all starts with keeping your pet healthy and being a responsible pet owner.

How can you keep your pet healthy?

- Adopt your pet from an animal shelter or purchase it from a reputable pet store or breeder.

- Have your new companion checked out right away by a veterinarian.
- Keep your pet under a veterinarian's care for regularly scheduled shots and treatment for worms. This reduces the chance that your pet could get sick and pass an infection to you or your family. Since the cost of veterinary care may not be within everyone's reach, the local animal shelter or humane society may have information about low-cost clinics.
- Give your pet a balanced diet and do not allow it to eat raw food or drink out of the toilet.
- Clean your pet's living area at least once a week. Bury the feces, or place them in a plastic bag and then put it in the trash.
- Litter boxes should be cleaned daily and the dirty litter placed in a plastic bag. To prevent infectious diseases that may cause birth defects, pregnant women should not change cat litter boxes. A child's sandbox can become a cat's litter box so cover it when not in use. Areas that have been contaminated with dog or cat feces should be off limits to children—not only at home but also in public areas such as parks or playgrounds. And because toddlers naturally explore their environment, teach children not to eat dirt.
- Wash your hands with soap and water after handling or cleaning up after animals, especially reptiles. Teach your children to do the same. This is also important after contacting dirt because hookworms from animal feces in the soil can enter through your skin.

What about having a wild animal as a pet?

In general, wild animals do not make good pets because they are not tame and do not adapt well to living in a house. But if you must have one make sure you know about any special needs the animal has or diseases it can transmit before buying it from a pet store.

What's the most serious disease that animals can transmit to people?

The most serious disease that animals can transmit to people is rabies. But, because responsible pet owners are keeping their animals immunized each year, the number of rabies cases in the United States has been drastically reduced. However, rabies is still found in wild animals. Cats, as well as dogs, should be immunized against rabies.

Why should you have your pet immunized against rabies?

Having your pet immunized protects it against rabies if it's attacked by a rabid animal. But if your pet is not immunized, it could get rabies and then give it to you or your family. So obey local leash laws and control your pets so that they do not come into contact with, or prey on, wild animals.

What should you do if you are bitten or scratched by an animal?

Each year almost 800,000 persons bitten by dogs or cats require medical attention. So, never approach an unfamiliar animal. If you do get bitten or scratched always

- Wash the area with soap and water,
- Apply anti-bacterial medication, and
- Bandage the wound, and consider medical attention.
- Teach your children to tell you about any animal bite or scratch that they receive.

Avoid Contact with Wild Animals

Wild animals can transmit deadly diseases to you and your pets. Keep your house free of wild animals by not leaving any food around and by eliminating possible nesting sites.

Basically, you and your pets need to avoid contact with rodents and other wild animals because they can carry some very deadly diseases. For example:

- Rodents can transmit hantavirus and plague.
- Ticks can transmit Rocky Mountain spotted fever and Lyme disease.
- Mammals such as raccoons, skunks, and foxes can transmit rabies. In fact, bats cause most of the human rabies cases in this country.

When are most wild animals active?

Most wild animals come out at night and are afraid of people. So, if you see a wild animal during the day, you should avoid having contact with it and notify animal control authorities because it may have rabies.

How can you discourage animals from nesting in your house?

- Keep your home clean.
- At night when insects, rodents and other animals search for food, keep tight-fitting lids on food containers and on the garbage containers.
- Discard any excess food and take up pet water bowls when not in use.

How can you discourage animals from entering your house?

The closer wild animals live to your house, the more likely they are to find a way inside.

- Eliminate any possible nesting sites and items that provide a water source.
- Seal entrances on the inside and the outside of your home because a mouse can squeeze through an opening as small as a dime.
- One pair of mice can produce over 15,000 offspring a year. You can keep rodent populations low by continually setting traps inside and outside your home.
- Keep baits and traps out of reach of children and pets.
- Natural predators also help control rodent populations in the wild.

What should you do if you find a dead animal?

- If you find a dead animal, spray it and any nesting materials with disinfectant before moving it. This reduces the risk of exposure to deadly viruses.
- Use protective measures when moving the carcass and dispose of the animal according to local regulations.
- Remember to wash your hands afterwards.
- If your home is infested with rodents, contact animal control authorities.

What precautions should you take against ticks and mosquitoes?

- In wooded areas and high grass, take extra precautions against ticks and mosquitoes.

- It helps to wear light-colored clothing that covers as much exposed skin as possible.
- Use an insect repellent containing DEET.
- Carefully check yourself and your family for ticks. Use tweezers to remove them.

What should you do if you are bitten or scratched by a wild animal?

- Apply first aid treatment as quickly as possible, and
- Immediately notify your health care provider.

Wild animals can carry fatal diseases and we have to keep them out of our homes. But we also need to take certain precautions with those endearing pets that we enjoy close at hand.

Chapter 4

Disease Risks Associated with Blood Transfusion

Testing of Donor Blood for Infectious Disease

The American Association of Blood Banks (AABB) and its members are committed to ensuring a safe blood supply for everyone who may need transfusions. An important step in ensuring safety is the screening of donated blood for infectious diseases. Today, nine tests for infectious diseases are conducted on each unit of donated blood. Tests for hepatitis B and syphilis were in place before 1985. Since then, tests for human immunodeficiency virus (HIV-1 and HIV-2), human T-lymphotropic virus (HTLV-I and -II) and the hepatitis C virus (HCV) have been added. The following tests are performed on each unit of blood.

Hepatitis B Surface Antigen (HBsAg)

The hepatitis B virus, which mainly infects the liver, has an inner core and an outer envelope (the surface). The HBsAg test detects the outer envelope, identifying an individual infected with the hepatitis B virus. Hepatitis B can cause inflammation of the liver, and in the earliest stage of the disease, infected people may feel ill or even have yellow discoloration of the skin or eyes, a condition known as jaundice. Fortunately, most patients recover completely and test negative

---

for HBsAg within a few months after the illness. A small percentage of people become chronic carriers of the virus, and in these cases, the test may remain positive for years. Chronically infected people can develop severe liver disease as time passes, and need to be followed carefully by an experienced doctor.

Antibodies to the Hepatitis B Core (Anti-HBc)

The anti-HBc test detects an antibody to the hepatitis B virus that is produced during and after infection. If an individual has a positive anti-HBc test, but the HBsAg test is negative, it may mean that the person once had hepatitis B, but has recovered from the infection. Of the individuals with a positive test for anti-HBc, many have not been exposed to the hepatitis B virus. This kind of test result is called a false positive, and although the individual may be permanently deferred from donating blood, it is unlikely that the person's health will be negatively affected. (Note: This antibody is not produced following vaccination against hepatitis B. Hepatitis B vaccination, by itself, will rarely cause the HbsAg test to be positive for a few days after the shots.)

Antibodies to the Hepatitis C Virus (Anti-HCV)

This test is used to screen donors for the hepatitis C virus (HCV). It works by detecting antibodies manufactured by the body in reaction to portions of the virus called antigens. HCV causes inflammation of the liver, and up to 80 percent of those exposed to the virus develop chronic infection. Eventually, up to 20 percent of people with HCV may develop cirrhosis of the liver or other severe liver diseases. As in other forms of hepatitis, individuals may be infected with the virus, but may not realize they are carriers since they do not have any symptoms. Because of the risk of serious illness, people with HCV need to be followed closely by a physician with experience evaluating this infection.

Antibodies to the Human Immunodeficiency Virus, Types 1 and 2 (Anti-HIV-1, -2)

This test is designed to detect antibodies directed against antigens of the HIV-1 or HIV-2 viruses. HIV-1 is much more common in the United States, while HIV-2 is prevalent in Western Africa. Donors are tested for both viruses because both are transmitted by infected blood, and a few cases of HIV-2 have been identified in U.S. residents. Both of these viruses can cause acquired immunodeficiency syndrome, or AIDS.

Antibodies to Human T-Lymphotropic Virus, Types I and II (Anti-HTLV-I, -II)

This test screens for antibodies directed against portions of the HTLV-I and HTLV-II viruses. Both of these viruses are relatively uncommon in the United States, but do occur more frequently in certain populations. HTLV-I is more common in Japan and the Caribbean. The infection can persist for a lifetime, but rarely causes major illnesses in most people who are infected. In rare instances, the virus may, after many years of infection, cause nervous system disease or an unusual type of leukemia. HTLV-II infections are usually associated with intravenous drug usage, especially among people who share needles or syringes. Disease associations with HTLV-II have been hard to confirm, but the virus may cause subtle abnormalities of immunity that lead to frequent infections, or rare cases of neurological disease.

Syphilis

This test is done to detect evidence of infection with the spirochete that causes syphilis. Blood centers began testing for this shortly after World War II, when syphilis rates in the general population were much higher. The risk of transmitting syphilis through a blood transfusion is exceedingly small (no cases have been recognized in this country for many years) because the infection is very rare in blood donors, and because the spirochete is fragile and unlikely to survive blood storage conditions.

Nucleic Acid Amplification Testing (NAT)

NAT employs testing technology that directly detects the genetic material of viruses. Because NAT detects a virus's genetic material—instead of waiting for the body's response, the formation of antibodies, as with many current tests—it offers the opportunity to reduce the window period during which an infecting agent is undetectable by traditional tests, thus further improving blood safety.

NAT is being used to detect HIV-1 and HCV, and this technology is under investigation for detecting other infectious disease agents.

Confirmatory Testing

All of the above tests are referred to as screening tests, and are designed to detect as many infections as possible. Because these tests are so sensitive, some donors may have a false positive result, even when the donor was never exposed to the particular infection. In order to sort out true infections from false positive test results, screening tests that are reactive may be followed up with more specific tests called confirmatory tests. Thus, confirmatory tests help determine whether a donor is truly infected.

If the test result from a donated unit of blood is abnormal for any of these disease markers, the unit is discarded and the donor is notified. The donor's name is then added to a donor deferral list and is prohibited from donating blood indefinitely.

Transfusion-Transmitted Diseases

Viruses

Cytomegalovirus (CMV): Cytomegalovirus (CMV) is a virus belonging to the herpes group that is rarely transmitted by blood transfusion. According to the Centers for Disease Control and Prevention (CDC), about 50 to 85 percent of adults in the United States are infected with CMV by the age of 40. CMV infection is usually mild, but it may be serious or fatal in those who are immunocompromised. Particularly at risk are low-birth weight infants and bone marrow and organ transplant patients. If a patient is at high risk of getting CMV diseases, blood that tests negative for CMV can be transfused. Alternatively, blood that has been filtered to decrease the number of white blood cells—the cells that carry CMV—will protect patients from getting a CMV infection from transfusion.

Hepatitis: Hepatitis was the first documented transfusion-transmitted disease. Many of the current practices for diminishing risk in transfusion medicine are based on the experiences of controlling the transmission of hepatitis.

Hepatitis viruses, which infect the liver, fall primarily into two groups: viruses with a chronic course that can readily be transmitted by blood transfusion (hepatitis B and C) and viruses that cause only acute disease and are rarely transmitted by transfusion (hepatitis A and E).

Hepatitis A Virus (HAV): Hepatitis A (HAV) infection is rarely transmitted through blood transfusion; it is usually spread by contaminated food and water. About 23,000 cases are reported annually in the US, but epidemiologists estimate that the virus infects 150,000 Americans each year. Hepatitis A is very prevalent in the developing world, including Mexico and parts of the Caribbean. Because HAV antibodies are present in approximately 20 percent of the population, many with no history of hepatitis, it is assumed that many people experience unrecognized infection. There have been occasional reports in the U.S. of transfusion-transmitted HAV, but little can be done to prevent this rare occurrence. A vaccine recently developed for HAV has replaced immune globulin as a pre-exposure prophylactic measure for people at a high risk for acquiring this infection, although the latter remains useful after exposure.

Hepatitis B Virus (HBV): Transmission of hepatitis B virus (HBV) is rare because of routine testing of blood for the HBsAg and hepatitis B core antibody, donor screening and deferral for risk of HBV infection, and the use of only altruistic volunteer blood donors. HBV is a major cause of acute and chronic hepatitis. Each year in the U.S., an estimated 300,000 persons are infected with HBV. More than 10,000 patients require hospitalization, and an average of 350 die from the disease. There is an estimated pool of 750,000–1,000,000 chronically infected HBV carriers in the U.S. Approximately 25 percent of carriers have active hepatitis that can progress to cirrhosis of the liver. An estimated 4,000 people die each year from hepatitis B-related cirrhosis, and more than 800 die from hepatitis B-related liver cancer. The number of HBV infections in the U.S. is falling because hepatitis B vaccinations of health care professionals and school-age children has become nearly universal.

Screening blood donors for HBV began in 1969 and became mandatory in 1972. By the mid-1970s, testing and an all-volunteer blood donor supply reduced the rate of post-transfusion hepatitis B to between 0.3 and 0.9 percent. From 1982 to 1985, an average of 3.0 percent of hepatitis B cases in the U.S. were related to blood transfusion. During the period from 1986 to 1988, the percentage of reported cases related to blood transfusion declined to 1.0 percent, possibly as a consequence of the donor screening questions that were instituted to identify persons at increased risk for HIV infection. In 2000, the frequency of post-transfusion hepatitis B developing after a blood transfusion was estimated at perhaps 1 in 137,000 screened units of blood.

Hepatitis C Virus (HCV): Hepatitis C, formerly known as non-A, non-B hepatitis, was discovered in the late 1980s, and all blood donations have been screened for it since 1990. Acute hepatitis C virus (HCV) is a relatively mild infection, and most people are unaware they have become infected; however, HCV becomes chronic in 80 percent of those infected. In the general population, 1.8 percent of the population has some evidence of HCV-infection. While the rate of new HCV infections is falling rapidly due to behavior changes and blood screening, HCV is an important source of serious chronic liver disease, which often develops decades after the initial exposure to the virus.

Antibody screening was started in 1990, and the test has undergone significant improvement since. In 1999, NAT testing was added in the U.S. After more than 10 years of testing for HCV, the risk of HCV transmission through transfusion is less than 1 per 1,000,000-screened units of blood.

HIV (Human Immunodeficiency Virus): Transfusion transmission of HIV, the virus that causes AIDS, has been almost completely eradicated, since blood banks began interviewing donors about at-risk behaviors and a blood test became available in early 1985. The HIV antibody tests, used on every blood donation since then, have undergone continuous improvement. Starting in 1999 nucleic acid amplification testing (NAT) has been used to directly detect the genetic material of the HIV virus in blood, and current estimates are that fewer than 1 in 1,900,000 blood components is capable of transmitting HIV. Transfusion medicine specialists are continually researching new technologies to further reduce the transmission of HIV. Examples of technologies on the horizon include methods to kill viruses in donated blood (called viral inactivation) and blood component substitutes.

Human T Lymphotropic Virus I, -II (HTLV-I, -II): HTLV-I and -II are viruses that are not related to HIV. HTLV-I is found mainly in Southwestern Japan and Caribbean islands. The viruses can cause blood or nervous system diseases in a small number of infected people (less than 5 percent lifetime risk). HTLV-II is endemic in the Americas (including the U.S.), and also may infrequently cause slightly increased susceptibility to infections. Both of these viruses, although rare, were found in the U.S. blood donor population in the 1980s. Few people have gotten HTLV as a result of transfusion, but because of the small transfusion risk that existed in the 1980s, tests to detect HTLV-I antibodies were developed and quickly implemented; these tests also detected many, but not all, HTLV-II infections. Tests specifically designed to detect both viruses are now available and are used by blood centers to screen every donation.

West Nile virus (WNV): West Nile virus (WNV) is spread by the bite of an infected mosquito. The virus can infect people, horses, many types of birds, and some other animals.

WNV was first detected in the United States in 1999 and has since been detected in many parts of the U.S. The first documented cases of WNV transmission through organ transplantation and transfusion were noted in 2002. The most common symptoms of transfusion-transmitted cases of WNV were fever and headache.

The preclinical incubation period is thought to range from 2 to 14 days following a bite from an infected mosquito. Approximately 80% of people infected with WNV remain without symptoms, while 20% develop mild symptoms, including fever, headache, eye pain, body aches, gastrointestinal complaints, and occasionally a generalized rash or swollen lymph nodes. One in 150 to 200 persons infected with WNV develops a more severe form of the disease that may be fatal.

FDA is allowing national deployment of investigational nucleic acid tests (NAT) to screen blood for West Nile virus (WNV), until FDA-licensed tests become available. Blood centers have implemented precautionary measures to protect the blood supply from WNV, including stockpiling frozen blood components before the start of mosquito season.

Because WNV can be transmitted through a blood transfusion, potential donors will be asked orally or in writing about history of fever and headache. A blood collection facility must implement the questioning of all donors by June 1 of each year and continue until November 30, or until there have been two consecutive weeks without any report of human WNV infection in the state in which the facility is located. Blood centers may decide to begin questioning earlier than June 1 in areas where they are aware of reports of epizootic (epidemic among wild animals) activity or human transmission of WNV. Depending on an individual's response to questioning, that individual may be requested not to donate blood for an interval of time called a deferral period. That person is said to be "deferred."

Although there are limited data on the natural course of WNV infection, the deferral periods recommended are based on the longest known viremic period (the length of time a virus remains in the blood stream), with an extra safety margin added.

Who will be deferred?

- A potential donor who has been diagnosed with WNV infection (including diagnoses based on symptoms and laboratory results) will be deferred for 28 days from the onset of symptoms or until the patient has been without symptoms for 14 days.
- A potential donor who responds positively to the question: "In the past week, have you had a fever with headache?" will be deferred for 28 days.

- A donor whose blood or components potentially were associated with a transfusion-related WNV transmission will be deferred 28 days from the date of the implicated donation.

Donors are encouraged to report unexplained post-donation febrile illness with headache or other symptoms suggestive of WNV infection that occur within one week after blood donation.

Parasitic Infections

Babesiosis: Babesiosis is a parasitic infection carried by the white-footed mouse and transmitted by tick bites. It appears primarily in the northeastern U.S., in coastal areas that are home to the white-footed mouse. Cases also have been identified in the Upper Midwest and Pacific Northwest. About 30 transfusion-associated cases have been reported in the U.S. While babesiosis is often quite mild, some patients, including those without a spleen, the elderly, or the immunocompromised, may be at risk of serious illness. There are no useful tests available for screening blood donors, although testing strategies are being developed and discussed. The AABB requires that all donors be asked if they have a history of babesiosis. Those individuals with a history of the disease are permanently deferred from donating blood.

Chagas' Disease: A Brazilian doctor, Carlos Chagas, discovered Chagas' disease almost 100 years ago. This disease is caused by a parasite that infects as many as 18 million people worldwide. Once infection is established, it is life-long. Each year, several thousand South and Central Americans die of heart and digestive problems caused by the disease. Up to 20 percent of infected people never exhibit symptoms. This infection is rare in the U.S., but because of recent global population shifts, individuals from countries where this disease is common now reside in the U.S. To date, there have been only five cases of transfusion-transmitted Chagas' disease reported in North America. The AABB requires that blood centers permanently prohibit blood donation from anyone who has had Chagas' disease, and tests are being developed and screening strategies discussed.

Lyme Disease: Although transfusion-related cases have not been reported, public health agencies and the AABB are monitoring this disease because of the remote chance that it could affect transfusion safety. Lyme disease is associated with the bite of certain species of the deer tick, and can cause an illness that affects many systems within the body. Donors with a history of Lyme disease can donate, provided they have undergone a full course of antibiotic treatment and no longer have any symptoms.

Malaria: Between 1958 and 1998, the CDC recorded 103 cases of transfusion-transmitted malaria. These cases were most likely caused by donations from people who felt well and were not aware that they were carrying malaria. Although exceedingly rare in the U.S., malaria can cause serious consequences, including fatalities. There is no practical test available to screen donors so AABB requires blood centers to temporarily defer blood donations from people who have visited malarial areas in the past year or who emigrated from a malarial area within the past three years.

Creutzfeldt-Jakob Disease (CJD)

CJD is a rare degenerative and fatal nervous system disorder. It is diagnosed in about one person per million per year in the U.S. and worldwide. There are three forms of CJD that can affect humans: sporadic CJD has no known risk factors and accounts for 85 percent of CJD cases; hereditary CJD occurs only in individuals with a family history of the disease and/or tests positive for specific genetic mutations; and acquired CJD is transmitted by exposure to brain or nervous system tissue. Acquired CJD accounts for less than 1 percent of CJD cases and can occur in individuals who have received injections of human pituitary gland growth hormone, or who have had their brain's outer lining (dura mater) repaired with dura mater from someone else who had CJD.

Individuals who will develop CJD can remain without symptoms for decades and then progress rapidly to dementia, severe loss of coordination and death. Scientists believe abnormal brain proteins that have undergone a peculiar shape change can cause other brain proteins to do the same and cause CJD.

Currently, there is no screening test for the disease, and while blood transfusions have never been shown to transmit any form of the disease, as a precaution the Food and Drug Administration (FDA) prohibits blood donation by individuals who may be at risk. These include potential donors who have received injections of human-derived pituitary hormone, those with a family history of CJD, or those who have had surgeries that involved transplanted dura mater.

Variant Creutzfeldt-Jakob Disease (vCJD)

Similar to CJD, vCJD, commonly known as the human form of "mad cow" disease, is a rare degenerative and fatal nervous system disorder. There is reason to believe that vCJD occurs when humans eat beef contaminated with bovine spongiform encephalopathy (BSE or "mad cow"). This new form of CJD has appeared in residents of the United Kingdom, France, and a single individual in Hong Kong. There have been no cases of vCJD infection in humans or of BSE in cattle in the US. Currently, there is no screening test in humans for the disease.

Even though there is no evidence that vCJD has ever been transmitted through a blood transfusion, the FDA requires donor deferral policies for anyone who potentially could have been exposed to the disease, by eating contaminated beef products in areas of the world where BSE has been found. These policies are changing as we learn more about vCJD and BSE.

The FDA recommends that the following donors be deferred indefinitely due to vCJD risk:

- Donors who spent a total of three months or more in the United Kingdom (UK) from the beginning of 1980 through the end of 1996;
- Donors who have spent a total of five years or more in France from 1980 to the present;
- Current or former U.S. military personnel, civilian military employees and their dependents who resided at U.S. military bases in Northern Europe (Germany, UK, Belgium, and the Netherlands) for a total of six months or more from 1980 through 1990, or elsewhere in Europe (Greece, Turkey, Spain, Portugal, and Italy) from 1980 through 1996.
- Donors who have received any blood or blood component transfusions in the UK between 1980 and the present;
- Whole blood, but not source plasma, donors, who have lived cumulatively for five years or more in Europe from 1980 to the present, (which includes the aforementioned deferral periods applied to the UK and France). Unless deemed unsuitable for other reasons, these donors, although deferred from whole blood collection, remain eligible to serve as source plasma donors;
- Donors who have injected bovine insulin since 1980, unless it is possible to obtain confirmation that the product was not manufactured after 1980 from cattle in the UK.

Other organizations have slightly different policies summarized below.

Department of Defense (DoD)

The DoD implemented its set of donor deferral rules in October 2001. All active-duty military personnel, civil service employees, and these two groups' family members will be deferred indefinitely due to vCJD risk if they are:

- Donors who traveled or resided in the UK for a cumulative total of three months or more at any time from 1980 through the end of 1996;
- Donors who have received a blood transfusion in the UK at any time from 1980 to the present;
- Donors who have traveled to or resided anywhere in Europe for a cumulative total of six months or more at any time from 1980 through the end of 1996;
- Donors who traveled to or resided anywhere in Europe for a cumulative total of five years or more at any time from Jan. 1, 1997, to the present.

American Red Cross (ARC)

The ARC implemented its set of donor deferral rules in September 2001. Donors will be indefinitely deferred if, since 1980 they:

- Spent a total time of three months or more in any of these countries: England, Scotland, Wales, Northern Ireland, Isle of Man, Falkland Islands, Gibraltar, Channel Islands, or
- Spent a total time of six months or more in any combination of these countries: Albania, Andorra, Austria, Azores, Belarus, Belgium, Boznia/Herzegovina, Bulgaria, Channel Islands, Croatia, Czech Republic, Denmark, England, Estonia, Falkland Islands, Faroe Island, Finland, France, Germany, Gibraltar, Greece, Greenland, Hungary, Iceland, Ireland (Republic of), Isle of Man, Italy, Latvia, Liechtenstein, Lithuania, Luxembourg, Macedonia, Madeira Islands, Malta, Moldova, Monaco, Netherlands (Holland), Northern Ireland, Norway, Oman, Poland, Portugal, Romania, San Marino, Scotland, Slovak Republic (Slovakia), Slovenia, Spain, Svalbard, Sweden, Switzerland, Turkey,

Ukraine, Vatican City, Wales, Yugoslavia (includes Kosovo, Montenegro, and Serbia)

- Received blood transfusions in the UK.

SARS (Severe Acute Respiratory Syndrome)

Severe acute respiratory syndrome—or SARS—is a respiratory infection that can develop serious complications. Most of the cases identified have been in Asia, but there have been cases in other countries, including the United States and Canada.

There has been no evidence this infection is transmitted from blood donors to transfusion recipients, but the virus associated with SARS is present in the blood of people who are sick, and it is possible that the virus could be present in blood immediately before a person gets sick, so that an individual with infection but no symptoms possibly could transmit SARS through a blood donation.

To help determine whether or not an individual might be infected with SARS, a blood collection facility will ask a potential donor orally or in writing about any travel to a SARS-affected country or a history of SARS or possible exposure to SARS.

Because the risk of contracting SARS through a blood transfusion theoretically exists, anyone who might be at risk of being infected with SARS is requested not to donate blood for an interval of time called a deferral period. The individual is said to be "deferred."

Who will be deferred?

- Anyone who has traveled or lived in a SARS-affected area, will be deferred from making a donation for a period of 14 days after arrival in the United States.
- Anyone who has had close contact with a person with SARS or suspected SARS, will be deferred for 14 days after the last exposure to that individual. Close contact is defined as having cared for, having lived with, or having had direct contact with respiratory secretions and/or body fluids of a person known to have, or to have had, SARS or suspected of having, or having had, the illness.
- Anyone who has been ill with SARS or suspected SARS, will be deferred for 28 days from the last date of treatment AND the last date that the individual had symptoms.

Please note that as long as a donor is and remains well, no other measures are necessary. If a donor becomes ill with fever of 100.4° F accompanied by cough or trouble breathing, that person should see a doctor. Also, any donor who develops a fever in the 14 days after making a donation should call the blood center.

- Information about the definition of SARS cases and the identification of SARS-affected areas are updated regularly. This information is posted on the CDC website http://www.cdc.gov/ncidod/sars/casedefinition.htm or may be obtained by calling the CDC at (888) 246-2675, 8 A.M.–11 P.M. weekdays, 10 A.M.–8 P.M. weekends.

Smallpox

Due to concern that terrorists may have access to the smallpox virus and attempt to use it against the American public, the U.S. Department of Health and Human Services (HHS) has been working, in cooperation with state and local governments, to strengthen our preparedness for bioterror attacks, by expanding the national stockpile of smallpox vaccine. The vaccine, which was routinely administered to Americans until 1972, is a highly effective protection against smallpox when given before or shortly after exposure to the virus. Vaccinia is the live virus used in smallpox vaccinations.

It is possible that until the vaccination scab spontaneously separates from the skin, recipients of the vaccinia virus could inadvertently infect close contacts who touch the vaccination site or dressing. The scabs themselves contain infectious virus. In an effort to ensure that the virus is not transmitted through a blood donation, potential donors will be asked by blood collection facilities about history of vaccination or close contact with anyone who has been vaccinated. A vaccine recipient who has had no complications may donate after the vaccination scab has spontaneously separated, or 21 days after vaccination, whichever is the later date. Some individuals who have received a smallpox vaccination may be requested not to donate for an interval of time called a deferral period. Those persons are said to be "deferred."

Who will be deferred:

- A vaccine recipient whose scab was pulled off or knocked off, and did not spontaneously separate, will be deferred for two months after the date of vaccination.
- A vaccine recipient who has experienced complications will be deferred for 14 days after all vaccine complications are completely gone.

- If a potential donor has had close contact (defined as physical intimacy, touching the vaccination site, touching the bandages or covering of the vaccination site, or handling bedding or clothing that had been in contact with an unbandaged vaccination site) with a vaccine recipient and has developed localized skin lesions without any other symptoms or complications, blood collection facility personnel will visually verify the absence of a scab.
    - If a scab spontaneously separated and is no longer present, there will be no deferral.
    - If a scab was otherwise removed, the donor will be deferred for three months from the date when the contact (that is the vaccine recipient) was vaccinated.
- If the date when the contact received the vaccination is unknown, the potential donor will be deferred for two months from the time of the interview.
- If a potential donor has had contact with a vaccine recipient who has had complications, the donor will be deferred for 14 days from the time that all vaccine complications are gone.
- If a potential donor has had contact with a vaccine recipient who has had no symptoms, the donor will not be deferred and may make a donation.

The primary concern with the vaccination scab is to ensure that it is healed, not necessarily how it came off. It is possible to contract smallpox from the vaccination site until the scab is fully healed, which generally occurs when the scab spontaneously separates, or drops off, the skin, usually before 21 days have elapsed. Healing is considered complete when there is no scab, oozing or discharge, bleeding, or opening. Healing is evidenced by pink, uninterrupted skin at the inoculation site.

An individual who wants to receive a smallpox vaccination and who also wishes to donate blood may want to consider scheduling the blood donation before the vaccination.

Chapter 5

Disease Risks Associated with Drug Abuse

Drug abuse involves health risks that often are as dangerous as the physiological effects of the drugs themselves. Injecting drug users (IDUs) are at high risk for direct exposure to a variety of blood-borne bacterial and viral infections. As a result, drug users are more likely than nonusers to contract a variety of infectious diseases and, when infected, to progress to serious illness and death.

HIV/AIDS

Injection drug use has been responsible for more than one-third of all adult and adolescent AIDS cases reported in the U.S. since the beginning of the AIDS epidemic, according to the Centers for Disease Control and Prevention (CDC) in Atlanta. More than one-half of all preadolescent AIDS cases in the U.S. have resulted from a transmission chain whereby a woman contracts HIV as a result of injection drug use and passes the disease to her child during pregnancy or birth. Of adult and adolescent AIDS cases, approximately 32 percent were

---

"Infectious Diseases and Drug Abuse," National Institute on Drug Abuse (NIDA), National Institutes of Health (NIH), August 1999, updated with excerpts from "Drug-Associated HIV Transmission Continues in the United States," National Center for HIV, STD and TB Prevention, Centers for Disease Control and Prevention (CDC), March 2002; "Hepatitis C Risk Not Limited to Injection Drug Users," NIH News Release, National Institutes of Health, May 2001; and Tables 28 and 29 from *Reported Tuberculosis in the United States, 2002*. Atlanta, GA: U.S. Department of Health and Human Services, CDC, September 2003.

among IDUs, and another 4 percent involved heterosexual sex with an IDU. During 1998, approximately one-third of all new AIDS cases in the U.S. were related directly or indirectly to injection drug use. Of the 42,156 new cases of AIDS reported in 2000, 11,635 (28%) were IDU-associated. IDU-associated AIDS accounts for a larger proportion of cases among adolescent and adult women than among men. Since the epidemic began, 57% of all AIDS cases among women have been attributed to injection drug use or sex with partners who inject drugs, compared with 31% of cases among men.

Noninjection drug use can also contribute to HIV transmission. Studies have shown that inner-city youths who smoke crack cocaine are up to three times more likely to be infected with HIV than are inner-city youths who do not. Noninjecting drug users who trade sex for drugs or who engage in unprotected sex while under the influence of drugs increase their risk of infection.

Drug-Associated HIV Transmission Continues in the United States

Sharing syringes and other equipment for drug injection is a well known route of HIV transmission, yet injection drug use contributes to the epidemic's spread far beyond the circle of those who inject. People who have sex with an IDU also are at risk for infection through sexual transmission of HIV. Children born to mothers who contracted HIV through sharing needles or having sex with an IDU may become infected as well.

Hepatitis

Hepatitis B (HBV) and hepatitis C (HCV) are viral diseases that destroy liver cells and can lead to cirrhosis and liver cancer. People can become infected with HBV through sexual intercourse with an infected person or through exposure to an infected person's blood, as may happen when IDUs share needles. Blood transfusion and needle sharing are the most common routes of infection with HCV. National Institute on Drug Abuse (NIDA)-supported research has shown that the risk of infection by HBV and HCV is extremely high in the first year after beginning injection drug use. One study found overall HCV and HBV prevalences of 76.9 percent and 65.7 percent, respectively, in a group who had been injecting drugs for 6 years or less. A study in New York City found a higher than expected prevalence of hepatitis C infection among non-injecting drug users, raising a question as to whether hepatitis C can be transmitted through the sharing of non-injecting drug paraphernalia such as straws or pipes.

Tuberculosis

Tuberculosis (TB) is transmitted from person to person by airborne bacteria. This disease is most prevalent in crowded low-income areas with substandard health conditions. Drug users are from two to six times more likely to contract TB than nonusers. CDC estimated that 2.2% of tuberculosis cases in 2002 were in injecting drug users and 7.0% of cases were in noninjecting drug users. Compared to others with TB, IDUs are more likely to develop the disease in multiple organs and sites, rather than only in the lungs.

Other Infectious Diseases

Drug users have a high incidence not only of HIV/AIDS but also of other sexually transmitted diseases including syphilis, chlamydia, trichomoniasis, gonorrhea, and genital herpes. The geographic distribution of syphilis and gonorrhea infections across the U.S. reflect the geographical distribution of the use of crack cocaine and its associated high-risk behaviors, such as unprotected sex and the exchange of sex for drugs.

Among IDUs, the most common cause for medical treatment is skin infection at the site of injection. Complications from these infections range from skin ulcers and localized abscesses to stroke, botulism, tetanus, destruction of lung tissue, and infection of the heart valves.

Bacterial and viral infections associated with injection drug use can progress to systemic infections and damage any body system. Directly observed medication therapy, in which the patient takes medications in the presence of a health care provider, is generally recommended for addicts, many of whom may have difficulty following treatment regimens.

Chapter 6

Contagious Disease Risks for People with Immune System Deficiencies

Every day people are constantly exposed to an overabundance of bacteria, viruses, fungi, parasites, and other microscopic creatures. Some of these are beneficial, some neutral, and some potentially quite harmful. Usually, people are unaware of their body's immune system as it handles these encounters, distinguishing between the harmful and the helpful, to protect health. Often it is only when the immune system is not working properly that people begin to appreciate how sophisticated and important it is.

An increasing number of people find themselves living with immunocompromise (an impaired immune system). In some cases, this is a result of improved medical care. Many people now survive for years with diseases that would have been rapidly fatal not long ago. Other people become immunocompromised as a result of medical treatments for serious diseases (such as cancer) or maintenance of organ transplants. Finally, the global epidemic of human immunodeficiency virus has lead to a relatively new disease, acquired immunodeficiency syndrome (AIDS).

When someone becomes immunocompromised, it is important to understand how this affects resistance to disease. In most cases, special precautions become necessary to prevent the development of severe infections.

Text in this chapter is by David A. Cooke, M.D., Diplomate, American Board of Internal Medicine.

The Normal Immune System

The term "immune system" refers to a large number of interlocking and interdependent defense systems active within the human body. It involves several defensive cell types, and critical but nonliving proteins found in blood and other body fluids. Each has unique functions, and the overall operation of the whole depends upon the individual components.

- **Neutrophils:** Polymorphonuclear neutrophils, also known as neutrophils or PMNs, are the first line of cellular immune defense. Neutrophils rush to the site of infection, and engulf and digest any invading organisms (phagocytosis).
- **Macrophages:** These cells are larger than neutrophils, but share their ability to voraciously devour intruders. They also have important functions coordinating with lymphocytes and other immune cells.
- **Lymphocytes:** These are some of the most complex immune cells. There are several subtypes, including *B-cells*, *helper T-cells*, and *killer T-cells*. Depending upon their type, these cells produce antibodies, kill infected body cells, or orchestrate the actions of other immune cell types. They are particularly important in defense against viruses, as well as certain hardy bacteria that have evolved ways to evade other immune defenses.
- **Eosinophils:** Usually a minor cell type, these cells are important in defense against parasites. They also appear to play a major role in allergic diseases.
- **Antibodies:** These are complex, Y-shaped proteins produced by lymphocytes. They are present in blood, saliva, respiratory secretions, and certain other body fluids. Each antibody is designed to attach to a specific kind of invader. They act like guided missiles. Some antibodies kill or inactivate viruses or bacteria. Others stick to their targets, tagging them for later destruction by other components of the immune system.
- **Complement:** Another class of defensive proteins, complement deposits on the surfaces of certain bacteria. Additionally, the complement proteins attach to targets previously tagged by antibodies. Once attached, they drill holes in their targets and kill them.

The Abnormal Immune System

Immunocompromised patients do not have normal immune systems. This puts these patients at increased risk of infections.

Immunocompromising conditions are not all alike. Most conditions affect one part of the immune system more than the others. This may result in problems unique to the particular disease. Understanding how this applies to particular conditions helps explain why particular precautions may be necessary.

Common Immunosuppressive Conditions

Chemotherapy

Cancer chemotherapy is a form of selective poisoning, intended to damage cancerous cells more than normal cells. Most chemotherapy drugs target rapidly dividing cells. This damages cancer cells, which tend to divide more rapidly than normal cells. However, it also damages some kinds of immune cells, which normally have rapid turnover.

Following a round of chemotherapy, cancer patients will frequently develop a deficiency of neutrophils, known as neutropenia. This is often delayed by days to weeks after the last chemotherapy dose, depending on the medication used. This period of neutropenia is known as the nadir. Frequently, medications known as colony stimulating factors are given following chemotherapy to speed the growth of new immune cells, and shorten the period of the nadir.

Because of the critical importance of neutrophils in stopping infection from common bacteria, neutropenic patients can be extremely susceptible to minor bacterial infections. Bacterial infections tend to create the biggest problems for these patients; viruses and parasites tend to be far less of a problem than with other conditions.

It is important to get clear instructions from the doctor performing chemotherapy regarding the degree and timing of neutropenia that may occur with the particular medication being used.

With some medications, in-hospital isolation procedures are used to minimize exposure to infectious agents. Patients who develop signs of infection are usually placed immediately on powerful antibiotics.

While specifics will vary, the following measures are usually appropriate for patients undergoing chemotherapy that causes neutropenia:

- **Fever is a very dangerous sign in chemotherapy patients.** Call your doctor about **any** fever after a round of chemotherapy, even if it is mild.

- Frequent handwashing with soap and water or an alcohol-based disinfectant, for the patient and all visitors or caretakers.
- Avoid contact with sick individuals. If contact cannot be avoided, the sick person should wear a surgical mask while around the immunocompromised person, and wash hands frequently.
- For some patients, wearing a surgical mask is best when going out in public.
- Daily inspections of skin for signs of infection.
- Good dental care, preferably before starting chemotherapy. Patients with severe tooth decay may need to have their teeth pulled to avoid later serious infections.
- Avoid raw, undercooked, or "rare" meats, eggs, or seafood; these can carry bacteria that an immunocompromised person may have difficulty fighting.
- Flowers and plants are not good gifts for patients undergoing chemotherapy. Microorganisms in the soil can cause serious infection.

Organ Transplantation

Most patients who receive organ transplants, such as a kidney, liver, heart, lungs, or pancreas, need to remain on medications that impair the immune system. These drugs are necessary because without them, the recipient's immune system will attack the transplanted organ as "foreign," quickly destroying it. This sort of drug therapy is known as immunosuppression.

The drugs used in organ transplants are different than those typically used in chemotherapy. The most commonly used transplant drugs are prednisone, azathioprine, cyclosporine, tacrolimus, mycophenolate, and sirolimus. In contrast to cancer chemotherapy, these drugs have much less effect on neutrophils. As a result, transplant patients are not as prone as chemotherapy patients to severe infections from everyday bacteria. However, transplant patients still become ill from bacterial infections more easily than healthy people do.

Immunosuppressive drugs have their greatest effects on lymphocytes, which are important in fighting viruses, fungi, and some of the more aggressive bacteria. As a result, transplant patients may have more problems with unusual infections than with common ones.

Physicians who care for transplant patients are aware of the unique infectious problems that these patients may face, and monitor them closely for them.

Viruses often create problems for transplant patients. Cytomegalovirus (CMV) is among the most difficult. About 50% of healthy people carry this virus, and many transplant patients are already infected before they receive their transplants. Sometimes, it is transmitted by the transplant surgery, when the donor was infected with CMV but the recipient was not. In healthy people, the immune system prevents CMV from causing disease. However, in immunosuppressed transplant patients, the virus can run rampant, and can infect almost any organ of the body. Transplant patients are usually tested for CMV before and after their transplants, and if symptoms that could be CMV occur. The infection cannot be cured, but it can be controlled with antiviral drugs.

The risk of infection in transplant patients depends on how much immunosuppressive medication is being taken. Generally speaking, patients are treated with high doses around the time of transplantation, and the doses are then tapered to the lowest possible levels as the transplant stabilizes. However, some patients require high doses of medication long after transplantation due to recurrent organ rejection. Your doctor can usually tell you how immunocompromised you are on your drug regimen.

The following measures are advisable for most transplant patients:

- Give prompt attention to any signs of fever. Call your doctor immediately if your temperature exceeds 100 degrees Fahrenheit.
- If travel abroad is planned, consult with your doctor first. In many cases, consultation with an infectious disease specialist may be advisable to help reduce the risk of acquiring infections.
- Avoid exposure to people with known or suspected tuberculosis. Transplant patients are at increased risk of developing tuberculosis, and it may be difficult to control if it develops. Any possible exposure should be promptly investigated.
- Avoid eating raw, undercooked, or "rare" meat, eggs, or seafood. These can carry bacteria or parasites that cause serious infection in transplant patients.
- Discuss your pets with your doctor. Some kinds of pets require special precautions to prevent you from catching infections from them.

- Avoid live virus vaccines. While they are beneficial for most people, they can be dangerous in transplant patients as they may not be able to control the vaccine virus. Live virus vaccines in common use at present are measles-mumps-rubella (MMR) and the chickenpox vaccine (varicella vaccine).
- Keep up to date on all other recommended vaccines. Most transplant patients should receive annual influenza vaccines, as well as the 23-valent pneumococcal vaccine (Pneumovax). These vaccines, which do not contain live viruses, are safe in transplant patients and reduce the risk of life-threatening infections.
- Avoid prolonged sunlight exposure. Transplant patients are at unusually high risk of developing skin cancer, which may be more aggressive than in other patients. Tanning is a dangerous activity for transplant patients.

HIV Disease and AIDS

Patients with advanced HIV infection pose a special challenge, as they are prone to a variety of common and unusual infections. HIV primarily affects "helper" T-lymphocytes. This results in a loss of coordination of the different elements of the immune system, and a less effective immune response. As the disease progresses, infections are seen with viruses and bacteria that do not normally make people ill. These are known as opportunistic infections. Patients who have had opportunistic infections are said to have AIDS, to distinguish them from HIV-infected patients with less advanced disease.

All HIV patients are at increased risk of common infections. For example, HIV patients catch pneumonia much more often than people without HIV, although it is usually caused by the same bacteria that infect healthy people.

Tuberculosis is also a particular problem for HIV patients. HIV patients catch tuberculosis easily, and it can be quite severe. In fact, prior to the onset of the HIV epidemic, tuberculosis was largely disappearing from the United States, but it has had a sharp rebound due to spread among HIV patients. Tuberculosis is spread from person to person, usually by coughing. It is most common among the poor, the homeless, IV drug users, prisoners, recent immigrants from third world countries, hospitalized patients, and nursing home residents. HIV patients who work with any of these groups are at risk of exposure, so be sure to discuss any such contact with your doctor. All HIV patients should be regularly tested for tuberculosis.

Cryptosporidium is an intestinal parasite that is found in water contaminated by stool. While municipal water systems usually remove cryptosporidium, there have been outbreaks linked to city water. In HIV patients, it can cause severe and persistent diarrhea. To reduce risk of infection, all HIV patients should avoid drinking untreated water or stream water. Additionally, avoiding raw, undercooked, or "rare" meats or raw oysters is important, as these foods can also transmit the parasite.

There is a spectrum of immunocompromise in HIV disease. Patients with early stage disease may be at little more risk than non-HIV patients, while patients with advanced HIV may be extremely susceptible. Risk in HIV correlates well with a measurement known as the CD4 count. This is the number of helper T-cells per microliter of blood. Physicians caring for HIV patients check this number on a regular basis. As the disease becomes more severe, this number drops.

When CD4 counts become low enough, preventative drug treatment (prophylaxis) is usually recommended. This means taking certain medications regularly to prevent the development of serious opportunistic infections. If CD4 counts are very low, it may be necessary to take several different prophylactic drugs. Some of the more important thresholds are as follows:

- **CD4 < 200:** Patients in this range should be started on antibiotic prophylaxis against *Pneumocystis carinii*. This microorganism is present in the environment. It is harmless to normal people, but may cause fatal *Pneumocystis carinii* pneumonia (PCP) in patients with HIV.
- **CD4 <100:** Patients with HIV should be tested for prior immunity to *Toxoplasma gondii*. This is a parasite which may be caught by handling cat litter, or eating undercooked meats. The presence or absence of prior immunity to this organism influences treatment, but most HIV patients with CD4 counts <100 should be on antibiotic prophylaxis to prevent encephalitis (brain infection) due to Toxoplasmosis.
- **CD4 <50:** Patients in this range require prophylaxis against *Mycobacterium avium* complex (MAC). MAC is present in the environment, and is a distant relative of tuberculosis. In patients with AIDS, it can cause overwhelming infection in multiple organs, and can be fatal. Additionally, prophylaxis against cytomegalovirus (CMV) may also be appropriate at this CD4 count. This is a decision best made by a specialist in HIV disease.

With the newer, more potent, antiviral drugs that treat HIV, CD4 counts often rise during therapy. When they rise above these thresholds, prophylactic medications can often be stopped. Besides these specific measures, the following advice applies to most HIV patients:

- Pay close attention to fevers, especially if prolonged. This may be a sign of serious infection.
- Unexplained weight loss is another common sign of infection in HIV patients, and should prompt medical evaluation.
- Persistent cough can be a sign of tuberculosis or other chronic lung infections, and needs to be investigated.
- HIV patients should receive yearly influenza vaccines, and should also receive the 23-valent pneumococcal vaccine every five years. Live virus vaccines should be avoided.
- Discuss your pets with your doctors. Certain types of pets may increase risk for diseases that can infect HIV patients.
- Discuss any planned travel abroad. Your doctor may recommend special vaccinations or other measures to prevent infection.

Autoimmune Diseases

A substantial number of patients with autoimmune diseases are treated with immunosuppressive medications. Autoimmune diseases involve malfunction of the immune system, leading immune cells to attack normal body organs. Common examples of autoimmune conditions include systemic lupus erythematosus, rheumatoid arthritis, Wegener's granulomatosis, psoriatic arthritis, and scleroderma.

Many patients with autoimmune conditions appear to have subtle immunocompromise. Patients with lupus and rheumatoid arthritis have an increased frequency of infections, and are more prone to developing infections due to unusual agents.

Autoimmune conditions are often treated with immunosuppressive medications. Most of these medications are the same ones that transplant patients use to prevent organ rejection. These medications primarily affect lymphocytes, and can lead to the same sorts of infections as are seen in transplant patients.

You should discuss with your physician whether specific precautions are necessary for the medications you take to control an autoimmune disease. However, the precautions listed above for transplant patients are generally prudent for patients under treatment for autoimmune diseases as well.

For patients who are on high doses of immunosuppressive drugs for autoimmune disease, prophylactic antibiotic treatment similar to what HIV patients receive may be necessary.

Splenectomy

The spleen is a fist-sized organ on the left side of the abdomen, tucked underneath the ribs. It has a sponge-like structure, and is packed full of immune cells. When blood flows through the spleen, it acts as a filter. The spleen rapidly removes and destroys any bacteria which enter the blood stream.

While the spleen is not essential to immune function, it is important in dealing with certain types of bacteria. The most troublesome are *Streptococcus pneumoniae*, *Haemophilus influenza*, and *Meningococcus*. These species have developed thick outer capsules that resist attacks from the immune system.

Sometimes, the spleen needs to be removed (splenectomy). The spleen can be ruptured by auto accidents or other serious injury, and may need to be removed to stop bleeding. Removing the spleen can cure certain blood disorders such as idiopathic thrombotic purpura (ITP). In some cancers such as Hodgkin's disease, the spleen may be removed to determine how far the cancer has spread. In patients who are born with sickle cell anemia, the spleen disappears over time due to multiple tiny blood clots.

People who have lost their spleen are at risk for overwhelming bloodstream infections with bacteria (sepsis). Within minutes to hours, previously healthy splenectomized patients can die from sepsis. This is a special category of immunocompromise, and important precautions are necessary.

The following measures are recommended for most patients who have had a splenectomy:

- Prompt attention to fever, even if mild. Many splenectomy patients' physicians give them an antibiotic prescription to start immediately when fever occurs.
- Regular vaccination with the 23-valent pneumococcal vaccine (Pneumovax), *Haemophilus influenza* Type B vaccine (Hib), and the meningococcal vaccine. Most sepsis in splenectomy patients is due to these three bacteria, and vaccination can sharply cut this risk.

- Avoid eating raw, undercooked, or "rare" meats, eggs, and seafood. These may contain bacteria such as *Salmonella* that can cause severe infection.
- Take antibiotics as recommended by your doctor or dentist immediately prior to dental cleaning or other dental work. Dental procedures can push bacteria into the bloodstream.

Summary

Being immunocompromised can lead to becoming sick easily, or developing unusual infections. The level of risk depends on the cause and severity of the immunocompromise. Paying attention to measures discussed above, and those recommended by your doctor, gives you the best chance of remaining healthy.

Chapter 7

Does Exercise Help Immune Function?

Introduction

From birth, we are exposed to a continuous onslaught of bacteria, viruses, and other disease-causing organisms. Without an effective shield, each of us would soon succumb to infectious disease and cancer. In the battle with microbial invaders, we protect ourselves with a complex array of defensive measures collectively identified as the immune system.

The immune system is a remarkably adaptive defense entity. It is able to generate an enormous variety of cells and molecules capable of recognizing and eliminating a limitless variety of foreign invaders. There are two functional divisions: innate immunity, which refers to the basic resistance to disease that we are born with, acting as a first line of defense; and acquired immunity which, when activated, produces a specific reaction and immunological memory to each infectious agent.

- The innate immune system includes anatomic and physiologic barriers (skin, mucous membranes, body temperature, low pH, and special chemical mediators such as complement and interferon), specialized cells (natural killer cells, and phagocytes

---

Excerpted from "Does Exercise Alter Immune Function and Respiratory Infections?" *Research Digest*, President's Council on Physical Fitness and Sports, June 2001. The full text, including references, is available online at www.fitness.gov/June2001digest.pdf.

including neutrophils, monocytes, and macrophages which can engulf, kill, and digest whole microorganisms), and inflammatory barriers. When the innate immune system fails to effectively combat an invading pathogen, the body mounts an acquired (specific) immune response.

- The acquired immune system includes special cells called B- and T-lymphocytes that are capable of secreting a large variety of specialized chemicals (antibodies and cytokines) to regulate the immune response. T-lymphocytes can also engage in direct cell-on-cell warfare.

Does physical activity influence immune function and as a consequence risk of infection from the common cold and other upper respiratory tract infections (URTI)? Does the immune system respond differently to moderate compared to intense physical exertion? These important questions will be explored in this chapter, with physical activity and lifestyle guidelines provided to support augmentation of one's immunity and a lower risk of the common cold.

Moderate Physical Activity and Immune Function

People who exercise regularly report fewer colds than their sedentary peers. Numerous surveys of fitness enthusiasts, runners, and masters athletes indicate that between 60% and 90% feel that they experience fewer colds than their sedentary peers.

Data from three randomized studies support the viewpoint that near-daily physical activity reduces the number of days with sickness. In these studies, women in the exercise groups walked briskly 35–45 minutes, five days a week, for 12–15 weeks during the winter/spring or fall, while the control groups remained physically inactive. Fitness enthusiasts reported results in the same direction—walkers experienced about half the days with cold symptoms of the sedentary controls. A recent one-year epidemiological study of 547 adults demonstrated a 23% reduction in risk of upper respiratory tract infection (URTI) in those engaging in regular versus irregular moderate-to-vigorous physical activity. In healthy elderly subjects, URTI symptomatology during a one-year period was inversely related to energy expended during moderate physical activity. Other research has shown that during moderate exercise, several positive changes occur in the immune system. Stress hormones, which can suppress immunity, and pro- and anti-inflammatory cytokines, indicative of intense metabolic activity, are not elevated during moderate exercise. Although the immune system returns to pre-exercise levels very quickly after the exercise session is over, each session represents an augmentation in immune surveillance that appears to reduce the risk of infection over the long term.

Although public health recommendations must be considered tentative, the data on the relationship between moderate exercise, enhanced immunity, and lowered risk of sickness are consistent with guidelines urging the general public to engage in near-daily brisk walking.

Guidelines to Reduce the Risk of Infection

Nutrition impacts the development of the immune system, both in the growing fetus and in the early months of life. Nutrients are also necessary for the immune response to pathogens so that cells can divide and produce antibodies and cytokines. Many enzymes in immune cells require the presence of micronutrients, and critical roles have been defined for zinc, iron, copper, selenium, vitamins A, B_6, C, and E in the maintenance of optimum immune function. The earliest research on nutrition and immune function focused on malnutrition. It has long been known that malnourished children have a high risk of severe and life-threatening infections. Protein-energy malnutrition adversely affects virtually all components of the immune system.

Should fitness enthusiasts use nutrient and herbal supplements to enhance immune function above and beyond the effects of physical activity? Despite all of the hype about supplements such as phytochemicals, antioxidants, flavonoids, carotenoids, glutamine (an amino acid), ginseng, and echinacea, there is insufficient evidence to warrant taking high doses in the belief they will prevent or cure ailments ranging from the common cold to cancer. In fact, extremely large doses may lead to health problems rather than confer benefits. The best practice is to eat a varied and balanced diet in accordance with energy needs and the U.S. Food Guide Pyramid, and be assured that vitamin, mineral, and phytochemical intake is adequate for both health and immune function.

Whether one gets sick with a cold after a sufficient amount of the virus has entered the body depends on many factors that affect the immune system other than just physical activity and nutrition. Old age, cigarette smoking, mental stress, and lack of sleep have all been associated with impaired immune function, and an increased risk of infection.

Based on current knowledge, good immune function can be maintained by regular physical activity, eating a well-balanced diet, keeping life stresses to a minimum, avoiding chronic fatigue, and obtaining adequate sleep. Immune function is suppressed during periods of very low caloric intake and quick weight reduction, so weight loss should be gradual to maintain good immunity.

For athletes, the influence of a growing list of nutritional supplements on the immune and infection response to intense and prolonged exercise has been assessed. Supplements studied thus far include zinc, dietary fat, plant sterols, antioxidants (for example, vitamins C and ß-carotene, N-acetylcysteine, and butylated hydroxyanisole), glutamine, and carbohydrate. Of these, only carbohydrate has emerged as a useful nutritional countermeasure.

Several studies with runners and cyclists have shown that carbohydrate beverage ingestion plays a role in attenuating changes in immunity when the athlete experiences physiologic stress and depletion of carbohydrate stores in response to high intensity exercise bouts lasting longer than two hours. In particular, carbohydrate ingestion (about one liter per hour of a typical sports drink) compared to a placebo has been linked to significantly lower blood cortisol and epinephrine levels, a reduced change in blood immune cell counts, and lower pro- and anti-inflammatory cytokines. These data suggest that the endurance athlete ingesting carbohydrate during the race event should experience a much lower perturbation in hormonal and immune measures compared to the athlete largely avoiding carbohydrate.

Conclusions and Recommendations

By far, the most important finding that has emerged from exercise immunology studies is that positive immune changes take place during each bout of moderate physical activity. Over time, this translates to fewer days of sickness with the common cold and other upper respiratory tract infections. This is consistent with public health guidelines urging individuals to engage in near-daily physical activity of 30 minutes or greater. Other factors that help maintain good immune function include eating a well-balanced diet, keeping life stresses to a minimum, avoiding chronic fatigue, obtaining adequate sleep, and avoiding rapid weight loss.

Should the fitness enthusiast exercise when sick? In general, if the symptoms are from the neck up (for example, the common cold), moderate exercise is probably acceptable and some researchers would argue even beneficial, while bed rest and a gradual progression to normal training are recommended when the illness is systemic (for example, the flu). If in doubt as to the type of infectious illness, individuals should consult a physician.

Many components of the immune system exhibit adverse change after prolonged, heavy exertion lasting longer than 90 minutes. These immune changes occur in several compartments of the immune system and body (for example, the skin, upper respiratory tract mucosal tissue, lung, blood, and muscle). During this "open window" of impaired immunity (which may last between three and 72 hours, depending on the immune measure), viruses and bacteria may gain a foothold, increasing the risk of subclinical and clinical infection. Thus risk of upper respiratory tract infections can increase when athletes push beyond normal limits.

Chapter 8

Are Some Chronic Diseases Caused by Infectious Agents?

"We used to think that chronic and infectious diseases were separate. But we gradually also learned that infectious diseases play a significant role in the emergence of chronic diseases. This may provide new opportunities to address and counter a significant public health challenge."

—*Dr. Gro Harlem Brundtland, Director-General, World Health Organization, January 26, 1998*

Several chronic diseases once attributed to lifestyle, genetics, or environmental factors are now known to be caused or exacerbated by infectious agents. These include stomach ulcers and certain types of cancer and arthritis. Evidence is mounting for other, still unproven associations between infectious agents and chronic diseases. These findings are prompting health professionals to rethink ways of preventing or minimizing long-term illness and disability. In the future,

---

This chapter includes excerpts from "Addressing the Issues of Chronic Diseases Caused by Infectious Agents," *Emerging Infectious Diseases: A Strategy for the 21st Century*, National Center for Infectious Diseases, Centers for Disease Control and Prevention (CDC), 1998, reviewed May 2001, and excerpts from "Chronic Fatigue Syndrome," National Institute of Allergy and Infectious Diseases (NIAID), January 2001. "What Research Needs to Be Been Done to Investigate Whether or Not Microbial Agents Play a Role in CFS?" is excerpted from "National Institutes of Health Chronic Fatigue Syndrome State-of-the Science Consultation," Division of Microbiology and Infectious Diseases, NIAID, February 2000.

some chronic diseases may be treated with antibiotics, prevented by vaccines, or controlled by health education programs that enable susceptible people to avoid disease-causing microbes.

The discovery of *Helicobacter pylori* bacteria in most duodenal ulcers revolutionized medical management of this chronic disease. In most cases, ulcers can be cured following appropriate antibiotic therapy. On the heels of this remarkable finding, a strong but not yet proven association has been reported between the common respiratory bacterium *Chlamydia pneumoniae* and cardiovascular disease. Epidemiologic, pathologic, and laboratory studies have correlated *C. pneumoniae* infection with heart attacks, coronary artery disease, and strokes. Since coronary artery disease is responsible for almost 50% of all deaths in the U.S., determining whether a proportion might be attributed to infection is clearly worthwhile. If future research confirms that a microbe plays a causative role in some heart attacks, antibiotics or vaccines might be used for prevention of certain forms of cardiovascular disease.

Infectious agents are known to cause a wide spectrum of chronic outcomes. For example, Lyme disease from the tick-borne spirochete *Borrelia burgdorferi* can induce arthritis and neurologic disease. Hepatitis B and hepatitis C viruses can result in chronic liver disease and liver cancer. Hepatitis C virus is also associated with inflammation of joints (arthritis) and blood vessels (vasculitis), as well as with cryoglobulinemia (a blood disorder) and peripheral neuropathy (loss of sensation). At least 90% of invasive cervical cancers are associated with human papillomaviruses. Although much is known about these processes, research and guidelines for diagnosis, prevention, and treatment are still needed.

Many of the bacteria, parasites, and viruses linked to the development of chronic diseases are common throughout the world, but only some infected people develop severe outcomes. Genetic, behavioral, or environmental factors may influence the risk of disease. For example, while infection with foodborne and waterborne diarrhea-inducing bacteria such as *Salmonella*, *Shigella*, *Yersinia*, and *Campylobacter* can cause reactive arthritis, people with the HLA-B27 gene are more likely to develop this potentially preventable condition. Education on ways to avoid infection with these bacteria might decrease the number of cases, particularly when targeted to persons likely to carry the HLA-B27 gene. In the years to come, scientists will continue to investigate potential infectious causes of chronic diseases, to determine which individuals are at risk, and to design disease prevention programs.

Table 8.1. Examples of Infectious Agents Associated with Chronic Disease

Organism	Chronic Condition
Borrelia burgdorferi (Tick-borne Lyme disease)	Arthritis; Neurologic disease
Chlamydia trachomatis Sexually transmitted	Reactive arthritis
Helicobacter pylori	Peptic ulcer disease
Hepatitis B virus	Chronic liver disease; Liver cancer
Hepatitis C Virus	Chronic liver disease; Liver cancer
Human herpesvirus-8	Kaposi's sarcoma
Human papillomavirus	Cervical cancer
Schistosoma haematobium	Bladder cancer
Trypanosoma cruzi	Chagas; Cardiomyopathy

Chronic Fatigue Syndrome (CFS)

What is chronic fatigue syndrome?

We all get tired. Many of us at times have felt depressed. But the mystery known as chronic fatigue syndrome (CFS) is not like the normal ups and downs we experience in everyday life. The early sign of this illness is a strong and noticeable fatigue that comes on suddenly and often comes and goes or never stops. You feel too tired to do normal activities or are easily exhausted with no apparent reason. Unlike the mind fog of a serious hangover, to which researchers have compared CFS, the profound weakness of CFS does not go away with a few good nights of sleep. Instead, it slyly steals your energy and vigor over months and sometimes years.

How does CFS begins?

For many people, CFS begins after a bout with a cold, bronchitis, hepatitis, or an intestinal bug. For some, it follows a bout of infectious mononucleosis, or mono, which temporarily saps the energy of many teenagers and young adults. Often, people say that their illnesses started during a period of high stress. In others, CFS develops more gradually, with no clear illness or other event starting it. Unlike flu symptoms, which usually go away in a few days or weeks, CFS symptoms either hang on or come and go frequently for more than six months. CFS symptoms include:

- Headache
- Tender lymph nodes
- Fatigue and weakness
- Muscle and joint aches
- Inability to concentrate

What causes CFS?

While no one knows what causes CFS, for more than a century, doctors have reported seeing illnesses similar to it. In the 1860s, Dr. George Beard named the syndrome neurasthenia because he thought it was a nervous disorder with weakness and fatigue. Since then, health experts have suggested other explanations for this baffling illness.

- Iron-poor blood (anemia)
- Low blood sugar (hypoglycemia)
- Environmental allergy
- A body wide yeast infection (candidiasis)

In the mid-1980s, the illness became labeled "chronic EBV" when laboratory clues led scientists to wonder whether the Epstein-Barr virus (EBV) might be causing this group of symptoms. New evidence soon cast doubt on the theory that EBV could be the only thing causing CFS. High levels of EBV antibodies (disease-fighting proteins) have now been found in some healthy people as well as in some people with CFS. Likewise, some people who don't have EBV antibodies, and who thus have never been infected with the virus, can show CFS symptoms.

What is the CFS case definition?

The EBV work sparked new interest in the syndrome among a small group of medical researchers. They realized they needed a standard way to describe CFS so that they could more easily compare research results. In the late 1980s, CDC brought together a group of

CFS experts to tackle this problem. Based on the best information available at the time, this group published in the March 1988 issue of the scientific journal, *Annals of Internal Medicine*, strict symptom and physical criteria—the first case definition—by which scientists could evaluate CFS study patients.

Not knowing the cause or a specific sign for the disease, the group agreed to call the illness "chronic fatigue syndrome" after its primary symptom. "Syndrome" means a group of symptoms that occur together but can result from different causes. (Today, CFS also is known as myalgic encephalomyelitis, postviral fatigue syndrome, and chronic fatigue and immune dysfunction syndrome.)

After using this definition for several years, CFS researchers realized some criteria were unclear or redundant. An international group of CFS experts reviewed the criteria for CDC, which led to the first changes in the case definition. This new definition was published in the same journal in December 1994.

Besides revising the CFS case criteria—which reduced the required minimum number of symptoms to four out of a list of eight possible symptoms—the newer report also proposed a conceptual outline for studying the syndrome. This outline recognizes CFS as part of a range of illnesses that have fatigue as a major symptom. Although primarily intended for researchers, these guidelines should help doctors better diagnose CFS.

What research needs to be been done to investigate whether or not microbial agents play a role in CFS?

Although the evidence to date for a microbial cause of CFS is not strong, and the epidemiology is inconsistent with an infectious cause, newer differential display assays may allow the search for rarer microbes. Such studies would need incident case patients and thus interlink with the recommendation for investigations of CFS incidence. While the 6-month illness period of the case definition appears to be a time period that does clearly distinguish CFS from other types of fatigue, it means that an organism that triggers disease and then disappears will probably not be detected. Organisms whose persistence or expression perpetuates illness should remain, and presumably their nucleic acids could be detected. It is also noted that while it seems unlikely that infectious agents cause CFS, they may well be among a variety of stressors that precipitate it.

Chapter 9

What Are Antibiotics?

Antibiotic Safety

What are antibiotics?

Antibiotics are powerful medicines that help stop bacterial infections. They are used to kill germs that cause certain illnesses. Protect yourself and your family by learning how to take them correctly. Learn when you should and should not take antibiotics.

What are the two main types of germs that cause most infections?

Viruses and bacteria are the two types of germs that cause infections and illnesses. It is very important to know that antibiotics cannot kill virus germs but can kill bacteria germs.

Viral infections should not be treated with antibiotics. Some examples of viral illnesses include:

- Common cold—stuffy nose, sore throat, sneezing, cough, headache

---

This chapter includes text used with permission from *Antibiotic Safety*. Also included is "Common Antibiotics," reprinted with permission from the Alliance for the Prudent Use of Antibiotics (APUA). For additional information, visit the APUA website at www.apua.org.

- Influenza (flu)—fever, chills, body aches, headache, sore throat, dry cough
- Most coughs
- Acute bronchitis (cough, fever)—almost always caused by viruses
- Pharyngitis (sore throat)—most sore throats are caused by viruses and are not effectively treated with an antibiotic
- Viral gastroenteritis

Bacterial infections should be treated with antibiotics. Some examples of bacterial infections include:

- Ear infections—Antibiotics are used for most, but not all ear infections
- Severe sinus infections—lasting two or more weeks
- Strep throat
- Urinary tract infection

Can antibiotics sometimes be harmful?

Antibiotics are generally safe and very helpful in fighting disease, but there are certain cases where antibiotics can actually be harmful. These are some things to watch for while taking antibiotics:

- **Side effects of the antibiotics:** Some common side effects of antibiotics include nausea, diarrhea, and stomach pain. Sometimes these symptoms can lead to dehydration and other problems. Be sure that your doctor has told you about side effects. It is very important to notify your doctor if you have any side effects from your antibiotics.
- **Allergic reaction:** Some people may experience an allergic reaction characterized by rash, itching, and in severe cases difficulty breathing. Tell your doctor about any drug allergies you have had in the past.
- **Antibiotic resistance:** Antibiotic resistance has become a very big problem in the world today. This may result when antibiotics are used too often or inappropriately for viral infections.

When resistance develops, the antibiotic is not able to kill the germs causing the infection. Your infection may last longer, and instead of getting better you get worse. Every time you take an antibiotic when you really don't need it or if you take it incorrectly, you increase your chance of getting an illness someday that is resistant to antibiotics.

How do I take antibiotics safely and effectively?

Over half of the people who use medications don't use them as prescribed. Here are some tips to avoid misuse and/or overuse of antibiotics:

- Do not demand that your doctor give you antibiotics for a viral infection.
- Wash your hands properly to reduce the chance of getting sick and spreading infection.
- Wash fruits and vegetables thoroughly; avoid raw eggs and undercooked meat to help prevent food-borne infection.
- When caring for an ill person whose defenses are weakened, antibacterial soaps or products are helpful, but should be used as directed.
- Take all of your prescribed antibiotic, even if you start to feel better.
- Make sure you are current on all of your vaccinations. Ask your doctor if you have all of the vaccinations (shots) you need to protect yourself from illness. Getting vaccinated will help prevent having to take more medications.
- Do not take an antibiotic that has been prescribed for someone else. Do not let anyone take your antibiotic, even if the symptoms are the same.
- Keep a written record of when and how often to take the antibiotic. If you forget or miss a dose, ask your doctor or pharmacist what you should do.
- Keep a complete written history of your antibiotic use. Include dates taken, strength of antibiotic and side effects, and how effective the antibiotics were in treating your illness. Share this diary with your doctor each time antibiotics are prescribed. This

written history may help your doctor determine which antibiotic is best for you.

How can I properly communicate with my doctor?

If your doctor prescribes antibiotics, you should ask the following questions:

1. Why do I need the antibiotic?
2. What is the antibiotic suppose to do?
3. What are the side effects of the antibiotic?
4. Is there anything that can prevent the side effects?
5. Should the drug be taken at a special time? With or without food?
6. Does the antibiotic interfere with the effectiveness of other medications such as birth control pills?
7. Are there any possible adverse reactions if the antibiotic is taken with other medications, food, or alcohol?

Also, be sure to tell your doctor about any of the following:

- previous drug reactions
- special diet
- allergies to drugs or foods
- health problems
- chance of pregnancy
- medicines you are currently taking
- herbal supplements

Always keep your doctor's phone number nearby in case of an emergency. If you have any questions or problems regarding your antibiotic treatment or your illness, don't hesitate to call your doctor, nurse, or health care provider.

What issues related to antibiotic use are of special concern to women?

Antibiotics can lead to vaginal yeast infections. This happens because antibiotics kill the normal bacteria in the vagina and this causes yeast to grow rapidly. Symptoms of a yeast infection include one or all of the following symptoms: itching, burning, pain during sex, and vaginal discharge. Antibiotics may cause birth control pills to be less effective. Another method of birth control may be needed during antibiotic treatment. Some antibiotics may be passed on to a fetus and cause harm. Because of this, it is important to let your doctor know if you are pregnant or nursing.

Common Antibiotics

GROUP I: Ample Spectrum Penicillins

Generic Name	Trade Name
amoxicillin	Amoxil®
ampicillin	Omnipen®
bacampicillin	Spectrobid®
carbenicillin Indanyl	Pyopen®, Geopen®, Geocillin®
mezlocillin	Mezlin®
piperacillin*	Pipracil®
ticarcillin	Ticar®

GROUP II: Penicillins and Beta Lactamase Inhibitors

Generic Name	Trade Name
amoxicillin-clavulanic Acid	Augmentin®
ampicillin-sulbactam*	Unasyn®
cloxacillin	Tegopen®, Cloxapen®
dicloxacillin	Dycill®, Dynapen®, Pathocil®
methicillin	Staphcillin®
oxacillin	Prostaphlin®, Bactocill®
penicillin G (Benzathine, Potassium, Procaine)	Bicillin®C-R/L-A, Pfizerpen®, Wycillin®
penicillin V	Pen Vee K®, Beepen-VK®
piperacillin+tazobactam*	Zosyn®
ticarcillin+clavulnate	Timentin®
nafcillin	Unipen®, Nafcil®

GROUP III: Cephalosporins

Cephalosporin I Generation

Generic Name	**Trade Name**
cefadroxil	Duricef®
cefazolin	Ancef®, Kefzol®, Zolicef®
cephalexin	Keflex®, Keftab®
cephalothin	Keflin®
cephapirin	Cefadyl®
cephradine	Velosef®

Cephalosporin II Generation

Generic Name	**Trade Name**
cefaclor	Ceclor®, Ceclor CD®
cefamandole	Mandol®
cefonicid	Monocid®
cefotetan	Cefotan®
cefoxitin	Mefoxin®
cefprozil	Cefzil®
cefmetazole	Zefazone®
cefuroxime	Kefurox®, Zinacef®
cefuroxime axetil	Ceftin®
loracarbef	Lorabid®

Cephalosporin III Generation

Generic Name	**Trade Name**
cefdinir	Omnicef®
ceftibuten	Cedax®
cefoperazone	Cefobid®
cefixime*	Suprax®
cefotaxime*	Claforan®
cefpodoxime proxetil	Vantin®
ceftazidime*	Ceptaz®, Fortaz®, Tazicef®
ceftizoxime*	Cefizox®
ceftriaxone*	Rocephin®

Cephalosporin IV Generation

Generic Name	**Trade Name**
cefepime	Maxipime®

GROUP IV: Macrolides and Lincosamides

Generic Name	**Trade Name**
azithromycin*	Zithromax®
clarithromycin*	Biaxin®
clindamycin	Cleocin®
dirithromycin	Dynabac®
erythromycin	E-mycin®, Ery-Tab®, Benzamycin®
lincomycin	Lincocin®
troleandomycin	Tao®

GROUP V: Quinolones and Fluoroquinolones

Generic Name	**Trade Name**
cinoxacin	Cinoxacin®
ciprofloxacin*	Cipro®
enoxacin	Penetrex®
gatifloxacin	Tequin®
grepafloxacin	Raxar®, Out of Market in USA
levofloxacin	Levaquin®, Quixin®
lomefloxacin	Maxaquin®
moxifloxacin	Avelox®
nalidixic acid	NegGram®
norfloxacin*	Noroxin®
ofloxacin	Floxin®
sparfloxacin	Zagam®
trovafloxacin	Trovan®
oxolinic acid	Not licensed in USA
gemifloxacin	Not licensed in USA
pefloxacin	Not licensed in USA

GROUP VI: Carbapenems

Generic Name	**Trade Name**
imipenem-cilastatin*	Primaxin®
meropenem	Merrem®

GROUP VII: Monobactams

Generic Name	**Trade Name**
aztreonam*	Azactam®

GROUP VIII: Aminoglycosides

Generic Name	**Trade Name**
amikacin*	Amikin®
gentamicin	Garamycin®
kanamycin	Kantrex®
neomycin	Mycifradin®
netilmicin	Netromycin®
streptomycin	Streptomycin®
tobramycin*	Tobrex®, Nebcin®
paromomycin	Humatin®

GROUP IX: Glycopeptides

Generic Name	**Trade Name**
teicoplanin	Targocid®
vancomycin*	Vancocin®, Lyphocin®

GROUP X: Tetracyclines

Generic Name	**Trade Name**
demeclocycline	Declomycin®
doxycycline	Doxy®, Vibra-Tabs®, Vibramycin®
methacycline	Rondomycin®
minocycline	Minocin®
oxytetracycline	Terramycin®
tetracycline	Sumycin®
chlortetracycline	

GROUP XI: Sulfonamides

Generic Name	**Trade Name**
mafenide	Sulfamylon®
silver sulfadiazine	SSD®, Silvadene®
sulfadiazine	Sulfadiazine
sulfamethoxazole	Gantanol®
sulfasalazine	Sulfasalazine®, Azulfidine®
sulfisoxazole	Sulfisoxazole
trimethoprim-sulfamethoxazole	Bactrim®, Septra®, Cofatrim Forte®, Primsol®
sulfamethizole	Thiosulfil Forte®

GROUP XII: Rifampin

Generic Name	**Trade Name**
rifabutin	Mycobutin®
rifampin	Rifadin®
rifapentine	Priftin®

GROUP XIII: Oxazolidinones

Generic Name	**Trade Name**
linezolid*	Zyvox®

GROUP XIV: Streptogramins

Generic Name	**Trade Name**
quinupristin+dalfopristin*	Synercid®

GROUP XV: Cyclic Lipopeptides

Generic Name	**Trade Name**
daptomycin	Cubicin®

GROUP XVI: Others

Generic Name	**Trade Name**
bacitracin	Baci-IM
chloramphenicol*	Chloromycetin®

GROUP XVI: Others *(continued on next page)*

GROUP XVI: Others (*continued*)

colistimethate	Coly-Mycin® M & S
fosfomycin	Monurol®
isoniazid	Rifamate®
methenamine	Hiprex®, Mandelamine®
metronidazole	Flagyl®
mupirocin	Bactroban®
nitrofurantoin	Macrobid®, Macrodantin®, Furantoin®
nitrofurazone	Furacin®
novobiocin	Albamycin®
spectinomycin	Trobicin®
trimethoprim	Proloprim®, Trimpex®
colistin	
cycloserine	
capreomycin	
ethionamide	
pyrazinamide	
erythromycin ethylsuccinate +	
sulfisoxazole	

*Antibiotics marked with an asterisks are subject to restricted use in hospitals following guidelines of Infection Control Committee. Physicians should consult with an infectious disease specialist.

Chapter 10

Understanding Antimicrobial Resistance

Drug-resistant infectious agents—those that are not killed or inhibited by antimicrobial compounds—are an increasingly important public health concern. Tuberculosis, gonorrhea, malaria and childhood ear infections are just a few of the diseases that have become more difficult to treat due to the emergence of drug-resistant pathogens. Antimicrobial resistance is becoming a factor in virtually all hospital-acquired (nosocomial) infections. Many physicians are concerned that several bacterial infections soon may be untreatable.

In addition to its adverse effect on public health, antimicrobial resistance contributes to higher health care costs. Treating resistant infections often requires the use of more expensive or more toxic drugs and can result in longer hospital stays for infected patients. The Institute of Medicine, a part of the National Academy of Sciences, has estimated that the annual cost of treating antibiotic resistant infections in the United States may be as high as $30 billion.

A key factor in the development of antimicrobial resistance is the ability of infectious organisms to adapt quickly to new environmental conditions. Microbes generally are unicellular creatures that, compared with multicellular organisms, have a small number of genes. Even a single random gene mutation can have a large impact on their disease-causing properties; and since most microbes replicate very rapidly, they can evolve rapidly. Thus, a mutation that helps a microbe

---

"Antimicrobial Resistance," National Institute of Allergy and Infectious Diseases (NIAID), National Institutes of Health (NIH), June 2000.

survive in the presence of an antibiotic drug will quickly become predominant throughout the microbial population. Microbes also commonly acquire genes, including those encoding for resistance, by direct transfer from members of their own species or from unrelated microbes.

The innate adaptability of microbes is complemented by the widespread and sometimes inappropriate use of antimicrobials. Ideal conditions for the emergence of drug-resistant microbes result when drugs are prescribed for the common cold and other conditions for which they are not indicated or when individuals do not complete their prescribed treatment regimen. Hospitals also provide a fertile environment for drug-resistant pathogens. Close contact among sick patients and extensive use of antimicrobials force pathogens to develop resistance.

Scope of the Problem

Antimicrobial resistance has been recognized since the introduction of penicillin nearly 50 years ago when penicillin-resistant infections caused by *Staphylococcus aureus* rapidly appeared. Today, hospitals worldwide are facing unprecedented crises from the rapid emergence and dissemination of other microbes resistant to one or more antimicrobial agents.

- Strains of *Staphylococcus aureus* resistant to methicillin and other antibiotics are endemic in hospitals. Infection with methicillin-resistant *S. aureus* (MRSA) strains may also be increasing in non-hospital settings. A limited number of drugs remain effective against these infections. *S. aureus* strains with reduced susceptibility to vancomycin have emerged recently in Japan and the United States. The emergence of vancomycin-resistant strains would present a serious problem for physicians and patients.

- Increasing reliance on vancomycin has led to the emergence of vancomycin-resistant enterococci (VRE), bacteria that infect wounds, the urinary tract and other sites. Until 1989, such resistance had not been reported in U.S. hospitals. By 1993, however, more than 10 percent of hospital-acquired enterococci infections reported to the CDC were resistant.

- *Streptococcus pneumoniae* causes thousands of cases of meningitis and pneumonia, and 7 million cases of ear infection in the

United States each year. Currently, about 30 percent of *S. pneumoniae* isolates are resistant to penicillin, the primary drug used to treat this infection. Many penicillin-resistant strains are also resistant to other antimicrobial drugs.

- In sexually transmitted disease clinics that monitor outbreaks of drug-resistant infections, doctors have found that more than 30 percent of gonorrhea isolates are resistant to penicillin or tetracycline, or both.
- An estimated 300 to 500 million people worldwide are infected with the parasites that cause malaria. Resistance to chloroquine, once widely used and highly effective for preventing and treating malaria, has emerged in most parts of the world. Resistance to other antimalaria drugs also is widespread and growing.
- Strains of multidrug-resistant tuberculosis (MDR-TB) have emerged over the last decade and pose a particular threat to people infected with HIV. Drug-resistant strains are as contagious as those that are susceptible to drugs. MDR-TB is more difficult and vastly more expensive to treat, and patients may remain infectious longer due to inadequate treatment.
- Diarrheal diseases cause almost 3 million deaths a year—mostly in developing countries, where resistant strains of highly pathogenic bacteria such as *Shigella dysenteriae*, *Campylobacter*, *Vibrio cholerae*, *Escherichia coli* and *Salmonella* are emerging. Recent outbreaks of *Salmonella* food poisoning have occurred in the United States. A potentially dangerous "superbug" known as *Salmonella typhimurium*, resistant to ampicillin, sulfa, streptomycin, tetracycline and chloramphenicol, has caused illness in Europe, Canada and the United States.
- Fungal pathogens account for a growing proportion of nosocomial infections. Fungal diseases such as candidiasis and *Pneumocystis carinii* pneumonia are common among AIDS patients, and isolated outbreaks of other fungal diseases in people with normal immune systems have occurred recently in the United States. Scientists and clinicians are concerned that the increasing use of antifungal drugs will lead to drug-resistant fungi. In fact, recent studies have documented resistance of *Candida* species to fluconazole, a drug used widely to treat patients with systemic fungal diseases.

- Recent years have seen the introduction of powerful new drugs and drug combinations against HIV. Although treatments that combine new protease inhibitor drugs with other anti-HIV medications often effectively suppress HIV production in infected individuals, results from recent clinical studies suggest that many treatment failures occur due to the development of resistance by the virus.

National Institute of Allergy and Infectious Diseases (NIAID) Research

Scientists and health professionals agree that decreasing the incidence of antimicrobial resistance will require improved systems for monitoring outbreaks of drug-resistant infections and a more judicious use of antimicrobial drugs. They also recognize the critical role that basic research plays in responding to this problem. For example, studies of microbial physiology help scientists understand the biological processes that pathogens use to resist drug treatment. This knowledge can lead to the development of novel strategies to overcome or reverse these processes.

Investigations in molecular genetics and biochemistry identify critical pathways and functions in how microbes replicate. Rapid improvements in gene sequencing technology are making it faster and easier to pinpoint the actual molecules involved in these pathways, which in turn could serve as targets for new antimicrobial drugs. Basic research like this has already yielded practical results. For example, studies of the molecular basis of drug resistance in parasites have led to:

- the development of molecular tools to identify drug-resistant parasites;
- the identification of the genetic basis of resistance and resulting biochemical alterations in several parasite species;
- the identification of methods to reverse resistance; and
- the synthesis of drugs that are effective against drug-resistant strains of malaria.

NIAID funding for antimicrobial resistance research has risen dramatically in recent years, from $7.8 million in 1992 to an estimated $13.8 million in 1998, an increase of more than 75 percent. NIAID supports investigator-initiated research on the molecular mechanisms responsible for drug resistance, as well as research to develop and evaluate new or improved therapeutics for disease intervention and prevention. These efforts include epidemiologic research on major nosocomial pathogens such as *Staphylococcus aureus*, *E. coli* species associated with urinary tract infections, the *enterococci*, *staphylococci* and *Streptococcus pyogenes*. These studies seek to define how bacterial pathogens acquire, maintain and transfer antibiotic-resistance genes. In collaboration with investigators from malaria endemic areas, NIAID-supported investigators are conducting field studies on the distribution of drug-resistant malaria parasites.

In 1996, NIAID alerted the scientific community with a Program Announcement to encourage investigators to submit grant applications to support basic and applied research on emerging infectious diseases, including fungal diseases and those due to bacteria that are resistant to antibiotics. Last year, NIAID released a Program Announcement to encourage basic research on the molecular biology and genetics of resistance among bacteria and fungi, development of new tests for detecting resistance, identification of new classes of antimicrobial agents, and evaluation of alternative treatments of drug-resistant infections.

In conjunction with the National Aeronautics and Space Administration, the Defense Advanced Research Projects Agency and the University of Alabama, NIAID recently co-sponsored a meeting on emerging infections and antimicrobial resistance to examine rational approaches to drug design and stimulate research in these areas. Scientists discussed strategies for developing new drugs against bacteria, fungi, parasites, and viruses.

About NIAID

NIAID is a component of the National Institutes of Health (NIH), which is an agency of the Department of Health and Human Services. NIAID supports basic and applied research to prevent, diagnose, and treat infectious and immune-mediated illnesses, including HIV/AIDS and other sexually transmitted diseases, illness from potential agents of bioterrorism, tuberculosis, malaria, autoimmune disorders, asthma, and allergies.

Chapter 11

What Can Be Done about Antibiotic Resistance?

An antibiotic may be classified as "narrow-spectrum" or "broad-spectrum" depending on the range of bacterial types that it affects. Narrow-spectrum antibiotics are active against a select group of bacterial types. Broad-spectrum antibiotics are active against a wider number of bacterial types and, thus, may be used to treat a variety of infectious diseases. Broad-spectrum antibiotics are particularly useful when the infecting agent (bacteria) is unknown. Examples of narrow-spectrum antibiotics are the older penicillins (penG), the macrolides and vancomycin. Examples of broad-spectrum antibiotics are the aminoglycosides, the 2nd and 3rd generation cephalosporins, the quinolones, and some synthetic penicillins.

What can I do?

Use good hygiene! By washing your hands often and thoroughly with soap and water, you are helping to prevent disease—and therefore the need for antibiotics. Additionally, cooking meat thoroughly and handling food hygienically will help to prevent food-borne illnesses. Also, you should take antibiotics only when necessary.

"What Can Be Done about Antibiotic Resistance?" Reprinted with permission from the Alliance for the Prudent Use of Antibiotics (APUA). For additional information, visit the APUA website at www.apua.org.

Are antibacterial agents, such as antibacterial soaps, a solution?

In institutions such as hospitals and nursing homes, these agents are useful and appropriate when used under strict guidelines for specific purposes. However, there is some concern that antibacterials could promote antibiotic resistance, and their usefulness by the general public is unproven.

Are antibiotics regulated?

Some institutions, such as hospitals, have 'Antibiotic Policy' guidelines and antibiotic review committees, to ensure that antibiotic use in their institution is rational and does not compound the antibiotic resistance problem.

Governmental oversight of antibiotics varies widely from country to country. In some countries, antibiotics can be purchased 'over-the-counter,' that is, without a prescription from a doctor. Other countries require a doctor's prescription before a patient is allowed to purchase an antibiotic, although these laws are not always enforced. Antibiotics have also been sold over the Internet, a commerce mechanism with little governmental oversight that reaches across national borders.

Furthermore, food animals (animals raised for human consumption) are often given long-term, low-levels of antibiotics to promote growth. This antibiotic use represents a large fraction of the total antibiotic use in the industrialized world. A few governments restrict which antibiotics can be used for food animals, with the goal of preserving the most powerful antibiotics for treating human disease.

Is there any international action on the antibiotic resistance issue?

The World Health Organization (WHO) has become quite concerned about the rising levels of resistant bacteria in all areas of the world. To provide some global coordination, WHO issued its Global Strategy for Containment of Antimicrobial Resistance, a document aimed at policy-makers that urges governments to take action to help contain antibiotic resistance.

Developing nations need to focus on eliminating uncontrolled access to antibiotics and prevention measures such as improving sanitation, cleaning up water supplies and relieving overcrowding. These preventative measures, along with frequent hand washing, would ensure that people get sick less often, and would therefore pass on fewer resistant infections to others.

Industrialized countries need to focus on prevention measures such as frequent handwashing and limiting antibacterial use, developing vaccines that can protect certain vulnerable populations such as young children, controlling multi-resistant bacteria in hospitals and in the community, and reducing antibiotic use in animal farming and agriculture.

Experts agree that a global system for tracking antibiotic resistance is needed. It would serve as an indicator for recognizing "hot-spots" of resistance and measuring trends that can tell us if our educational programs or other solutions are having positive effects.

Can the effectiveness of existing antibiotics be preserved?

To preserve the potency of existing antibiotics, overall antibiotic use must be decreased. Physicians, pharmacists, and the general public must avoid careless use of these valuable drugs. Antibiotics must be prescribed only for bacterial infections and in the proper dose for the correct amount of time. Narrow spectrum drugs should be chosen by doctors whenever possible to avoid destroying populations of beneficial bacteria along with the disease-causing bacteria. In addition, non-therapeutic uses of antibiotics in farm animals and agriculture should be eliminated.

Can new antibiotics be developed?

The epidemic of resistant bacteria has spurred renewed interest in finding novel antibiotics. The process of producing a new antibiotic, however, is long and expensive, requiring approximately ten years and $300 million to bring a new antibiotic to market. Many efforts to find novel drugs in fungi and soil result in compounds that are the same or very similar to previously discovered antibiotics. Thus, resistance eventually develops to these new antibiotics. Heavy use of the latest antibiotic can lead to the emergence of resistance in as little as two years. Nonetheless, scientists are still searching for new antibiotics by looking in unusual places such as in bacteria living deep below the earth's surface, in the skin of frogs and in certain insects.

Can antibiotic resistance be overcome?

One approach taken by scientists to combat antibiotic resistance is to strengthen the action of existing antibiotics by modifying them so the bacterial enzymes that cause resistance cannot attack them. Alternately, "decoy" molecules can be used along with the antibiotic, so that the bacterium's resistance enzyme attacks the decoy molecule rather than the antibiotic. Decoy molecules such as clavulanic acid or sulbactam are already in use for blocking the beta-lactamase enzymes that destroy the penicillin family of drugs.

An alternative approach to the antibiotic resistance problem is to interfere with the mechanisms that promote resistance, rather than to attempt to kill the bacteria. For example, interfering with the duplication or movement of a bacterium's genetic material would eliminate the transfer of resistance genes between bacteria.

Part Two

Bacterial Diseases

Chapter 12

Chlamydia

What is chlamydial infection?

Chlamydial ("kla-MID-ee-uhl") infection is a curable sexually transmitted disease (STD), which is caused by a bacterium called *Chlamydia trachomatis*. You can get genital chlamydial infection during oral, vaginal, or anal sexual contact with an infected partner. It can cause serious problems in men and women as well as in newborn babies of infected mothers.

Chlamydial infection is one of the most widespread bacterial STDs in the United States. The U.S. Centers for Disease Control and Prevention (CDC) estimates that more than 4 million people are infected each year. Health economists estimate that chlamydial infections and the other problems they cause cost Americans more than $2 billion a year.

What are the symptoms of this STD?

Because chlamydial infection does not make most people sick, you can have it and not know it. Those who do have symptoms may have an abnormal discharge (mucus or pus) from the vagina or penis or pain while urinating. These early symptoms may be very mild. Symptoms usually appear within one to three weeks after being infected. Because the symptoms may be mild or not exist at all, you might not seek care and get treated.

"Chlamydial Infection," National Institute of Allergy and Infectious Diseases (NIAID), National Institutes of Health (NIH), May 2002.

The infection may move inside the body if it is not treated. There, it can cause pelvic inflammatory disease (PID) in women and epididymitis in men, two very serious illnesses.

C. trachomatis can cause inflamed rectum and inflammation of the lining of the eye ("pink eye"). The bacteria also can infect the throat from oral sexual contact with an infected partner.

How does the doctor diagnose chlamydial infection?

Chlamydial infection is easily confused with gonorrhea because the symptoms of both diseases are similar and the diseases can occur together, though rarely.

The most reliable ways to find out whether the infection is chlamydial are through laboratory tests. Usually, a doctor or other health care worker will send a sample of pus from the vagina or penis to a laboratory that will look for the bacteria.

The urine test does not require a pelvic exam or swabbing of the penis. Results from the urine test are available within 24 hours.

How is chlamydial infection treated?

If you are infected with *C. trachomatis*, your doctor or other health care worker will probably give you a prescription for an antibiotic such as azithromycin (taken for one day only) or doxycycline (taken for seven days) to treat people with chlamydial infection. Or, you might get a prescription for another antibiotic such as erythromycin or ofloxacin.

Doctors may treat pregnant women with azithromycin or erythromycin, or sometimes, with amoxicillin. Penicillin, which doctors often use to treat some other STDs, won't cure chlamydial infections.

If you have chlamydial infection:

- Take all of the prescribed medicine, even after symptoms disappear.
- If the symptoms do not disappear within one to two weeks after finishing the medicine, go to your doctor or clinic again.
- It is very important to tell your sex partners that you have chlamydial infection so that they can be tested and treated.

What can happen if the infection is not treated?

In women, untreated chlamydial infections can lead to PID. In men, untreated chlamydial infections may lead to pain or swelling in the scrotal area, which is a sign of inflammation of a part of the male reproductive system located near the testicles known as the epididymis. Left untreated, these complications can prevent people from having children.

Each year up to 1 million women in the United States develop PID, a serious infection of the reproductive organs. As many as half of all cases of PID may be due to chlamydial infection, and many of these don't have symptoms. PID can cause scarring of the fallopian tubes, which can block the tubes and prevent fertilization from taking place. Researchers estimate that 100,000 women each year become infertile because of PID.

In other cases, scarring may interfere with the passage of the fertilized egg to the uterus during pregnancy. When this happens, the egg may attach itself to the fallopian tube. This is called ectopic or tubal pregnancy. This very serious condition results in a miscarriage and can cause death of the mother.

Can chlamydial infection affect a newborn baby?

A baby who is exposed to *C. trachomatis* in the birth canal during delivery may develop an eye infection or pneumonia. Symptoms of conjunctivitis or "pink eye," which include discharge and swollen eyelids, usually develop within the first 10 days of life.

Symptoms of pneumonia, including a cough that gets steadily worse and congestion, most often develop within three to six weeks of birth. Doctors can treat both conditions successfully with antibiotics. Because of these risks to the newborn, many doctors recommend that all pregnant women get tested for chlamydial infection.

How can I prevent getting chlamydial infection?

You can reduce your chances of getting chlamydia or of giving it to your partner by using male latex condoms correctly every time you have sexual intercourse.

If you are infected but have no symptoms, you may pass the bacteria to your sex partners without knowing it. Therefore, any doctors recommend that anyone who has more than one sex partner, especially women under 25 years of age, be tested for chlamydial infection regularly, even if they don't have symptoms.

What research is going on?

Scientists are looking for better ways to diagnose, treat, and prevent chlamydial infections. NIAID-supported scientists recently completed sequencing the genome for *C. trachomatis*. The sequence represents an encyclopedia of information about the organism. This accomplishment will give scientists important information as they try to develop a safe and effective vaccine. Developing topical microbicides (preparations that can be inserted into the vagina to prevent infection) that are effective and easy for women to use is also a major research focus.

Chapter 13

Diphtheria

What is diphtheria?

Diphtheria is an acute bacterial disease that usually affects the tonsils, throat, nose or skin. It is extremely rare in the United States. The bacteria that causes diphtheria is called *Corynebacterium diphtheriae*.

Who gets diphtheria?

Diphtheria is most common where people live in crowded conditions. Unimmunized children under 15 years of age are likely to contract diphtheria. The disease is often found among adults whose immunization was neglected, and is most severe in unimmunized or inadequately immunized individuals.

How is diphtheria spread?

Diphtheria is transmitted to others through close contact with discharge from an infected person's nose, throat, skin, eyes, and lesions.

This chapter begins with "Diphtheria," © 2003 New York State Health Department, which is reprinted with permission from the New York State Department of Health. These pages, and any updates to them, are available to the public on the New York State Department of Health website, www.health .state.ny.us. "Facts about Diphtheria for Adults," is reprinted with permission from the National Foundation for Infectious Diseases - National Coalition for Adult Immunization. © 2003. For additional information visit the National Foundation for Infectious Diseases website at www.nfid.org, or the National Coalition for Adult Immunization at http://www.nfid.org/ncai.

What are the symptoms of diphtheria?

There are two types of diphtheria. One type involves the nose and throat, and the other involves the skin. Symptoms include sore throat, low-grade fever, and enlarged lymph nodes located in the neck. Skin lesions may be painful, swollen, and reddened.

How soon do symptoms appear?

Symptoms usually appear two to four days after infection, with a range of one to ten days.

When and for how long is a person able to spread diphtheria?

People who are infected with the diphtheria germ may be contagious for up to two weeks, but seldom more than four weeks. If the patient is treated with appropriate antibiotics, the contagious period can be limited to less than four days.

Does past infection with diphtheria make a person immune?

Recovery from diphtheria is not always followed by lasting immunity.

Is there a vaccine for diphtheria?

Diphtheria vaccine is usually combined with tetanus vaccine and acellular pertussis vaccine to form a triple vaccine known as DTaP. This vaccine should be given at two, four, six and 15–18 months of age, and between four and six years of age. A combination of tetanus vaccine and diphtheria vaccine (Td) should be given every 10 years to maintain immunity.

How can diphtheria be prevented?

The single most effective control measure is maintaining the highest possible level of immunization in the community. Other methods of control include prompt treatment of cases and a community surveillance program.

What is the treatment for diphtheria?

Certain antibiotics, such as penicillin and erythromycin, can be prescribed for the treatment of diphtheria. A diphtheria antitoxin is also used for treatment.

What can be the effect of not being treated for diphtheria?

If diphtheria goes untreated, serious complications such as paralysis, heart failure, and blood disorders may occur. Death occurs in approximately 5 to 10 percent of all cases.

Facts about Diphtheria for Adults

- Diphtheria can be prevented with a safe and effective vaccine.
- You cannot get diphtheria from the vaccine.
- Diphtheria is transmitted to others through close contact with discharges from an infected person's nose, throat, eyes, and/or skin lesions.
- Nearly one out of every 10 people who get diphtheria will die from it.
- Diphtheria can lead to breathing problems, heart failure, paralysis, and sometimes death.
- Most cases of diphtheria occur among unvaccinated or inadequately vaccinated people.
- Recovery from diphtheria is not always followed by lasting immunity, so even those persons who have survived the disease need to be immunized.
- A tetanus-diphtheria (Td) shot every 10 years gives protection against these two diseases.
- Although no longer a very common disease in the United States, diphtheria remains a large problem in other countries and can pose a serious threat to United States citizens who may not be fully immunized and who travel to other countries or have contact with immigrants or international travelers coming to the U.S.
- An epidemic of diphtheria in Eastern Europe and the New Independent States of the former Soviet Union resulted in over 5,000 deaths between 1990 and 1995.

Prevention

There is a vaccine for diphtheria. Most people receive their first dose as children in the form of a combined vaccine called DTP (diphtheria-tetanus-pertussis).

For adults, a combination shot, called a Td booster, protects against both tetanus and diphtheria. It should be administered once every 10 years after age 7 to maintain immunity.

Symptoms

In its early stages, diphtheria may be mistaken for a severe sore throat. Other symptoms include a low-grade fever and enlarged lymph nodes (swollen glands) located in the neck. Another presentation of diphtheria can be skin lesions that may be painful, red, and swollen. Symptoms usually appear 2 to 4 days after infection, with a range of 1 to 6 days. People carrying diphtheria germs are contagious for up to 4 weeks without antibiotic therapy, even if they themselves do not develop symptoms.

Who Should Get Td Vaccine?

- All persons who did not receive a primary series of immunization against tetanus and diphtheria during childhood.
- Persons who have not received a booster dose within the past 10 years.
- All adolescents and adults who deferred their regular booster during 2001–2002 because of shortages of the vaccine—the supply problems have been resolved.

Vaccine Safety

The tetanus-diphtheria (Td) vaccine is very safe. When side effects do occur, they are usually soreness, redness or swelling at the injection site, and a slight fever. As with any medicine, there are very small risks that serious problems, such as an allergic reaction or neurologic condition, could occur after getting a vaccine. However, the potential risks associated with diphtheria are much greater than the potential risks associated with the diphtheria vaccine. You cannot get diphtheria from the vaccine.

Chapter 14

Gonorrhea

What is gonorrhea?

Gonorrhea is a curable sexually transmitted disease (STD) caused by a bacterium called *Neisseria gonorrhoeae*. These bacteria can infect the genital tract, the mouth, and the rectum. In women, the opening to the uterus, the cervix, is the first place of infection.

The disease however can spread into the uterus and fallopian tubes, resulting in pelvic inflammatory disease (PID). PID affects more than 1 million women in this country every year and can cause infertility in as many as 10 percent of infected women and tubal (ectopic) pregnancy.

In 2000, 358,995 cases of gonorrhea were reported to the U.S. Centers for Disease Control and Prevention (CDC). In the United States, approximately 75 percent of all reported cases of gonorrhea is found in younger persons aged 15 to 29 years. The highest rates of infection are usually found in 15 to 19-year old women and 20 to 24-year-old men. Health economists estimate that the annual cost of gonorrhea and its complications is close to $1.1 billion.

Gonorrhea is spread during sexual intercourse. Infected women also can pass gonorrhea to their newborn infants during delivery, causing eye infections in their babies. This complication is rare because newborn babies receive eye medicine to prevent infection. When the infection occurs in the genital tract, mouth, or rectum of a child, it is due most commonly to sexual abuse.

"Gonorrhea," National Institute of Allergy and Infectious Diseases (NIAID), National Institutes of Health (NIH), May 2002.

What are the symptoms of gonorrhea?

The early symptoms of gonorrhea often are mild. Symptoms usually appear within 2 to 10 days after sexual contact with an infected partner. A small number of people may be infected for several months without showing symptoms.

When women have symptoms, the first ones may include:

- Bleeding associated with vaginal intercourse
- Painful or burning sensations when urinating
- Vaginal discharge that is yellow or bloody

More advanced symptoms, which may indicate development of PID, include cramps and pain, bleeding between menstrual periods, vomiting, or fever.

Men have symptoms more often than women, including:

- Pus from the penis and pain
- Burning sensations during urination that may be severe

Symptoms of rectal infection include discharge, anal itching, and occasional painful bowel movements with fresh blood on the feces.

How is gonorrhea diagnosed?

Doctors or other health care workers usually use three laboratory techniques to diagnose gonorrhea: staining samples directly for the bacterium, detection of bacterial genes or DNA in urine, and growing the bacteria in laboratory cultures. Many doctors prefer to use more than one test to increase the chance of an accurate diagnosis.

The staining test involves placing a smear of the discharge from the penis or the cervix on a slide and staining the smear with a dye. Then the doctor uses a microscope to look for bacteria on the slide. You usually can get the test results while in the office or clinic. This test is quite accurate for men but is not good in women. Only one in two women with gonorrhea have a positive stain.

More often, doctors use urine or cervical swabs for a new test that detects the genes of the bacteria. These tests are as accurate or more so than culturing the bacteria, and many doctors use them.

The culture test involves placing a sample of the discharge onto a culture plate and incubating it up to 2 days to allow the bacteria to grow. The sensitivity of this test depends on the site from which the sample is taken. Cultures of cervical samples detect infection approximately 90 percent of the time. The doctor also can take a culture to detect gonorrhea in the throat. Culture allows testing for drug-resistant bacteria.

How is gonorrhea treated?

Doctors usually prescribe a single dose of one of the following antibiotics to treat gonorrhea:

- Cefixime
- Ceftriaxone
- Ciprofloxacin
- Ofloxacin
- Levofloxacin

If you have gonorrhea and are pregnant or are younger than 18 years old, you should not take ciprofloxacin or ofloxacin. Your doctor can prescribe the best and safest antibiotic for you.

Gonorrhea and chlamydial infection, another common STD, often infect people at the same time. Therefore, doctors usually prescribe a combination of antibiotics, such as ceftriaxone and doxycycline or azithromycin, which will treat both diseases.

If you have gonorrhea, all of your sexual partners should get tested and then treated if infected, whether or not they have symptoms of infection.

What can happen if gonorrhea is not treated?

In untreated gonorrhea infections, the bacteria can spread up into the reproductive tract, or more rarely, can spread through the blood stream and infect the joints, heart valves, or the brain.

The most common result of untreated gonorrhea is PID, a serious infection of the female reproductive tract. Gonococcal PID often appears immediately after the menstrual period. PID causes scar tissue to form in the fallopian tubes. If the tube is partially scarred, the fertilized egg may not be able to pass into the uterus. If this happens, the embryo may implant in the tube causing a tubal (ectopic) pregnancy. This serious complication may result in a miscarriage and can cause death of the mother.

Rarely, untreated gonorrhea can spread through the blood to the joints. This can cause an inflammation of the joints which is very serious.

If you are infected with gonorrhea, your risk of getting HIV infection increases (HIV, human immunodeficiency virus, causes AIDS). Therefore, it is extremely important for you to either prevent yourself from getting gonorrhea or get treated early if you already are infected with it.

Can gonorrhea affect a newborn baby?

If you are pregnant and have gonorrhea, you may give the infection to your baby as it passes through the birth canal during delivery. A doctor can prevent infection of your baby's eyes by applying silver nitrate or other medications to the eyes immediately after birth. Because of the risks from gonococcal infection to both you and your baby, doctors recommend that pregnant women have at least one test for gonorrhea during pregnancy.

How can I prevent getting infected with gonorrhea?

By using latex condoms correctly and consistently during vaginal or rectal sexual activity, you can reduce your risk of getting gonorrhea and its complications.

What research is going on?

The National Institute of Allergy, Immunology and Infectious Diseases (NIAID) continues to support a comprehensive, multidisciplinary program of research on *N. gonorrhoeae* (gonococci). Researchers are trying to understand how gonococci infect cells while evading human immune defenses (immune response). Studies are ongoing to determine

1. How this bacterium attaches to host cells
2. How it gets inside them
3. Gonococcal surface structures and how they can change
4. Human response to infection by gonococci

All of these efforts, together, will eventually lead to development of an effective vaccine against gonorrhea. They also have led to, and will lead to further, improvements in diagnosis and treatment of gonorrhea.

Another important area of gonorrhea research concerns antibiotic resistance. This is particularly important because strains of *N. gonorrhoeae* that are resistant to recommended antibiotic therapies have spread from Southeast Asia to Hawaii and are now starting to appear on the West Coast. These events add urgency to NIAID efforts to develop effective microbicides (antimicrobial preparations that can be applied inside the vagina) to prevent infections.

Recently, scientists have determined the sequence of the *N. gonorrhoeae* genome. They are using this information to find promising new leads to help us better understand how the organism causes disease and becomes resistant to antibiotics.

Chapter 15

Group A Streptococcal (GAS) Disease

What is group A streptococcus (GAS)?

Group A streptococcus is a bacterium often found in the throat and on the skin. People may carry group A streptococci in the throat or on the skin and have no symptoms of illness. Most GAS infections are relatively mild illnesses such as "strep throat," or impetigo. On rare occasions, these bacteria can cause other severe and even life-threatening diseases.

How are group A streptococci spread?

These bacteria are spread through direct contact with mucus from the nose or throat of persons who are infected or through contact with infected wounds or sores on the skin. Ill persons, such as those who have strep throat or skin infections, are most likely to spread the infection. Persons who carry the bacteria but have no symptoms are much less contagious. Treating an infected person with an antibiotic for 24 hours or longer generally eliminates their ability to spread the bacteria. However, it is important to complete the entire course of antibiotics as prescribed. It is not likely that household items like plates, cups, or toys spread these bacteria.

"Group A Streptococcal (GAS) Disease," Division of Bacterial and Mycotic Diseases, Centers for Disease Control and Prevention (CDC), reviewed December 2003.

What kind of illnesses are caused by group A streptococcal infection?

Infection with GAS can result in a range of symptoms:

- No illness
- Mild illness (strep throat or a skin infection such as impetigo)
- Severe illness (necrotizing fasciitis, streptococcal toxic shock syndrome)

Severe, sometimes life-threatening, GAS disease may occur when bacteria get into parts of the body where bacteria usually are not found, such as the blood, muscle, or the lungs. These infections are termed "invasive GAS disease." Two of the most severe, but least common, forms of invasive GAS disease are necrotizing fasciitis and streptococcal toxic shock syndrome. Necrotizing fasciitis (occasionally described by the media as "the flesh-eating bacteria") destroys muscles, fat, and skin tissue. Streptococcal toxic shock syndrome (STSS), causes blood pressure to drop rapidly and organs (e.g., kidney, liver, lungs) to fail. STSS is not the same as the "toxic shock syndrome" frequently associated with tampon usage. About 20% of patients with necrotizing fasciitis and more than half with STSS die. About 10%–15% of patients with other forms of invasive group A streptococcal disease die.

How common is invasive group A streptococcal disease?

About 9,400 cases of invasive GAS disease occurred in the United States in 1999. Of these, about 300 were STSS and 600 were necrotizing fasciitis. In contrast, there are several million cases of strep throat and impetigo each year.

Why does invasive group A streptococcal disease occur?

Invasive GAS infections occur when the bacteria get past the defenses of the person who is infected. This may occur when a person has sores or other breaks in the skin that allow the bacteria to get into the tissue, or when the person's ability to fight off the infection is decreased because of chronic illness or an illness that affects the immune system. Also, some virulent strains of GAS are more likely to cause severe disease than others.

Who is most at risk of getting invasive group A streptococcal disease?

Few people who come in contact with GAS will develop invasive GAS disease. Most people will have a throat or skin infection, and some may have no symptoms at all. Although healthy people can get invasive GAS disease, people with chronic illnesses like cancer, diabetes, and kidney dialysis, and those who use medications such as steroids have a higher risk.

What are the early signs and symptoms of necrotizing fasciitis and streptococcal toxic shock syndrome?

Early signs and symptoms of necrotizing fasciitis:

- Fever
- Severe pain and swelling
- Redness at the wound site

Early signs and symptoms of STSS:

- Fever
- Dizziness
- Confusion
- A flat red rash over large areas of the body

How is invasive group A streptococcal disease treated?

GAS infections can be treated with many different antibiotics. Early treatment may reduce the risk of death from invasive group A streptococcal disease. However, even the best medical care does not prevent death in every case. For those with very severe illness, supportive care in an intensive care unit may be needed. For persons with necrotizing fasciitis, surgery often is needed to remove damaged tissue.

What can be done to help prevent group A streptococcal infections?

The spread of all types of GAS infection can be reduced by good hand washing, especially after coughing and sneezing and before preparing foods or eating. Persons with sore throats should be seen by a doctor who can perform tests to find out whether the illness is strep throat. If the test result shows strep throat, the person should stay home from work, school, or day care until 24 hours after taking an antibiotic. All wounds should be kept clean and watched for possible signs of infection such as redness, swelling, drainage, and pain at the wound site. A person with signs of an infected wound, especially if fever occurs, should seek medical care. It is not necessary for all persons exposed to someone with an invasive group A strep infection (necrotizing fasciitis or strep toxic shock syndrome) to receive antibiotic therapy to prevent infection. However, in certain circumstances, antibiotic therapy may be appropriate. That decision should be made after consulting with your doctor.

Chapter 16

Group B Streptococcal (GBS) Disease

Group B streptococcus (GBS) is a type of bacterium that causes illness in newborn babies, pregnant women, the elderly, and adults with other illnesses, such as diabetes or liver disease. GBS is the most common cause of life-threatening infections in newborns.

Frequently Asked Questions about GBS

How common is GBS disease?

GBS is the most common cause of sepsis (blood infection) and meningitis (infection of the fluid and lining surrounding the brain) in newborns.

GBS is a frequent cause of newborn pneumonia and is more common than other, better known, newborn problems such as rubella, congenital syphilis, and spina bifida.

Before prevention methods were widely used, approximately 8,000 babies in the United States would get GBS disease each year. One of every 20 babies with GBS disease dies from infection. Babies that survive, particularly those who have meningitis, may have long-term problems, such as hearing or vision loss or learning disabilities.

In pregnant women, GBS can cause bladder infections, womb infections (amnionitis, endometritis), and stillbirth. Among men and among

---

"Group B Streptococcal Disease (GBS)," Division of Bacterial and Mycotic Diseases, Centers for Disease Control and Prevention (CDC), reviewed February 2004; and "Group B Strep Disease: Frequently Asked Questions," Centers for Disease Control and Prevention (CDC), reviewed November 8, 2002.

women who are not pregnant, the most common diseases caused by GBS are blood infections, skin or soft tissue infections, and pneumonia.

Approximately 20% of men and nonpregnant women with GBS disease die of the disease.

Does everyone who has GBS get sick?

Many people carry GBS in their bodies but do not become ill. These people are considered to be "carriers." Adults can carry GBS in the bowel, vagina, bladder, or throat. One of every four or five pregnant women carries GBS in the rectum or vagina. A fetus may come in contact with GBS before or during birth if the mother carries GBS in the rectum or vagina. People who carry GBS typically do so temporarily—that is, they do not become lifelong carriers of the bacteria.

How is GBS disease diagnosed and treated?

GBS disease is diagnosed when the bacterium is grown from cultures of sterile body fluids, such as blood or spinal fluid. Cultures take a few days to complete. GBS infections in both newborns and adults are usually treated with antibiotics (for example, penicillin or ampicillin) given through a vein.

What research is being done on prevention of GBS disease?

In spite of testing and antibiotic treatment, some babies still get GBS disease. Vaccines to prevent GBS disease are being developed. In the future, women who are vaccinated may make antibodies that cross the placenta and protect the baby during birth and early infancy.

Who is at higher risk for GBS disease?

Pregnant women with the following conditions are at higher risk of having a baby with GBS disease:

- previous baby with GBS disease
- urinary tract infection due to GBS
- GBS carriage late in pregnancy
- fever during labor
- rupture of membranes 18 hours or more before delivery
- labor or rupture of membranes before 37 weeks

Questions about Newborns and Group B Strep

How common is group B strep disease in newborns?

Group B strep is the most common cause of sepsis (blood infection) and meningitis (infection of the fluid and lining around the brain) in newborns. Group B strep is a frequent cause of newborn pneumonia and is more common than other, more well-known, newborn problems such as rubella, congenital syphilis, and spina bifida.

In the year 2001, there were about 1,700 babies in the U.S. less than one week old who got early-onset group B strep disease.

How does group B strep disease affect newborns?

About half of the cases of group B strep disease among newborns happen in the first week of life ("early-onset disease"), and most of these cases start a few hours after birth. Sepsis, pneumonia (infection in the lungs), and meningitis (infection of the fluid and lining around the brain) are the most common problems. Premature babies are more at risk of getting a group B strep infection, but most babies who become sick from group B strep are full-term.

Group B strep disease may also develop in infants one week to several months after birth ("late-onset disease"). Meningitis is more common with late-onset group B strep disease. Only about half of late-onset group B strep disease among newborns comes from a mother who is a group B strep carrier; the source of infection for others with late-onset group B strep disease can be hard to figure out. Late-onset disease is slightly less common than early-onset disease.

Can group B strep disease among newborns be prevented?

Yes. Most early-onset group B strep disease in newborns can be prevented by giving pregnant women antibiotics (medicine) through the vein (IV) during labor. Antibiotics help to kill some of the strep bacteria that are dangerous to the baby during birth. The antibiotics help during labor only—they can't be taken before labor, because the bacteria can grow back quickly. Any pregnant woman who had a baby with group B strep disease in the past, or who now has a bladder (urinary tract) infection caused by group B strep should receive antibiotics during labor.

Pregnant women who carry group B strep (test positive during this pregnancy) should be given antibiotics at the time of labor or when their water breaks. GBS carriers at highest risk are those with any of the following conditions:

- fever during labor
- rupture of membranes (water breaking) 18 hours or more before delivery
- labor or rupture of membranes before 37 weeks

Because women who carry GBS but do not develop any of these three complications have a relatively low risk of delivering an infant with GBS disease, the decision to take antibiotics during labor should balance risks and benefits. Penicillin is very effective at preventing GBS disease in the newborn and is generally safe. A GBS carrier with none of the conditions above has the following risks:

- 1 in 200 chance of delivering a baby with GBS disease if antibiotics are not given
- 1 in 4000 chance of delivering a baby with GBS disease if antibiotics are given
- 1 in 10 chance, or lower, of experiencing a mild allergic reaction to penicillin (such as rash)
- 1 in 10, 000 chance of developing a severe allergic reaction—anaphylaxis—to penicillin. Anaphylaxis requires emergency treatment and can be life-threatening.

If a prenatal culture for GBS was not done or the results are not available, physicians may give antibiotics to women with one or more of the risk conditions listed above.

What are the symptoms of group B strep in a newborn?

The symptoms for early-onset group B strep can seem like other problems in newborns. Some symptoms are fever, difficulty feeding, irritability, or lethargy (limpness or hard to wake up the baby). If you think your newborn is sick, get medical help right away.

How is group B strep disease diagnosed and treated in babies?

If a mother received antibiotics for group B strep during labor, the baby will be observed to see if he or she should get extra testing or treatment. If the doctors suspect that a baby has group B strep infection, they will take a sample of the baby's sterile body fluids, such as blood or spinal fluid. Group B strep disease is diagnosed when the bacteria are grown from cultures of those fluids. Cultures take a few days to grow. Group B strep infections in both newborns and adults are usually treated with antibiotics (for example, penicillin or ampicillin) given through a vein (IV).

Questions about Pregnancy and Group B Strep Prevention

How will I know if I need antibiotics to prevent passing group B strep to my baby?

You should get a screening test late in pregnancy to see if you carry group B strep. If your test comes back positive, you should get antibiotics through the vein (IV) during labor.

If you had a previous baby who got sick with group B strep disease, or if you had a urinary tract infection (bladder infection) during this pregnancy caused by group B strep, you also need to get antibiotics through the vein (IV) when your labor starts.

How do you find out if you carry group B strep during pregnancy?

GBS carriage can be detected during pregnancy by taking a swab of both the vagina and rectum for special culture. Physicians who culture for GBS carriage during prenatal visits should do so late in pregnancy (35–37 weeks' gestation); cultures collected earlier do not accurately predict whether a mother will have GBS at delivery.

A positive culture result means that the mother carries GBS—not that she or her baby will definitely become ill. Women who carry GBS should not be given oral antibiotics before labor because antibiotic treatment at this time does not prevent GBS disease in newborns. An exception to this is when GBS is identified in urine during pregnancy. GBS in the urine should be treated at the time it is diagnosed. Carriage of GBS, in either the vagina or rectum, becomes important at the time of labor and delivery—when antibiotics are effective in preventing the spread of GBS from mother to baby.

What happens if my pregnancy screening test is positive for group B strep?

To prevent group B strep bacteria from being passed to the newborn, pregnant women who carry group B strep should be given antibiotics through the vein (IV) at the time of labor or when their water breaks.

Are there any symptoms if you are a group B strep carrier?

Most pregnant women have no symptoms when they are carriers for group B strep bacteria.

Sometimes, group B strep can cause bladder infections during pregnancy, or infections in the womb during labor or after delivery.

Being a carrier (testing positive for group B strep, but having no symptoms) is quite common. Around 25% of women may carry the bacteria at any time. This doesn't mean that they have group B strep disease, but it does mean that they are at higher risk for giving their baby a group B strep infection during birth.

What if I don't know whether or not I am group B strep positive when my labor starts?

Talk to your doctor about your group B strep status. Pregnant women who do not know whether or not they are group B strep positive when labor starts should be given antibiotics if they have:

- labor starting at less than 37 weeks (preterm labor);
- prolonged membrane rupture (water breaking more than 18 hours before labor starts);
- fever during labor.

What are the risks of taking antibiotics to prevent group B strep disease in my newborn?

Penicillin is the most common antibiotic that is given. If you are allergic to penicillin, there are other antibiotics that can be given. Penicillin is very safe and effective at preventing group B strep disease in newborns. There can be side effects from penicillin for the woman, including a mild reaction to penicillin (about a 10% chance). There is a rare chance (about 1 in 10,000) of the mother having a severe allergic reaction that requires emergency treatment.

However, a pregnant woman who is a group B strep carrier (tested positive) at full-term delivery who gets antibiotics can feel confident knowing that she has only a 1 in 4000 chance of delivering a baby with group B strep disease. If a pregnant woman who is a group B strep carrier does not get antibiotics at the time of delivery, her baby has a 1 in 200 chance of developing group B strep disease. This means that those infants whose mothers are group B strep carriers and do not get antibiotics have over 20 times the risk of developing disease than those who do receive treatment.

Can group B strep cause stillbirth, pre-term delivery, or miscarriage?

There are many different factors that lead to stillbirth, pre-term delivery, or miscarriage. Most of the time, the cause is not known. Group B strep can cause some stillbirths, and pre-term babies are at greater risk of group B strep infections. However, the relationship between group B strep and premature babies is not always clear.

Will a C-section prevent group B strep in a newborn?

A C-section should not be used to prevent early-onset group B strep infection in infants. If you need to have a C-section for other reasons, and you are group B strep positive, you will not need antibiotics for group B strep only, unless you begin labor or your water breaks before the surgery begins.

What should I do if my water breaks early?

If your water breaks before term, get to the hospital right away. If your group B strep test has not been done, or if you don't know if you have been tested, you should talk with your doctor about group B strep disease prevention. If you have already tested positive for group B strep, remind the doctors and nurses during labor.

Can I breastfeed my baby if I am group B strep positive?

Yes. Women who are group B strep positive can breastfeed safely. There are many benefits for both the mother and child.

More Questions about Group B Strep

How does someone get group B strep?

The bacteria that cause group B strep disease normally live in the intestine, vagina, or rectal areas.

Group B strep colonization is not a sexually transmitted disease (STD). Approximately 25% (1 in 4) of pregnant women carry group B strep bacteria in their vagina or rectum. For most women there are no symptoms of carrying group B strep bacteria.

Will group B strep go away with antibiotics?

Antibiotics that are given when labor starts help to greatly reduce the number of group B strep bacteria present during labor.

This reduces the chances of the newborn becoming exposed and infected.

However, for women who are group B strep carriers, antibiotics before labor starts are not a good way to get rid of group B strep bacteria. Since they naturally live in the gastrointestinal tract (guts), the bacteria can come back after antibiotics. A woman may test positive at certain times and not at others. That's why it's important for all pregnant women to be tested for group B strep carriage between 35 to 37 weeks of every pregnancy. Talk to your doctor or nurse about the best way to prevent group B strep disease, or review the revised group B strep guidelines to learn more.

What if I'm allergic to some antibiotics?

Tell your doctor or nurse about your allergies during your checkup. Try to make a plan for delivery. When you get to the hospital, remind your doctor if you are allergic to any medicines. There are a variety of different antibiotics that can be used, even if you are allergic to some.

Is there a vaccine for group B strep?

There is not a vaccine right now to prevent group B strep. The federal government is supporting research on a vaccine for the prevention of group B strep disease.

Are yeast infections caused by group B strep?

Yeast infections are not caused by group B strep bacteria. Taking antibiotics can sometimes increase the chances of having a yeast infection. When bacteria that are normally found in the vagina are killed by antibiotics, yeast may have a chance to grow more quickly than usual.

Is group B strep the same as strep throat?

No. Strep throat is caused by group A streptococcus bacteria. Group A and group B streptococcus are different kinds of bacteria. They both belong to the same family, but they are different species.

Chapter 17

Haemophilus Influenzae *Type B (Hib) Disease*

What is Haemophilus influenzae *type B (Hib)?*

Hib are bacteria that may cause a variety of diseases including blood infection and meningitis (inflammation of the lining of the brain).

How common is Hib disease?

Since thc introduction of the Hib vaccine in 1988, Hib cases have declined by 95% in infants and young children. Before the use of an effective vaccine, Hib was the most common cause of bacterial meningitis in children.

Who gets Hib infection?

Anyone can get Hib infection, but it is most common in children between the ages of three months and three years. The elderly and persons with weakened immune systems are also at a higher risk of developing the disease.

How is Hib infection spread?

Hib infection is spread by inhalation of droplets that contain the bacteria from the nose and throat. Although not common, some individuals

---

Reprinted with permission from "Haemophilus Influenzae Type B," Wisconsin Department of Health and Family Services, revised December 2003; available online at http://www.dhfs.state.wi.us/healthtips/BCD/HaemophilusInfluenzaeTypeB.htm.

may carry Hib in their nose and throat without becoming ill and potentially spread the bacteria to others.

What are the symptoms of Hib infection?

Fever is present in all forms of Hib infection. Other symptoms of Hib infection depend on the part of the body affected. Hib can result in sinus infections, earaches, and skin infections. Hib may also cause serious illnesses like meningitis, (characterized by the usually sudden onset of fever, lethargy, vomiting, and a stiff and/or rigid neck and back), pneumonia, epiglottitis (inflammation of upper airway), and blood stream infections.

How soon do the symptoms appear?

The period between exposure to Hib and the beginning of symptoms is unknown, but is probably short (2–4 days).

Does past infection with Hib make a person immune?

Children who develop Hib infection before 24 months of age may not develop immunity and should still be immunized with the Hib vaccine. If Hib infection occurs in an unimmunized child after 24 months of age, the child generally develops future immunity and vaccination is not necessary.

What is the treatment for Hib infection?

Hib infections are treated with antibiotics. Patients are no longer infectious 24–48 hours after receiving effective antimicrobial therapy.

What can be done to prevent the spread of Hib infection?

All children should be immunized with Hib conjugate vaccine beginning at approximately two months of age. Close contacts of a person infected with Hib may require immediate preventative antibiotics depending on circumstances.

For more information contact your Local Public Health Department.

Chapter 18

Hansen's Disease (Leprosy)

What is Hansen's disease?

Hansen's disease (HD), erroneously associated with biblical leprosy, is a complex infectious disease. Although recognized for more than two thousand years and found over a century ago to be caused by a bacterium, the disease is still not completely understood. Dr. Gerhard Armauer Hansen, a Norwegian scientist, first discovered the HD bacillus in 1873. Considerable progress has been made over the last 40 years so that today we can treat the majority of cases without undue difficulty and counteract most of the fears generated by the folklore surrounding this disease.

HD is in the same bacterial family as *Mycobacterium tuberculosis* but is uniquely a disease of the peripheral nerves. It also affects the skin and sometimes other tissues, notably the eye, the mucosa of the upper respiratory tract, muscles, bone and testes.

There are both localized and disseminated forms of HD. If left untreated, HD causes nerve damage, which can result in loss of muscle control and crippling of hands and feet. Eye involvement can result in blindness.

"Frequently Asked Questions," National Hansen's Disease Programs (NHDP), Bureau of Primary Health Care (BPHC), Health Resources and Services Administration, 2001.

Where is Hansen's disease found?

In 1994 the World Health Organization estimated that there were 2.4 million cases of HD worldwide with 1.7 million cases registered on treatment. The estimates for 1985 were 10–12 million and 5.4 million respectively. According to these estimates, in 1994, 70% of those who should be on treatment are now being treated. In 1992 there were 690,000 new cases reported and in 1993, 591,00 cases. There are also an estimated 2–3 million cases who have completed treatment but still have residual disabilities. These cases are not included in the 1994 totals. The largest numbers of Hansen's disease patients continue to be in Southeast Asia and Central Africa with smaller numbers in South and Central America. The largest number of patients in the Western Hemisphere are in Brazil.

In the United States there are approximately 6,500 cases on the registry which includes all cases reported since the registry began and still living. The number of cases with active disease and requiring drug treatment is approximately 600. There are 200–250 new cases reported to the registry annually with about 175 of these being new cases diagnosed for the first time. The largest number of cases in the United States (U.S.) are in California, Texas, Hawaii, Louisiana, Florida, New York, and Puerto Rico.

The National Hansen's Disease Programs in Baton Rouge, Louisiana, is the only institution in the United States (U.S.) exclusively devoted to Hansen's disease. The center functions as a referral and consulting center with related research and training activities. Most patients in the U.S. are treated under U.S. Public Health Service grants at clinics in major cities or by private physicians.

How does HD spread?

The most commonly accepted theory is that it is transmitted by way of the respiratory tract since large numbers of bacteria can be found in the nose of some untreated patients. The degree of susceptibility of the person, the extent of exposure and environmental conditions are among factors probably of great importance in transmission.

Is Hansen's disease contagious?

Yes, but far less so than other infectious diseases. Most specialists agree that more than 95% of the world's population has a natural immunity to the disease. Healthcare workers rarely contract the disease. Cases of HD which respond satisfactorily to treatment become noninfectious within a short time.

Is there effective treatment?

Although the sulfone drugs, introduced at Carville in 1941, continue to be an important weapon against the Hansen bacillus, the rising incidence of sulfone resistant disease necessitates treating all patients with more than one drug. There is very effective treatment for Hansen's disease in the form of antibiotics. The three most commonly used are Dapsone, Rifampin and Clofazimine. Other antibiotics such as Clarithromycin, Ofloxacin, Levofloxacin and Minocycline also have excellent antibacterial activity against *M. leprae*. Treatment rapidly renders the disease non-communicable by killing nearly all the bacilli. These dead bacilli are then cleared from the body within a variable number of years. Treatment regimens differ depending upon the form of the disease. Information on treatment can be obtained by contacting NHDP.

Are there different forms of Hansen's disease?

Yes. There is a limited form of the disease called tuberculoid or paucibacillary (few bacilli) and a more generalized form called lepromatous or multibacillary (many bacilli).

Are both forms of Hansen's disease contagious?

No. The tuberculoid or paucibacillary form is not contagious.

How do I know if I have Hansen's disease?

Pale or slightly red areas on the skin which have lost feeling, or loss of feeling of the hands or feet may be the first signs of HD. Your doctor can make the diagnosis by doing a test called a skin biopsy.

Who is at greatest risk of contacting the disease?

Those at greatest risk are the household contacts of the untreated case possibly because of genetic factors relating to susceptibility and/or the prolonged intimate contact. The spouse is the least at risk familial member. The greatest risk is for the children, brothers or sisters, or parents of someone with HD.

Must a patient be treated for life for Hansen's disease?

No. Clinicians now use fixed duration treatment. Treatment will generally continue for 1 year for tuberculoid or paucibacillary disease and 2 years for lepromatous or multibacillary disease.

Is it passed on during pregnancy or through sex?

HD is not passed on from a mother to her unborn baby. You also do not get it through sexual contact.

What effects does it have on the body?

Because the bacteria like the cooler parts of the body, the skin and its nerves are affected. This can cause dryness and stiffness of the skin. In some cases affected nerves can swell, causing pain, loss of feeling and weakness in the muscles of the hands or feet.

Are all patients disfigured with loss of fingers and toes?

No. Early diagnosis and treatment is very important and can prevent many of the complications associated with the disease. Many patients with tuberculoid or paucibacillary disease can even self heal without benefit of treatment, but it is the standard of care to treat all patients identified with the disease. Problems with fingers or toes can be prevented by avoiding injury and infections to these areas, and by taking the HD medicines.

Some patients report that they get worse after treatment has begun. How can that happen?

Some patients experience what is called reaction after treatment has begun. This is a response of the immune system to dead or dying bacteria and can cause worsening of the rash or a painful neuritis which can affect sensation and/or strength.

Is reaction harmful?

Reaction can be mild or severe. If mild, no treatment or only over the counter anti-inflammatory medication may be sufficient. More severe reaction can be harmful to nerves and should be promptly treated by a physician. If you think you are having a reaction of any type, it is best to notify your physician so that he can decide on appropriate treatment.

Why is diagnosis difficult and often delayed?

Unfortunately, the rash caused by Hansen's disease often resembles other skin diseases. Lack of experience with this disease, because of its infrequent occurrence in our population, occasionally leads to lack of recognition and delay in diagnosis. Further complicating diagnosis is the inability to grow or culture this bacteria in the laboratory as we would do with other infections such as pneumonia or pharyngitis.

How does Hansen's disease present itself?

Hansen's disease mainly presents as a rash on the trunk or extremities. Frequently there is an associated decrease in light touch sensation in the area of the rash but not always. This change in sensation can be a valuable clue to diagnosis. Nasal congestion may be a sign of infection but infection is usually associated with changes of the skin on the face, and perhaps thinning of the eyebrows or eyelashes.

How is diagnosis made?

The diagnosis is made by a combination of the characteristic clinical picture of rash with change in sensation plus a skin biopsy which reveals a particular pathologic pattern and demonstrates the specific "red" staining bacteria. By far the most important diagnostic tool is the biopsy of the rash.

Is there any medicine that I should take if I think I have been exposed to the disease?

No! Household contacts of patients with HD need only a good examination by a physician. These examinations should be repeated annually for 5 years. The degree of natural immunity is very high and there is no need for prophylaxis. Household contacts who have a questionable skin rash should have a skin biopsy to determine whether or not Hansen's disease is present.

Is there any test that will tell if I have been exposed or if I have early disease?

No. Unfortunately there is no blood or skin test that will tell if you have been exposed or if you have pre-clinical disease.

Is there any way to prevent the disease such as a vaccine that would protect against exposure?

No. We do not as yet have a suitable vaccine to prevent Hansen's disease, but it is an area of very active research.

Can I continue to work?

A person with HD can continue to work and lead an active life.

Where is treatment available?

Medicine for HD can be provided at no cost to patients by their family doctor or through the Hansen's Disease Clinic closest to them. A directory of clinics is available online at www.bphc.hrsa.gov/nhdp/DIRECTORY_OF_CLINICS_AMBULATORY_CARE.htm

Chapter 19

Lymphogranuloma Venereum and Granuloma Inguinale

Lymphogranuloma Venereum

What is lymphogranuloma venereum (LGV)?

LGV is a sexually transmitted disease (STD) or infection involving the lymph glands in the genital area. It is caused by a specific strain of chlamydia.

Who gets LGV?

The incidence is highest among sexually active people living in tropical or subtropical climates. It has also occurred in some areas of the southern United States.

How is LGV spread?

The infection is spread by sexual contact.

What are the symptoms of LGV?

The first symptom may be a small, painless pimple or lesion occurring on the penis or vagina. It is often unnoticed. The infection then

---

"Lymphogranuloma Venereum," March 2003, and "Granuloma Inguinale," March 2003, are reprinted with permission from the New York State Department of Health. These pages, and any updates to them, are available to the public on the New York State Department of Health website, www.health.state.ny.us.

spreads to the lymph nodes in the groin area and from there to the surrounding tissue. Complications may include inflamed and swollen lymph glands which may drain and bleed.

How soon do symptoms appear?

The onset of symptoms varies widely. The initial lesion may appear from three to 30 days after exposure.

When and for how long is a person able to spread LGV?

An individual remains infectious as long as there are active lesions.

What is the treatment for LGV?

Treatment involves the use of certain antibiotics, specifically tetracycline or sulfamethoxazole.

What can be done to prevent the spread of LGV?

There are a number of ways to prevent the spread of LGV:

- Limit your number of sex partners.
- Use a male or female condom.
- Carefully wash genitals after sexual relations.
- If you think you are infected, avoid any sexual contact and visit your local STD clinic, a hospital, or your doctor.
- Notify all sexual contacts immediately so they can obtain examination and treatment.

Granuloma Inguinale

What is granuloma inguinale?

Granuloma inguinale is a chronic bacterial infection of the genital region, generally regarded to be sexually transmitted.

Who gets granuloma inguinale?

Granuloma inguinale is a relatively rare disease occurring in people living in tropical and subtropical areas. It occurs more frequently in males. In the United States, while homosexuals are at greater risk, it is relatively rare in heterosexual partners of those infected.

How is granuloma inguinale spread?

Granuloma inguinale is thought to be spread by sexual contact with an infected individual.

What are the symptoms of granuloma inguinale?

The disease begins with the appearance of lumps or blisters in the genital area. The blister becomes a slowly enlarging open sore.

How soon do symptoms appear?

The incubation period appears to be between eight and 80 days after infection.

When and for how long is a person able to spread granuloma inguinale?

Granuloma inguinale is communicable as long as the infected person remains untreated and bacteria from lesions are present.

Does past infection with granuloma inguinale make a person immune?

Past infection does not make a person immune. Susceptibility is variable. There is no evidence of natural resistance.

What is the treatment for granuloma inguinale?

There are several antibiotics that will effectively cure granuloma inguinale. Response to the antibiotic should be evident within seven days and total healing usually occurs within three to five weeks.

What complications can result from granuloma inguinale?

If left untreated, granuloma inguinale can result in extensive destruction of genital organs and may also spread to other parts of the body.

How can the spread of granuloma inguinale be prevented?

- Limit the number of your sex partners.
- Use a condom.

- Carefully wash the genitals after sexual relations.
- If you think you are infected, avoid any sexual contact and visit your local sexually transmitted disease (STD) clinic, a hospital, or your doctor.
- Notify all sexual contacts immediately so they can obtain medical care.

Chapter 20

Meningococcal Disease

What is meningitis?

Meningitis is an infection of the fluid of a person's spinal cord and the fluid that surrounds the brain. People sometimes refer to it as spinal meningitis. Meningitis is usually caused by a viral or bacterial infection. Knowing whether meningitis is caused by a virus or bacterium is important because the severity of illness and the treatment differ. Viral meningitis is generally less severe and resolves without specific treatment, while bacterial meningitis can be quite severe and may result in brain damage, hearing loss, or learning disability. For bacterial meningitis, it is also important to know which type of bacteria is causing the meningitis because antibiotics can prevent some types from spreading and infecting other people. Before the 1990s, *Haemophilus influenzae* type b (Hib) was the leading cause of bacterial meningitis, but new vaccines being given to all children as part of their routine immunizations have reduced the occurrence of invasive disease due to *H. influenzae*. Today, *Streptococcus pneumoniae* and *Neisseria meningitidis* are the leading causes of bacterial meningitis.

What are the signs and symptoms of meningitis?

High fever, headache, and stiff neck are common symptoms of meningitis in anyone over the age of 2 years. These symptoms can develop

"Meningococcal Disease," Division of Bacterial and Mycotic Diseases, Centers for Disease Control and Prevention (CDC), reviewed April 3, 2003.

over several hours, or they may take 1 to 2 days. Other symptoms may include nausea, vomiting, discomfort looking into bright lights, confusion, and sleepiness. In newborns and small infants, the classic symptoms of fever, headache, and neck stiffness may be absent or difficult to detect, and the infant may only appear slow or inactive, or be irritable, have vomiting, or be feeding poorly. As the disease progresses, patients of any age may have seizures.

How is meningitis diagnosed?

Early diagnosis and treatment are very important. If symptoms occur, the patient should see a doctor immediately. The diagnosis is usually made by growing bacteria from a sample of spinal fluid. The spinal fluid is obtained by performing a spinal tap, in which a needle is inserted into an area in the lower back where fluid in the spinal canal is readily accessible. Identification of the type of bacteria responsible is important for selection of correct antibiotics.

Can meningitis be treated?

Bacterial meningitis can be treated with a number of effective antibiotics. It is important, however, that treatment be started early in the course of the disease. Appropriate antibiotic treatment of most common types of bacterial meningitis should reduce the risk of dying from meningitis to below 15%, although the risk is higher among the elderly.

Is meningitis contagious?

Yes, some forms of bacterial meningitis are contagious. The bacteria are spread through the exchange of respiratory and throat secretions (i.e., coughing, kissing). Fortunately, none of the bacteria that cause meningitis are as contagious as things like the common cold or the flu, and they are not spread by casual contact or by simply breathing the air where a person with meningitis has been.

However, sometimes the bacteria that cause meningitis have spread to other people who have had close or prolonged contact with a patient with meningitis caused by *Neisseria meningitidis* (also called meningococcal meningitis) or Hib. People in the same household or day-care center, or anyone with direct contact with a patient's oral secretions (such as a boyfriend or girlfriend) would be considered at increased risk of acquiring the infection. People who qualify as close contacts of a person with meningitis caused by *N. meningitidis* should receive antibiotics to prevent them from getting the disease. Antibiotics for contacts of a person with Hib meningitis disease are no longer recommended if all contacts 4 years of age or younger are fully vaccinated against Hib disease.

Are there vaccines against meningitis?

Yes, there are vaccines against Hib and against some strains of *N. meningitidis* and many types of *Streptococcus pneumoniae*. The vaccines against Hib are very safe and highly effective.

There is also a vaccine that protects against four strains of *N. meningitidis*, but it is not routinely used in the United States. The vaccine against *N. meningitidis* is sometimes used to control outbreaks of some types of meningococcal meningitis in the United States. Meningitis cases should be reported to state or local health departments to assure follow-up of close contacts and recognize outbreaks. College freshman, especially those who live in dormitories are at higher risk for meningococcal disease and should be educated about the availability of a safe and effective vaccine which can decrease their risk. Although large epidemics of meningococcal meningitis do not occur in the United States, some countries experience large, periodic epidemics. Overseas travelers should check to see if meningococcal vaccine is recommended for their destination. Travelers should receive the vaccine at least 1 week before departure, if possible. Information on areas for which meningococcal vaccine is recommended can be obtained by calling the Centers for Disease Control and Prevention at 404-332-4565.

There are vaccines to prevent meningitis due to *S. pneumoniae* (also called pneumococcal meningitis) which can also prevent other forms of infection due to *S. pneumoniae*. The pneumococcal polysaccharide vaccine is recommended for all persons over 65 years of age and younger persons at least 2 years old with certain chronic medical problems. There is a newly licensed vaccine (pneumococcal conjugate vaccine) that appears to be effective in infants for the prevention of pneumococcal infections and is routinely recommended for all children greater than 2 years of age.

Chapter 21

Mycoplasma Infection

What is mycoplasma infection?

Mycoplasma infection is respiratory illness caused by *Mycoplasma pneumoniae*, a microscopic organism related to bacteria. It is also called walking pneumonia or atypical pneumonia.

Who gets mycoplasma infection?

Anyone can get the disease, but it most often affects older children and young adults.

When do mycoplasma infections occur?

Mycoplasma infections occur sporadically throughout the year. Widespread community outbreaks may occur at intervals of four to eight years. Mycoplasma infection is most common in late summer and fall.

How is mycoplasma spread?

Mycoplasma is spread through contact with droplets from the nose and throat of infected people especially when they cough and sneeze. Transmission is thought to require prolonged close contact with an

---

"Mycoplasma Infection," March 2003, reprinted with permission from the New York State Department of Health. These pages, and any updates to them, are available to the public on the New York State Department of Health website, www.health.state.ny.us.

infected person. Spread in families, schools, and institutions occurs slowly. The contagious period is probably fewer than 10 days and occasionally longer.

What are the symptoms of mycoplasma infection?

Typical symptoms include fever, cough, bronchitis, sore throat, headache, and tiredness. A common result of mycoplasma infection is pneumonia (sometimes called "walking pneumonia" because it is usually mild and rarely requires hospitalization). Infections of the middle ear (otitis media) also can result. Symptoms may persist for a few days to more than a month.

How soon after exposure do symptoms appear?

Symptoms generally begin 15–25 days after exposure. The symptoms generally develop slowly, over a period of two to four days.

How is mycoplasma infection diagnosed?

Mycoplasma infection is usually diagnosed on the basis of typical symptoms. A nonspecific blood test (cold agglutinins) is helpful in definitive diagnosis, but is not always positive. The use of more specific laboratory tests is often limited to special outbreak investigations.

Does past infection with mycoplasma make a person immune?

Immunity after mycoplasma infection does occur, but is not lifelong. Second infections are known to occur, although they may be milder. The duration of immunity is unknown.

What is the treatment for mycoplasma infection?

Antibiotics such as erythromycin, clarithromycin, or azithromycin are effective treatment. However, because mycoplasma infection usually resolves on its own, antibiotic treatment of mild symptoms is not always necessary.

What can be done to prevent the spread of mycoplasma?

At this time, there are no vaccines for the prevention of mycoplasma infection and there are no reliably effective measures for control. As with any respiratory disease, all people should cover their face when coughing or sneezing.

Chapter 22

Pertussis (Whooping Cough)

Basic Information about Pertussis

Signs and Symptoms

The first symptoms of whooping cough are similar to those of a "common cold," with a runny nose, dry cough and mild fever. After about 1 to 2 weeks, coughing begins to occur in spells that may last for over a minute. Between coughing spells, the child may gasp for air with a characteristic "whooping" sound—although infants may not "whoop" as do older children. Severe coughing spells can cause a child to turn blue in the face or vomit. Infants may actually stop breathing for a few seconds. Although the severe spells usually improve in about a week, coughing can continue for several weeks.

Because adults and adolescents with whooping cough may have milder symptoms, their whooping cough infection may be more likely to be misdiagnosed.

This chapter begins with "Pertussis (Whooping Cough)," reviewed by Kim Rutherford, M.D. This information was provided by KidsHealth, one of the largest resources online for medically reviewed health information written for parents, kids, and teens. For more articles like this one, visit www.KidsHealth.org, or www.TeensHealth.org. © 2003 The Nemours Center for Children's Health Media, a division of The Nemours Foundation. Information under the heading "Improved Pertussis Vaccines: Enhancing Protection," is from *NIAID Research: Stories of Discovery*, February 1999, National Institutes of Health, National Institute of Allergy and Infectious Diseases (NIAID).

Description

Whooping cough is a serious infection of the respiratory system caused by *Bordetella pertussis* bacteria. People become infected with *B. pertussis* by inhaling contaminated droplets of an infected person's cough or sneeze.

Before a vaccine was available, whooping cough killed 5,000 to 10,000 people in the United States each year. Now, the whooping cough vaccine has reduced the annual number of deaths to less than 20. Currently, about 50% of all whooping cough infections occur in children less than 1 year old, and only 15% occur in children over than 15 years old.

Duration

Whooping cough can cause prolonged symptoms. There are usually 1 to 2 weeks of "common cold" symptoms, followed by 2 to 4 weeks of severe coughing, followed by 3 to 4 weeks of a convalescent period when coughing is less severe. In some children, the convalescent stage may last for months.

Contagiousness

Whooping cough is a highly contagious bacterial infection. Whooping cough bacteria spread from person to person through the air—as when a susceptible person inhales airborne droplets from an infected person's sneeze or cough.

Experts believe that 70% to 100% of nonimmunized family members will probably develop whooping cough if they live in the same household as someone who has the infection. For this reason, persons living in the same household are also usually given prophylactic (disease-preventing) antibiotics and/or booster doses of the vaccine.

Incubation

The incubation period for whooping cough is usually 7 to 10 days, with a range of 5 to 21 days.

Prevention

Infections can be prevented by the whooping cough vaccine, which is part of the DTaP (diphtheria, tetanus, pertussis) immunization.

DTaP immunizations are routinely given in five doses before a child's sixth birthday.

Some children may experience mild side effects, including fever, irritability, and soreness at the injection site.

When to Call Your Child's Doctor

Call your child's doctor immediately if you suspect that your child has whooping cough. Also, call your child's doctor if your child has been exposed to someone with whooping cough, even if your child has already received all of the scheduled whooping cough immunizations (DTaP).

Call your child's doctor immediately if your child has prolonged coughing spells, especially if these spells:

- make your child turn red or blue
- are followed by vomiting
- occur together with a "whooping" sound when your child breathes in following coughing episodes

Professional Treatment

If you think that your child has whooping cough, consult your child's doctor immediately. Your child's doctor can confirm that the illness is whooping cough and can prescribe treatment that may lessen symptoms and prevent the spread of illness to others. He or she will guide you in watching for complications. Your child's doctor will also notify those health authorities who keep track of whooping cough outbreaks.

Your child may need treatment in a hospital. About 75% of infants with whooping cough who are less than 6 months old receive hospital treatment for their illness, and about 40% of older babies are also hospitalized. Hospital treatment helps to decrease the risk of complications. Pneumonia occurs in about 20% of children with whooping cough who are less than 1 year old.

While in the hospital, your child may need suctioning of thick respiratory secretions. Breathing will be monitored and oxygen may be needed. For several days, your child will be isolated from other patients, with special precautions to prevent the infection from spreading to others, including hospital staff and visitors.

Whooping cough is treated with antibiotics, usually for 2 weeks. Most experts believe that these medicines are most effective when they are given in the first stage of the illness before coughing spells begin. Antibiotics are mostly important in stopping the spread of whooping cough infection.

Your child's doctor can confirm the diagnosis of whooping cough by taking cultures of respiratory fluids for examination in the laboratory. This involves taking swabs or suction samples from your child's nose or throat and checking the samples for growth of whooping cough bacteria. Blood tests and a chest x-ray may also be done.

Cough medicines often do not relieve whooping cough coughing spells, so your child's doctor will probably recommend other forms of home treatment to help manage the cough. He or she will help you monitor your child's progress and watch for the development of complications like pneumonia or ear infection.

Home Treatment

Because infants and younger children are at greater risk of complications from whooping cough infection, they are more likely to be treated in a hospital.

If your child is being treated for whooping cough at home, follow your child's doctor's schedule for giving antibiotics. Ask your child's doctor about the need for prophylactic antibiotics or vaccine boosters to others in your household.

Let your child rest in bed, and use a cool-mist vaporizer to help soothe irritated lungs and breathing passages. A vaporizer also will help loosen respiratory secretions. (If you do use a vaporizer, be sure to follow directions for keeping it clean and mold-free—usually with small amounts of bleach.)

Your child's doctor will tell you how to best position your child to help drain secretions and aid breathing.

Because even strong cough medicines usually cannot relieve the coughing spells of whooping cough, parents often need to use other ways of treating their child's cough. This includes keeping the home environment free of irritants that can trigger coughing spells: aerosol sprays, tobacco smoke, smoke from cooking, and fumes from fireplaces and wood-burning stoves.

Whooping cough can cause your child to vomit and/or decrease her ability to take adequate food and fluid needed to support recovery. To help decrease vomiting, give your child more frequent meals with smaller portions. Encourage your child to drink fruit juice and other clear fluids and soups. Watch for signs of dehydration: dry lips and tongue, dry skin, crying without tears, and infrequent urination.

Improved Pertussis Vaccines: Enhancing Protection

The National Institute of Allergies and Infectious Diseases (NIAID) devotes substantial resources to developing improved vaccines that are more effective and have fewer side effects than currently used vaccines. Using powerful new technologies and knowledge gained from basic research, NIAID has been instrumental in the development of second-generation vaccines that protect against important childhood diseases. The story of NIAID's role in the development of acellular pertussis vaccines for infants exemplifies the public health benefits of the Institute's investment in basic research and its international collaborations with partners in government, industry, and academia. The new acellular (non-whole cell) pertussis vaccines are safer and cause fewer side effects because they use select parts of the disease-causing microbe that are important for immunity. The traditional whole-cell vaccines, by contrast, use the entire, killed cell of the infectious microbe.

The First Pertussis Vaccine

Pertussis, also known as whooping cough, is a highly contagious respiratory disease that affects more than 50 million people worldwide and causes an estimated 350,000 deaths each year, primarily among infants. Before pertussis vaccines were available, more than 200,000 cases of the disease were reported annually in the United States. The search for a pertussis vaccine began in 1906, when two French bacteriologists isolated *Bordetella pertussis*, the bacterium that causes infection. In the 1940s, experimental vaccines using whole-cell *B. pertussis* were successful in mimicking infection and producing a protective immune response in humans. The first whole-cell pertussis vaccine was licensed for use in the United States in 1948. Subsequent widespread use of the vaccine contributed to a dramatic decline in the U.S. incidence of the disease, which reached an all-time low of approximately 1,010 cases in 1976.

Although the whole-cell vaccine was extremely effective in controlling pertussis, it was associated with side effects ranging from fever and inflammation at the injection site to rare but more serious events such as seizures. Concerns about these side effects discouraged some parents from having their children immunized against pertussis. As a result, by the early 1980s the number of pertussis cases was increasing in the United States.

The side effects associated with the whole-cell pertussis vaccine were also commonly seen with whole-cell vaccines for other types of bacteria. These bacteria had something in common with *B. pertussis*. They all belonged to a subgroup called gram negative bacteria. Specific molecules unique to the gram negative bacteria were believed to be responsible for the inflammatory response that caused the side effects.

In response to public concerns about the safety of the whole-cell vaccine, NIAID set out to develop an improved vaccine that would be equally effective but that caused fewer and less harmful side effects. As an initial step in this process, NIAID-supported scientists began to conduct more basic research to thoroughly analyze the biology of *B. pertussis* and to learn more about how the bacterium causes disease.

New Vaccine Technology

As early as 1975, basic researchers at NIAID's Rocky Mountain Laboratories were characterizing the properties of a protein called pertussigen, or pertussis toxin (PT), secreted by *B. pertussis*, which triggered an immune response. PT became the cornerstone of second-generation pertussis vaccine development, and all future acellular pertussis vaccines contained an inactivated form of PT that was no longer capable of causing harmful effects. With information gained from this basic research, NIAID scientists and other researchers began to design acellular vaccines that excluded *B. pertussis* bacterium molecules that were likely to cause side effects and used only purified *B. pertussis* products, such as pertussis toxin or other antibody-producing components, that would invoke an immune response against the bacterium while producing minimal side effects.

Testing the New Vaccine

In the early 1980s, NIAID-supported researchers began collaborating with vaccine manufacturers and investigators around the world to speed the development of acellular pertussis vaccines. A large Swedish study supported by NIAID in the mid-1980s tested the disease-preventing effectiveness of two acellular pertussis vaccines. In 1989, the Institute invited manufacturers of acellular pertussis vaccines to participate in further studies. The following year, NIAID initiated a multicenter trial that compared the effectiveness of 13 acellular pertussis vaccine candidates with two whole-cell vaccines. The trial was the first to compare acellular and whole-cell vaccines among infants. It was also a significant collaborative venture involving government agencies, manufacturers in five countries, and the NIAID-supported network of university-based Vaccine and Treatment Evaluation Units.

Encouraging findings from the multicenter study prompted NIAID to support two large clinical trials in Sweden and Italy. Begun in 1991–1992, these landmark international studies demonstrated that acellular vaccines are as effective in protecting infants against pertussis but cause fewer side effects than whole-cell vaccines. These positive results were instrumental in the 1996 licensure of the first children's diphtheria-tetanus-pertussis (DTaP) vaccine that includes an acellular, rather than a whole-cell, pertussis component. NIAID's collaborations with the Food and Drug Administration, the Centers for Disease Control and Prevention, and the pharmaceutical industry were crucial to the expedited approval of DTaP vaccines. Widespread use of these safer, well-tolerated vaccines is expected to promote rates of immunization against pertussis and reduce related illness and death.

NIAID is now applying the success of acellular pertussis vaccines for children to the development of similar vaccines for adolescents and adults. Because vaccine-induced immunity weakens after 6 to 10 years, adults have become a major source of pertussis transmission, particularly to unvaccinated infants. Adult formulations being developed with NIAID support could increase booster immunization of adolescents and adults, thereby helping to reduce the incidence of pertussis in young infants as well as adults. The Institute also is continuing efforts to improve pertussis vaccines further by finding ways to reduce the number of vaccine doses required and to lengthen the period of immunity produced by the vaccine.

Chapter 23

Pneumococcal Pneumonia

What is pneumonia?

Pneumonia is a lung disease that can be caused by a variety of viruses, bacteria, and sometimes fungi. The U.S. Centers for Diseases Control and Prevention (CDC) estimate nearly 90,000 people in the United States died from one of several kinds of pneumonia in 1999. In the United States, pneumonia is the fifth leading cause of death. Rates of infection are three-times higher in African Americans than in whites and are 5- to 10-times higher in Native American adults and 10-times higher in Native American children.

On an international scale, acute respiratory infection ranks as the third most frequent cause of death among children less than 5 years old and was responsible for approximately 3.5 million deaths in 1998.

What is pneumococcal pneumonia?

Pneumococcal pneumonia is an infection in the lungs caused by bacteria called *Streptococcus pneumoniae*. *S. pneumoniae*, also called pneumococcus, can infect the upper respiratory tracts of adults and children and can spread to the blood, lungs, middle ear, or nervous system. CDC estimates *S. pneumoniae* causes 40,000 deaths and

---

"Pneumococcal Pneumonia," National Institute of Allergy and Infectious Diseases (NIAID), National Institutes of Health (NIH), August 2001; and "Drug-resistant *Streptococcus pneumoniae* Disease," Division of Bacterial and Mycotic Diseases, Centers for Disease Control and Prevention (CDC), December 2003, reviewed February 2004.

500,000 cases of pneumonia annually in the United States. The yearly incidence of pneumococcal pneumonia is twice as high in African Americans than in whites and is responsible for 3,000 cases of meningitis (inflammation of spinal cord membranes), 50,000 cases of bacteremia (bacteria in the blood), and 7 million cases of otitis media (inner ear infection).

According to the World Health Organization, *S. pneumoniae* is the leading cause of severe pneumonia worldwide in children younger than 5 years old, causing more than 1 million deaths in children each year.

Pneumococcal pneumonia primarily causes illness in children younger than 2 years old and adults 65 years of age or older. The elderly are especially vulnerable to getting seriously ill and dying from this disease. In addition, people with certain medical conditions such as chronic heart, lung, or liver diseases or sickle cell anemia are also at increased risk for getting pneumococcal pneumonia as are people with HIV infection or AIDS or people who have had organ transplants and are taking medicines that lower their resistance to infection.

How is pneumococcus spread?

The noses and throats of up to 70 percent of healthy people contain pneumococcus at any given time. It is spread from person to person by coughing, sneezing, or close contact. Researchers don't know why it suddenly invades the lungs and the bloodstream to cause disease.

What are the symptoms of pneumococcal pneumonia?

Pneumococcal pneumonia may begin suddenly, with a severe shaking chill usually followed by:

- High fever
- Cough
- Shortness of breath
- Rapid breathing
- Chest pains

There may be other symptoms as well:

- Nausea
- Vomiting
- Headache

- Tiredness
- Muscle aches

In an otherwise healthy adult, pneumococcal pneumonia usually involves one or more parts of the lungs, known as lobes. Thus, it is sometimes called lobar pneumonia. The remainder of the respiratory system is comparatively not affected. In contrast, infants, young children, and elderly people more commonly develop a relatively mild infection in other parts of the lungs, such as around the air vessels (bronchi) causing bronchopneumonia.

How is pneumococcal pneumonia diagnosed?

A doctor or other health care provider diagnoses pneumonia based on:

- Symptoms
- Physical examination
- Laboratory tests
- Chest x-ray

Because a number of bacteria, viruses, and other infectious agents can cause pneumonia, if you have any of the symptoms, you should get diagnosed early and start taking the right medicine if you have any of the symptoms. The presence of *S. pneumoniae* in the blood, saliva, or lung fluid helps lead to a diagnosis of pneumococcal pneumonia.

How is pneumococcal pneumonia treated?

Health care providers usually prescribe antibiotics, such as penicillin, to treat this bacterial disease. The symptoms of pneumococcal pneumonia usually subside within 12 to 36 hours after treatment has begun. Bacteria such as *S. pneumoniae*, however, are resisting and fighting off the powers of antibiotics to destroy them. Such antibiotic resistance is increasing worldwide because these medicines have been overused or misused. Therefore, if you are at risk of getting pneumococcal pneumonia, you should talk with your doctor about taking steps to prevent it.

Can pneumococcal pneumonia be prevented?

The pneumococcal vaccine is the only way to prevent getting pneumococcal pneumonia. Vaccines are available for children and adults.

The CDC National Immunization Program (NIP) recommends that you get immunized against pneumococcal pneumonia if you are in any of the following groups.

- You are 65 years old or older.
- You have a serious long-term health problem such as heart disease, sickle cell disease, alcoholism, leaks of cerebrospinal fluid, lung disease (not including asthma), diabetes, or liver cirrhosis.
- Your resistance to infection is lowered due to HIV infection or AIDS; lymphoma, leukemia, or other cancers; cancer treatment with x-rays or drugs; treatment with long-term steroids; bone marrow or organ transplant; kidney failure; nephrotic (kidney) syndrome; damaged spleen or no spleen.
- You are an Alaskan-Native or from certain Native American populations.

In February 2000, the U.S. Food and Drug Administration approved a pneumococcal vaccine for use in toddlers and children. It is the first pneumococcal vaccine approved for children younger than 2 years old. NIP recommends that all children ages 2 to 23 months old get this vaccine.

Does pneumococcal pneumonia cause complications?

In about 30 percent of people with pneumococcal pneumonia, the bacteria invade the blood stream from the lungs. This causes bacteremia, a very serious Pneumococcal pneumonia also can cause other lung problems and certain heart problems.

What research is going on?

The National Institute of Allergy and Infectious Diseases (NIAID) supports research on more effective prevention and treatment approaches to control pneumonia and its causes. These include:

- Developing and licensing vaccines and treatments for the disease-causing microbes (pathogens) that cause pneumonia
- Stimulating research on the structure and function of these pathogens
- Developing better and more rapid diagnostic tools

- Understanding the long-term health impact respiratory pathogens have in various populations
- Examining the effect of vaccines in high-risk populations
- Determining how pneumococcus becomes resistant to antibiotics

The recently approved pneumococcal conjugate vaccine for children is partially the result of crucial NIAID research in the early development of the vaccine. This vaccine helps prevent pneumococcal diseases in babies and toddlers and is the latest advance in developing vaccines against common bacterial infections. This effort was led in large part by NIAID for more than 30 years.

NIAID supports studies to develop improved pneumococcal conjugate vaccines for children worldwide. In one such study, NIAID researchers are working with The Gambia Government and scientists from several international research institutions to test a pneumococcal conjugate vaccine in The Gambia, West Africa. Health care experts have consistently identified pneumococcus as the most common cause of bacterial pneumonia in The Gambia. In a pattern typical of many developing areas, infant and child mortality rates in The Gambia are high, acute respiratory infections are a leading cause of death, and pneumococcus is the most common cause of these infections.

Drug-resistant Streptococcus Pneumoniae *Disease*

Some types of *Streptococcus pneumoniae* are resistant to one or more commonly used antibiotics.

Until 2000, *S. pneumoniae* infections caused 60,000 cases of invasive disease each year and up to 40% of these were caused by pneumococci non-susceptible to at least one drug. These figures have decreased substantially following the introduction of the pneumococcal conjugate vaccine for children. In the year 2002, there were 37,000 cases of invasive pneumococcal disease. Of these, 34% were caused by pneumococci non-susceptible to at least one drug and 17% were due to a strain non-susceptible to 3 or more drugs. Prevalence of drug-resistant *Streptococcus pneumoniae* (DRSP) shows geographic variation.

Death occurs in 14% of hospitalized adults with invasive disease. Neurologic sequelae occur in meningitis patients. Hearing impairment can result from recurrent otitis media. Resistance has led to treatment failures.

DRSP is associated with increased costs due to use of antimicrobial agents, recurrent disease, surveillance, education, and new antimicrobial drug development.

Persons who attend or work at child-care centers and persons who recently used antimicrobial agents are at increased risk for infection with DRSP.

The new pneumococcal conjugate vaccine is preventing many infections due to drug-resistant pneumococci. Outbreaks of DRSP have been reported in nursing homes, institutions for HIV-infected persons, and child-care centers.

Widespread overuse of antimicrobial agents and the spread of resistant strains has contributed to emerging resistance. The 23-valent vaccine is underused. Supplies of the new conjugate vaccine for children are inadequate. Some clinical laboratories have not adopted standard methods (NCCLS [formerly National Committee for Clinical Laboratory Standards] guidelines) for identifying and defining DRSP.

Campaigns for more judicious use of antibiotics and use of the new conjugate vaccine may slow or reverse emerging drug resistance. Prevention of infections could improve through expanded use of 23-valent polysaccharide vaccine and the new conjugate vaccine. Among children 5 years of age, the conjugate vaccine elicits protection against about 80% of invasive pneumococcal isolates that are not susceptible to penicillin.

Chapter 24

Shigellosis

What is shigellosis?

Shigellosis is an infectious disease caused by a group of bacteria called *Shigella*. Most who are infected with *Shigella* develop diarrhea, fever, and stomach cramps starting a day or two after they are exposed to the bacterium. The diarrhea is often bloody. Shigellosis usually resolves in 5 to 7 days. In some persons, especially young children and the elderly, the diarrhea can be so severe that the patient needs to be hospitalized. A severe infection with high fever may also be associated with seizures in children less than 2 years old. Some persons who are infected may have no symptoms at all, but may still pass the *Shigella* bacteria to others.

What sort of germ is Shigella?

The *Shigella* germ is actually a family of bacteria that can cause diarrhea in humans. They are microscopic living creatures that pass from person to person. *Shigella* were discovered over 100 years ago by a Japanese scientist named Shiga, for whom they are named. There are several different kinds of *Shigella* bacteria: *Shigella sonnei*, also known as "Group D" *Shigella*, accounts for over two-thirds of the shigellosis in the United States. A second type, *Shigella flexneri*, or "group B" *Shigella*, accounts for almost all of the rest. Other types of

---

"Shigellosis," Division of Bacterial and Mycotic Diseases, Centers for Disease Control and Prevention (CDC), reviewed March 7, 2003.

Shigella are rare in this country, though they continue to be important causes of disease in the developing world. One type found in the developing world, *Shigella dysenteriae* type 1, causes deadly epidemics there.

How can Shigella *infections be diagnosed?*

Many different kinds of diseases can cause diarrhea and bloody diarrhea, and the treatment depends on which germ is causing the diarrhea. Determining that *Shigella* is the cause of the illness depends on laboratory tests that identify *Shigella* in the stools of an infected person. These tests are sometimes not performed unless the laboratory is instructed specifically to look for the organism. The laboratory can also do special tests to tell which type of *Shigella* the person has and which antibiotics, if any, would be best to treat it.

How can Shigella *infections be treated?*

Shigellosis can usually be treated with antibiotics. The antibiotics commonly used for treatment are ampicillin, trimethoprim/sulfamethoxazole (also known as Bactrim® or Septra®), nalidixic acid, or ciprofloxacin. Appropriate treatment kills the *Shigella* bacteria that might be present in the patient's stools, and shortens the illness. Unfortunately, some *Shigella* bacteria have become resistant to antibiotics and using antibiotics to treat shigellosis can actually make the germs more resistant in the future. Persons with mild infections will usually recover quickly without antibiotic treatment. Therefore, when many persons in a community are affected by shigellosis, antibiotics are sometimes used selectively to treat only the more severe cases. Antidiarrheal agents such as loperamide (Imodium®) or diphenoxylate with atropine (Lomotil®) are likely to make the illness worse and should be avoided.

Are there long term consequences to a Shigella *infection?*

Persons with diarrhea usually recover completely, although it may be several months before their bowel habits are entirely normal. About 3% of persons who are infected with one type of *Shigella*, *Shigella flexneri*, will later develop pains in their joints, irritation of the eyes, and painful urination. This is called Reiter's syndrome. It can last for months or years, and can lead to chronic arthritis which is difficult to treat. Reiter's syndrome is caused by a reaction to *Shigella* infection that happens only in people who are genetically predisposed to it.

Once someone has had shigellosis, they are not likely to get infected with that specific type again for at least several years. However, they can still get infected with other types of *Shigella*.

How do people catch Shigella?

The *Shigella* bacteria pass from one infected person to the next. *Shigella* are present in the diarrheal stools of infected persons while they are sick and for a week or two afterwards. Most *Shigella* infections are the result of the bacterium passing from stools or soiled fingers of one person to the mouth of another person. This happens when basic hygiene and handwashing habits are inadequate. It is particularly likely to occur among toddlers who are not fully toilet-trained. Family members and playmates of such children are at high risk of becoming infected.

Shigella infections may be acquired from eating contaminated food. Contaminated food may look and smell normal. Food may become contaminated by infected food handlers who forget to wash their hands with soap after using the bathroom. Vegetables can become contaminated if they are harvested from a field with sewage in it. Flies can breed in infected feces and then contaminate food. *Shigella* infections can also be acquired by drinking or swimming in contaminated water. Water may become contaminated if sewage runs into it, or if someone with shigellosis swims in it.

What can a person do to prevent this illness?

There is no vaccine to prevent shigellosis. However, the spread of *Shigella* from an infected person to other persons can be stopped by frequent and careful handwashing with soap. Frequent and careful handwashing is important among all age groups. Frequent, supervised handwashing of all children should be followed in day care centers and in homes with children who are not completely toilet-trained (including children in diapers). When possible, young children with a *Shigella* infection who are still in diapers should not be in contact with uninfected children.

People who have shigellosis should not prepare food or pour water for others until they have been shown to no longer be carrying the *Shigella* bacterium.

If a child in diapers has shigellosis, everyone who changes the child's diapers should be sure the diapers are disposed of properly in a closed-lid garbage can, and should wash his or her hands carefully with soap and warm water immediately after changing the diapers.

After use, the diaper changing area should be wiped down with a disinfectant such as household bleach, Lysol® or bactericidal wipes.

Basic food safety precautions and regular drinking water treatment prevents shigellosis. At swimming beaches, having enough bathrooms near the swimming area helps keep the water from becoming contaminated.

Simple precautions taken while traveling to the developing world can prevent getting shigellosis. Drink only treated or boiled water, and eat only cooked hot foods or fruits you peel yourself. The same precautions prevent traveler's diarrhea in general.

How common is shigellosis?

Every year, about 18,000 cases of shigellosis are reported in the United States. Because many milder cases are not diagnosed or reported, the actual number of infections may be twenty times greater. Shigellosis is particularly common and causes recurrent problems in settings where hygiene is poor and can sometimes sweep through entire communities. Shigellosis is more common in summer than winter. Children, especially toddlers aged 2 to 4, are the most likely to get shigellosis. Many cases are related to the spread of illness in child-care settings, and many more are the result of the spread of the illness in families with small children.

In the developing world, shigellosis is far more common and is present in most communities most of the time.

What else can be done to prevent shigellosis?

It is important for the public health department to know about cases of shigellosis. It is important for clinical laboratories to send isolates of *Shigella* to the City, County or State Public Health Laboratory so the specific type can be determined and compared to other *Shigella*. If many cases occur at the same time, it may mean that a restaurant, food or water supply has a problem which needs correction by the public health department. If a number of cases occur in a day-care center, the public health department may need to coordinate efforts to improve handwashing among the staff, children, and their families. When a community-wide outbreak occurs, a community-wide approach to promote handwashing and basic hygiene among children can stop the outbreak. Improvements in hygiene for vegetables and fruit picking and packing may prevent shigellosis caused by contaminated produce.

Some prevention steps occur everyday, without you thinking about it. Making municipal water supplies safe and treating sewage are highly effective prevention measures that have been in place for many years.

What is the government doing about shigellosis?

The Centers for Disease Control and Prevention (CDC) monitors the frequency of *Shigella* infections in the country, and assists local and State health departments to investigate outbreaks, determine means of transmission and devise control measures. CDC also conducts research to better understand how to identify and treat shigellosis. The Food and Drug Administration inspects imported foods, and promotes better food preparation techniques in restaurants and food processing plants. The Environmental Protection Agency regulates and monitors the safety of our drinking water supplies. The government has also maintained active research into the development of a *Shigella* vaccine.

How can I learn more about this and other public health problems?

You can discuss any medical concerns you may have with your doctor or other heath care provider. Your local city or county health department can provide more information about this and other public health problems that are occurring in your area. General information about the public health of the nation is published every week in the *Morbidity and Mortality Weekly Report*, by the CDC in Atlanta, GA. Epidemiologists in your local and State Health Departments are tracking a number of important public health problems, investigating special problems that arise, and helping to prevent them form occurring in the first place, or from spreading if they do occur.

Some tips for preventing the spread of shigellosis:

- wash hands with soap carefully and frequently, especially after going to the bathroom, after changing diapers, and before preparing foods or beverages
- dispose of soiled diapers properly
- disinfect diaper changing areas after using them
- keep children with diarrhea out of child care settings

- supervise handwashing of toddlers and small children after they use the toilet
- persons with diarrheal illness should not prepare food for others
- if you are traveling to the developing world, "boil it, cook it, peel it, or forget it"
- avoid drinking pool water (See more information about this.)

Chapter 25

Strep Throat and Scarlet Fever

Strep Throat/Strep Tonsillitis (Streptococcal Pharyngitis)

What causes strep throat?

- Strep throat is a throat infection caused by bacteria called streptococcus.

Who can get strep throat?

- Getting strep throat is common for school-age children and children in daycare.
- Strep throat is common in the winter months.

What are the symptoms of strep throat?

- Strep throat can cause a sore throat or a tickling feeling in the throat.
- Strep throat can cause pain when swallowing and bad breath.

This chapter includes "Strep Throat/Strep Tonsillitis (Streptococcal Pharyngitis)," by Donna D'Alessandro, M.D. and Lindsay Huth, B.A. © 2002. Copyright protected material used with permission of the author and the University of Iowa's Virtual Children's Hospital, www.vh.org/VCH. "Scarlet Fever" is from the Division of Bacterial and Mycotic Diseases, Centers for Disease Control and Prevention, reviewed October 2002.

- Strep throat can cause a fever, headache, earache, or stomach-ache.
- The tonsils may be swollen and bright red. Neck glands could be swollen.
- There might be yellow or white spots of pus on the back of the throat.
- The roof of the mouth may be red or have red spots.
- Infants may have a runny nose, crusty nose, and little appetite.

Is strep throat contagious?

- Yes. Strep throat is contagious.
- Strep bacteria are spread through coughing, sneezing, and direct contact.
- Children with strep throat are contagious until 24 hours after their first dose of antibiotics.

How is strep throat treated?

- The doctor will take a throat culture, a painless swab of the throat, to see if your child has strep.
- Test results will come back in 1 or 2 days.
- If the doctor uses a rapid strep test, it will take about 10 minutes to get results.
- Strep throat is treated with antibiotics (usually penicillin) taken by shot or mouth.
- Antibiotics taken by mouth have to be taken for a full 10 days to clear the infection.
- Acetaminophen (such as Tylenol, Panadol, or Liquiprin) or Ibuprofen can be given to ease aches, pain, and fever.
- Throat lozenges, hard candy, cool drinks, and ice cream can help ease throat pain.
- Your child should drink lots of fluids. Avoid acidic juices (orange juice) and spicy food.
- Older children can drink tea with honey or gargle warm salt water (one teaspoon of table salt in one cup water) to ease throat pain.

- A cool mist humidifier or a warm, damp towel can help throat pain and swollen glands.

How long does strep throat last?

- When strep throat is treated, pain lasts 1 to 3 days.
- Children can return to school or daycare 24 hours after the start of antibiotic treatment and if their temperature and energy are normal.

Can strep throat be prevented?

- You can prevent the spread of infection by washing dishes and glasses in hot soapy water.
- Wash your hands often, especially after caring for the sick person.
- Avoid close contact with the infected person.

When should I call the doctor?

- Go to the emergency room if your child has a hard time breathing, swallowing, or keeps drooling.
- Call the doctor if your child has a fever over 104 degrees F (or 40 degrees C) or a fever that lasts for many days.
- Call the doctor if your child can't open her mouth or drink liquids.
- Call the doctor if your child has joint pain or is very weak.
- Call the doctor if your child has a rash, earache, or glands that are swollen, red, or tender.

Quick Answers

- Strep throat is a throat infection caused by bacteria.
- Getting strep throat is common for school-age children and children in daycare.
- Strep throat can cause a sore throat, fever, headache, earache, and pain when swallowing.
- Strep bacteria are spread through coughing, sneezing, and direct contact.

- Strep throat is treated with antibiotics.
- Children can return to school or daycare 24 hours after the start of antibiotic treatment.
- One way to prevent the spread of infection is to wash hands and dishes with hot soapy water.
- Call the doctor if your child has a rash, earache, or glands that are swollen, red, or tender.

References

- Casano, PJ, MD, Sore Throats: Causes and Cures. American Academy of Otolaryngology: Head and Neck Surgery Public Service Brochure. (cited 2001 July 27). Available from: URL: http://www.sinuscarecenter.com/throaaao.html
- Marsocci SM, MD, Pichichero ME, MD. Streptococcal Pharyngitis (Strep Throat, Strep Tonsillitis). *Pediatric Infectious Diseases Journal* 1992–2001 (cited 2001 July 27). URL: http://www.vh.org/Patients/IHB/Peds/Infectious/Strep.html
- Rutherford K, MD. KidsHealth. Strep Throat (Group A Streptococci Infections). 2001 May (cited 2001 July 27). URL: http://www.kidshealth.org/pageManager.jsp?dn=KidsHealth&lic=1&ps=107&cat_id=&article_set=941

Scarlet Fever

What is scarlet fever?

Scarlet fever is a disease caused by a bacteria called group A streptococcus, the same bacteria that causes strep throat. Scarlet fever is a rash that sometimes occurs in people that have strep throat. The rash of scarlet fever is usually seen in children under the age of 18.

How do you get scarlet fever?

This illness can be caught from other people if you come in contact with the sick person because this germ is carried in the mouth and nasal fluids. If you touch your mouth, nose or eyes after touching something that has these fluids on them, you may become ill. Also, if you drink from the same glass or eat from the same plate as the sick person, you could also become ill. The best way to keep from getting sick is to wash your hands often and avoid sharing eating utensils.

What are the symptoms of scarlet fever?

The most common symptoms of scarlet fever are:

- A rash first appears as tiny red bumps on the chest and abdomen. This rash may then spread all over the body. It looks like a sunburn and feels like a rough piece of sandpaper. It is usually redder in the arm pits and groin areas. The rash lasts about 2–5 days. After the rash is gone, often the skin on the tips of the fingers and toes begins to peel.
- The face is flushed with a pale area around the lips.
- The throat is very red and sore. It can have white or yellow patches.
- A fever of 101 degrees Fahrenheit (38.3 degrees Celsius) or higher is common. Chills are often seen with the fever.
- Glands in the neck are often swollen.
- A whitish coating can appear on the surface of the tongue. The tongue itself looks like a strawberry because the normal bumps on the tongue look bigger.

Other less common symptoms include:

- Nausea and vomiting
- Headache
- Body aches

How is scarlet fever diagnosed?

Your doctor or health care provider will examine your child and swab the back of the throat with a cotton swab to see if there is a streptococcus infection.

What is the treatment for scarlet fever?

If the swab test (throat culture) shows that there is streptococcus, you will be given an antibiotic prescription for your child. Give this medicine exactly as you are told. It is very important to finish all of the medicine. Never share any of this medicine with family or friends. Ask your doctor or health care provider about over-the-counter medicine to lessen sore throat pain.

Is there anything else I can do to make my child feel better?

Warm liquids like soup or cold foods like popsicles or milkshakes help to ease the pain of the sore throat. Offer these to your child often, especially when he/she has a fever since the body needs a lot of fluid when it is sick with a fever. A cool mist humidifier will help to keep the air in your child's room moist which will keep the throat from getting too dry and more sore. Rest is important.

What should I do if I think my child has scarlet fever?

The best thing to do if you think your child may be ill is to call your doctor or health care provider.

Chapter 26

Syphilis

What is syphilis?

Syphilis is a sexually transmitted disease (STD), once responsible for devastating epidemics. It is caused by a bacterium called *Treponema pallidum*. The rate of primary and secondary syphilis in the United States declined by 89.2 percent from 1990 to 2000. The number of cases rose, however, from 5,979 in 2000 to 6,103 in 2001. The U.S. Centers for Disease Control and Prevention reported in November 2002 that this was the first increase since 1990.

Of increasing concern is the fact that syphilis increases by 3- to 5-fold the risk of transmitting and acquiring HIV (human immunodeficiency virus), the virus that causes AIDS (acquired immunodeficiency syndrome).

How is syphilis transmitted?

The syphilis bacterium is very fragile, and the infection is almost always transmitted by sexual contact with an infected person. The bacterium spreads from the initial ulcer (sore) of an infected person to the skin or mucous membranes (linings) of the genital area, mouth, or anus of an uninfected sexual partner. It also can pass through broken skin on other parts of the body.

"Syphilis," National Institute of Allergy and Infectious Diseases (NIAID), National Institutes of Health (NIH), November 2002.

In addition, a pregnant woman with syphilis can pass *T. pallidum* to her unborn child, who may be born with serious mental and physical problems as a result of this infection.

What are the symptoms of syphilis?

The initial infection causes an ulcer at the site of infection. The bacteria, however, move throughout the body, damaging many organs over time. Medical experts describe the course of the disease by dividing it into four stages-primary, secondary, latent, and tertiary (late). An infected person who has not been treated may infect others during the first two stages, which usually last 1 to 2 years. In its late stages, untreated syphilis, although not contagious, can cause serious heart abnormalities, mental disorders, blindness, other neurologic problems, and death.

Primary syphilis: The first symptom of primary syphilis is an ulcer called a chancre ("shan-ker"). The chancre can appear within 10 days to 3 months after exposure, but it generally appears within 2 to 6 weeks. Because the chancre may be painless and may occur inside the body, the infected person might not notice it. It usually is found on the part of the body exposed to the infected partner's ulcer, such as the penis, vulva, or vagina. A chancre also can develop on the cervix, tongue, lips, or other parts of the body. The chancre disappears within a few weeks whether or not a person is treated. If not treated during the primary stage, about one-third of people will go on to the chronic stages.

Secondary syphilis: A skin rash, with brown sores about the size of a penny, often marks this chronic stage of syphilis. The rash appears anywhere from 3 to 6 weeks after the chancre appears. While the rash may cover the whole body or appear only in a few areas, it is almost always on the palms of the hands and soles of the feet.

Because active bacteria are present in the sores, any physical contact—sexual or nonsexual—with the broken skin of an infected person may spread the infection at this stage. The rash usually heals within several weeks or months.

Other symptoms also may occur, such as mild fever, fatigue, headache, sore throat, patchy hair loss, and swollen lymph glands throughout the body. These symptoms may be very mild and, like the chancre of primary syphilis, will disappear without treatment. The signs of secondary syphilis may come and go over the next 1 to 2 years of the disease.

Latent syphilis: If untreated, syphilis may lapse into a latent stage during which the disease is no longer contagious and no symptoms are present. Many people who are not treated will suffer from no further signs and symptoms of the disease.

Tertiary syphilis: Approximately one-third of people who have had secondary syphilis go on to develop the complications of late, or tertiary, syphilis, in which the bacteria damage the heart, eyes, brain, nervous system, bones, joints, or almost any other part of the body. This stage can last for years, or even for decades. Late syphilis can result in mental illness, blindness, other neurologic problems, heart disease, and death.

How is syphilis diagnosed?

Syphilis is sometimes called "the great imitator" because its early symptoms are similar to those of many other diseases. Sexually active people should consult a doctor or other health care worker about any rash or sore in the genital area. Those who have been treated for another STD, such as gonorrhea, should be tested to be sure they do not also have syphilis.

There are three ways to diagnose syphilis:

- Recognizing the signs and symptoms
- Examining blood samples
- Identifying syphilis bacteria under a microscope

The doctor usually uses all these approaches to diagnose syphilis and decide upon the stage of infection.

Blood tests also provide evidence of infection, although they may give false-negative results (not show signs of an infection despite its presence) for up to 3 months after infection. False-positive tests (showing signs of an infection when it is not present) also can occur. Therefore, two blood tests are usually used. Interpretation of blood tests for syphilis can be difficult, and repeated tests are sometimes necessary to confirm the diagnosis.

How is syphilis treated?

Unfortunately, the early symptoms of syphilis can be very mild, and many people do not seek treatment when they first become infected.

Doctors usually treat patients with syphilis with penicillin, given by injection. They use other antibiotics for patients allergic to penicillin. A person usually can no longer transmit syphilis 24 hours after starting treatment. Some people, however, do not respond to the usual doses of penicillin. Therefore, it is important that people being treated for syphilis have periodic blood tests to check that the infectious agent has been completely destroyed.

People with neurosyphilis may need to be retested for up to 2 years after treatment. In all stages of syphilis, proper treatment will cure the disease. But in late syphilis, damage already done to body organs cannot be reversed.

What are the effects of syphilis in pregnant women?

A pregnant woman with untreated, active syphilis is likely to pass the infection to her unborn child. In addition, miscarriage may occur in as many as 25 to 50 percent of women acutely infected with syphilis during pregnancy. Between 40 to 70 percent of women with active syphilis will give birth to a syphilis-infected infant.

Some infants with congenital syphilis may have symptoms at birth, but most develop symptoms between 2 weeks and 3 months later. These symptoms may include:

- Skin ulcers
- Rashes
- Fever
- Weakened or hoarse crying sounds
- Swollen liver and spleen
- Yellowish skin (jaundice)
- Anemia (low red blood cell count)
- Various deformities

People who care for infants with congenital syphilis must use special cautions because the moist sores are infectious.

Rarely, the symptoms of syphilis go undetected in infants. As infected infants become older children and teenagers, they may develop the symptoms of late-stage syphilis, including damage to their bones, teeth, eyes, ears, and brains.

Can syphilis cause other complications?

Syphilis bacteria frequently invade the nervous system during the early stages of infection. Approximately 3 to 7 percent of persons with untreated syphilis develop neurosyphilis, a sometimes serious disorder of the nervous system. In some instances, the time from infection to developing neurosyphilis may be up to 20 years.

Some people with neurosyphilis never develop any symptoms. Others may have headache, stiff neck, and fever that result from an inflammation of the lining of the brain. Some people develop seizures. People whose blood vessels are affected may develop symptoms of stroke with numbness, weakness, or visual problems. Neurosyphilis may be more difficult to treat, and its course may be different, in people with HIV infection or AIDS.

How can syphilis be prevented?

The open sores of syphilis may be visible and infectious during the active stages of infection. Any contact with these infectious sores and other infected tissues and body fluids must be avoided to prevent spread of the disease. As with many other STDs, using latex male condoms properly during sexual intercourse may give some protection from the disease.

Screening and treatment of infected individuals, or secondary prevention, is one of the few options for preventing the advanced stages of the disease. Testing and treatment early in pregnancy are the best ways to prevent syphilis in infants and should be a routine part of prenatal care.

What research is going on?

Developing better ways to diagnose and treat syphilis is an important research goal of scientists supported by the National Institute of Allergy and Infectious Diseases (NIAID). New tests are being developed that may provide better ways to diagnose syphilis and define the stage of infection.

In an effort to stem the spread of syphilis, scientists are conducting research on the development of a vaccine. Molecular biologists are learning more about the various surface components of the syphilis bacterium that stimulate the immune system to respond to the invading organism. This knowledge will pave the way for development of an effective vaccine that can ultimately prevent this STD.

A high priority for researchers is developing a diagnostic test that does not require a blood sample. Saliva and urine are being evaluated to see whether they would work as well as blood. Researchers also are trying to develop other diagnostic tests for detecting infection in babies.

Another high research priority is the development of a safe, effective single-dose oral antibiotic therapy for syphilis. Many patients do not like getting an injection for treatment, and about 10 percent of the general population is allergic to penicillin.

The genome of the bacterium that causes syphilis has been sequenced through NIAID-funded research. The DNA sequence represents an encyclopedia of information about the bacterium. Clues as to how to diagnose, treat, and vaccinate against syphilis have been identified and are fueling intensive research efforts on this ancient but intractable disease.

Chapter 27

Tuberculosis

Many people think tuberculosis (TB) is a disease of the past. But, TB is still a leading killer of young adults worldwide. Some 2 billion people—one-third of the world's population—are infected with the TB bacterium, *M. tuberculosis*. TB is a chronic bacterial infection. It is spread through the air and usually infects the lungs, although other organs are sometimes involved. Most persons that are infected with *M. tuberculosis* harbor the bacterium without symptoms but many develop active TB disease. Each year, 8 million people worldwide develop active TB and 3 million die.

This chapter begins with "Tuberculosis," a fact sheet produced by the National Institute of Allergy and Infectious Diseases (NIAID), March 2002 with additional information regarding vaccines and vaccine development excerpted from "Tuberculosis Vaccines: State of The Science," Division of Microbiology and Infectious Diseases, 2001, and "First U.S. Tuberculosis Vaccine Trial in 60 Years Begins," NIH News, National Institutes of Health, January 2004. Remaining text in this chapter is from, "American Lung Association® Fact Sheet: Tuberculosis Skin Test," "American Lung Association® Fact Sheet: Pediatric Tuberculosis," "American Lung Association® Fact Sheet: Tuberculosis and HIV," and "American Lung Association® Fact Sheet: Multidrug-Resistant Tuberculosis," are reprinted with permission. For more information on how you can support the fight against lung disease, the third leasing cause of death in the U.S., please contact The American Lung Association at 1-800-LUNG-USA (1-800-586-4872) or visit the website at www.lungusa.org. The information contained in American Lung Association® website is not a substitute for medical advice or treatment, and the American Lung Association recommends consultation with your doctor or health care professional.

Is TB a problem in the United States?

In the United States, TB has re-emerged as a serious public health problem. In 2001, based on provisional data reported to the U.S. Centers for Disease Control and Prevention, the number of cases has decreased for the ninth straight year to 15,991 cases of active TB (infection with full-blown disease symptoms). This all-time low is due largely to improved public health control measures. In addition to those with active TB, however, an estimated 10 to 15 million people in the United States are infected with *M. tuberculosis* without displaying symptoms (latent TB) and about one in ten of these individuals will develop active TB at some time in their lives.

Minorities are affected disproportionately by TB: 54 percent of active TB cases in 1999 were among African-American and Hispanic people, with an additional 20 percent found in Asians.

What caused TB to return?

Cases of TB dropped rapidly in the 1940s and 1950s when the first effective antibiotic therapies for TB were introduced. In 1985, however, the decline ended and the number of active TB cases in the United States began to rise again. Several forces, often interrelated, were behind TB's resurgence:

- The HIV/AIDS epidemic. People with HIV are particularly vulnerable to turn infection with *M. tuberculosis* into active TB and are also more sensitive to developing active TB when they are first infected with the TB germ.
- Increased numbers of foreign-born nationals from countries where many cases of TB occur, such as Africa, Asia, and Latin America. TB cases among those persons now living in the U.S. account for nearly half of the national total.
- Increased poverty, injection drug use, and homelessness. TB transmission is rampant in crowded shelters and prisons where people weakened by poor nutrition, drug addiction, and alcoholism are exposed to *M. tuberculosis*.
- Failure of patients to take their prescribed antibiotics against TB as directed.
- Increased numbers of residents in long-term care facilities such as nursing homes. Many develop active TB from infections with *M. tuberculosis* that occurred much earlier in life because their

general health has declined. Other elderly people, especially those with weak immune systems, become newly infected with *M. tuberculosis* and can rapidly develop active TB.

How do people catch TB?

TB is primarily an airborne disease. The disease is spread from person to person in tiny microscopic droplets when a TB sufferer coughs, sneezes, speaks, sings, or laughs. Only people with active disease are contagious.

It usually takes lengthy contact with someone with active TB before a person can become infected. On average, people have a 50 percent chance of becoming infected with *M. tuberculosis* if they spend eight hours a day for six months or 24 hours a day for two months working or living with someone with active TB. However, people with TB who have been treated with appropriate drugs for at least two weeks are no longer contagious and do not spread the germ to others.

Adequate ventilation is the most important measure to prevent the transmission of TB.

What happens when someone gets infected with M. tuberculosis?

Between two to eight weeks after being infected with *M. tuberculosis*, a person's immune system responds to the TB germ by walling off infected cells. From then on the body maintains a standoff with the infection, sometimes for years. Most people undergo complete healing of their initial infection, and the bacteria eventually die off. A positive TB skin test, and old scars on a chest x-ray, may provide the only evidence of the infection.

If, however, the body's resistance is low because of aging, infections such as HIV, malnutrition, or other reasons, the bacteria may break out of hiding and cause active TB.

What is "active" disease?

One in ten people who are infected with *M. tuberculosis* may develop active TB at some time in their lives. The risk of developing active disease is greatest in the first year after infection, but active disease often does not occur until many years later.

Early symptoms of active TB can include weight loss, fever, night sweats, and loss of appetite, or they may be vague and go unnoticed by the affected individual. One in three patients with TB will die within weeks to months if the disease is not treated. For the rest, their disease either goes into remission (halts) or becomes chronic and more debilitating with cough, chest pain, and bloody sputum.

Symptoms of TB involving areas other than the lungs vary, depending upon the organ affected.

How is TB diagnosed?

Doctors can identify most people infected with *M. tuberculosis* with a skin test. They will inject a substance under the skin of the forearm. If a red welt forms around the injection site within 72 hours, the person may have been infected. This doesn't necessarily mean he or

Table 27.1. Difference between Latent TB Infection and TB Disease

Latent TB Infection

- Have no symptoms
- Do not feel sick
- Cannot spread TB to others
- Usually have a positive skin test
- Chest x-ray and sputum test normal

TB Disease

- Symptoms include:
  - a bad cough that lasts longer than 2 weeks
  - pain in the chest
  - coughing up blood or sputum
  - weakness or fatigue
  - weight loss
  - no appetite
  - chills
  - fever
  - sweating at night
- May spread TB to others
- Usually have a positive skin test
- May have abnormal chest x-ray, and/or positive sputum smear or culture

Source: Excerpted from "Questions and Answers about TB," Division of Tuberculosis Elimination, National Center for HIV, STD, and TB Prevention, Centers for Disease Control and Prevention.

she has active disease. Most people with previous exposure to *M. tuberculosis* will test positive on the tuberculin test, as will some people exposed to bacteria that are related to the TB germ.

If a person has an obvious reaction to the skin test, other methods can help to show if the individual has active TB. In making a diagnosis, doctors rely on symptoms and other physical signs, a person's history of exposure to TB, and x-rays that may show evidence of *M. tuberculosis* infection.

The doctor also will take sputum and other samples, to see if the TB bacteria will grow in the lab. If bacteria are growing, this positive culture confirms the diagnosis of TB. Because *M. tuberculosis* grows very slowly, it can take four weeks to confirm the diagnosis. An additional two to three weeks usually are needed to determine which antibiotics the bacteria are susceptible to.

Can TB be cured?

With appropriate antibiotic treatment, TB can be cured in more than nine out of ten patients.

Successful treatment of TB depends on close cooperation between the patient and doctor and other health care workers. Treatment usually combines several different antibiotic drugs which are given for at least six months, sometimes for as long as 12 months.

Patients must take their medicine on time every day for the 6 to 12 months. Some TB patients stop taking their prescribed medicines because they may feel better after only a couple of weeks of treatment. Another reason they may stop taking their medicine is because TB drugs can have unpleasant side effects.

Why is it so important to finish all of the TB medicine?

If patients don't take all their medicine the way their doctor tells them, they can become sick again and spread TB to their friends and family. Additionally, when patients do not take all the drugs the doctor has prescribed or skip times when they are supposed to take them, the TB bacteria learn to outwit the TB antibiotics, and soon those medications no longer work against the disease. If this happens, the person now has resistant TB infection. Some patients have disease that is resistant to two or more drugs. This is called multidrug-resistant TB or MDR-TB because the TB germ, *M. tuberculosis* resists eradication with more than drug. This form of TB is much more difficult to cure.

Can MDR-TB be treated?

Treatment for MDR-TB often requires the use of special TB drugs, all of which can produce serious side effects. To cure MDR-TB, patients may have to take several antibiotics, at least three to which the bacteria still respond, every day for up to two years. However, even with this treatment, between four and six out of ten patients with MDR-TB will die, which is the same as for patients with normal TB who do not receive treatment.

How is TB prevented?

TB is largely a preventable disease. In the United States, doctors try to identify persons infected with *M. tuberculosis* as early as possible, before they have developed active TB. They will give a drug called isoniazid (INH) to prevent the active disease. This drug is given every day for 6 to 12 months. INH can cause hepatitis in a small percentage of patients, especially those older than 35 years. A nurse may watch the patients take their medicine to make sure all pills are taken.

Hospitals and clinics can take precautions to prevent the spread of TB. Precautions include using ultraviolet light to sterilize the air, special filters, and special respirators and masks. Until they can no longer spread the TB germs, TB patients in hospitals should be isolated in special rooms with controlled ventilation and airflow.

Is there a vaccine for TB?

In those parts of the world where the disease is common, the World Health Organization (WHO) recommends that infants receive a vaccine called BCG (bacille Calmette-Guerin) made from a live weakened bacterium related to *M. tuberculosis*. BCG vaccine prevents *M. tuberculosis* from spreading within the body, thus preventing TB from developing.

However, the vaccine has its drawbacks. It does not protect adults very well against TB. In addition, BCG interferes with the TB skin test, showing a positive skin test reaction in people who have received BCG vaccine. In countries where BCG vaccine is used, the ability of the skin test to identify persons that are infected with *M. tuberculosis* is limited. Because of these limitations, more effective vaccines are needed and BCG is not recommended for general use in the United States.

What research is underway regarding TB vaccines?

BCG represents the only vaccine currently available against tuberculosis. It has been shown to protect against disseminated and meningeal TB in young children and to provide some protection against leprosy, but its efficacy in preventing adult pulmonary TB, which carries the major burden of morbidity and mortality from this disease, has varied dramatically in carefully conducted studies throughout the world—from 77% in the UK to 0% in Chingleput, India. As a result of this variability in efficacy, the impact of BCG on the global TB epidemic has been negligible. Current models predict that an effective TB vaccine would save tens of millions of lives over the next three decades, and that the beneficial effects of combining effective vaccination and treatment of active disease would be multiplicative.

Relatively large numbers of potential vaccine candidates have been and continue to be developed and screened in small animal models. In addition, a whole genome screen of *M. tuberculosis* for protective antigens is being conducted.

Significant challenges to TB vaccine development remain, however. One study suggests that in areas with high prevalence of tuberculosis, there may be higher than previously expected rates of exogenous re-infection in humans cured of primary tuberculosis. This result remains somewhat controversial, but an accumulating number of documented cases of re-infection confirm that complete natural protective immunity following cure of primary tuberculosis is not universal.

TB vaccine development would be greatly advanced by an improved understanding of the human protective immune response to *M. tuberculosis* infection, including the potential role(s) of various T cell populations and the molecular signals that activate the protective immune response. Low cost, simple diagnostics that could effectively distinguish *M. tuberculosis* infection from vaccination or exposure to environmental mycobacteria and from TB disease would be enormously useful both clinically and to facilitate clinical trials. Additional research is also required to further define the antigens of *M. tuberculosis* that induce human protective immunity, develop improved animal models that better mimic the realities of human tuberculosis (including persistent infection and reactivation, and effects of non-pathogenic, environmental mycobacteria and BCG vaccination), and identification of the optimal route of human immunization.

Are any new TB vaccines currently being tested?

A new vaccine, made with several proteins from the bacterium that causes tuberculosis (TB), will soon enter the first phase of human safety testing. The trial will be conducted in the United States by

Seattle biotechnology company Corixa and GlaxoSmithKline Biologicals, a vaccine manufacturer headquartered in Belgium.

The vaccine combines two TB proteins known to stimulate strong immune responses in humans. The proteins were initially identified by screening blood taken from volunteers who never became ill with tuberculosis despite long-term infection with *Mycobacterium tuberculosis* bacteria. Using recombinant DNA technology, the TB proteins were fused and then combined with adjuvants, substances that further boost the immune system's response to the vaccine.

The Phase I trial will enroll 20 volunteers at a single site in the United States and will assess the vaccine's safety. Researchers will examine blood from the volunteers to determine which dosage of vaccine promotes the greatest anti-TB immune response. If the vaccine proves safe in this initial stage of testing, it will be further tested for evidence of efficacy in larger clinical trials.

How is M. tuberculosis *infection different in people with HIV infection?*

One of the first indications that a person is infected with HIV may be that he or she suddenly develops TB. This form of TB often occurs in areas outside the lungs, particularly when the patient is in the later stages of AIDS.

In the United States, it is much more likely for persons infected with *M. tuberculosis* and HIV to develop active TB than it is for someone that is only infected with *M. tuberculosis*. However, TB disease can be prevented and cured, even in people with HIV infection.

People with MDR-TB that are also infected with HIV appear to have a more rapid and deadly disease course than do those patients with MDR-TB who are otherwise healthy. If no medicines are available for these patients as many as eight out of ten may die, often within months of diagnosis.

Diagnosing TB in HIV-infected people is often difficult. HIV infected patients frequently have disease symptoms similar to those of TB, and may not react to the standard TB skin test because their immune system does not work properly. X-rays, sputum tests, and physical exams may also fail to provide evidence of infection with *M. tuberculosis* in HIV-infected individuals.

How is research helping the fight against TB?

The National Institute of Allergy and Infectious Diseases (NIAID) leads TB research at the National Institutes of Health. NIAID supports not only studies to better understand how *M. tuberculosis* infects and causes disease in humans but also how the human immune system responds to it. This research will help to develop new tools to diagnose TB, find better vaccines, and new medicines against TB. Below are some important advances that have been made in TB research:

- **Diagnosis:** Potential new tests to speed the diagnosis of TB from four weeks to two days; differences found in the DNA of *M. tuberculosis* and the bacterium used in the BCG vaccine may lead to a test to tell the difference between people who really have TB and those who only react to previous BCG vaccination.
- **Treatment:** Discovery of the molecules responsible for drug resistance, knowledge that will help doctors quickly select the best treatments for their patients; a new drug under study can be taken less often to help patients comply with their treatment regimen.
- **Vaccines:** More than 90 vaccine candidates have been developed and tested in animals.
- **Training:** An innovative TB telemedicine program where NIAID physicians share their expertise with doctors in Texas; an urban program in Washington, DC where NIAID TB clinical trials are made more accessible to inner city patients; international collaborations with investigators to help them build research capabilities, and carry out research that will benefit populations in countries where TB disease is most common.

Recognizing that disease knows no borders, NIAID has developed a global TB research agenda. A concerted global effort will require collaborations with sister agencies and other organizations with similar goals such as the Global Alliance for TB Drug Development and the STOP TB initiative, as well as partnerships with governments and scientists from countries where the burden of tuberculosis is greatest.

Tuberculosis Skin Test

Tuberculosis (TB) is an infectious disease caused by the bacterium *Mycobacterium tuberculosis*, which primarily affects the lungs. TB is spread by an airborne germ. Someone with pulmonary TB can spread the germs by coughing, sneezing, laughing, or singing; however, repeated and/or prolonged exposure to someone with TB disease is generally necessary before a person will become infected. TB infection is most commonly diagnosed through the TB skin test.

- A person recently infected with TB may not react to the TB skin test. This is also true of elderly, debilitated, and immunocompromised (for example, AIDS) patients. In the case of patients who fit into these categories and who are suspected to be infected with tuberculosis, other tests including a chest x-ray or a skin test at a later date may be used to determine the presence or absence of TB infection and disease.
- A positive (now called "significant") reaction indicates infection with TB. It is important to understand that there is a difference between being infected with TB and having TB disease. Someone who is infected with TB has the TB germs, or bacteria, in their body. The body's defenses are protecting them from the germs, and they are not sick. Someone with TB disease is sick and may be able to spread the disease to other people. A person with a significant skin test needs to see a doctor to determine what further tests and treatment may be necessary. Chest x-rays, sputum tests, and other tests are used to determine whether the positive reaction is associated with TB disease.
- In countries other than the U.S., many people are vaccinated against tuberculosis using the BCG (bacillus Calmette-Guerin) vaccine. BCG can cause a positive skin test, especially if it has been recently administered. There is no reliable method of distinguishing tuberculin reactions caused by vaccination with BCG from those caused by natural mycobacterial infections. CDC [Centers for Disease Control and Prevention] and ATS [American Thoracic Society] recommend, however, that large reactions to a TB skin test in BCG-vaccinated persons be considered as indicating TB infection.
- In the United States, a so-called "false positive" result, especially after repeated tests, can also occur from exposure to "atypical" mycobacteria, which cause different patterns of infection and disease. These non-tuberculous forms of mycobacteria are most often found in patients who are HIV positive, although they infrequently cause disease in non-HIV infected individuals.
- Two types of skin tests are currently available in the U.S.: the recommended Mantoux skin test, which uses a needle to place a standard dose of tuberculin just under the surface of the skin.

The multi-puncture or "tine" test uses multiple tines (pins) dipped in tuberculin. This test is not considered as accurate as the Mantoux test because the quantity of the tuberculin administered cannot be precisely controlled. The Mantoux test should be used for screening and diagnosis.

- A person who has become infected with TB and is not yet sick may be advised to have preventive therapy. Preventive therapy aims to kill germs that are not causing damage to the body but could eventually become active.
- Individuals with TB symptoms should receive medical attention immediately. A skin test will frequently be prescribed. But in some patients, the test may not be significant even though TB disease is present. TB symptoms include: prolonged cough; night sweats; unexplained weight loss; loss of appetite; weakness; fever/chills; occasionally coughing up blood.
- Individuals in high risk populations should be tested regularly if they have not previously had a positive skin test. These groups include: people who interact with persons with active TB disease; poor and medically under-served people; homeless people; those who come from countries with high TB incidence rates; nursing home residents; alcoholics and intravenous drug users; people with HIV or AIDS, or who are otherwise immune-suppressed; people in jail or prison; the elderly; health care workers and others such as prison guards and teachers who work with high-risk populations.

For more information call the American Lung Association at 1-800-LUNG-USA (1-800-586-4872), or visit our web site at http://www.lungusa.org.

Pediatric Tuberculosis

Tuberculosis (TB) is an airborne infection caused by the bacterium *Mycobacterium tuberculosis*. Although TB primarily affects the lungs, other organs and tissues may be affected as well. For decades the incidence of TB had been on the decline. It increased, however, in the late 1980s and early 1990s. Since 1992, the trend has reversed, and the rate has begun to decline again.

- In 2001, 931 children 14 and younger had TB, a case rate of 1.5 per 100,000. Between 1992 and 2001 the incidence of tuberculosis cases among children 14 and younger decreased 52 percent, while the total number of cases in all ages decreased 47 percent.

- Cases of active tuberculosis and asymptomatic TB infection in children are of great concern. They indicate that transmission of tuberculosis has occurred recently. Many adults who develop active tuberculosis were infected many years ago, when their immune systems were stronger and able to protect them. Children, particularly infants, could have been infected only recently because of their age. When a child is diagnosed with active tuberculosis, it means that someone close to them, almost always an adult, must have active tuberculosis and is possibly transmitting the disease to others as well.
- Diagnosis of tuberculosis in children is difficult and poses problems that are not present in adults. Children are less likely to have obvious symptoms of tuberculosis. In addition, sputum samples are difficult to collect from children. Culture and drug susceptibility results from tests of the adult source case often have to be relied upon for diagnosing and properly treating tuberculosis in a child.
- Tuberculosis in infants and children younger than 4 years of age is much more likely to spread throughout the body through the bloodstream. Because of this, children are at much greater risk of developing tuberculous meningitis, a very dangerous form of the disease that affects the central nervous system. For these reasons, prompt diagnosis and immediate treatment of tuberculosis are critical in pediatric cases.
- In general, the same methods are used in treating tuberculosis in children as are used in treating tuberculosis in adults. The primary difference between treatment for adults and children is the use of ethambutol. One of the side effects of ethambutol is impaired vision. Because this effect is difficult to monitor in young children, ethambutol is not routinely recommended for children under eight years old.
- The best method to prevent cases of pediatric tuberculosis is to find, diagnose, and treat cases of active tuberculosis among adults. Children do not usually contract tuberculosis from other children or transmit it themselves. Adults are usually the ones who pass tuberculosis on to children. Improved contact investigations and use of directly observed therapy should improve the success

rate of finding and treating adult cases of tuberculosis and therefore reduce the number of cases of pediatric tuberculosis.

- Some groups of children are at greater risk for tuberculosis than others. These include: children living in a household with an adult who has active tuberculosis; children living in a household with an adult who is at high risk for contracting TB; children infected with HIV or another immunocompromising condition; children born in a country that has a high prevalence of tuberculosis; children from communities that are medically underserved.

Tuberculosis and HIV

Human immunodeficiency virus (HIV) infection is a major risk factor for the development of tuberculosis (TB). The increase in reported cases of TB since the mid-1980s is attributed, in part, to TB occurring in persons infected with HIV, the virus that causes AIDS. AIDS robs the body of its natural ability to fight infection, making people with AIDS more likely to develop TB.

- Tuberculosis is caused by the bacillus *Mycobacterium tuberculosis*. Many Americans—as many as 10 to 15 million—have latent TB infection; they are not sick but carry the bacterium. Only one in 10 infected individuals will develop active TB disease. Because HIV-infected people have weakened immune systems, they have much greater chances of developing active TB disease, either by activation of latent infection or by being newly infected.
- It has been estimated that an individual who is infected with both HIV and TB has a seven to ten percent chance per year of developing active TB, as opposed to the 10 percent lifetime chance of someone who is infected with tuberculosis but not HIV.
- An estimated 12 million people worldwide are infected with both HIV and TB. Estimates of the proportions of individuals similarly infected in the United States have varied greatly. Worldwide, TB is the leading cause of death among people who are HIV positive, accounting for 11% of AIDS deaths, 50% in Africa. However, this is not the case in the U.S. TB is a much less common cause of death in HIV infected individuals.
- An annual TB skin test (tuberculin test) is recommended for all persons who are HIV-positive. If the test is positive, TB is highly

suspected. Many HIV-positive patients will have a negative skin test despite TB infection or disease.

- Preventive treatment is recommended for someone who has tested positive for both HIV and TB bacteria and does not have the active disease.
- Multidrug-resistant TB (MDR-TB) is dangerous for all people but is especially dangerous for individuals who are HIV-infected. MDR-TB can develop when a patient with TB does not complete his or her full drug therapy. If patients stop taking their medicine or are inadequately treated, the TB bacteria may become resistant to those drugs. Some people may catch already resistant TB from others.
- TB sometimes affects parts of the body other than the lungs. This is called extrapulmonary TB, and it may affect bones, joints, the nervous system, urinary tract, and other areas. This happens more frequently in persons with HIV infection.
- Treatment of TB in HIV-infected individuals is most likely to be successful when it is begun early. Recent evidence also suggests that the presence of TB in HIV-infected individuals may hasten the progression of AIDS. It is therefore essential for a person who is HIV-positive or who has AIDS to be alert for respiratory symptoms such as coughing or shortness of breath, as well as any other symptoms, such as fever, weight loss and night sweats, that may suggest active infection.
- In 1995 and 1996, the FDA approved three new protease inhibitors, the most potent antiretroviral agents available to treat patients with HIV diseases. Protease inhibitors, however, interact with rifampin and other drugs used to treat TB, reducing the efficacy of both the protease inhibitors and the drugs treating the TB.
- To reduce the likelihood of drug interactions while providing optimal anti-TB care for HIV infected persons, the CDC recommends that health-care workers treating TB and those involved in HIV clinical care coordinate their efforts to ensure the best outcome for their patients.

For more information call the American Lung Association at 1-800-LUNG-USA (1-800-586-4872), or visit our website at http://www.lungusa.org.

Multidrug-Resistant Tuberculosis

Multidrug-resistant tuberculosis (MDR-TB) is a form of tuberculosis that is resistant to two or more of the primary drugs used for the treatment of tuberculosis. Resistance to one or several forms of treatment occurs when the bacteria develops the ability to withstand antibiotic attack and relay that ability to their progeny. Since that entire strain of bacteria inherits this capacity to resist the effects of the various treatments, resistance can spread from one person to another. On an individual basis, however, inadequate treatment or improper use of the anti-tuberculosis medications remains an important cause of drug-resistant tuberculosis.

- In 2001, the CDC reported that 7.4% of U.S. tuberculosis cases were resistant to isoniazid, the first line drug used to treat TB.
- The CDC also reported that 1 percent of tuberculosis cases (in U.S.) were resistant to both isoniazid and rifampin. Certain areas, however, have been shown to have much higher rates. Over 30 percent of all MDR-TB cases were reported from New York City and California.
- The World Health Organization estimates that up to 50 million persons worldwide may be infected with drug resistant strains of TB.
- A strain of MDR-TB originally develops when a case of drug-susceptible tuberculosis is improperly or incompletely treated. This occurs when a physician does not prescribe proper treatment regimens or when a patient is unable to adhere to therapy. Improper treatment allows individual TB bacilli that have natural resistance to a drug to multiply. Eventually the majority of bacilli in the body are resistant.
- Once a strain of MDR-TB develops it can be transmitted to others just like a normal drug-susceptible strain. Airborne transmission has been the cause of several well-publicized cases of nosocomial (hospital-based) outbreaks of MDR-TB in New York City and Florida. These outbreaks were responsible for the deaths of several patients and health care workers, a majority of whom were co-infected with HIV.
- Persons at risk for MDR-TB include: persons who have been exposed to someone with active MDR-TB, especially if they are immunocompromised; TB patients who have failed to take

medications as prescribed; TB patients who have been prescribed an ineffective treatment regimen; persons who have been previously treated for TB and experience a recurrence; persons from other countries and areas in the U.S. with a high incidence of MDR-TB.

- MDR-TB has been a particular concern among HIV-infected persons. Some of the factors that have contributed to the number of cases of MDR-TB, both in general and among HIV-infected individuals are: delayed diagnosis and delayed determination of drug susceptibility, which may take several weeks; susceptibility of immunosuppressed individuals for not only acquiring MDR-TB but for rapid disease progression, which may result in rapid transmission of the disease to other immunosuppressed patients; inadequate respiratory isolation procedures and other environmental safety conditions, especially in confined areas such as prisons; noncompliance or intermittent compliance with antituberculosis drug therapy.
- MDR-TB is more difficult to treat than drug-susceptible strains of TB. The success of treatment depends upon how quickly a case of TB is identified as drug resistant and whether an effective drug therapy is available. The second-line drugs used in cases of MDR-TB are often less effective and more likely to cause side effects.
- Tests to determine the resistance of a particular strain to various drugs usually take several weeks to complete. During the delay the patient may be treated with a drug regimen that is ineffective. Once a strain's drug resistance is known, an effective drug regimen must be identified and begun. Some strains of MDR-TB are resistant to seven or more drugs, making the identification of effective drugs difficult. To deal with this problem, it is recommended that newly discovered cases of TB in populations at high risk for MDR-TB be treated with four drugs rather than the standard three as part of initial treatment.
- Treatment for MDR-TB involves drug therapy over many months or years. Despite the longer course of treatment, the cure rate decreases from over 90 percent for nonresistant strains of TB to 50 percent or less for MDR-TB.
- Because it is difficult for some people to successfully complete their tuberculosis treatment, several innovations have been

developed. One of these is the use of incentives and enablers, which may be transportation, tokens or food coupons that are given to patients each time they appear at the clinic or doctor's office for treatment. Incentives and enablers are combined with the use of directly observed therapy (DOT). DOT is a system of treatment in which the patient is administered his or her medication by a nurse or health worker and observed taking the medication.

- Another innovation in TB treatment was the FDA approval of Rifater. Rifater is a medication that combines the three main drugs (isoniazid, rifampin, and pyrazinamide) used to treat tuberculosis into one pill. This reduces the number of pills a patient has to take each day and makes it impossible for the patient to take only one of the three medications, a common path to the development of MDR-TB.
- In June 1998, the U.S. Food and Drug Administration approved the first new drug for pulmonary tuberculosis in 25 years. The drug, rifapentine (Priftin), has been approved for use with other drugs to fight TB. One potential advantage of rifapentine is that it can be taken less often in the final four months of treatment—once a week compared with twice a week for the standard regimen.

For more information call the American Lung Association at 1-800-LUNG-USA (1-800-586-4872), or visit our web site at http://www.lungusa.org.

Chapter 28

Typhoid Fever

Typhoid fever is a life-threatening illness caused by the bacterium *Salmonella typhi*. In the United States about 400 cases occur each year, and 70% of these are acquired while traveling internationally. Typhoid fever is still common in the developing world, where it affects about 12.5 million persons each year.

Typhoid fever can be prevented and can usually be treated with antibiotics. If you are planning to travel outside the United States, you should know about typhoid fever and what steps you can take to protect yourself.

How is typhoid fever spread?

Salmonella typhi lives only in humans. Persons with typhoid fever carry the bacteria in their bloodstream and intestinal tract. In addition, a small number of persons, called carriers, recover from typhoid fever but continue to carry the bacteria. Both ill persons and carriers shed *S. typhi* in their feces (stool).

You can get typhoid fever if you eat food or drink beverages that have been handled by a person who is shedding *S. typhi* or if sewage contaminated with *S. typhi* bacteria gets into the water you use for drinking or washing food. Therefore, typhoid fever is more common in areas of the world where handwashing is less frequent and water is likely to be contaminated with sewage.

"Typhoid Fever," Division of Bacterial and Mycotic Diseases, Centers for Disease Control and Prevention (CDC), reviewed February 2004.

Once *S. typhi* bacteria are eaten or drunk, they multiply and spread into the bloodstream. The body reacts with fever and other signs and symptoms.

Where in the world do you get typhoid fever?

Typhoid fever is common in most parts of the world except in industrialized regions such as the United States, Canada, western Europe, Australia, and Japan. Therefore, if you are traveling to the developing world, you should consider taking precautions. Over the past 10 years, travelers from the United States to Asia, Africa, and Latin America have been especially at risk.

How can you avoid typhoid fever?

Two basic actions can protect you from typhoid fever:

1. Avoid risky foods and drinks.
2. Get vaccinated against typhoid fever.

It may surprise you, but watching what you eat and drink when you travel is as important as being vaccinated. This is because the vaccines are not completely effective. Avoiding risky foods will also help protect you from other illnesses, including travelers' diarrhea, cholera, dysentery, and hepatitis A.

"Boil it, cook it, peel it, or forget it"

- If you drink water, buy it bottled or bring it to a rolling boil for 1 minute before you drink it. Bottled carbonated water is safer than uncarbonated water.
- Ask for drinks without ice unless the ice is made from bottled or boiled water. Avoid popsicles and flavored ices that may have been made with contaminated water.
- Eat foods that have been thoroughly cooked and that are still hot and steaming.
- Avoid raw vegetables and fruits that cannot be peeled. Vegetables like lettuce are easily contaminated and are very hard to wash well.
- When you eat raw fruit or vegetables that can be peeled, peel them yourself. (Wash your hands with soap first.) Do not eat the peelings.

- Avoid foods and beverages from street vendors. It is difficult for food to be kept clean on the street, and many travelers get sick from food bought from street vendors.

When should you get vaccinated against typhoid?

If you are traveling to a country where typhoid is common, you should consider being vaccinated against typhoid. Visit a doctor or travel clinic to discuss your vaccination options.

Remember that you will need to complete your vaccination at least 1 week before you travel so that the vaccine has time to take effect. Typhoid vaccines lose effectiveness after several years; if you were vaccinated in the past, check with your doctor to see if it is time for a booster vaccination. Taking antibiotics will not prevent typhoid fever; they only help treat it.

Table 28.1 provides basic information on typhoid vaccines that are available in the United States.

What are the signs and symptoms of typhoid fever?

Persons with typhoid fever usually have a sustained fever as high as 103° to 104° F (39° to 40° C). They may also feel weak, or have stomach pains, headache, or loss of appetite. In some cases, patients have

Table 28.1. Typhoid vaccines

Vaccine Name	**Ty21a (Vivotif Berna, Swiss Serum and Vaccine Institute)**	**ViCPS Typhim Vi, (Pasteur Merieux)**
How given	1 capsule by mouth	Injection
Number of doses necessary	4	1
Time between doses	2 days	N/A
Total time needed to set aside for vaccination	2 weeks	1 week
Minimum age for vaccination	6 years	2 years
Booster needed every...	5 years	2 years

The parenteral heat-phenol-inactivated vaccine (manufactured by Wyeth-Ayerst) has been discontinued.

a rash of flat, rose-colored spots. The only way to know for sure if an illness is typhoid fever is to have samples of stool or blood tested for the presence of *S. typhi*.

What do you do if you think you have typhoid fever?

If you suspect you have typhoid fever, see a doctor immediately. If you are traveling in a foreign country, you can usually call the U.S. consulate for a list of recommended doctors.

You will probably be given an antibiotic to treat the disease. Three commonly prescribed antibiotics are ampicillin, trimethoprim-sulfamethoxazole, and ciprofloxacin. Persons given antibiotics usually begin to feel better within 2 to 3 days, and deaths rarely occur. However, persons who do not get treatment may continue to have fever for weeks or months, and as many as 20% may die from complications of the infection.

Does typhoid fever's danger end when symptoms disappear?

Even if your symptoms seem to go away, you may still be carrying *S. typhi*. If so, the illness could return, or you could pass the disease to other people. In fact, if you work at a job where you handle food or care for small children, you may be barred legally from going back to work until a doctor has determined that you no longer carry any typhoid bacteria.

If you are being treated for typhoid fever, it is important to do the following:

- Keep taking the prescribed antibiotics for as long as the doctor has asked you to take them.
- Wash your hands carefully with soap and water after using the bathroom, and do not prepare or serve food for other people. This will lower the chance that you will pass the infection on to someone else.
- Have your doctor perform a series of stool cultures to ensure that no *S. typhi* bacteria remain in your body.

Chapter 29

Vaginal Infections

Vaginitis Due to Vaginal Infections

Vaginitis is an inflammation of the vagina characterized by discharge, odor, irritation, and/or itching. The cause of vaginitis may not always be determined adequately solely on the basis of symptoms or a physical examination. For a correct diagnosis, a doctor should perform laboratory tests including microscopic evaluation of vaginal fluid. A variety of effective drugs are available for treating vaginitis.

Vaginitis often is caused by infections, which cause distress and discomfort. Some infections are associated with more serious diseases. The most common vaginal infections are bacterial vaginosis, trichomoniasis, and vaginal yeast infection or candidiasis. Some vaginal infections are transmitted through sexual contact, but others such as yeast infections probably are not, depending on the cause.

Bacterial Vaginosis

Bacterial vaginosis (BV) is the most common cause of vaginitis symptoms among women of childbearing age. Previously called nonspecific vaginitis or *Gardnerella*-associated vaginitis, BV is associated with sexual activity. BV reflects a change in the vaginal ecosystem. This imbalance, including pH changes, occurs when different types

---

"Vaginitis Due to Vaginal Infections," National Institute of Allergy and Infectious Diseases (NIAID), National Institutes of Health (NIH), June 1998. Reviewed by David A. Cooke, M.D., April 2004.

of bacteria outnumber the normal ones. Instead of *Lactobacillus* bacteria being the most numerous, increased numbers of organisms such as *Gardnerella vaginalis*, *Bacteroides*, *Mobiluncus*, and *Mycoplasma hominis* are found in the vaginas of women with BV. Investigators are studying the role that each of these microbes may play in causing BV, but they do not yet understand the role of sexual activity in developing BV. A change in sexual partners and douching may increase the risk of acquiring bacterial vaginosis.

Symptoms

The primary symptom of BV is an abnormal, odorous vaginal discharge. The fish-like odor is noticeable especially after intercourse. Nearly half of the women with clinical signs of BV, however, report no symptoms. A physician may observe these signs during a physical examination and may confirm the diagnosis by doing tests of vaginal fluid.

Diagnosis

A healthcare worker can examine a sample of vaginal fluid under a microscope, either stained or in special lighting, to detect the presence of the organisms associated with BV. They can make a diagnosis based on the absence of lactobacilli, the presence of numerous "clue cells" (cells from the vaginal lining that are coated with BV organisms), a fishy odor, and decreased acidity or change in pH of vaginal fluid.

Treatment

All women with BV should be informed of their diagnoses, including the possibility of sexual transmission, and offered treatment. They can be treated with antibiotics such as metronidazole or clindamycin. Generally, male sex partners are not treated. Many women with symptoms of BV do not seek medical treatment, and many asymptomatic women decline treatment.

Complications

Researchers have shown an association between BV and pelvic inflammatory disease (PID), which can cause infertility and tubal (ectopic) pregnancy. BV also can cause adverse outcomes of pregnancy such as premature delivery and low-birth-weight infants. Therefore, the U.S. Centers for Disease Control and Prevention (CDC) recommends that doctors check all pregnant women for BV who previously have delivered a premature baby, whether or not the women have symptoms. If these women have BV, they should be treated with oral metronidazole or oral clindamycin. A pregnant woman who has not delivered a premature baby should be treated if she has symptoms and laboratory evidence of BV. BV is also associated with increased risk of gonorrhea and HIV infection (HIV, human immunodeficiency virus, causes AIDS).

Trichomoniasis

Trichomoniasis, sometimes referred to as "trich," is a common STD that affects 2 to 3 million Americans yearly. It is caused by a single-celled protozoan parasite called *Trichomonas vaginalis*. Trichomoniasis is primarily an infection of the urogenital tract; the urethra is the most common site of infection in man, and the vagina is the most common site of infection in women.

Symptoms

Trichomoniasis, like many other STDs, often occurs without any symptoms. Men almost never have symptoms. When women have symptoms, they usually appear within four to 20 days of exposure. The symptoms in women include a heavy, yellow-green or gray vaginal discharge, discomfort during intercourse, vaginal odor, and painful urination. Irritation and itching of the female genital area, and on rare occasions, lower abdominal pain also can be present. The symptoms in men, if present, include a thin, whitish discharge from the penis and painful or difficult urination.

Treatment

Because men can transmit the disease to their sex partners even when symptoms are not present, it is preferable to treat both partners to eliminate the parasite. Metronidazole is the drug used to treat people with trichomoniasis. It usually is administered in a single dose. People taking this drug should not drink alcohol because mixing the two substances occasionally can cause severe nausea and vomiting.

Complications

Research has shown a link between trichomoniasis and two serious sequelae. Data suggest that trichomoniasis is associated with increased risk of transmission of HIV and may cause a woman to deliver a low-birth-weight or premature infant. Additional research is needed to fully explore these relationships.

Prevention

Use of male condoms may help prevent the spread of trichomoniasis, although careful studies have never been done that focus on how to prevent this infection.

Vaginal Yeast Infection

Vaginal yeast infection or vulvovaginal candidiasis is a common cause of vaginal irritation. Doctors estimate that approximately 75 percent of all women will experience at least one symptomatic yeast infection during their lifetimes. Yeast are always present in the vagina in small numbers, and symptoms only appear with overgrowth. Several factors are associated with increased symptomatic infection in women, including pregnancy, uncontrolled diabetes mellitus, and the use of oral contraceptives or antibiotics. Other factors that may increase the incidence of yeast infection include using douches, perfumed feminine hygiene sprays, and topical antimicrobial agents, and wearing tight, poorly ventilated clothing and underwear. Whether or not yeast can be transmitted sexually is unknown. Because almost all women have the organism in the vagina, it has been difficult for researchers to study this aspect of the natural history.

Symptoms

The most frequent symptoms of yeast infection in women are itching, burning, and irritation of the vagina. Painful urination and/or intercourse are common. Vaginal discharge is not always present and may be minimal. The thick, whitish-gray discharge is typically described as cottage-cheese-like in nature, although it can vary from watery to thick in consistency. Most male partners of women with yeast infection do not experience any symptoms of the infection. A transient rash and burning sensation of the penis, however, have been reported after intercourse if condoms were not used. These symptoms are usually self-limiting.

Diagnosis

Because few specific signs and symptoms are usually present, this condition cannot be diagnosed by the patient's history and physical examination. The doctor usually diagnoses yeast infection through microscopic examination of vaginal secretions for evidence of yeast forms.

Scientists funded by the National Institute of Allergy and Infectious Diseases (NIAID) have developed a rapid simple test for yeast infection, which will soon be available for use in doctors' offices. If such a test were available for home screening, it would help them to appropriately use yeast medication.

Treatment

Various antifungal vaginal medications are available to treat yeast infection. Women can buy some antifungal creams, tablets, or suppositories (butoconazole, miconazole, clotrimazole, and tioconazole) over the counter for use in the vagina. But because BV, trichomoniasis, and yeast infection are difficult to distinguish on the basis of symptoms alone, a woman with vaginal symptoms should see her physician for an accurate diagnosis before using these products.

Other products available over the counter contain antihistamines or topical anesthetics that only mask the symptoms and do not treat the underlying problem. Women who have chronic or recurring yeast infections may need to be treated with vaginal creams for extended periods of time. Recently, effective oral medications have become available. Women should work with their physicians to determine possible underlying causes of their chronic yeast infections. HIV-infected women may have severe yeast infections that are often unresponsive to treatment.

Other Causes of Vaginitis

Although most vaginal infections in women are due to bacterial vaginosis, trichomoniasis, or yeast, there may be other causes as well. These causes may include allergic and irritative factors or other STDs. Noninfectious allergic symptoms can be caused by spermicides, vaginal hygiene products, detergents, and fabric softeners. Cervical inflammation from these products often is associated with abnormal vaginal discharge, but can be distinguished from true vaginal infections by appropriate diagnostic tests.

In an effort to control vaginitis, research is under way to determine the factors that promote the growth and disease-causing potential of vaginal microbes. No longer considered merely a benign annoyance, vaginitis is the object of serious investigation as scientists attempt to clarify its role in such conditions as pelvic inflammatory disease and pregnancy-related complications.

Part Three

Viral Diseases

Chapter 30

Adenoviruses

Clinical Features

Adenoviruses most commonly cause respiratory illness; however, depending on the infecting serotype, they may also cause various other illnesses, such as gastroenteritis, conjunctivitis, cystitis, and rash illness. Symptoms of respiratory illness caused by adenovirus infection range from the common cold syndrome to pneumonia, croup, and bronchitis. Patients with compromised immune systems are especially susceptible to severe complications of adenovirus infection. Acute respiratory disease (ARD), first recognized among military recruits during World War II, can be caused by adenovirus infections during conditions of crowding and stress.

The Viruses

Adenoviruses are medium-sized (90–100 nanometers), nonenveloped icosahedral viruses containing double-stranded DNA. There are 49 immunologically distinct types (6 subgenera: A through F) that can cause human infections. Adenoviruses are unusually stable to chemical or physical agents and adverse pH conditions, allowing for prolonged survival outside of the body.

"Adenoviruses," National Center for Infectious Diseases, Centers for Disease Control and Prevention (CDC), reviewed August 2003.

Epidemiologic Features

Although epidemiologic characteristics of the adenoviruses vary by type, all are transmitted by direct contact, fecal-oral transmission, and occasionally waterborne transmission. Some types are capable of establishing persistent asymptomatic infections in tonsils, adenoids, and intestines of infected hosts, and shedding can occur for months or years. Some adenoviruses (e.g., serotypes 1, 2, 5, and 6) have been shown to be endemic in parts of the world where they have been studied, and infection is usually acquired during childhood. Other types cause sporadic infection and occasional outbreaks; for example, epidemic keratoconjunctivitis is associated with adenovirus serotypes 8, 19, and 37. Epidemics of febrile disease with conjunctivitis are associated with waterborne transmission of some adenovirus types, often centering around inadequately chlorinated swimming pools and small lakes. ARD is most often associated with adenovirus types 4 and 7 in the United States. Enteric adenoviruses 40 and 41 cause gastroenteritis, usually in children. For some adenovirus serotypes, the clinical spectrum of disease associated with infection varies depending on the site of infection; for example, infection with adenovirus 7 acquired by inhalation is associated with severe lower respiratory tract disease, whereas oral transmission of the virus typically causes no or mild disease. Outbreaks of adenovirus-associated respiratory disease have been more common in the late winter, spring, and early summer; however, adenovirus infections can occur throughout the year.

Diagnosis

Antigen detection, polymerase chain reaction assay, virus isolation, and serology can be used to identify adenovirus infections. Adenovirus typing is usually accomplished by hemagglutination-inhibition and/or neutralization with type-specific antisera. Since adenovirus can be excreted for prolonged periods, the presence of virus does not necessarily mean it is associated with disease.

Treatment

Most infections are mild and require no therapy or only symptomatic treatment. Because there is no virus-specific therapy, serious adenovirus illness can be managed only by treating symptoms and complications of the infection.

Prevention

Vaccines were developed for adenovirus serotypes 4 and 7, but were available only for preventing ARD among military recruits. Strict attention to good infection-control practices is effective for stopping nosocomial outbreaks of adenovirus-associated disease, such as epidemic keratoconjunctivitis. Maintaining adequate levels of chlorination is necessary for preventing swimming pool-associated outbreaks of adenovirus conjunctivitis.

References

American Academy of Pediatrics. Adenovirus Infections. In: Peter G, ed. *1997 Red Book: Report of the Committee on Infectious Diseases. 24th ed.* Elk Grove Village, IL: American Academy of Pediatrics; 1997: 131.

Horwitz MS. Adenoviruses. In: Fields BN, Knipe DM, Howley PM, eds. *Fields Virology. 3rd ed.* Philadelphia: Lippincott-Raven; 1995: 2149-71.

Foy HM. Adenoviruses. In: Evans A, Kaslow R, eds. *Viral Infections in Humans: epidemiology and control. 4th ed.* New York: Plenum; 1997:119-38.

Chapter 31

Chickenpox (Varicella) and Shingles

Varicella Disease (Chickenpox)

What is varicella (chickenpox)?

Chickenpox is an infectious disease caused by the varicella-zoster virus which results in a blister-like rash, itching, tiredness, and fever.

The rash appears first on the trunk and face, but can spread over the entire body causing between 250 to 500 itchy blisters. Most cases of chickenpox occur in persons less than 15 years old. Prior to the use of varicella vaccine, the disease had annual cycles, peaking in the spring of each year.

How do you get chickenpox?

Chickenpox is highly infectious and spreads from person to person by direct contact or through the air from an infected person's coughing or sneezing. A persons with chickenpox is contagious 1–2 days before the rash appears and until all blisters have formed scabs. It takes from 10–21 days after contact with an infected person for someone to develop chickenpox.

This chapter includes text from "Varicella Disease," December 20, 2001, "Varicella Treatment," February 15, 2001, "Varicella Vaccine," December 20, 2001, and "Shingles (Herpes Zoster)," February 15, 2001, National Immunization Program, Centers for Disease Control and Prevention (CDC); and "Facts about Shingles (Varicella-Zoster Virus)," National Institute of Allergy and Infectious Diseases (NIAID), National Institutes of Health (NIH), June 2003.

What is the chickenpox illness like?

In children, chickenpox most commonly causes an illness that lasts about 5–10 days. Children usually miss 5 or 6 days of school or childcare due to their chickenpox. About half of all children with chickenpox visit a health care provider due to symptoms of their illness such as high fever, severe itching, an uncomfortable rash, dehydration, or headache. In addition, about 1 child in 10 has a complication from chickenpox serious enough to visit a health care provider including infected skin lesions, other infections, dehydration from vomiting or diarrhea, exacerbation of asthma, or more serious complications such as pneumonia.

Certain groups of persons are more likely to have more serious illness with complications. These include adults, infants, adolescents, and people with weak immune systems from either illnesses or from medications such a long-term steroids.

What are the serious complications from chickenpox?

Serious complications from chickenpox include bacterial infections which can involve many sites of the body including the skin, tissues under the skin, bone, lungs (pneumonia), joints, and the blood. Other serious complications are due directly to the virus infection and include viral pneumonia, bleeding problems, and infection of the brain (encephalitis). Many people are not aware that, before a vaccine was available, there were approximately 11,000 hospitalizations and 100 deaths from chickenpox in the U.S. every year. One child and one adult died each week. For information about serious infections following chickenpox visit the following site: Complications from Group A Streptococcus: http://www.cdc.gov/epo/mmwr/preview/mmwrhtml/00049535.htm.

Can a healthy person with varicella die from the disease?

Yes, many of the deaths and complications from chickenpox occur in previously healthy children and adults. From 1990 to 1994, before there was a vaccine available, there were about 50 chickenpox deaths in children and 50 chickenpox deaths in adults every year; most of these persons were healthy or did not have a medical illness (such as cancer) that placed them at higher risk of getting severe chickenpox. Since 1999, states have been encouraged to report chickenpox deaths to CDC. In 1999 and 2000, CDC received reports that showed that deaths from chickenpox continue to occur in healthy, unvaccinated children and adults. Most of the healthy adults who died from chickenpox contracted the disease from their unvaccinated children.

Can chickenpox be prevented?

Yes, chickenpox can now be prevented by vaccination.

Can you get chickenpox more than once?

Yes, but it is uncommon to do so. For most people, one infection is thought to confer lifelong immunity.

Chickenpox in children is usually not serious. Why not let children get the disease?

It is never possible to predict who will have a mild case of chickenpox and who will have a serious or even deadly case of disease. Now that there is a safe and effective vaccine available, it is not worth taking this chance.

Varicella Treatment

What home treatments are available for chickenpox?

Scratching the blisters may cause them to become infected. Therefore, keep fingernails trimmed short. Calamine lotion and Aveeno (oatmeal) baths may help relieve some of the itching. Do not use aspirin or aspirin-containing products to relieve your child's fever. The use of aspirin has been associated with development of Reye syndrome (a severe disease affecting all organs, but most seriously affecting the liver and brain, that may cause death). Use non aspirin medications such as acetaminophen (commonly known as Tylenol®).

Are there any treatments that my doctor can prescribe for chickenpox?

Your health care provider will advise you on options for treatment. Acyclovir (a medicine that works against herpes viruses) is recommended for persons who are more likely to develop serious disease including persons with chronic skin or lung disease, otherwise healthy individuals 13 years of age or older, and those persons receiving steroid therapy. In order for acyclovir to be effective it must be administered within 24 hours of the onset of the chickenpox rash. Persons with weakened immune systems from disease or medication should contact their doctor immediately if they are exposed to or develop chickenpox. If you are pregnant and are either exposed to, or develop chickenpox, you should immediately discuss prevention and treatment options with your doctor.

When is it necessary to go to the doctor for treatment?

If a fever lasts longer than 4 days or rises above 102° F, call your health care provider. Also take note of areas of the rash or any part of your body which become very red, warm, tender, or is leaking pus (thick, discolored fluid) as this may mean there is a bacterial infection. Call your doctor immediately if the individual with chickenpox seems extremely ill, is difficult to wake up, or is confused, has difficulty walking, has a stiff neck, is vomiting repeatedly, has difficulty breathing, or has a severe cough.

Is there any preventive treatment available after exposure to chickenpox for susceptible persons who are not eligible to receive chickenpox vaccine?

Yes, varicella zoster immune globulin (VZIG) can prevent or modify disease after exposure (coming into close contact with a case). However because it is costly and only provides temporary protection, VZIG is only recommended for persons at high risk of developing severe disease. Such persons are not eligible to receive chickenpox vaccine. They include:

- Newborns whose mothers have chickenpox 5 days prior to 2 days after delivery;
- Children with leukemia or lymphoma who have not been vaccinated;
- Persons with cellular immunodeficiencies or other immune problems;
- Persons receiving drugs, including steroids, that suppress the immune system; and,
- Pregnant women.

VZIG should be administered as soon as possible, but no later than 96 hours after exposure to chickenpox. If you have had a varicella exposure and you fit into one of these groups, contact your doctor.

Varicella (Chickenpox) Vaccine

Why get vaccinated?

Chickenpox vaccine is the best way to prevent chickenpox, therefore protecting children and adults from the severe complications and death associated with the disease. Even with uncomplicated chickenpox cases, lost time from school and work and the cost of medications or treatment that may be needed can result in a significant cost for the family.

Do children prefer vaccination over having chickenpox?

In a recent study, 7 out of 10 children said given the choice, they'd rather have the shot than have the natural disease. Seven out of 10 children also considered chickenpox to be worse than many other common childhood ailments, including colds, earaches, sore throat, and fever. The study also found that 3 out of 4 parents are unaware that death is a potential complication of chickenpox.

How long has chickenpox vaccine been available?

Chickenpox vaccine was licensed by the Food and Drug Administration in 1995 and is now widely available in private doctors' offices and public health clinics.

Who should be vaccinated?

- All children between 12 and 18 months of age should have one dose of chickenpox vaccine. Children who have had chickenpox do not need the vaccine. No tests need to be administered to determine immune status—a parent's recollection of the disease is considered a reliable measure of previous infection and therefore immunity.
- Children between 19 months and their 13th birthday who have not had chickenpox should be vaccinated with a single dose.
- People 13 and older who have not had chickenpox should get two doses of the vaccine 4 to 8 weeks apart.

Is the chickenpox vaccine required for child care and school entry?

Yes, more than 20 states have passed such requirements—children entering child care and school must have a history of chickenpox, serological (blood) evidence of immunity or evidence of receiving chickenpox vaccine. Many other states are in the process of enacting such requirements.

What are the benefits of having chickenpox vaccination requirements for child care and school entry?

The decision to vaccinate an individual child benefits both the individual and the wider community. Having school requirements for vaccination achieves high levels of protection in schools, pre-schools, and child care centers resulting in less illness and school time missed by healthy children (some of whom may have serious complications) and less danger of severe infection among children who cannot be vaccinated. Persons who are not able to receive chickenpox vaccine include children with leukemia and other cancers, persons taking high doses of steroid medications for a variety of medical conditions (including asthma), pregnant women, and infants less than 1 year of age. These people have a higher risk of developing severe chickenpox with complications. The only way to protect them is to achieve high levels of vaccination coverage among persons in the community so that they are less likely to come in contact with a person with chickenpox.

How important is it for adults to be vaccinated for chickenpox?

All adults who have never had chickenpox should be vaccinated. Immunity is especially important for adolescents and adults who have close contact with persons at high risk for serious complications and for those who are likely to come in close contact with children. CDC's Advisory Committee on Immunization Practices especially recommends vaccination for the following susceptible adolescents and adults:

- Persons who live or work in environments in which chickenpox transmission is likely (for example teachers of young children, day-care employees, and residents/staff in institutional settings)
- Persons who live or work in places where chickenpox transmission can occur (for example college students, inmates and staff of correctional institutions, and military personnel)
- Nonpregnant women of childbearing age (women should avoid pregnancy for 1 month following each vaccine dose)
- Adolescents and adults living in households with children
- International travelers

Is the vaccine effective in preventing chickenpox all the time?

No vaccine is 100% effective in preventing disease. For chickenpox vaccine, about 8 to 9 out of every 10 people who are vaccinated are completely protected from chickenpox. The vaccine almost always prevents against severe disease. If a vaccinated person does get chickenpox, it is usually a very mild case with fewer skin lesions (usually less than 50) lasting only a few days, no fever or a low fever, and few other symptoms.

I don't think I have had chickenpox, but I am not sure. Is there a blood test available to determine whether or not I have had the disease?

Yes, a blood test is available to check immunity. Since 70% to 90% of adults who do not remember having chickenpox actually have protection in their blood when tested, blood testing before vaccination can be cost saving. Ask your doctor about this blood test. If it is not available, it is still safe to receive the vaccine even if you have previously had chickenpox.

Is there anyone who should not receive the chickenpox vaccine?

Yes, certain persons should not receive the chickenpox vaccine. These persons are those who:

- Ever had a serious allergic reaction to chickenpox vaccine, neomycin, or gelatin (note: chickenpox vaccine does not contain egg),
- Now have moderate or serious illness (note: vaccine may be given to persons with a mild fever, cold, or diarrhea),
- Are pregnant,
- Are unable to fight serious infections because of:
    - any kind of cancer or cancer treatment with x-rays or drugs, (note: if your child has leukemia in remission he/she may be eligible to receive the vaccine, ask your doctor)
    - a disease that depresses cellular immune function (note: if your child has HIV infection but has normal immune function he/she may receive the vaccine, ask your doctor)

- treatment with drugs such as long-term steroids
- Have gotten blood products (such as immune globulin or a transfusion) during the past five months.

If you are not sure, ask your doctor or nurse.

What problems can occur after chickenpox vaccination?

- Soreness, redness, or swelling where the shot was given is the most common side effect, occurring about 20% of the time.
- A very mild rash or several small bumps can result in about 1% to 4% of vaccine recipients. (NOTE: In very rare instances, it may be possible for someone who gets a rash from chickenpox vaccine to give vaccine strain chickenpox to another person. Persons developing a rash after vaccination should take extra precautions to avoid contact with anyone whose immune system is not working properly.)
- In children, the vaccine does not cause fever. There have not been studies comparing fever following vaccination in adults who were vaccinated with adults who were not vaccinated. The vaccine may cause a mild fever 2 weeks after vaccination.
- A seizure (jerking and staring spell) usually caused by fever may occur in less than 1 in 1000 vaccine recipients. This may not be related to the vaccine.

Have serious reactions ever occurred from the chickenpox vaccine?

As with any vaccine, there is a very small chance that serious problems could occur after getting chickenpox vaccine. However, after distribution of the first 10 million doses of the vaccine, reports of serious adverse events after vaccination for example, seizures, brain infection (encephalitis), pneumonia, loss of balance (ataxia) and severe allergic reactions (anaphylaxis) have been very rare, occurring approximately 1 for every 50,000 doses given. Adverse events that are reported following vaccination may not always be caused by the vaccine. Some may be caused by natural chickenpox virus which is still common in most communities and some may be caused by other viruses that happened to be circulating in the community at the time of vaccination. It is important to note that the risks from the vaccine remain much lower than the risks from the disease.

What should I do if there is a serious reaction after chickenpox vaccination?

- Call a doctor or get the person to a doctor right away.
- Write down what happened and the date and time it happened.
- Ask your doctor, nurse, or health department to file a Vaccine Adverse Event Report form, or you can call 800-822-7967 (toll-free).

Can the varicella vaccine virus be transmitted (caught from a person who was vaccinated)?

Yes; however, transmission of the varicella vaccine virus is very rare. It has only been documented in healthy persons on three occasions out of the 21 million doses of vaccine distributed. All three cases resulted in mild disease without complications.

I recently got vaccinated and then found out I was pregnant. What should I do?

If you discovered that you were pregnant when you got the chickenpox vaccine, or if you get pregnant within 1 month after getting the vaccine, contact your doctor or call 800-986-8999 (toll-free). The vaccine manufacturer (Merck) and CDC maintain a registry for reports of women inadvertently vaccinated prior to or during pregnancy. There is a theoretical risk that when administered one month prior to, or during, pregnancy, the vaccine may cause birth defects similar to those that can occur from natural chickenpox (for example, limb abnormalities including absence or underdevelopment; abnormal brain development; mental retardation; scarring of the skin; eye abnormalities). So far, there have been no cases reported to the registry of birth defects in babies born to mothers vaccinated during pregnancy similar to those that can occur from having natural chickenpox during pregnancy.

Have cases of chickenpox declined in the United States since chickenpox vaccine became available?

Yes, cases have declined dramatically. Since 1995, CDC, in collaboration with Los Angeles County, Texas, and Philadelphia health departments, has been monitoring chickenpox cases in these 3 areas in the United States. As use of the vaccine has increased, chickenpox cases have declined substantially.

Shingles (Herpes Zoster)

Shingles is caused by the varicella-zoster virus, the same virus that causes chickenpox. After an attack of chickenpox, the virus lies dormant in the nerve tissue. As we get older, it is possible for the virus to reappear in the form of shingles. Shingles is estimated to affect 2 in every 10 persons in their lifetime. This year, more than 500,000 people will develop shingles. Fortunately, there is currently research being done to find a vaccine to prevent the disease.

What is shingles?

Shingles, or herpes zoster, is caused by the chickenpox virus that remains in the nerve roots of all persons who had chickenpox and can come out in your body again years later to cause illness.

Shingles is more common after the age of 50 and the risk increases with advancing age. Shingles causes numbness, itching, or severe pain followed by clusters of blister-like lesions in a strip-like pattern on one side of your body. The pain can persist for weeks, months, or years after the rash heals and is then known as post-herpetic neuralgia.

Who is at risk for developing shingles?

Although it is most common in people over age 50, anyone who has had chickenpox is at risk for developing shingles. Shingles is also more common in people with weakened immune systems from HIV infection, chemotherapy, or radiation treatment, transplant operations, and stress.

What are the symptoms of shingles?

Early signs of shingles include burning or shooting pain and tingling or itching generally located on one side of the body or face. The rash or blisters are present anywhere from one to 14 days.

Are other complications associated with shingles?

Yes. If shingles appears on the face, it can lead to complications in hearing and vision. For instance, if shingles affects the eye, the cornea can become infected and lead to temporary or permanent blindness. Another complication of the virus is postherpetic neuralgia (PHN), a condition where the pain from shingles persists for months, sometimes years, after the shingles rash has healed.

Is shingles contagious?

Yes, people with shingles are contagious to persons who have not had chickenpox. Therefore, people who have not had chickenpox can catch chickenpox if they have close contact with a person who has shingles. However, you can not catch shingles itself from someone else. Shingles is caused by the chickenpox virus which has been dormant (staying quiet) in your body ever since you had chickenpox. So, you get shingles from your own chickenpox virus, not from someone else.

What should I do if I get shingles?

Contact your health care provider as soon as possible to discuss treatment with antiviral medications. These medications are most effective if given as soon as possible after rash onset.

Can someone who has been vaccinated for chickenpox develop shingles?

Yes. However, a study conducted among children with leukemia determined that after receiving the vaccine these children were much less likely to develop shingles than children who had prior natural chickenpox. Available information from healthy children and adults suggest that shingles is less common in vaccinated healthy persons compared with persons who have had natural chickenpox.

Is there a vaccine available to prevent or modify shingles?

No; however, a study is currently underway with a new formulation of the chickenpox vaccine to determine whether vaccination of persons older than 55 years of age will reduce the frequency and/or severity of shingles in adults. Results from this study will be available in about 5 years.

Is any research being done to prevent shingles?

There is a national, multicenter study under way of an experimental vaccine to prevent shingles, called the Shingles Prevention Study. The Shingles Prevention Study is a Department of Veterans Affairs (VA) cooperative study representing a scientific collaboration among the VA, National Institute of Allergy and Infectious Diseases, and Merck & Co., Inc., the vaccine's producer.

Chapter 32

The Common Cold: Rhinoviruses, Coronaviruses, and Others

The Common Cold

Sneezing, scratchy throat, runny nose—everyone knows the first signs of a cold, probably the most common illness known. Although the common cold is usually mild, with symptoms lasting one to two weeks, it is a leading cause of doctor visits and of school and job absenteeism.

The Problem

In the course of a year, individuals in the United States suffer 1 billion colds, according to some estimates.

Colds are most prevalent among children, and seem to be related to youngsters' relative lack of resistance to infection and to contacts with other children in day-care centers and schools. Children have about six to ten colds a year. In families with children in school, the number of colds per child can be as high as 12 a year. Adults average about two to four colds a year, although the range varies widely. Women, especially those aged 20 to 30 years, have more colds than men, possibly because of their closer contact with children. On average, individuals older than 60 have fewer than one cold a year.

"The Common Cold," March 2001 and "Is It a Cold or the Flu?" April 2001, National Institute of Allergy and Infectious Diseases (NIAID), National Institutes of Health (NIH); "What to Do for Colds and Flu," Food and Drug Administration (FDA), May 2000.

The economic impact of the common cold is enormous. The National Center for Health Statistics (NCHS) estimates that, in 1996, 62 million cases of the common cold in the United States required medical attention or resulted in restricted activity. In 1996, colds caused 45 million days of restricted activity and 22 million days lost from school, according to NCHS.

The Causes

The Viruses. More than 200 different viruses are known to cause the symptoms of the common cold. Some, such as the rhinoviruses, seldom produce serious illnesses. Others, such as parainfluenza and respiratory syncytial virus, produce mild infections in adults but can precipitate severe lower respiratory infections in young children.

Rhinoviruses (from the Greek *rhin*, meaning "nose") cause an estimated 30 to 35 percent of all adult colds, and are most active in early fall, spring and summer. More than 110 distinct rhinovirus types have been identified. These agents grow best at temperatures of 33 degrees Celsius (about 91 degrees Fahrenheit), the temperature of the human nasal mucosa.

Coronaviruses are believed to cause a large percentage of all adult colds. They induce colds primarily in the winter and early spring. Of the more than 30 isolated strains, three or four infect humans. The importance of coronaviruses as causative agents is hard to assess because, unlike rhinoviruses, they are difficult to grow in the laboratory.

Approximately 10 to 15 percent of adult colds are caused by viruses also responsible for other, more severe illnesses: adenoviruses, coxsackieviruses, echoviruses, orthomyxoviruses (including influenza A and B viruses), paramyxoviruses (including several parainfluenza viruses), respiratory syncytial virus and enteroviruses.

The causes of 30 to 50 percent of adult colds, presumed to be viral, remain unidentified. The same viruses that produce colds in adults appear to cause colds in children. The relative importance of various viruses in pediatric colds, however, is unclear because of the difficulty in isolating the precise cause of symptoms in studies of children with colds.

Does cold weather cause a cold? Although many people are convinced that a cold results from exposure to cold weather, or from getting chilled or overheated, NIAID grantees have found that these conditions have little or no effect on the development or severity of a cold. Nor is susceptibility apparently related to factors such as exercise, diet, or enlarged tonsils or adenoids. On the other hand, research suggests that psychological stress, allergic disorders affecting the nasal passages or pharynx (throat), and menstrual cycles may have an impact on a person's susceptibility to colds.

The Cold Season

In the United States, most colds occur during the fall and winter. Beginning in late August or early September, the incidence of colds increases slowly for a few weeks and remains high until March or April, when it declines. The seasonal variation may relate to the opening of schools and to cold weather, which prompt people to spend more time indoors and increase the chances that viruses will spread from person to person.

Seasonal changes in relative humidity also may affect the prevalence of colds. The most common cold-causing viruses survive better when humidity is low—the colder months of the year. Cold weather also may make the nasal passages' lining drier and more vulnerable to viral infection.

Cold Symptoms

Symptoms of the common cold usually begin two to three days after infection and often include nasal discharge, obstruction of nasal breathing, swelling of the sinus membranes, sneezing, sore throat, cough, and headache. Fever is usually slight but can climb to 102° F in infants and young children. Cold symptoms can last from two to 14 days, but two-thirds of people recover in a week. If symptoms occur often or last much longer than two weeks, they may be the result of an allergy rather than a cold.

Colds occasionally can lead to secondary bacterial infections of the middle ear or sinuses, requiring treatment with antibiotics. High fever, significantly swollen glands, severe facial pain in the sinuses, and a cough that produces mucus, may indicate a complication or more serious illness requiring a doctor's attention.

How Cold Viruses Cause Disease

Viruses cause infection by overcoming the body's complex defense system. The body's first line of defense is mucus, produced by the membranes in the nose and throat. Mucus traps the material we inhale: pollen, dust, bacteria, and viruses. When a virus penetrates the mucus and enters a cell, it commandeers the protein-making machinery to manufacture new viruses which, in turn, attack surrounding cells.

Cold symptoms: The body fights back. Cold symptoms are probably the result of the body's immune response to the viral invasion. Virus-infected cells in the nose send out signals that recruit specialized white blood cells to the site of the infection. In turn, these cells emit a range of immune system chemicals such as kinins. These chemicals probably lead to the symptoms of the common cold by causing swelling and inflammation of the nasal membranes, leakage of proteins and fluid from capillaries and lymph vessels, and the increased production of mucus.

Kinins and other chemicals released by immune system cells in the nasal membranes are the subject of intensive research. Researchers are examining whether drugs to block them, or the receptors on cells to which they bind, might benefit people with colds.

How Colds Are Spread

Depending on the virus type, any or all of the following routes of transmission may be common:

- Touching infectious respiratory secretions on skin and on environmental surfaces and then touching the eyes or nose.
- Inhaling relatively large particles of respiratory secretions transported briefly in the air.
- Inhaling droplet nuclei: smaller infectious particles suspended in the air for long periods of time.

Research on rhinovirus transmission. Much of the research on the transmission of the common cold has been done with rhinoviruses, which are shed in the highest concentration in nasal secretions. Studies suggest a person is most likely to transmit rhinoviruses in the second to fourth day of infection, when the amount of virus in nasal secretions is highest. Researchers also have shown that using aspirin to treat colds increases the amount of virus shed in nasal secretions, possibly making the cold sufferer more of a hazard to others.

Prevention

Hand washing is the simplest and most effective way to keep from getting rhinovirus colds. Not touching the nose or eyes is another.

Individuals with colds should always sneeze or cough into a facial tissue, and promptly throw it away. If possible, one should avoid close, prolonged exposure to persons who have colds.

Because rhinoviruses can survive up to three hours outside the nasal passages on inanimate objects and skin, cleaning environmental surfaces with a virus-killing disinfectant might help prevent spread of infection.

A cold vaccine? The development of a vaccine that could prevent the common cold has reached an impasse because of the discovery of many different cold viruses. Each virus carries its own specific antigens, substances that induce the formation of specific protective proteins (antibodies) produced by the body. Until ways are found to combine many viral antigens in one vaccine, or take advantage of the antigenic cross-relationships that exist, prospects for a vaccine are dim. Evidence that changes occur in common-cold virus antigens further complicate development of a vaccine. Such changes occur in some influenza virus antigens and make it necessary to alter the influenza vaccine each year.

Treatment

Only symptomatic treatment is available for uncomplicated cases of the common cold: bed rest, plenty of fluids, gargling with warm salt water, petroleum jelly for a raw nose, and aspirin or acetaminophen to relieve headache or fever.

Nonprescription cold remedies, including decongestants and cough suppressants, may relieve some cold symptoms but will not prevent, cure, or even shorten the duration of illness. Moreover, most have some side effects, such as drowsiness, dizziness, insomnia, or upset stomach, and should be taken with care.

Nonprescription antihistamines may have some effect in relieving inflammatory responses such as runny nose and watery eyes that are commonly associated with colds.

Antibiotics do not kill viruses. These prescription drugs should be used only for rare bacterial complications, such as sinusitis or ear infections, that can develop as secondary infections. The use of antibiotics "just in case" will not prevent secondary bacterial infections.

A word of caution: Several studies have linked the use of aspirin to the development of Reye's syndrome in children recovering from influenza or chickenpox. Reye's syndrome is a rare but serious illness that usually occurs in children between the ages of three and 12 years.

It can affect all organs of the body, but most often injures the brain and liver. While most children who survive an episode of Reye's syndrome do not suffer any lasting consequences, the illness can lead to permanent brain damage or death. The American Academy of Pediatrics recommends children and teenagers not be given aspirin or any medications containing aspirin when they have any viral illness, particularly chickenpox or influenza. Many doctors recommend these medications be used for colds in adults only when headache or fever is present. Researchers, however, have found that aspirin and acetaminophen can suppress certain immune responses and increase nasal stuffiness in adults.

Does vitamin C have a role? Many people are convinced that taking large quantities of vitamin C will prevent colds or relieve symptoms.

Table 32.1. Is It a Cold or the Flu?

Symptoms	**Cold**	**Flu**
Fever	Rare	Characteristic, high (102–104°F); lasts 3–4 days
Headache	Rare	Prominent
General Aches, Pains	Slight	Usual; often severe
Fatigue, Weakness	Quite mild	Can last up to 2–3 weeks
Extreme Exhaustion	Never	Early and prominent
Stuffy Nose	Common	Sometimes
Sneezing	Usual	Sometimes
Sore Throat	Common	Sometimes
Chest Discomfort, Cough	Mild to moderate; hacking cough	Common; can become severe
Complications	Sinus congestion or earache	Bronchitis, pneumonia; can be life-threatening
Prevention	None	Annual vaccination; antiviral medicines—see your doctor
Treatment	Only temporary relief of symptoms	Antiviral medicines—see your doctor

Source: National Institute of Allergy and Infectious Diseases, April 2001.

To test this theory, several large-scale, controlled studies involving children and adults have been conducted. To date, no conclusive data has shown that large doses of vitamin C prevent colds. The vitamin may reduce the severity or duration of symptoms, but there is no definitive evidence.

Taking vitamin C over long periods of time in large amounts may be harmful. Too much vitamin C can cause severe diarrhea, a particular danger for elderly people and small children. In addition, too much vitamin C distorts results of tests commonly used to measure the amount of glucose in urine and blood. Combining oral anticoagulant drugs and excessive amounts of vitamin C can produce abnormal results in blood-clotting tests.

Other treatments. Inhaling steam also has been proposed as a treatment of colds on the assumption that increasing the temperature inside the nose inhibits rhinovirus replication. Recent studies found that this approach had no effect on the symptoms or amount of viral shedding in individuals with rhinovirus colds. But steam may temporarily relieve symptoms of congestion associated with colds.

Interferon-alpha has been studied extensively for the treatment of the common cold. Investigators have shown interferon, given in daily doses by nasal spray, can prevent infection and illness. Interferon, however, causes unacceptable side effects such as nosebleeds and does not appear useful in treating established colds. Most cold researchers are concentrating on other approaches to combating cold viruses.

The Outlook

Thanks to basic research, scientists know more about the rhinovirus than almost any other virus, and have powerful new tools for developing antiviral drugs. Although the common cold may never be uncommon, further investigations offer the hope of reducing the huge burden of this universal problem.

What to Do for Colds

Know When to Call Your Doctor

You usually do not have to call your doctor right away if you have signs of a cold or flu. But you should call your doctor in these situations:

- Your symptoms get worse.

- Your symptoms last a long time.
- After feeling a little better, you develop signs of a more serious problem. Some of these signs are a sick-to-your-stomach feeling, vomiting, high fever, shaking chills, chest pain, or coughing with thick, yellow-green mucus.

Try to Avoid Getting a Cold

- Wash your hands often. You can pick up cold germs easily, even when shaking someone's hand or touching doorknobs or handrails.
- Avoid people with colds when possible.
- If you sneeze or cough, do it into a tissue and then throw the tissue away.
- Clean surfaces you touch with a germ-killing disinfectant.
- Don't touch your nose, eyes, or mouth. Germs can enter your body easily by these paths.

Do Not Take Antibiotics for a Cold

Antibiotics won't work against cold and flu germs. Antibiotics should be taken only when really needed.

Help Yourself Feel Better while You Are Sick

A cold usually lasts only a couple of days to a week. To feel better while you are sick:

- Drink plenty of fluids.
- Get plenty of rest.
- Use a humidifier—an electric device that puts water into the air.
- A cough and cold medicine you buy without a prescription may help.

Choose the Right Medicines for Your Symptoms

Make sure the label states that it treats your symptoms. See Table 32.2 for a list of symptoms and corresponding medicines.

Protect Your Children from "Salicylates" in Cold Medicines

Do not give aspirin or other "salicylates" to children or teenagers with symptoms of a cold or flu. If you aren't sure whether a product has salicylates, ask your doctor or pharmacist. Young people can get sick or die from a rare condition called Reye syndrome if they take these medicines while they have these symptoms.

Table 32.2. Choose the Right Medicine

If You Want to Do This	Choose Medicine With This
Unclog a stuffy nose	Nasal decongestant
Quiet a cough	Cough suppressant
Loosen mucus so you can cough it up	Expectorant
Stop runny nose and sneezing	Antihistamine
Ease fever, headaches, minor aches and pains	Pain Reliever (Analgesic)

Chapter 33

Coxsackie and Other Non-Polio Enteroviruses

Coxsackie Viruses

The coxsackie viruses are part of the enterovirus family of viruses (including echoviruses, polio, and hepatitis A viruses) that live in the human digestive tract. They can spread from person to person, usually on unwashed hands and surfaces contaminated by feces, where they can live for several days. In tropical parts of the world, they infect humans year-round, but in cooler climates, outbreaks of coxsackie virus most often occur in the summer and fall.

Signs and Symptoms

About half of all children with coxsackie virus infection have no symptoms. Some children suddenly develop fevers of 101 to 104 degrees Fahrenheit (38.3 to 40 degrees Celsius), headache, and muscle aches. Some also develop a mild sore throat, abdominal discomfort, or nausea. A child with coxsackie virus may simply feel hot but have no other symptoms. In most children, the fever lasts about 3 days, then

---

"Coxsackie Viruses," originally reviewed by Joel Klein, MD, updated and reviewed by Mary Gavin, MD, was provided by KidsHealth, one of the largest resources online for medically reviewed health information written for parents, kids, and teens. For more articles like this one, visit www.KidsHealth.org, or www.TeensHealth.org. © 2003 The Nemours Center for Children's Health Media, a division of The Nemours Foundation. "Non-Polio Enterovirus Infections," is from the National Center for Infectious Diseases, Centers for Disease Control and Prevention, reviewed August 2001.

disappears; in others, the fever is biphasic: it appears for 1 day, then disappears for 2 to 3 days, then returns for 2 to 4 days more.

Besides causing a simple fever, coxsackie viruses can cause several different patterns of symptoms that affect different body parts:

- hand, foot, and mouth disease, a type of coxsackie virus syndrome, causes painful red blisters on the tongue, gums, and inside the cheeks, and on the palms of hands and soles of feet
- herpangina, a coxsackie virus infection of the throat, causes red-ringed blisters and ulcers on the tonsils and soft palate, the fleshy back portion of the roof of the mouth
- pleurodynia (also called Bornholm disease) is a related coxsackie virus infection that causes painful spasms in the muscles of the chest and upper abdomen. Boys with pleurodynia may also have pain in the testicles beginning about 2 weeks after the chest pain starts.
- hemorrhagic conjunctivitis is an infection that affects the whites of the eyes. In hemorrhagic conjunctivitis, eye pain usually begins suddenly followed by red, watery eyes, swelling, light sensitivity, and blurry vision.

Coxsackie viruses can also cause meningitis, an infection of the membranes that cover the brain, and rarely, encephalitis, a brain infection. They may also cause myocarditis, an infection of the heart muscle.

Newborns, who can be infected from their mothers during or shortly after birth, are more at risk for developing serious infections like meningitis or sepsis (an overwhelming blood infection). Symptoms usually occur within 2 weeks after birth and can include fever, poor feeding, irritability, and lethargy. Infants with coxsackie myocarditis have trouble breathing and sometimes develop cyanosis, a bluish color of the skin, lips, and nails caused by too little oxygen in the blood.

Contagiousness

Coxsackie viruses are very contagious. They are usually passed from person to person on unwashed hands and surfaces contaminated by feces. They can also be spread through droplets of fluid sprayed into the air when someone sneezes or coughs.

When an outbreak of coxsackie virus affects a community, risk for infection is highest among infants and children younger than 5. The virus spreads easily in group settings like schools, child care centers, or summer camp. People who are infected with a coxsackie virus are most contagious the first week they are sick.

Incubation

The incubation period (the time between infection and the onset of symptoms) for most coxsackie virus infections is about 2 to 10 days.

Diagnosis

Doctors diagnose a coxsackie virus by performing a physical exam and looking for any of the telltale symptoms, such as rash or blisters. They might also test stool or fluids from the back of the throat to see if the virus is present.

Treatment

Depending on the type of infection and symptoms, your child's doctor may prescribe medications to make her feel more comfortable. Antibiotics can't be used to fight a coxsackie virus infection because they work only against bacteria.

The most severe forms of coxsackie virus infection, myocarditis and encephalitis, can be fatal, especially in newborns. Even older children with coxsackie myocarditis or encephalitis may need special care in a hospital. However, these complications are rare.

Most children with a simple coxsackie infection recover completely after a few days at home. If your child has a fever without any other symptoms, she should rest in bed or play quietly indoors. Offer plenty of fluids to prevent dehydration. Acetaminophen (such as Tylenol) may be given to relieve any minor aches and pains. If the fever lasts for more than 24 hours or if your child has any symptoms of a more serious coxsackie infection, call your child's doctor.

Duration

The duration of coxsackie virus infection varies, depending on the specific type. For coxsackie fever without other symptoms, a child's temperature may return to normal within 24 hours, although the average fever lasts 3 to 4 days. In pleurodynia, fever and muscle pain usually last 1 to 2 days, and in herpangina, symptoms generally last 3 to 6 days.

Complications

Children with coxsackie virus may become dehydrated because mouth sores can make it painful to eat and drink. If the dehydration is severe, intravenous (IV) fluids may be necessary.

Prevention

There is no vaccine to prevent coxsackie virus infection. Hand washing is the best prevention. Remind the members of your family to wash their hands frequently, particularly after using the toilet (especially those in public places), after changing a diaper, before meals, and before preparing food. Shared toys in child care centers should be routinely cleaned with a disinfectant because the virus can live on these objects for days.

Children who are sick with a coxsackie virus should be kept out of school or day care for a few days to avoid spreading the infection.

When to Call Your Child's Doctor

Call your child's doctor immediately if your child develops any of the following symptoms:

- fever (higher than 100.4 degrees Fahrenheit for infants younger than 6 months of age and higher than 102 degrees Fahrenheit for an older child)
- poor appetite
- trouble feeding
- vomiting
- diarrhea
- difficulty breathing
- convulsions
- unusual sleepiness

Even if your child doesn't have a fever, call your child's doctor for any of the following:

- pain in the chest or abdomen
- sores on the skin or inside the mouth
- difficulty breathing

- severe sore throat
- severe headache, especially with vomiting, confusion, unusual sleepiness, or convulsions
- neck stiffness
- red, swollen, and watery eyes
- pain in one or both testicles

If you are pregnant and have a fever, call your doctor immediately, especially if you are near your due date.

Non-Polio Enterovirus Infections

What are enteroviruses?

Enteroviruses are small viruses that are made of ribonucleic acid (RNA) and protein. This group includes the polioviruses, coxsackieviruses, and echoviruses. In addition to the three different polioviruses, there are 61 non-polio enteroviruses that can cause disease in humans: 23 coxsackie A viruses, 6 coxsackie B viruses, 28 echoviruses, and 4 other enteroviruses.

How common are infections with these viruses?

Non-polio enteroviruses are second only to the "common cold" viruses, the rhinoviruses, as the most common viral infectious agents in humans. The enteroviruses cause an estimated 10–15 million or more symptomatic infections a year in the United States. All three types of polioviruses have been eliminated from the Western Hemisphere by the widespread use of vaccines.

Who is at risk of infection and illness from these viruses?

Everyone is at risk. Infants, children, and adolescents are more likely to be susceptible to infection and illness from these viruses, but adults can also become infected and ill if they do not have immunity to a specific enterovirus.

How does someone become infected with one of these viruses?

Enteroviruses can be found in the respiratory secretions (e.g., saliva, sputum, or nasal mucus) and stool of an infected person. Other persons may become infected by direct contact with secretions from an infected person or by contact with contaminated surfaces or objects, such as a drinking glass or telephone. Parents, teachers, and child care center workers may also become infected by contamination of the hands with stool from an infected infant or toddler during diaper changes.

What time of year is someone at risk for infection/illness?

In the United States, infections caused by the enteroviruses are most likely to occur during the summer and fall.

What illnesses do these viruses cause?

Most people who are infected with an enterovirus have no disease at all. Infected persons who become ill usually develop either mild upper respiratory symptoms (a "cold"), a flu-like illness with fever and muscle aches, or an illness with rash. Less commonly, some persons have aseptic or viral meningitis. Rarely, a person may develop an illness that affects the heart (myocarditis) or the brain (encephalitis) or causes paralysis. Enterovirus infections are suspected to play a role in the development of juvenile-onset diabetes mellitus (sugar diabetes). Newborns who become infected with an enterovirus may rarely develop an overwhelming infection of many organs, including liver and heart, and die from the infection.

Are there any long-term complications from these illnesses?

Usually, there are no long-term complications from the mild illnesses or from aseptic meningitis. Some patients who have paralysis or encephalitis, however, do not fully recover. Persons who develop heart failure (dilated cardiomyopathy) from myocarditis require long-term care for their conditions.

What are the health care costs of these infections?

The health care costs from enterovirus infections are unknown, but a large portion of the costs may come from use of over-the-counter medications to treat symptoms for millions of cases of "summer colds and flu". There are also significant costs associated with the 30,000 to 50,000 hospitalizations for aseptic meningitis each year in the United States.

Are these infections more severe in some years than in others?

There are no predictable patterns of circulation of these viruses or of diseases such as aseptic meningitis. There are occasional national or regional outbreaks of aseptic meningitis, such as the echovirus 30 outbreaks in the United States between 1989 and 1992. However, there is significant yearly variation, and no long-term trends have been identified.

Can these infections be prevented?

No vaccine is currently available for the non-polio enteroviruses. General cleanliness and frequent handwashing are probably effective in reducing the spread of these viruses.

Do CDC and state health departments keep track of these viruses?

State health department laboratories report to CDC the enteroviruses they identify by testing specimens from patients. Aseptic meningitis is no longer a nationally notifiable disease in the United States. Other forms of meningitis and poliomyelitis are notifiable, which means that any doctor or laboratory that diagnoses a case must report it to the public health department.

Chapter 34

Epstein-Barr Virus and Infectious Mononucleosis

Disease Information

Epstein-Barr virus, frequently referred to as EBV, is a member of the herpesvirus family and one of the most common human viruses. The virus occurs worldwide, and most people become infected with EBV sometime during their lives. In the United States, as many as 95% of adults between 35 and 40 years of age have been infected. Infants become susceptible to EBV as soon as maternal antibody protection (present at birth) disappears. Many children become infected with EBV, and these infections usually cause no symptoms or are indistinguishable from the other mild, brief illnesses of childhood. In the United States and in other developed countries, many persons are not infected with EBV in their childhood years. When infection with EBV occurs during adolescence or young adulthood, it causes infectious mononucleosis 35% to 50% of the time.

Symptoms of infectious mononucleosis are fever, sore throat, and swollen lymph glands. Sometimes, a swollen spleen or liver involvement may develop. Heart problems or involvement of the central nervous system occurs only rarely, and infectious mononucleosis is almost never fatal. There are no known associations between active EBV infection and problems during pregnancy, such as miscarriages or birth defects. Although the symptoms of infectious mononucleosis usually

---

"Epstein-Barr Virus and Infectious Mononucleosis," National Center for Infectious Diseases, Centers for Disease Control and Prevention (CDC), updated October 26, 2002.

resolve in 1 or 2 months, EBV remains dormant or latent in a few cells in the throat and blood for the rest of the person's life. Periodically, the virus can reactivate and is commonly found in the saliva of infected persons. This reactivation usually occurs without symptoms of illness.

EBV also establishes a lifelong dormant infection in some cells of the body's immune system. A late event in a very few carriers of this virus is the emergence of Burkitt's lymphoma and nasopharyngeal carcinoma, two rare cancers that are not normally found in the United States. EBV appears to play an important role in these malignancies, but is probably not the sole cause of disease.

Most individuals exposed to people with infectious mononucleosis have previously been infected with EBV and are not at risk for infectious mononucleosis. In addition, transmission of EBV requires intimate contact with the saliva (found in the mouth) of an infected person. Transmission of this virus through the air or blood does not normally occur. The incubation period, or the time from infection to appearance of symptoms, ranges from 4 to 6 weeks. Persons with infectious mononucleosis may be able to spread the infection to others for a period of weeks. However, no special precautions or isolation procedures are recommended, since the virus is also found frequently in the saliva of healthy people. In fact, many healthy people can carry and spread the virus intermittently for life. These people are usually the primary reservoir for person-to-person transmission. For this reason, transmission of the virus is almost impossible to prevent.

The clinical diagnosis of infectious mononucleosis is suggested on the basis of the symptoms of fever, sore throat, swollen lymph glands, and the age of the patient. Usually, laboratory tests are needed for confirmation. Serologic results for persons with infectious mononucleosis include an elevated white blood cell count, an increased percentage of certain atypical white blood cells, and a positive reaction to a "mono spot" test.

There is no specific treatment for infectious mononucleosis, other than treating the symptoms. No antiviral drugs or vaccines are available. Some physicians have prescribed a 5-day course of steroids to control the swelling of the throat and tonsils. The use of steroids has also been reported to decrease the overall length and severity of illness, but these reports have not been published.

It is important to note that symptoms related to infectious mononucleosis caused by EBV infection seldom last for more than 4 months. When such an illness lasts more than 6 months, it is frequently called chronic EBV infection. However, valid laboratory evidence for continued active EBV infection is seldom found in these patients. The illness should be investigated further to determine if it meets the criteria for chronic fatigue syndrome, or CFS. This process includes ruling out other causes of chronic illness or fatigue. For additional information about chronic fatigue syndrome, please call CDC's toll-free line at 888-232-3228; after the call goes through, press 22136 to get the CFS menu.

Diagnosis of EBV Infections

In most cases of infectious mononucleosis, the clinical diagnosis can be made from the characteristic triad of fever, pharyngitis, and lymphadenopathy lasting for 1 to 4 weeks. Serologic test results include a normal to moderately elevated white blood cell count, an increased total number of lymphocytes, greater than 10% atypical lymphocytes, and a positive reaction to a "mono spot" test. In patients with symptoms compatible with infectious mononucleosis, a positive Paul-Bunnell heterophile antibody test result is diagnostic, and no further testing is necessary. Moderate-to-high levels of heterophile antibodies are seen during the first month of illness and decrease rapidly after week 4. False-positive results may be found in a small number of patients, and false-negative results may be obtained in 10% to 15% of patients, primarily in children younger than 10 years of age. True outbreaks of infectious mononucleosis are extremely rare. A substantial number of pseudo-outbreaks have been linked to laboratory error, as reported in CDC's *Morbidity and Mortality Weekly Report*, vol. 40, no. 32, on August 16, 1991.

When "mono spot" or heterophile test results are negative, additional laboratory testing may be needed to differentiate EBV infections from a mononucleosis-like illness induced by cytomegalovirus, adenovirus, or *Toxoplasma gondii*. Direct detection of EBV in blood or lymphoid tissues is a research tool and is not available for routine diagnosis. Instead, serologic testing is the method of choice for diagnosing primary infection.

EBV-Specific Laboratory Tests

Laboratory tests are not always foolproof. For various reasons, false-positive and false-negative results can occur for any test. However, the laboratory tests for EBV are for the most part accurate and specific. Because the antibody response in primary EBV infection appears to be quite rapid, in most cases testing paired acute- and convalescent-phase serum samples will not demonstrate a significant change in antibody level. Effective laboratory diagnosis can be made on a single acute-phase serum sample by testing for antibodies to several EBV-associated antigens simultaneously. In most cases, a distinction can be made as to whether a person is susceptible to EBV, has had a recent infection, has had infection in the past, or has a reactivated EBV infection.

Antibodies to several antigen complexes may be measured. These antigens are the viral capsid antigen, the early antigen, and the EBV nuclear antigen (EBNA). In addition, differentiation of immunoglobulin G (IgG) and M (IgM) subclasses to the viral capsid antigen can often be helpful for confirmation. When the "mono spot" test is negative, the optimal combination of EBV serologic testing consists of the antibody titration of four markers: IgM and IgG to the viral capsid antigen, IgM to the early antigen, and antibody to EBNA.

IgM to the viral capsid antigen appears early in infection and disappears within 4 to 6 weeks. IgG to the viral capsid antigen appears in the acute phase, peaks at 2 to 4 weeks after onset, declines slightly, and then persists for life. IgG to the early antigen appears in the acute phase and generally falls to undetectable levels after 3 to 6 months. In many people, detection of antibody to the early antigen is a sign of active infection, but 20% of healthy people may have this antibody for years.

Antibody to EBNA determined by the standard immunofluorescent test is not seen in the acute phase, but slowly appears 2 to 4 months after onset, and persists for life. This is not true for some EBNA enzyme immunoassays, which detect antibody within a few weeks of onset.

Finally, even when EBV antibody tests, such as the early antigen test, suggest that reactivated infection is present, this result does not necessarily indicate that a patient's current medical condition is caused by EBV infection. A number of healthy people with no symptoms have antibodies to the EBV early antigen for years after their initial EBV infection.

Therefore, interpretation of laboratory results is somewhat complex and should be left to physicians who are familiar with EBV testing and who have access to the entire clinical picture of a person. To determine if EBV infection is associated with a current illness, consult with an experienced physician.

Additional Information about EBV Antibody Tests and Interpretation

Antibody tests for EBV can measure the presence and/or the concentration of at least six specific EBV antibodies. By evaluating the results of these different tests, the stage of EBV infection can be determined. However, these tests are expensive and not usually needed for the diagnosis of infectious mononucleosis.

It is not appropriate for CDC to interpret test results or to handle counseling for the public. We suggest that questions be directed to a local physician who is familiar with the patient's history and laboratory test results. In addition, CDC cannot recommend specific physicians for referral. Our general recommendation is for patients to consult with an infectious disease specialist or their local or state public health department.

Summary of Interpretation

The diagnosis of EBV infection is summarized as follows.

Susceptibility

If antibodies to the viral capsid antigen are not detected, the patient is susceptible to EBV infection.

Primary Infection

Primary EBV infection is indicated if IgM antibody to the viral capsid antigen is present and antibody to EBV nuclear antigen, or EBNA, is absent. A rising or high IgG antibody to the viral capsid antigen and negative antibody to EBNA after at least 4 weeks of illness is also strongly suggestive of primary infection. In addition, 80% of patients with active EBV infection produce antibody to early antigen.

Past Infection

If antibodies to both the viral capsid antigen and EBNA are present, then past infection (from 4 to 6 months to years earlier) is indicated. Since 95% of adults have been infected with EBV, most adults will show antibodies to EBV from infection years earlier. High or elevated antibody levels may be present for years and are not diagnostic of recent infection.

Reactivation

In the presence of antibodies to EBNA, an elevation of antibodies to early antigen suggests reactivation. However, when EBV antibody to the early antigen test is present, this result does not automatically indicate that a patient's current medical condition is caused by EBV. A number of healthy people with no symptoms have antibodies to the EBV early antigen for years after their initial EBV infection. Many times reactivation occurs subclinically.

Chronic EBV Infection

Reliable laboratory evidence for continued active EBV infection is very seldom found in patients who have been ill for more than 4 months. When the illness lasts more than 6 months, it should be investigated to see if other causes of chronic illness or CFS are present.

Chapter 35

Fifth Disease and Parvovirus B19

What is fifth disease?

Fifth disease is a mild rash illness that occurs most commonly in children. The ill child typically has a "slapped-cheek" rash on the face and a lacy red rash on the trunk and limbs. Occasionally, the rash may itch. An ill child may have a low-grade fever, malaise, or a "cold" a few days before the rash breaks out. The child is usually not very ill, and the rash resolves in 7 to 10 days.

What causes fifth disease?

Fifth disease is caused by infection with human parvovirus B19. This virus infects only humans. Pet dogs or cats may be immunized against "parvovirus," but these are animal parvoviruses that do not infect humans. Therefore, a child cannot "catch" parvovirus from a pet dog or cat, and a pet cat or dog cannot catch human parvovirus B19 from an ill child.

Can adults get fifth disease?

Yes, they can. An adult who is not immune can be infected with parvovirus B19 and either have no symptoms or develop the typical rash of fifth disease, joint pain or swelling, or both. Usually, joints on

---

"Fifth Disease," National Center for Infectious Diseases, Centers for Disease Control and Prevention (CDC), reviewed September 7, 2000

both sides of the body are affected. The joints most frequently affected are the hands, wrists, and knees. The joint pain and swelling usually resolve in a week or two, but they may last several months. About 50% of adults, however, have been previously infected with parvovirus B19, have developed immunity to the virus, and cannot get fifth disease.

Is fifth disease contagious?

Yes. A person infected with parvovirus B19 is contagious during the early part of the illness, before the rash appears. By the time a child has the characteristic "slapped cheek" rash of fifth disease, for example, he or she is probably no longer contagious and may return to school or child care center. This contagious period is different than that for many other rash illnesses, such as measles, for which the child is contagious while he or she has the rash.

How does someone get infected with parvovirus B19?

Parvovirus B19 has been found in the respiratory secretions (e.g., saliva, sputum, or nasal mucus) of infected persons before the onset of rash, when they appear to "just have a cold." The virus is probably spread from person to person by direct contact with those secretions, such as sharing drinking cups or utensils. In a household, as many as 50% of susceptible persons exposed to a family member who has fifth disease may become infected. During school outbreaks, 10% to 60% of students may get fifth disease.

How soon after infection with parvovirus B19 does a person become ill?

A susceptible person usually becomes ill 4 to 14 days after being infected with the virus, but may become ill for as long as 20 days after infection.

Does everyone who is infected with parvovirus B19 become ill?

No. During outbreaks of fifth disease, about 20% of adults and children who are infected with parvovirus B19 do not develop any symptoms. Furthermore, other persons infected with the virus will have a non-specific illness that is not characteristic of fifth disease. Persons infected with the virus, however, do develop lasting immunity that protects them against infection in the future.

How is fifth disease diagnosed?

A physician can often diagnose fifth disease by seeing the typical rash during a physical examination. In cases in which it is important to confirm the diagnosis, a blood test may be done to look for antibodies to parvovirus. Antibodies are proteins produced by the immune system in response to parvovirus B19 and other germs. If immunoglobulin M (IgM) antibody to parvovirus B19 is detected, the test result suggests that the person has had a recent infection.

Is fifth disease serious?

Fifth disease is usually a mild illness that resolves on its own among children and adults who are otherwise healthy. Joint pain and swelling in adults usually resolve without long-term disability.

Parvovirus B19 infection may cause a serious illness in persons with sickle-cell disease or similar types of chronic anemia. In such persons, parvovirus B19 can cause an acute, severe anemia. The ill person may be pale, weak, and tired, and should see his or her physician for treatment. (The typical rash of fifth disease is rarely seen in these persons.) Once the infection is controlled, the anemia resolves. Furthermore, persons who have problems with their immune systems may also develop a chronic anemia with parvovirus B19 infection that requires medical treatment. People who have leukemia or cancer, who are born with immune deficiencies, who have received an organ transplant, or who have human immunodeficiency virus (HIV) infection are at risk for serious illness due to parvovirus B19 infection.

Occasionally, serious complications may develop from parvovirus B19 infection during pregnancy.

How are parvovirus B19 infections treated?

Treatment of symptoms such as fever, pain, or itching is usually all that is needed for fifth disease. Adults with joint pain and swelling may need to rest, restrict their activities, and take medicines such as aspirin or ibuprofen to relieve symptoms. The few people who have severe anemia caused by parvovirus B19 infection may need to be hospitalized and receive blood transfusions. Persons with immune problems may need special medical care, including treatment with immune globulin (antibodies), to help their bodies get rid of the infection.

Can parvovirus B19 infection be prevented?

There is no vaccine or medicine that prevents parvovirus B19 infection. Frequent handwashing is recommended as a practical and probably effective method to decrease the chance of becoming infected. Excluding persons with fifth disease from work, child care centers, or schools is not likely to prevent the spread of the virus, since people are contagious before they develop the rash.

Chapter 36

Genital Warts (Human Papillomavirus)

What is human papillomavirus?

Human papillomavirus (HPV) is one of the most common causes of sexually transmitted disease (STD) in the world. Health experts estimate that there are more cases of genital HPV infection than of any other STD in the United States. According to the American Social Health Association, approximately 5.5 million new cases of sexually transmitted HPV infections are reported every year. At least 20 million Americans are already infected.

Scientists have identified more than 100 types of HPV, most of which are harmless. About 30 types are spread through sexual contact. Some types of HPV that cause genital infections can also cause cervical cancer and other genital cancers.

Like many STDs, genital HPV infections often do not have visible signs and symptoms. One study sponsored by the National Institute of Allergy and Infectious Diseases (NIAID) reported that almost half of the women infected with HPV had no obvious symptoms. People who are infected but who have no symptoms may not know they can transmit HPV to others or that they can develop complications from the virus.

"Human Papillomavirus and Genital Warts," National Institute of Allergy and Infectious Diseases (NIAID), National Institutes of Health (NIH), March 2001.

What are genital warts?

Genital warts (condylomata acuminata or venereal warts) are the most easily recognized sign of genital HPV infection. Many people, however, have a genital HPV infection without genital warts.

Can HPV cause other kinds of warts?

Some types of HPV cause common skin warts, such as those found on the hands and soles of the feet. These types of HPV do not cause genital warts.

How are genital warts spread?

Genital warts are very contagious and are spread during oral, genital, or anal sex with an infected partner. About two-thirds of people who have sexual contact with a partner with genital warts will develop warts, usually within three months of contact.

In women, the warts occur on the outside and inside of the vagina, on the opening (cervix) to the womb (uterus), or around the anus. In men, genital warts are less common. If present, they usually are seen on the tip of the penis. They also may be found on the shaft of the penis, on the scrotum, or around the anus. Rarely, genital warts also can develop in the mouth or throat of a person who has had oral sex with an infected person.

Genital warts often occur in clusters and can be very tiny or can spread into large masses in the genital or anal area.

How are genital warts diagnosed?

A doctor or other health care worker usually can diagnose genital warts by seeing them on a patient. Women with genital warts also should be examined for possible HPV infection of the cervix.

The doctor may be able to identify some otherwise invisible warts in the genital tissue by applying vinegar (acetic acid) to areas of suspected infection. This solution causes infected areas to whiten, which makes them more visible, particularly if a procedure called colposcopy is performed. During colposcopy, the doctor uses a magnifying instrument to look at the vagina and cervix. In some cases, the doctor takes a small piece of tissue from the cervix and examines it under the microscope.

A Pap smear test also may indicate the possible presence of cervical HPV infection. In a Pap smear, a laboratory worker examines cells scraped from the cervix under a microscope to see if they are cancerous. If a woman's Pap smear is abnormal, she might have an HPV infection. If a woman has an abnormal Pap smear, she should have her doctor examine her further to look for and treat any cervical problems.

What is the treatment for genital warts?

Genital warts often disappear even without treatment. In other cases, they eventually may develop a fleshy, small raised growth that looks like cauliflower. There is no way to predict whether the warts will grow or disappear. Therefore, if you suspect you have genital warts, you should be examined and treated, if necessary.

Depending on factors such as the size and location of the genital warts, a doctor will offer you one of several ways to treat them.

- Imiquimod, an immune response cream which you can apply to the affected area
- A 20 percent podophyllin anti-mitotic solution, which you can apply to the affected area and later wash off
- A 0.5 percent podofilox solution, applied to the affected area but shouldn't be washed off
- A 5 percent 5-fluorouracil cream
- Trichloroacetic acid (TCA)

If you are pregnant, you should not use podophyllin or podofilox because they are absorbed by the skin and may cause birth defects in your baby. In addition, you should not use 5-fluorouracil cream if you are expecting.

If you have small warts, the doctor can remove them by freezing (cryosurgery), burning (electrocautery), or laser treatment. Occasionally, the doctor will have to use surgery to remove large warts that have not responded to other treatment.

Some doctors use the antiviral drug alpha interferon, which they inject directly into the warts, to treat warts that have returned after removal by traditional means. The drug is expensive, however, and does not reduce the rate that the genital warts return.

Although treatments can get rid of the warts, none gets rid of the virus. Because the virus is still present in your body, warts often come back after treatment.

How can HPV infection be prevented?

The only way you can prevent getting an HPV infection is to avoid direct contact with the virus, which is transmitted by skin-to-skin contact. If you or your sexual partner have warts that are visible in the genital area, you should avoid any sexual contact until the warts are treated. Studies have not confirmed that male latex condoms prevent transmission of HPV itself, but results do suggest that condom use may reduce the risk of developing diseases linked to HPV, such as genital warts and cervical cancer.

Can HPV and genital warts cause complications?

Cancer. Some types of HPV can cause cervical cancer. Others, however, cause cervical cancer and also are associated with vulvar cancer, anal cancer, and cancer of the penis (a rare cancer).

Most HPV infections do not progress to cervical cancer. If a woman does have abnormal cervical cells, a Pap test will detect them. It is particularly important for women who have abnormal cervical cells to have regular pelvic exams and Pap tests so that they can be treated early, if necessary.

Pregnancy and Childbirth. Genital warts may cause a number of problems during pregnancy. Sometimes they get larger during pregnancy, making it difficult to urinate. If the warts are in the vagina, they can make the vagina less elastic and cause obstruction during delivery.

Rarely, infants born to women with genital warts develop warts in their throats (laryngeal papillomatosis). Although uncommon, it is a potentially life-threatening condition for the child, requiring frequent laser surgery to prevent obstruction of the breathing passages. Research on the use of interferon therapy in combination with laser surgery indicates that this drug may show promise in slowing the course of the disease.

What research is going on?

Scientists are doing research on two types of HPV vaccines. One type would be used to prevent infection or disease (warts or precancerous tissue changes). The other type would be used to treat cervical cancers. Researchers are testing both types of vaccines in people.

Chapter 37

Hepatitis

The ABCs of Hepatitis

Hepatitis Facts: Worldwide Snapshot

Hepatitis A Virus (HAV) Infection

- Medical care alone for hepatitis A can cost $2,800 for each hospitalized case.
- Approximately 100 Americans die each year from Hepatitis A.
- The annual cost associated with Hepatitis A is estimated at $200 million in the U.S.

Hepatitis B Virus (HBV) Infection

- HBV is 100 times more infectious than HIV, the virus that can cause AIDS.
- Hepatitis B vaccine can provide immunity in over 95% of young healthy adults.
- An estimated 350 million people are infected globally with HBV.

- Approximately 1 million die each year from complications from HBV.
- 70% of new cases occur among people between the ages of 15–39.
- Every year 5,000 Americans die from cirrhosis and 1,000 from liver cancer due to HBV infections.
- 22,000 pregnant women in the U.S. are infected with HBV and can transmit it to their newborns.
- HBV can live on a dry surface for at least 7 days.

Hepatitis C Virus (HCV) Infection

- 3% of the world's population is infected with HCV, or approximately 170 million people. 90% of HCV patients who are in need of treatment today cannot afford it.
- 80% of affected people can become chronically infected and risk serious long-term clinical disease including cirrhosis and liver cancer.
- 8 countries—Bolivia, Burundi, Cameroon, Egypt, Guinea, Mongolia, Rwanda, and Tanzania—have an HCV prevalence above 10%.
- 7 countries/areas—Gabon, Libya, Papua New Guinea, Suriname, Vietnam, Zaire, and the United Nations Relief and Works Agency for Palestine Refugees in the Near East—have an HCV prevalence between 5 and 10%.
- In developing countries, the primary sources of HCV infection include transfusion of blood or blood products from unscreened donors; transfusion of blood products that have not undergone viral inactivation; parenteral exposure to blood through the use of contaminated or adequately sterilized instruments and needles used in medical and dental procedures; the use of unsterilized objects for rituals (for example, circumcision, scarification), traditional medicine (for example, blood-letting) or other activities that break the skin (for example, tattooing, ear or body-piercing); and intravenous drug use. Household or sexual contacts of HCV-infected persons are marginally at risk.
- In developed countries, persons at risk of HCV infection include recipients of previously unscreened blood, blood products, and

organs; intravenous drug users; individuals undergoing chronic hemodialysis; health care workers with percutaneous exposure from contaminated needles or sharps; persons who participate in high-risk sexual practices; and persons undergoing medical or dental procedures with inadequately sterilized instruments. Sexual and household transmission are uncommon.

Basics: Hepatitis A (HAV)

What Is Hepatitis A?

Hepatitis A is one of many hepatitis viruses causing inflammation of the liver.

Who Is at Risk?

Hepatitis A can affect anyone. In the U.S., hepatitis A can occur in situations ranging from isolated cases of disease to widespread epidemics. Hepatitis A is one of the most frequently reported vaccine-preventable diseases in the U.S. Some of the higher-risk groups are: travelers to countries with high rates of hepatitis A, men who have sex with men, injecting-drug users, people with clotting-factor disorders, people with chronic liver disease, and children living in communities with high rates of disease.

Symptoms

Children with hepatitis A usually have no symptoms. Adults may become quite ill suddenly, experiencing jaundice, fatigue, nausea, vomiting, abdominal pain, dark urine/light stools, and fever. The incubation period averages 30 days. However, an infected individual can transmit the virus to others as early as two weeks before symptoms appear. Symptoms will disappear over a 6–12-month period until complete recovery occurs.

Diagnosis

Your doctor can't single out Hepatitis A from other types of viral hepatitis based upon your physical symptoms alone. The only way to diagnose HAV is to do a blood test seeking to find IgM antibodies. In most people, these antibodies become detectable 5–10 days before the onset of symptoms and can persist for up to 6 months after infection.

How Does It Spread?

Hepatitis A is most often spread from person to person through situations such as these:

- Food preparers who are infected can pass the virus on if they do not wash their hands with soap and water after having a bowel movement, especially when they prepare uncooked foods.
- Fecal contamination of food and water.
- Anal/oral contact, by putting something in the mouth that had been contaminated with infected feces.
- Diaper changing tables, if not cleaned properly or changed after each use, may facilitate the spread of HAV.
- Fecal residue may remain on the hands of people changing soiled diapers.
- Eating raw or partially cooked shellfish contaminated with HAV.

Treatment

No specific treatment is necessary for hepatitis A disease.

Outcome

Hepatitis A will clear up on its own in a few weeks or months with no serious after effects. Once recovered, an individual is then immune for life to HAV through the presence of the IgG antibody. About 1 in 100 HAV sufferers may experience a sudden and severe (that is, "fulminant") infection.

Preventing HAV

Infection HAV infection is preventable. Here's how you do it:

- Get an immune globulin (IG) shot. An IG shot can provide temporary immunity to the virus for 2 to 3 months when given prior to exposure to HAV or within 2 weeks after exposure.
- Ask for the HAV vaccine. The HAV vaccine, made from inactive hepatitis A virus (synthetic), is highly effective in preventing the hepatitis A infection. However, its safety when given during pregnancy has not been determined. Check with your doctor to determine how many shots you need. The vaccine provides

protection for about four weeks after the first injection; a second injection protects you longer, possibly up to 20 years.

Who Should Have the HAV Vaccine?

- Users of illegal drugs.
- Individuals who have chronic liver disease or blood clotting disorders (for example, hemophilia).
- Those who have close physical contact with people who live in areas with poor sanitary conditions.
- Those who travel or work in developing countries. This includes all countries except northern and western Europe, Japan, Australia, New Zealand, and North America except Mexico.
- Men who have sex with other men.
- Children in populations that have repeated epidemics of hepatitis A (for example, Alaska natives, American Indians, and certain closed religious communities).
- People who have chronic lever disease.

Basics: Hepatitis B (HBV)

What Is Hepatitis B?

Hepatitis B is an inflammatory liver disease caused by the hepatitis B virus (HBV) that results in liver cell damage. This damage can lead to scarring of the liver (cirrhosis) and increased risk of liver cancer in some people. About 80,000 Americans were newly infected with HBV in 1999.

Who Is at Risk?

One out of every 20 people in the U. S. will become infected with HBV sometime during their lives. Your risk is higher if you:

- Have sex with someone infected with HBV.
- Have sex with more than one partner.
- Are a man and have sex with a man.
- Live in the same house with someone who has chronic HBV infection.
- Have a job that involves contact with human blood.

- Inject illegal substances/drugs. Have hemophilia.
- Travel to areas where HBV is common (this includes all countries except northern and western Europe, Japan, Australia, New Zealand, and North America except Mexico).

Symptoms

Many people with newly acquired hepatitis B have no symptoms at all, or they may be very mild and flu-like—loss of appetite, nausea, fatigue, muscle or joint aches, mild fever, and possibly jaundice (yellowish tinge to the skin). The only way to know if you are currently infected with HBV—or if you still carry the virus—is to ask your doctor to do a specific blood test for hepatitis B (it may not be included in a routine blood test). The test may not show positive during the incubation period (45–180 days).

Diagnosis

There are three standard blood tests for HBV:

- HBsAG (hepatitis B surface antigen): When this test is positive or reactive, you are infected with HBV and can pass it on to others.
- Anti-HBc (antibody to hepatitis B core antigen): When you test positive, it means you are currently infected with HBV or have been infected at some point in the past.
- Anti-HBs (antibody to HbsAg): When this test is positive, it means that you are immune to hepatitis B either as a result of having had the disease or from having been given the vaccine.

How Does It Spread?

HBV is found in blood, seminal fluid, and vaginal secretions. The risk of transmission is increased in these situations:

- Sexual contact with an infected person.
- Living in the same household with an infected individual.
- Contact with infected blood or seminal fluid and contaminated needles, including tattoo/body piercing instruments.
- HBV-infected mother to her newborn at time of delivery (prenatal blood tests for HBV should always be done if there is a suspicion of HBV).

Treating HBV

There are two medications to treat chronic HBV—Interferon (IFN) and Lamivudine. Less than 50% of patients with chronic HBV are candidates for interferon therapy. Initially, 40% of HBV patients who are treated with IFN will respond. However, some will relapse when the treatment is stopped. Overall, about 35% of the eligible patients will benefit. IFN treatments may have a number of side effects, including flu-like symptoms, headache, nausea, vomiting, loss of appetite, depression, diarrhea, fatigue, and thinning hair. Interferon may lower the production of white blood cells and platelets by depressing the bone marrow. Thus, blood tests are needed to monitor blood cells, platelets, and liver enzymes. The response to oral Lamivudine, given for at least one year, may be somewhat lower. In addition, those who are chronically infected with HBV should be vaccinated against hepatitis A. There is no treatment for acute Hepatitis B.

Disease Outcome

- Either you develop immunity to HBV—95% of adults infected develop antibodies and recover spontaneously within six months. Upon recovery, they develop immunity to the virus and they are not infectious to others. Blood tests will always test positive for the HBV antibody. Blood banks will not accept donations of blood from HBV-immune people.
- OR you become chronically infected. About 5% of the time, the virus clear the body within six months. If so, a person is considered a carrier—or chronically infected. Chronically infected people may or may not show outward signs or symptoms. The HBV virus remains in blood and body fluids, and can infect others.

Preventing HBV Infection

Things you can do:

- Practice safe sex (use latex condoms).
- Don't share anything that could have an infected person's blood on it, such as toothbrushes, razors, nail clippers, body piercing instruments.
- Don't share drug needles, cocaine straws or any drug paraphernalia.

- Cover all sores and rashes and do not touch them.
- Clean up any blood spills with a 10% solution of household bleach. Infected persons should not pre-chew food for babies.
- If exposed to hepatitis B, get an HBIG (hepatitis B immune globulin) injection within 14 days following exposure.

Get an HBV Vaccination

Here's who should be vaccinated without fail:

- All individuals living in the same household with a chronically infected individual.
- All newborns and children up to the age of 19.
- Those who are in positions where they are exposed to blood at work, through drug use, or who have multiple sex partners.
- Individuals with hepatitis C and other chronic liver diseases.

Vaccination provides protection for more than 15 years, and possibly a lifetime. HBV booster shots are not recommended.

Newborn Vaccination

All newborns should get three vaccination doses of the HBV vaccine—the first within 12 hours of birth, the second at 1–2 months, and the third at 6 months. In addition, babies born to infected mothers should receive a shot called H-BIG within 12 hours of delivery. Without the above intervention, 90% of babies born to infected mothers will become chronically infected, reducing their life expectancies. A few months after the last dose is given, the doctor will test to see if the baby is making HBV antibodies. If so, the baby will be safe from hepatitis B for life. HBV-infected mothers may nurse their babies.

Basics: Hepatitis C (HCV)

What Is Hepatitis C?

Hepatitis C virus (HCV) causes inflammation of the liver. A national U. S. survey found that 1.8 percent of Americans—about 3.9 million—have been infected with HCV, of whom most—about 2.7 million—are chronically infected with HCV, with many showing no signs or symptoms. The good news is that, in 1995, a reliable antibody test for HCV was finally implemented nationwide. About 41,000 new cases occurred in 1998 with 15–25% recovering spontaneously. Hepatitis C is a slow-progressing disease that may take 10–40 years to cause serious liver damage in some people.

Who Is at Risk?

Since about four million Americans are infected with HCV and most don't know it, you should have a blood test for hepatitis C—whether you feel sick or not. About one in ten people infected with HCV have had no identifiable exposure to HCV. That said, here are several obvious risk factors:

- Intravenous (IV) drug users—even IV use in the distant past.
- Those with multiple sex partners or sex with partners who have other sexually transmitted diseases.
- Those with tattoos or body piercing done with unsterile instruments. Anyone who has had a blood transfusion prior to 1992 or clotting factors produced before 1987.
- Hemodialysis (diabetes) patients.
- The potential for transmission from an HCV-infected mother to her newborn appears to be about 5%.

How Does It Spread?

- Injection drug use is the primary risk for HCV infection. Injection drug use accounts for about 60% of all new cases of hepatitis C and is a major risk factor for infection with hepatitis B virus. Among frequent drug users, 50–80% are infected by HCV within the first 12 months of beginning injecting.
- Straws shared in snorting drugs are also a potential source of infection of HCV. The hepatitis C virus is found mainly in blood.
- HCV is not spread through kissing or casual contact.
- In relationships where there is one steady partner, sexual transmission is low (under 5%). Transmission is estimated to be about 15% among those who have multiple sex partners or where there is a history of sexually transmitted diseases.
- HCV may be transmitted by using razors, needles, toothbrushes, nail files, a barber's scissors, tattooing equipment, body

piercing or acupuncture needles if these items are contaminated by blood of an infected person.

- Healthcare workers have a 2% risk of acquiring HCV after a needle stick contaminated with HCV-positive blood.
- There is no evidence indicating that HCV is transmitted through breast milk.
- The current transmission rate through blood transfusions is estimated at less than 1 per 1,000,000 units transfused.

Symptoms

Most people who are infected with the HCV do not have symptoms and are leading normal lives. If symptoms are present, they may be very mild and flu-like—nausea, fatigue, loss of appetite, fever, headaches, and abdominal pain. Most people do not have jaundice although jaundice can sometimes occur along with dark urine.

The incubation period varies from 2–26 weeks. Liver enzyme tests may range from being elevated to being normal for weeks to as long as a year. The virus is in the blood and may be causing liver cell damage, and the infected person can transmit the disease to others.

Diagnosis

Test for HCV antibodies: HCV infection can be determined by a simple and specific blood test that detects antibodies against HCV. The current enzyme immunoassay test (EIA) that detects anti-HCV has a sensitivity of about 95% in chronic HCV. HCV infection may be identified by anti-HCV testing in approximately 80% of people as early as five weeks after exposure. This test is not a part of a routine physical examination, and people must ask their doctor for a hepatitis C antibody test. (Note: The antibody itself does not provide immunity, and the test does not distinguish between acute or chronic infection.) If the initial test is positive, it test should be repeated to confirm the diagnosis (and exclude possible laboratory error). If the initial test is negative, but the infection could have occurred within the last six months and HCV is suspected, antibody levels may not be high enough yet to be detectable (antibodies may not be present in the first 4 weeks of infection in about 30% of patients) or you may lack immune response. Under these circumstances, ask you doctor about repeating the test and about alternative test methods.

Test liver enzyme levels: If you may already have chronic infection, your doctor will test the levels of two liver enzymes. These are alanine aminotransferase (ALT) and aspartate aminotransferase (AST). Both are released when liver cells are injured or die. Elevated ALT and AST levels may appear and disappear throughout the course of the HCV infection. If the liver enzyme levels are normal with chronic HCV, they should be re-checked several times over a 6–12 month period. If the liver enzyme levels remain normal, your doctor may check them less frequently, such as once a year.

Treating HCV

- There are three types of interferon, plus a combination of interferon and ribavirin, used to treat hepatitis C. Blood tests and liver biopsy findings may determine the need for treatment.
- Interferon must be given by injection, and may have a number of side effects, including flu-like symptoms—headaches, fever, fatigue, loss of appetite, nausea, vomiting, and thinning of hair.
- Ribavirin, given by mouth, can have additional side effects including depression, severe anemia and especially birth defects. Women or the male partners of women, who are pregnant or who are planning pregnancy, should not take ribavirin. Pregnancy should not be attempted until six months after treatment is ended. Ribavirin may also interfere with the production of red blood cells and platelets by depressing bone marrow. Patients should be monitored frequently.
- While 50–60% of patients respond to treatment initially, sustained response occurs in up to 40%.
- Treatment of children with HCV is under investigation.
- Researchers are re-examining when treatment should begin, for how long it should continue, and its effectiveness.
- Many pharmaceutical companies and NIH are conducting research to find more effective treatments and cures.
- Currently, almost 1/2 of all liver transplants in the U.S. are performed for end-stage hepatitis C. However, re-infection of the transplanted liver by the virus usually occurs and may require a second transplant.

- Try to maintain as normal a life as possible, eating a well-balanced diet, exercising and keeping a positive attitude. Avoid depressing or overwhelming tasks and learn how to pace yourself. Rest when you feel tired. Plan physically exhausting tasks in the morning when your energy level is at its peak.

Disease Outcomes

Between 20–30% of HCV sufferers are able to become virus-free with proper treatment. Between 70–80% of the HCV infections reported each year become classified as chronic. Chronic HCV refers to infections that do not clear up within 6 months after the acute infection. Within the chronically infected group, about 20% go on to develop cirrhosis (scarring of the liver). Of this group, 25% may develop liver failure, even though this may take 30–40 years. Cirrhosis slows the blood flow through the liver and causes increased pressure in the vein that carries blood from the stomach and the intestines to the liver. As a result, varicose veins ("varices") may develop in the stomach and esophagus. Without warning these large veins can break causing a person to vomit blood or have black, tarry stools. An estimated 8,000–10,000 deaths occur each year resulting from the complications of HCV.

Preventing HCV Infection

- There is NO vaccine to prevent HCV. Vaccines for Hepatitis A and B do not provide immunity against hepatitis C. There are various genotypes of HCV and the virus undergoes mutations making it difficult to develop a vaccine.
- Avoid handling anything that may have the blood of an infected person on it, such as razors, scissors, toothbrushes, nail clippers or files, tampons or sanitary napkins, etc. Detergent and a 10% solution of household bleach is believed to kill the virus.
- Don't share drug needles, cocaine straws, or any drug paraphernalia.
- Practice safe sex (use latex condoms).
- Notify your physician and dentist that you have hepatitis.
- Get vaccinated against hepatitis A and B.
- Those infected with hepatitis C should not drink alcohol, as it accelerates the liver damage.

Caring for Your Liver

Most people know that the liver acts as a filter and can be badly damaged by too much drinking of alcohol. Other than that they have little knowledge of the complexities and importance of the many thousands of vital functions it performs 24 hours each day.

The liver is about the size of a football is the largest organ in the body. The liver plays a vital role in regulating life processes. Its primary functions are to refine and detoxify everything you eat, breathe, and absorb through your skin. It is your body's internal chemical power plant, converting nutrients in the food you eat into muscles, energy, hormones, clotting factors, and immune factors. It stores certain vitamins, minerals and sugars, regulates fat stores, and controls the production and excretion of cholesterol. The bile, produced by liver cells, helps you to digest your food and absorb important nutrients. It neutralizes and destroys poisonous substances and metabolizes alcohol. Before you were born it served as the main organ of blood formation. It helps you resist infection and removes bacteria from the blood stream, helping you to stay healthy. Storing iron is another important task it performs.

In essence your liver serves as your engine, pantry, refinery, food processor, garbage disposal, and "guardian angel." Your liver is your silent partner, your internal chemical power plant, and a non-complaining organ. Unfortunately, it doesn't usually let you know it is in trouble until the damage is far advanced. It needs your help to keep it healthy.

One of the most remarkable accomplishments of this miraculous organ is its ability to regenerate. Three quarters of the liver can be removed and it will grow back in the same shape and form within a few weeks. However, overworking your liver can cause liver cells, the employees in your power plant, to become permanently damaged or scarred. This is called cirrhosis. Alcohol, drugs, and even some prescribed and over the counter drugs such as acetaminophen, as well as viruses, environmental pollutants and some metabolic disorders can cause liver cell damage. Liver specialists suggest that more than two drinks a day for men and one drink a day for women may even be too much for some people. Medicine should never be taken with alcoholic beverages. Remember they are all made up of chemicals and could be potentially hazardous to your precious liver cells.

Fumes from paint thinners, bug sprays, and other aerosol sprays are picked up by the tiny blood vessels in your lungs and carried to your liver where they are detoxified and discharged in your bile. The amount and concentration of those chemicals should be controlled to prevent liver damage. Make certain you have good ventilation, use a mask, cover your skin and wash off any chemicals you get on your skin with soap and water as soon as possible.

- **Hepatitis A (HAV).** There are safe and effective vaccines for hepatitis A. If you eat raw shellfish frequently you may want to discuss being vaccinated with your physician. If you work in a health care facility or day-care center you may be at risk. Children who attend day-care centers are also at risk. Food handlers, travelers to developing countries, and young people living in dorms or in close contact with others should consider being vaccinated. There is a risk of contracting hepatitis A through anal/oral contact. Good hygiene, washing hands with soap and water after using the toilet, and good common sense are essential.
- **Hepatitis B (HBV).** Hepatitis B can cause severe liver damage and even death. Safe and effective vaccines can prevent hepatitis B. Currently the Centers for Disease Control and Prevention recommend that all newborns, infants and children up to 19 years of age be vaccinated. If you have more than one sex partner within a six-month period or engage in high-risk behavior, you should consider vaccination. Everyone who handles blood or blood products in their daily activities should be vaccinated.
- **Hepatitis C (HCV).** Hepatitis C poses a more difficult problem. There is no vaccine available, so precautionary measures are very important. HCV is transmitted through blood and possibly other body fluids. Body piercing, tattooing and sharing razor blades, nail files, scissors, clippers, or toothbrushes with an infected person can result in the transmission of HCV However, the mode of transmission is uncertain in about 10% of the cases.

Caring for your liver means eating a good healthy diet, exercising, and getting lots of fresh air, and avoiding things that can cause liver damage. Your liver has to depend on you to take care of it… so it can take care of you.

About Hepatitis Foundation International

Hepatitis Foundation International (HFI) provides educational materials and training to the public, patients, health educators, and medical professionals about the prevention, diagnosis, and treatment of viral hepatitis, and also provides support to hepatitis patients and researchers. HFI has a variety of materials available through its Liver Wellness/Hepatitis Education program including:

- Videos for lending library
- Brochures on liver wellness and hepatitis
- Posters on hepatitis prevention
- Workplace programs
- Teacher and parent information
- Coloring books for children

For more information contact:

Hepatitis Foundation International
504 Blick Drive
Silver Spring, MD 20904-2901
Phone: 301-622-4200
Toll Free Hotline: 800-891-0707
Fax: 301-622-4702
Website: http://www.HepFI.org

Chapter 38

Herpes

Genital Herpes

What is genital herpes?

Genital herpes is an infection caused by the herpes simplex virus or HSV. There are two types of HSV, and both can cause genital herpes. HSV type 1 most commonly infects the lips, causing sores known as fever blisters or cold sores, but it also can infect the genital area and produce sores. HSV type 2 is the usual cause of genital herpes, but it also can infect the mouth. A person who has genital herpes infection can easily pass or transmit the virus to an uninfected person during sex.

Both HSV 1 and 2 can produce sores (also called lesions) in and around the vaginal area, on the penis, around the anal opening, and on the buttocks or thighs. Occasionally, sores also appear on other parts of the body where the virus has entered through broken skin.

HSV remains in certain nerve cells of the body for life, and can produce symptoms off and on in some infected people.

According to the U.S. Centers for Disease Control and Prevention, 45 million people in the United States ages 12 and older, or 1 out of 5 of the total adolescent and adult population, are infected with HSV-2.

"Genital Herpes," National Institute of Allergy and Infectious Diseases, September 2003; and "Herpes Labialis (Oral Herpes Simplex)," © 2002 A.D.A.M., Inc.; reprinted with permission.

Nationwide, since the late 1970s, the number of people with genital herpes infection has increased 30 percent. The largest increase is occurring in young teens. HSV-2 infection is more common in three of the youngest age groups which include people aged 12 to 39 years.

How does someone get genital herpes?

Most people get genital herpes by having sex with someone who is having a herpes "outbreak." This outbreak means that HSV is active. When active, the virus usually causes visible lesions in the genital area. The lesions shed (cast off) viruses that can infect another person. Sometimes, however, a person can have an outbreak and have no visible sores at all. People often get genital herpes by having sexual contact with others who don't know they are infected or who are having outbreaks of herpes without any sores.

A person with genital herpes also can infect a sexual partner during oral sex. The virus is spread only rarely, if at all, by touching objects such as a toilet seat or hot tub.

What are the symptoms?

Unfortunately, most people who have genital herpes don't know it because they never have any symptoms, or they do not recognize any symptoms they might have. When there are symptoms, they can be different in each person. Most often, when a person becomes infected with herpes for the first time, the symptoms will appear within 2 to 10 days. These first episodes of symptoms usually last 2 to 3 weeks.

Early symptoms of a genital herpes outbreak include

- Itching or burning feeling in the genital or anal area
- Pain in the legs, buttocks, or genital area
- Discharge of fluid from the vagina
- Feeling of pressure in the abdomen

Within a few days, sores appear near where the virus has entered the body, such as on the mouth, penis, or vagina. They also can occur inside the vagina and on the cervix in women, or in the urinary passage of women and men. Small red bumps appear first, develop into blisters, and then become painful open sores. Over several days, the sores become crusty and then heal without leaving a scar.

Other symptoms that may go with the first episode of genital herpes are fever, headache, muscle aches, painful or difficult urination, vaginal discharge, and swollen glands in the groin area.

Can outbreaks recur?

If you have been infected by HSV 1 and/or 2, you will probably have symptoms or outbreaks from time to time. After the virus has finished being active, it then travels to the nerves at the end of the spine where it stays for a while. Even after the lesions are gone, the virus stays inside the nerve cells in a still and hidden state, which means that it's inactive.

In most people, the virus can become active several times a year. This is called a recurrence. But scientists do not yet know why this happens. When it becomes active again, it travels along the nerves to the skin, where it makes more viruses near the site of the very first infection. That is where new sores usually will appear.

Sometimes, the virus can become active but not cause any sores that can be seen. At these times, small amounts of the virus may be shed at or near places of the first infection, in fluids from the mouth, penis, or vagina, or from barely noticeable sores. You may not notice this shedding because it often does not cause any pain or feel uncomfortable. Even though you might not be aware of the shedding, you still can infect a sex partner during this time.

After the first outbreak, any future outbreaks are usually mild and last only about a week. An infected person may know that an outbreak is about to happen by a tingling feeling or itching in the genital area, or pain in the buttocks or down the leg. For some people, these early symptoms can be the most painful and annoying part of an episode. Sometimes, only the tingling and itching are present and no visible sores develop. At other times, blisters appear that may be very small and barely noticeable, or they may break into open sores that crust over and then disappear.

The frequency and severity of recurrent episodes vary greatly. While some people have only one or two outbreaks in a lifetime, others may have several outbreaks a year. The number and pattern of repeat outbreaks often change over time for a person. Scientists do not know what causes the virus to become active again. Although some people with herpes report that their outbreaks are brought on by another illness, stress, or having a menstrual period, outbreaks often are not predictable. In some cases, outbreaks may be connected to exposure to sunlight.

How is genital herpes diagnosed?

Because the genital herpes sores may not be visible to the naked eye, a doctor or other health care worker may have to do several laboratory tests to try to prove that symptoms are caused by the herpes virus. A person may still have genital herpes, however, even if the laboratory tests do not show the virus in the body.

A blood test cannot show whether a person can infect another with the herpes virus. A blood test, however, can show if a person has been infected at any time with HSV. There are also newer blood tests that can tell whether a person has been infected with HSV 1 and/or 2.

How is genital herpes treated?

Although there is no cure for genital herpes, your health care worker might prescribe one of three medicines to treat it as well as to help prevent future episodes.

- Acyclovir (Zovirax)
- Famciclovir (Famvir)
- Valacyclovir (Valtrex)

Recently, the Food and Drug Administration approved Valtrex for use in preventing transmission of genital herpes. (See section below: "How can I protect myself or my sexual partner?")

During an active herpes episode, whether the first episode or a repeat one, you should follow a few simple steps to speed healing and avoid spreading the infection to other places on the body or to other people.

- Keep the infected area clean and dry to prevent other infections from developing.
- Try to avoid touching the sores.
- Wash your hands after contact with the sores.
- Avoid sexual contact from the time you first feel any symptoms until the sores are completely healed, that is, the scab has fallen off and new skin has formed where the sore was.

Can genital herpes cause any other problems?

Usually, genital herpes infections do not cause major problems in healthy adults. In some people whose immune systems do not work properly, genital herpes episodes can last a long time and be unusually severe. (The body's immune system fights off foreign invaders such as viruses.)

If a woman has her first episode of genital herpes while she is pregnant, she can pass the virus to her unborn child and may deliver a premature baby. Half of the babies infected with herpes either die or suffer from damage to their nerves. A baby born with herpes can develop serious problems that may affect the brain, the skin, or the eyes. If babies born with herpes are treated immediately with acyclovir, their chances of being healthy are increased.

If a pregnant woman has an outbreak, which is not the first episode, her baby's risk of being infected during delivery is very low. In either case, if you are pregnant and infected with genital herpes, you should stay in close touch with your doctor before, during, and after your baby is born.

If a woman is having an outbreak during labor and delivery and there are herpes lesions in or near the birth canal, the doctor will do a cesarean section to protect the baby. Most women with genital herpes, however, do not have signs of active infection with the virus during this time, and can have a normal delivery.

Is genital herpes worse in a person with HIV infection or AIDS?

Genital herpes, like other genital diseases that produce lesions, increases a person's risk of getting HIV, the virus that causes AIDS. Also, prior to better treatments for AIDS, persons infected with HIV had severe herpes outbreaks, which may have helped them pass both genital herpes and HIV infection to others.

How can I protect myself or my sexual partner?

If you have early signs of a herpes outbreak or visible sores, you should not have sexual intercourse or oral sex until the signs are gone and/or the sores have healed completely. Between outbreaks, using male latex condoms during sexual intercourse may offer some protection from the virus. When used with these precautions, Valtrex can also help prevent infecting your partner during heterosexual sex.

Is any research going on?

The National Institute of Allergy and Infectious Diseases (NIAID) supports research on genital herpes and on herpes simplex virus

(HSV-1 and HSV-2). Studies are currently underway to develop better treatments for the millions of people who suffer from genital herpes.

While some scientists are carrying out clinical trials to determine the best way to use existing drugs, others are studying the biology of herpes simplex virus. NIAID scientists have identified certain genes and enzymes that the virus needs to survive. They are hopeful that drugs aimed at disrupting these viral targets might lead to the design of more effective treatments.

Meanwhile, other researchers are devising methods to control the virus' spread. Two important means of preventing HSV infection are vaccines and topical microbicides. Several different vaccines are in various stages of development. These include vaccines made from proteins on the HSV cell surface, peptides or chains of amino acids, and the DNA of the virus itself.

NIAID and GlaxoSmithKline Biologicals are supporting a large clinical trial in women of an experimental vaccine that may help prevent transmission of genital herpes. The trial is being conducted at more than 20 sites in 15 states nationwide.

Topical microbicides, preparations containing microbe-killing compounds, are also in various stages of development and testing. These include gels, creams, or lotions that a woman could insert into the vagina prior to intercourse to prevent infection.

Where can I get help if I'm upset about having genital herpes or I have an infected partner?

Genital herpes outbreaks can be distressing, inconvenient, and sometimes painful. Concern about transmitting the disease to others and disruption of sexual relations during outbreaks can affect personal relationships. If you or your partner has genital herpes, you can learn to cope with and treat the disease effectively by getting proper counseling and medicine, and by using ways to prevent getting infected or infecting someone else, as mentioned above.

Herpes Labialis (Oral Herpes Simplex)

Alternative Names

- Cold sore
- Fever blister
- Herpes simplex—oral

Definition

Herpes labialis is an infection caused by the herpes simplex virus, characterized by an eruption of small and usually painful blisters on the skin of the lips, mouth, gums, or the skin around the mouth. These blisters are commonly called cold sores or fever blisters.

Causes, Incidence, and Risk Factors

Herpes labialis is an extremely common disease caused by infection of the mouth area with herpes simplex virus, most often type 1. Most Americans are infected with the type 1 virus by the age of 20.

The initial infection may cause no symptoms or mouth ulcers. The virus remains in the nerve tissue of the face. In some people, the virus reactivates and produces recurrent cold sores that are usually in the same area, but are not serious. Herpes virus type 2 usually causes genital herpes and infection of babies at birth but can also cause herpes labialis.

Herpes viruses are contagious. Contact can occur directly, or through contact with infected razors, towels, dishes, etc. Occasionally, oral/genital contact can spread oral herpes to the genitals (and vice versa), so people with active herpes lesions on or around their mouths or on their genitals should avoid oral sex.

The first symptoms usually appear within 1 or 2 weeks, and as late as 3 weeks, after contact with an infected person. The lesions of herpes labialis usually last for 7 to 10 days, then begin to resolve. The virus may become latent, residing in the nerve cells, with recurrence at or near the original site.

Recurrence is usually milder. It may be triggered by menstruation, sun exposure, illness with fever, stress, or other unknown causes.

Symptoms

Warning symptoms of itching, burning, increased sensitivity, or tingling sensation may occur about 2 days before lesions appear.

- Skin lesion/rash located around the lips, mouth, and gums
- Small blisters (vesicles), filled with clear yellowish fluid
  - blisters appear on a raised, red, painful skin area
  - blisters form, break, and ooze
  - yellow crusts slough to reveal pink, healing skin
  - several smaller blisters may merge to form a larger blister
- Mild fever (may occur)

Signs and Tests

Diagnosis is made on the basis of the appearance and/or culture of the lesion. Examination may also show enlargement of lymph nodes in the neck or groin.

Viral culture or Tzanck test of the skin lesion may reveal the herpes simplex virus.

Treatment

Untreated, the symptoms will generally subside in 1 to 2 weeks. Antiviral medications may be given by mouth to may shorten the course of the symptoms and decrease pain.

Wash blisters gently with soap and water to minimize the spread of the virus to other areas of skin. An antiseptic soap may be recommended. Applying ice or warmth to the area may reduce pain.

Take precautions to avoid infecting others (see Prevention).

Expectations (Prognosis)

Herpes labialis usually disappears spontaneously in 1 to 2 weeks. It may recur. Infection may be severe and dangerous if it occurs in or near the eye, or if it happens in immunosuppressed people.

Complications

- Spread of herpes to other skin areas
- Secondary bacterial skin infections
- Recurrence of herpes labialis
- Generalized infection—may be life-threatening in immunosuppressed people, including those with atopic dermatitis, cancer, HIV infections
- Blindness

Herpes infection of the eye is a leading cause of blindness in the U.S., causing scarring of the cornea.

Calling Your Health Care Provider

Call for an appointment with your health care provider if symptoms indicate herpes labialis and symptoms persist for longer than 1 or 2 weeks.

Also call if symptoms are severe, or if you have a disorder associated with immunosuppression and you develop herpes symptoms.

Prevention

Avoid direct contact with cold sores or other herpes lesions. Minimize the risk of indirect spread by thoroughly washing items in hot (preferably boiling) water before re-use. Do not share items with an infected person, especially when herpes lesions are active. Avoid precipitating causes (especially sun exposure) if prone to oral herpes.

Avoid performing oral sex when you have active herpes lesions on or near your mouth and avoid passive oral sex with someone who has active oral or genital herpes lesions. Condoms can help reduce, but do not entirely eliminate, the risk of transmission via oral or genital sex with an infected person.

Unfortunately, both oral and genital herpes viruses can sometimes be transmitted even when the person does not have active lesions.

Chapter 39

Human Immunodeficiency Virus (HIV)

HIV Infection and AIDS: An Overview

AIDS—acquired immunodeficiency syndrome—was first reported in the United States in 1981 and has since become a major worldwide epidemic. AIDS is caused by the human immunodeficiency virus (HIV). By killing or damaging cells of the body's immune system, HIV progressively destroys the body's ability to fight infections and certain cancers. People diagnosed with AIDS may get life-threatening diseases called opportunistic infections, which are caused by microbes such as viruses or bacteria that usually do not make healthy people sick.

More than 830,000 cases of AIDS have been reported in the United States since 1981. As many as 950,000 Americans may be infected with HIV, one-quarter of whom are unaware of their infection. The epidemic is growing most rapidly among minority populations and is a leading killer of African-American males ages 25 to 44. According to the U.S. Centers for Disease Control and Prevention (CDC), AIDS affects nearly seven times more African Americans and three times more Hispanics than whites.

This chapter includes "HIV Infection and AIDS: An Overview," October 2003, "How HIV Causes AIDS," October 2001, "Treatment of HIV Infection," October 2003, and "HIV/AIDS Statistics," January 2004, National Institute of Allergy and Infectious Diseases (NIAID), National Institutes of Health (NIH).

How HIV Is Transmitted

HIV is spread most commonly by having unprotected sex with an infected partner. The virus can enter the body through the lining of the vagina, vulva, penis, rectum, or mouth during sex.

HIV also is spread through contact with infected blood. Before donated blood was screened for evidence of HIV infection and before heat-treating techniques to destroy HIV in blood products were introduced, HIV was transmitted through transfusions of contaminated blood or blood components. Today, because of blood screening and heat treatment, the risk of getting HIV from such transfusions is extremely small.

HIV frequently is spread among injection drug users by the sharing of needles or syringes contaminated with very small quantities of blood from someone infected with the virus. It is rare, however, for a patient to give HIV to a health care worker or vice-versa by accidental sticks with contaminated needles or other medical instruments.

Women can transmit HIV to their babies during pregnancy or birth. Approximately one-quarter to one-third of all untreated pregnant women infected with HIV will pass the infection to their babies. HIV also can be spread to babies through the breast milk of mothers infected with the virus. If the mother takes the drug AZT during pregnancy, she can significantly reduce the chances that her baby will get infected with HIV. If health care providers treat mothers with AZT and deliver their babies by cesarean section, the chances of the baby being infected can be reduced to a rate of 1 percent.

A study sponsored by the National Institute of Allergy and Infectious Diseases (NIAID) in Uganda found a highly effective and safe drug for preventing transmission of HIV from an infected mother to her newborn. This regimen is more affordable and practical than any other examined to date. Results from the study show that a single oral dose of the antiretroviral drug nevirapine (NVP) given to an HIV-infected woman in labor and another to her baby within three days of birth reduces the transmission rate of HIV by half compared with a similar short course of AZT.

Although researchers have found HIV in the saliva of infected people, there is no evidence that the virus is spread by contact with saliva. Laboratory studies reveal that saliva has natural properties that limit the power of HIV to infect. Research studies of people infected with HIV have found no evidence that the virus is spread to others through saliva by kissing. No one knows, however, whether so-called "deep" kissing, involving the exchange of large amounts of saliva, or oral intercourse increase the risk of infection. Scientists also have found no evidence that HIV is spread through sweat, tears, urine, or feces.

Studies of families of HIV-infected people have shown clearly that HIV is not spread through casual contact such as the sharing of food utensils, towels and bedding, swimming pools, telephones, or toilet seats. HIV is not spread by biting insects such as mosquitoes or bedbugs.

HIV can infect anyone who practices risky behaviors such as:

- Sharing drug needles or syringes
- Having sexual contact with an infected person without using a condom
- Having sexual contact with someone whose HIV status is unknown

Having a sexually transmitted disease such as syphilis, genital herpes, chlamydial infection, gonorrhea, or bacterial vaginosis appears to make people more susceptible to getting HIV infection during sex with infected partners.

Symptoms of HIV Infection

Many people do not have any symptoms when they first become infected with HIV. Some people, however, have a flu-like illness within a month or two after exposure to the virus. This illness may include

- Fever
- Headache
- Tiredness
- Enlarged lymph nodes (glands of the immune system easily felt in the neck and groin)

These symptoms usually disappear within a week to a month and are often mistaken for those of another viral infection. During this period, people are very infectious, and HIV is present in large quantities in genital fluids.

More persistent or severe symptoms may not appear for 10 years or more after HIV first enters the body in adults, or within two years in children born with HIV infection. This period of "asymptomatic" infection is highly individual. Some people may begin to have symptoms within a few months, while others may be symptom-free for more than 10 years.

Even during the asymptomatic period, the virus is actively multiplying, infecting, and killing cells of the immune system. The most obvious effect of HIV infection is a decline in the number of CD4 positive T cells (also called T4 cells) found in the blood—the immune system's key infection fighters. At the beginning of its life in the human body, the virus disables or destroys these cells without causing symptoms.

As the immune system worsens, a variety of complications start to take over. For many people, the first signs of infection are large lymph nodes or "swollen glands" that may be enlarged for more than three months. Other symptoms often experienced months to years before the onset of AIDS include

- Lack of energy
- Weight loss
- Frequent fevers and sweats
- Persistent or frequent yeast infections (oral or vaginal)
- Persistent skin rashes or flaky skin
- Pelvic inflammatory disease in women that does not respond to treatment
- Short-term memory loss

Some people develop frequent and severe herpes infections that cause mouth, genital, or anal sores, or a painful nerve disease called shingles. Children may grow slowly or be sick a lot.

AIDS

The term AIDS applies to the most advanced stages of HIV infection. CDC developed official criteria for the definition of AIDS and is responsible for tracking the spread of AIDS in the United States.

CDC's definition of AIDS includes all HIV-infected people who have fewer than 200 CD4 positive T cells (abbreviated CD4+ T cells) per cubic millimeter of blood (Healthy adults usually have CD4 positive T-cell counts of 1,000 or more.). In addition, the definition includes 26 clinical conditions that affect people with advanced HIV disease. Most of these conditions are opportunistic infections that generally do not affect healthy people. In people with AIDS, these infections are often severe and sometimes fatal because the immune system is so ravaged by HIV that the body cannot fight off certain bacteria, viruses, fungi, parasites, and other microbes.

Symptoms of opportunistic infections common in people with AIDS include

- Coughing and shortness of breath
- Seizures and lack of coordination
- Difficult or painful swallowing
- Mental symptoms such as confusion and forgetfulness
- Severe and persistent diarrhea
- Fever
- Vision loss
- Nausea, abdominal cramps, and vomiting
- Weight loss and extreme fatigue
- Severe headaches
- Coma

Children with AIDS may get the same opportunistic infections as do adults with the disease. In addition, they also have severe forms of the bacterial infections all children may get, such as conjunctivitis (pink eye), ear infections, and tonsillitis.

People with AIDS are particularly prone to developing various cancers, especially those caused by viruses such as Kaposi's sarcoma and cervical cancer, or cancers of the immune system known as lymphomas. These cancers are usually more aggressive and difficult to treat in people with AIDS. Signs of Kaposi's sarcoma in light-skinned people are round brown, reddish, or purple spots that develop in the skin or in the mouth. In dark-skinned people, the spots are more pigmented.

During the course of HIV infection, most people experience a gradual decline in the number of CD4 positive T cells; although some may have abrupt and dramatic drops in their CD4 positive T-cell counts. A person with CD4 positive T cells above 200 may experience some of the early symptoms of HIV disease. Others may have no symptoms even though their CD4 positive T-cell count is below 200.

Many people are so debilitated by the symptoms of AIDS that they cannot hold steady employment or do household chores. Other people with AIDS may experience phases of intense life-threatening illness followed by phases in which they function normally.

A small number of people first infected with HIV 10 or more years ago have not developed symptoms of AIDS. Scientists are trying to determine what factors may account for their lack of progression to AIDS, such as particular characteristics of their immune systems or whether they were infected with a less aggressive strain of the virus, or if their genes may protect them from the effects of HIV. Scientists hope that understanding the body's natural method of control may lead to ideas for protective HIV vaccines and use of vaccines to prevent the disease from progressing.

Diagnosis

Because early HIV infection often causes no symptoms, a doctor or other health care provider usually can diagnose it by testing a person's blood for the presence of antibodies (disease-fighting proteins) to HIV. HIV antibodies generally do not reach detectable levels in the blood for one to three months following infection. It may take the antibodies as long as six months to be produced in quantities large enough to show up in standard blood tests.

People exposed to the virus should get an HIV test as soon as they are likely to develop antibodies to the virus—within 6 weeks to 12 months after possible exposure to the virus. By getting tested early, people with HIV infection can discuss with a health care provider when they should start treatment to help their immune systems combat HIV and help prevent the emergence of certain opportunistic infections. Early testing also alerts HIV-infected people to avoid high-risk behaviors that could spread the virus to others.

Most health care providers can do HIV testing and will usually offer counseling to the patient at the same time. Of course, individuals can be tested anonymously at many sites if they are concerned about confidentiality.

Health care providers diagnose HIV infection by using two different types of antibody tests, ELISA and Western Blot. If a person is highly likely to be infected with HIV and yet both tests are negative, the health care provider may request additional tests. The person also may be told to repeat antibody testing at a later date, when antibodies to HIV are more likely to have developed.

Babies born to mothers infected with HIV may or may not be infected with the virus, but all carry their mothers' antibodies to HIV for several months. If these babies lack symptoms, a doctor cannot make a definitive diagnosis of HIV infection using standard antibody tests until after 15 months of age. By then, babies are unlikely to still carry their mothers' antibodies and will have produced their own, if they are infected. Health care experts are using new technologies to detect HIV itself to more accurately determine HIV infection in infants between ages 3 months and 15 months. They are evaluating a number of blood tests to determine if they can diagnose HIV infection in babies younger than 3 months.

Prevention

Because no vaccine for HIV is available, the only way to prevent infection by the virus is to avoid behaviors that put a person at risk of infection, such as sharing needles and having unprotected sex.

Many people infected with HIV have no symptoms. Therefore, there is no way of knowing with certainty whether a sexual partner is infected unless he or she has repeatedly tested negative for the virus and has not engaged in any risky behavior.

People should either abstain from having sex or use male latex condoms or female polyurethane condoms, which may offer partial protection, during oral, anal, or vaginal sex. Only water-based lubricants should be used with male latex condoms.

Although some laboratory evidence shows that spermicides can kill HIV, researchers have not found that these products can prevent a person from getting HIV.

The risk of HIV transmission from a pregnant woman to her baby is significantly reduced if she takes AZT during pregnancy, labor, and delivery, and if her baby takes it for the first six weeks of life.

How HIV Causes AIDS

A significant component of the research effort of the National Institute of Allergy and Infectious Diseases (NIAID) is devoted to the pathogenesis of human immunodeficiency virus (HIV) disease. Studies on pathogenesis address the complex mechanisms that result in the destruction of the immune system of an HIV-infected person. A detailed understanding of HIV and how it establishes infection and causes the acquired immunodeficiency syndrome (AIDS) is crucial to identifying and developing effective drugs and vaccines to fight HIV and AIDS. This fact sheet summarizes the state of knowledge in this area and provides a brief glossary of terms.

Overview

HIV disease is characterized by a gradual deterioration of immune function. Most notably, crucial immune cells called CD4+ T cells are disabled and killed during the typical course of infection. These cells, sometimes called "T-helper cells," play a central role in the immune response, signaling other cells in the immune system to perform their special functions.

A healthy, uninfected person usually has 800 to 1,200 CD4+ T cells per cubic millimeter (mm^3) of blood. During HIV infection, the number of these cells in a person's blood progressively declines. When a person's CD4+ T cell count falls below 200/mm^3, he or she becomes particularly vulnerable to the opportunistic infections and cancers that typify AIDS, the end stage of HIV disease. People with AIDS often suffer infections of the lungs, intestinal tract, brain, eyes, and other organs, as well as debilitating weight loss, diarrhea, neurologic conditions and cancers, such as Kaposi's sarcoma and certain types of lymphomas.

Most scientists think that HIV causes AIDS by directly inducing the death of CD4+ T cells or interfering with their normal function, and by triggering other events that weaken a person's immune function. For example, the network of signaling molecules that normally regulates a person's immune response is disrupted during HIV disease, impairing a person's ability to fight other infections. The HIV-mediated destruction of the lymph nodes and related immunologic organs also plays a major role in causing the immunosuppression seen in people with AIDS.

HIV Is a Retrovirus

HIV belongs to a class of viruses called retroviruses. Retroviruses are ribonucleic acid (RNA) viruses, and in order to replicate they must make a deoxyribonucleic acid (DNA) copy of their RNA. It is the DNA genes that allow the virus to replicate.

Like all viruses, HIV can replicate only inside cells, commandeering the cell's machinery to reproduce. However, only HIV and other retroviruses, once inside a cell, use an enzyme called reverse transcriptase to convert their RNA into DNA, which can be incorporated into the host cell's genes.

Slow viruses. HIV belongs to a subgroup of retroviruses known as lentiviruses, or "slow" viruses. The course of infection with these viruses is characterized by a long interval between initial infection and the onset of serious symptoms.

Other lentiviruses infect nonhuman species. For example, the feline immunodeficiency virus (FIV) infects cats and the simian immunodeficiency virus (SIV) infects monkeys and other nonhuman primates. Like HIV in humans, these animal viruses primarily infect immune system cells, often causing immunodeficiency and AIDS-like symptoms. These viruses and their hosts have provided researchers with useful, albeit imperfect, models of the HIV disease process in people.

Early Events in HIV Infection

Once it enters the body, HIV infects a large number of CD4+ cells and replicates rapidly. During this acute or primary phase of infection, the blood contains many viral particles that spread throughout the body, seeding various organs, particularly the lymphoid organs. Lymphoid organs include the lymph nodes, spleen, tonsils, and adenoids.

Two to four weeks after exposure to the virus, up to 70 percent of HIV-infected persons suffer flu-like symptoms related to the acute infection. The patient's immune system fights back with killer T cells (CD8+ T cells) and B-cell-produced antibodies, which dramatically reduce HIV levels. A patient's CD4+ T cell count may rebound somewhat and even approach its original level. A person may then remain free of HIV-related symptoms for years despite continuous replication of HIV in the lymphoid organs that had been seeded during the acute phase of infection.

One reason that HIV is unique is the fact that despite the body's aggressive immune responses, which are sufficient to clear most viral infections, some HIV invariably escapes. This is due in large part to the high rate of mutations that occur during the process of HIV replication. Even when the virus does not avoid the immune system by mutating, the body's best soldiers in the fight against HIV—certain subsets of killer T cells that recognize HIV may be depleted or become dysfunctional.

In addition, early in the course of HIV infection, patients may lose HIV-specific CD4+ T cell responses that normally slow the replication of viruses. Such responses include the secretion of interferons and other antiviral factors, and the orchestration of CD8+ T cells.

Finally, the virus may hide within the chromosomes of an infected cell and be shielded from surveillance by the immune system. Such cells can be considered as a latent reservoir of the virus.

Course of HIV Infection

Among patients enrolled in large epidemiologic studies in western countries, the median time from infection with HIV to the development of AIDS-related symptoms has been approximately 10 to 12 years in the absence of antiretroviral therapy. However, researchers have observed a wide variation in disease progression. Approximately 10 percent of HIV-infected people in these studies have progressed to AIDS within the first two to three years following infection, while up to 5 percent of individuals in the studies have stable CD4+ T cell counts and no symptoms even after 12 or more years.

Factors such as age or genetic differences among individuals, the level of virulence of an individual strain of virus, and co-infection with other microbes may influence the rate and severity of disease progression. Drugs that fight the infections associated with AIDS have improved and prolonged the lives of HIV-infected people by preventing or treating conditions such as *Pneumocystis carinii* pneumonia, cytomegalovirus disease, and diseases caused by a number of fungi.

HIV co-receptors and disease progression. Recent research has shown that most infecting strains of HIV use a co-receptor molecule called CCR5, in addition to the CD4 molecule, to enter certain of its target cells. HIV-infected people with a specific mutation in one of their two copies of the gene for this receptor may have a slower disease course than people with two normal copies of the gene. Rare individuals with two mutant copies of the CCR5 gene appear—in most cases—to be completely protected from HIV infection. Mutations in the gene for other HIV co-receptors also may influence the rate of disease progression.

Viral burden predicts disease progression. Numerous studies show that people with high levels of HIV in their bloodstream are more likely to develop new AIDS-related symptoms or die than individuals with lower levels of virus. For instance, in the Multicenter AIDS Cohort Study (MACS), investigators demonstrated that the level of HIV in an untreated individual's plasma 6 months to a year after infection—the so-called viral "set point"—is highly predictive of the rate of disease progression; that is, patients with high levels of virus are much more likely to get sicker, faster, than those with low levels of virus. The MACS and other studies have provided the rationale for providing aggressive antiretroviral therapy to HIV-infected people, as well as for routinely using newly available blood tests to measure viral load when initiating, monitoring and modifying anti-HIV therapy.

Potent combinations of three or more anti-HIV drugs known as highly active antiretroviral therapy or HAART can reduce a person's "viral burden" to very low levels and in many cases delay the progression of HIV disease for prolonged periods. However, antiretroviral regimens have yet to completely and permanently suppress the virus in HIV-infected people. Recent studies have shown that HIV persists in a replication-competent form in resting CD4+ T cells even in patients receiving aggressive antiretroviral therapy who have no readily detectable HIV in their blood. Investigators around the world are working to develop the next generation of anti-HIV drugs.

HIV Is Active in the Lymph Nodes

Although HIV-infected individuals often exhibit an extended period of clinical latency with little evidence of disease, the virus is never truly completely latent although individual cells may be latently infected. Researchers have shown that even early in disease, HIV actively replicates within the lymph nodes and related organs, where large amounts of virus become trapped in networks of specialized cells with long, tentacle-like extensions. These cells are called follicular dendritic cells (FDCs).

FDCs are located in hot spots of immune activity in lymphoid tissue called germinal centers. They act like flypaper, trapping invading pathogens (including HIV) and holding them until B cells come along to initiate an immune response.

Close on the heels of B cells are CD4+ T cells, which rush into the germinal centers to help B cells fight the invaders. CD4+ T cells, the primary targets of HIV, may become infected as they encounter HIV trapped on FDCs. Research suggests that HIV trapped on FDCs remains infectious, even when coated with antibodies. Thus, FDCs are an important reservoir of HIV, and the large quantity of infectious HIV trapped on FDCs may explain in part how the momentum of HIV infection is maintained.

Once infected, CD4+ T cells may infect other CD4+ cells that congregate in the region of the lymph node surrounding the germinal center.

Over a period of years, even when little virus is readily detectable in the blood, significant amounts of virus accumulate in the lymphoid tissue, both within infected cells and bound to FDCs. In and around the germinal centers, numerous CD4+ T cells are probably activated by the increased production of cytokines such as TNF-alpha and IL-6 by immune system cells within the lymphoid tissue. Activation allows uninfected cells to be more easily infected and increases replication of HIV in already infected cells.

While greater quantities of certain cytokines such as TNF-alpha and IL-6 are secreted during HIV infection, other cytokines with key roles in the regulation of normal immune function may be secreted in decreased amounts. For example, CD4+ T cells may lose their capacity to produce interleukin 2 (IL-2), a cytokine that enhances the growth of other T cells and helps to stimulate other cells' response to invaders. Infected cells also have low levels of receptors for IL-2, which may reduce their ability to respond to signals from other cells.

Breakdown of FDC networks. Ultimately, accumulated HIV overwhelms the FDC networks. As these networks break down, their trapping capacity is impaired, and large quantities of virus enter the bloodstream.

Although it remains unclear why FDCs die and the FDC networks dissolve, some scientists think that this process may be as important in HIV pathogenesis as the loss of CD4+ T cells. The destruction of the lymphoid tissue structure seen late in HIV disease may preclude a successful immune response against not only HIV but other pathogens as well. This devastation heralds the onset of the opportunistic infections and cancers that characterize AIDS.

Role of CD8+ T Cells

CD8+ T cells are critically important in the immune response to HIV. These cells attack and kill infected cells that are producing virus. Thus, vaccine efforts are directed toward eliciting or enhancing these killer T cells, as well as eliciting antibodies that will neutralize the infectivity of HIV.

CD8+ T cells also appear to secrete soluble factors that suppress HIV replication. Several molecules, including RANTES, MIP-1alpha, MIP-1beta, and MDC appear to block HIV replication by occupying the co-receptors necessary for the entry of many strains of HIV into their target cells. There may be other immune system molecules—yet undiscovered—that can suppress HIV replication to some degree.

Rapid Replication and Mutation of HIV

HIV replicates rapidly; several billion new virus particles may be produced every day. In addition, the HIV reverse transcriptase enzyme makes many mistakes while making DNA copies from HIV RNA. As a consequence, many variants of HIV develop in an individual, some of which may escape destruction by antibodies or killer

T cells. Additionally, different strains of HIV can recombine to produce a wide range of variants or strains.

During the course of HIV disease, viral strains emerge in an infected individual that differ widely in their ability to infect and kill different cell types, as well as in their rate of replication. Scientists are investigating why strains of HIV from patients with advanced disease appear to be more virulent and infect more cell types than strains obtained earlier from the same individual.

Theories of Immune System Cell Loss in HIV Infection

Researchers around the world are studying how HIV destroys or disables CD4+ T cells, and many think that a number of mechanisms may occur simultaneously in an HIV-infected individual. Recent data suggest that billions of CD4+ T cells may be destroyed every day, eventually overwhelming the immune system's regenerative capacity.

Direct cell killing. Infected CD4+ T cells may be killed directly when large amounts of virus are produced and bud off from the cell surface, disrupting the cell membrane, or when viral proteins and nucleic acids collect inside the cell, interfering with cellular machinery.

Apoptosis. Infected CD4+ T cells may be killed when the regulation of cell function is distorted by HIV proteins, probably leading to cell suicide by a process known as programmed cell death or apoptosis. Recent reports indicate that apoptosis occurs to a greater extent in HIV-infected individuals, both in the bloodstream and lymph nodes. Apoptosis is closely correlated with the aberrant cellular activation seen in HIV disease.

Uninfected cells also may undergo apoptosis. Investigators have shown in cell cultures that the HIV envelope alone or bound to antibodies sends an inappropriate signal to CD4+ T cells causing them to undergo apoptosis, even if not infected by HIV.

Innocent bystanders. Uninfected cells may die in an innocent bystander scenario: HIV particles may bind to the cell surface, giving them the appearance of an infected cell and marking them for destruction by killer T cells after antibody attaches to the viral particle on the cell. This process is called antibody dependent cellular cytotoxicity.

Killer T cells also may mistakenly destroy uninfected cells that have consumed HIV particles and that display HIV fragments on their surfaces. Alternatively, because HIV envelope proteins bear some resemblance to certain molecules that may appear on CD4+ T cells, the body's immune responses may mistakenly damage such cells as well.

Anergy. Researchers have shown in cell cultures that CD4+ T cells can be turned off by activation signals from HIV that leaves them unable to respond to further immune stimulation. This inactivated state is known as anergy.

Damage to precursor cells. Studies suggest that HIV also destroys precursor cells that mature to have special immune functions, as well as the microenvironment of the bone marrow and the thymus needed for the development of such cells. These organs probably lose the ability to regenerate, further compounding the suppression of the immune system.

Central Nervous System Damage

Although monocytes and macrophages can be infected by HIV, they appear to be relatively resistant to killing by the virus. However, these cells travel throughout the body and carry HIV to various organs, including the brain, which may serve as a hiding place or "reservoir" for the virus that may be relatively impervious to most anti-HIV drugs.

Neurologic manifestations of HIV disease are seen in up to 50 percent of HIV-infected people, to varying degrees of severity. People infected with HIV often experience cognitive symptoms, including impaired short-term memory, reduced concentration, and mental slowing; motor symptoms such as fine motor clumsiness or slowness, tremor, and leg weakness; and behavioral symptoms including apathy, social withdrawal, irritability, depression, and personality change. More serious neurologic manifestations in HIV disease typically occur in patients with high viral loads, generally when an individual has advanced HIV disease or AIDS.

Neurologic manifestations of HIV disease are the subject of many research projects. Current evidence suggests that although nerve cells do not become infected with HIV, supportive cells within the brain, such as astrocytes and microglia (as well as monocyte/macrophages that have migrated to the brain) can be infected with the virus. Researchers postulate that infection of these cells can cause a disruption of normal neurologic functions by altering cytokine levels, by delivering aberrant signals, and by causing the release of toxic products in the brain. The use of anti-HIV drugs frequently reduces the severity of neurologic symptoms, but in many cases does not, for reasons that are unclear.

Role of Immune Activation in HIV Disease

During a normal immune response, many components of the immune system are mobilized to fight an invader. CD4+ T cells, for instance, may quickly proliferate and increase their cytokine secretion, thereby signaling other cells to perform their special functions. Scavenger cells called macrophages may double in size and develop numerous organelles, including lysosomes that contain digestive enzymes used to process ingested pathogens. Once the immune system clears the foreign antigen, it returns to a relative state of quiescence.

Paradoxically, although it ultimately causes immune deficiency, HIV disease for most of its course is characterized by immune system hyperactivation, which has negative consequences. As noted above, HIV replication and spread are much more efficient in activated CD4+ cells. Chronic immune system activation during HIV disease may also result in a massive stimulation of B cells, impairing the ability of these cells to make antibodies against other pathogens.

Chronic immune activation also can result in apoptosis, and an increased production of cytokines that may not only increase HIV replication but also have other deleterious effects. Increased levels of TNF-alpha, for example, may be at least partly responsible for the severe weight loss or wasting syndrome seen in many HIV-infected individuals.

The persistence of HIV and HIV replication plays an important role in the chronic state of immune activation seen in HIV-infected people. In addition, researchers have shown that infections with other organisms activate immune system cells and increase production of the virus in HIV-infected people. Chronic immune activation due to persistent infections, or the cumulative effects of multiple episodes of immune activation and bursts of virus production, likely contribute to the progression of HIV disease.

Treatment of HIV Infection

When AIDS was first recognized in 1981, patients with the disease were unlikely to live longer than a year or two. Since then, scientists have developed an effective arsenal of drugs that can help many people infected with HIV (human immunodeficiency virus) live longer and healthier lives. The treatment and prevention of HIV is a high priority for the National Institute of Allergy and Infectious Diseases (NIAID). Research supported by NIAID has greatly advanced our understanding of HIV and how it causes AIDS. This knowledge provides the foundation for NIAID's AIDS research effort and continues to support studies designed to further extend and improve the quality of life of those infected with HIV.

Drugs Developed for HIV Infection

Twenty drugs have been approved for treating individuals with HIV infection. They are called antiretroviral drugs because they attack HIV, which is a retrovirus.

Once inside the cell, HIV uses specific enzymes to survive. The first approved classes of antiretroviral drugs that were approved work by interfering with the virus' ability to use these enzymes. They fall into two categories:

- **Reverse transcriptase (RT) inhibitors.** RT inhibitors interfere with an enzyme called reverse transcriptase or RT that HIV needs to make copies of itself. There are two main types of RT inhibitors, and they each work differently.
    - Nucleoside/nucleotide drugs provide faulty DNA building blocks, halting the DNA chain that the virus uses to make copies of itself.
    - Non-nucleoside RT inhibitors bind RT so the virus cannot carry out its copying function.
- **Protease inhibitors (PI).** Protease Inhibitors interfere with the protease enzyme that HIV uses to produce infectious viral particles.

The newest class of antiretroviral drugs works by changing the shape of the gp41 envelope protein surrounding HIV. This class of drug is called fusion inhibitors. Fusion inhibitors interfere with the virus' ability to fuse with and enter the host cell.

Antiretroviral Drugs: Not a Cure for HIV Infection

The currently available drugs cannot cure HIV infection. This is because the current drugs can suppress HIV but are unable to eliminate it from the body. Since HIV can become resistant to any one drug, researchers use a combination of antiretroviral drugs to suppress the

Table 39.1. Drugs Approved for HIV Infection

Nucleoside/ Nucleotide RT Inhibitors	Non-nucleoside RT Inhibitors	Protease Inhibitors	Fusion Inhibitors
abacavir	delavirdine	ritonavir	pentafuside
ddC	nevirapine	saquinavir	
ddI	efavirenz	indinavir	
d4T		amprenavir	
3TC		nelfinavir	
ZDV		lopinavir	
tenofovir		atazanavir	
		emtricitabine	
		fosamprenavir calcium	

virus. By combining both RT inhibitors and protease inhibitors, NIAID-supported research groups and drug companies developed the potent and effective combination therapy called highly active antiretroviral therapy or HAART.

Although the use of HAART has greatly reduced the number of deaths due to AIDS, this powerful combination of drugs cannot suppress the virus indefinitely. In addition, while people with HIV are living longer, new medical problems are surfacing. Even those individuals who take antiretroviral drugs can pass on HIV to others through unprotected sex.

Problems Associated with Antiretroviral Drug Use

People with HIV must take medicines with complicated regimens, often taking several drugs per day, some of which may require the person to fast. Patients may have difficulty adhering to these complicated regimens, find the food restrictions difficult to deal with, and may experience unpleasant side effects such as nausea and vomiting.

Aside from the complicated dosing regimens, antiretroviral drugs themselves may cause significant medical problems. Metabolic changes occur in people with HIV infection. Some of these changes may be related to the antiretrovirals, and may include abnormal fat distribution, abnormal lipid and glucose metabolism, and bone loss.

Some anti-HIV drugs are toxic to mitochondria, the energy producers in cells. Tissues that require high levels of energy, like muscles and nerves, are most susceptible to the affects of damaged mitochondria. Muscle wasting, heart failure, nerve damage, degeneration of the liver, and inflammation of the pancreas may be associated with mitochondrial damage.

New Drugs in the Pipeline

- The Pharmaceutical Research and Manufacturers Association lists nearly two dozen new anti-HIV drugs now in development. They include new protease inhibitors and more potent, less toxic RT inhibitors, as well as drugs that interfere with entirely different steps in the virus' lifecycle. These new categories of drugs include:
    - Entry inhibitors—drugs that interfere with HIV's ability to enter cells.
    - Integrase inhibitors—drugs that interfere with HIV's ability to insert its genes into a cell's normal DNA.
    - Assembly and budding inhibitors—drugs that interfere with the final stage of the HIV life cycle, when new virus particles are released into the bloodstream.
    - Cellular metabolism modulators—drugs that interfere with the cellular processes needed for HIV replication.

In addition, scientists are learning how immune modulators help boost the immune system's response to the virus and may make the existing anti-HIV drugs more effective. Therapeutic vaccines are also being evaluated for this purpose and could help reduce the number of anti-HIV drugs needed or the duration of treatment.

HIV/AIDS Statistics

HIV/AIDS Worldwide

- As of the end of 2003, an estimated 40 million people worldwide—37 million adults and 2.5 million children younger than 15 years—were living with HIV/AIDS. Approximately two-thirds of these people (26.6 million) live in Sub-Saharan Africa; another 18 percent (7.4 million) live in Asia and the Pacific.[1]

- Worldwide, approximately 11 of every 1,000 adults aged 15 to 49 are HIV-infected. In Sub-Saharan Africa, about 8 percent of all adults in this age group are HIV-infected.[1]
- An estimated 5 million new HIV infections occurred worldwide during 2003; that is, about 14,000 infections each day. More than 95 percent of these new infections occurred in developing countries, and nearly 50 percent were among females.[1]
- In 2003, approximately 2,000 children under the age of 15 years, and 6,000 young people aged 15 to 24 years became infected with HIV every day.[1]
- In 2003 alone, HIV/AIDS-associated illnesses caused the deaths of approximately 3 million people worldwide, including an estimated 500,000 children younger than 15 years.[1]

HIV/AIDS in the United States

- The Centers for Disease Control and Prevention (CDC) estimate that 850,000 to 950,000 U.S. residents are living with HIV infection, one-quarter of whom are unaware of their infection.[2]
- Approximately 40,000 new HIV infections occur each year in the United States, about 70 percent among men and 30 percent among women. Of these newly infected people, half are younger than 25 years of age.[3,4]
- Of new infections among men in the United States, CDC estimates that approximately 60 percent of men were infected through homosexual sex, 25 percent through injection drug use, and 15 percent through heterosexual sex. Of newly infected men, approximately 50 percent are black, 30 percent are white, 20 percent are Hispanic, and a small percentage are members of other racial/ethnic groups.[4]
- Of new infections among women in the United States, CDC estimates that approximately 75 percent of women were infected through heterosexual sex and 25 percent through injection drug use. Of newly infected women, approximately 64 percent are black, 18 percent are white, 18 percent are Hispanic, and a small percentage are members of other racial/ethnic groups.[4]
- The estimated number of AIDS diagnoses through 2002 in the United States is 886,575. Adult and adolescent AIDS cases total 877,275, with 718,002 cases in males and 159,271 cases in

females. Through the same time period, 9,300 AIDS cases were estimated in children under age 13.[5]

- The estimated number of new adult/adolescent AIDS diagnoses in the United States was 43,225 in 1998, 41,134 in 1999, 42,239 in 2000, 41,227 in 2001, and 42,136 in 2002.[5]
- The estimated number of new pediatric AIDS cases (cases among individuals younger than age 13) in the United States fell from 952 in 1992 to 92 in 2002.[5]
- The estimated rate of adult/adolescent AIDS diagnoses in the United States in 2002 (per 100,000 population) was 76.4 among blacks, 26.0 among Hispanics, 11.2 among American Indians/ Alaska Natives, 7.0 among whites, and 4.9 among Asians/Pacific Islanders.[5]
- From 1985 to 2002, the proportion of adult/adolescent AIDS cases in the United States reported in women increased from 7 percent to 26 percent.[5]
- As of the end of 2002, an estimated 384,906 people in the United States were living with AIDS.[5]
- As of December 31, 2002, an estimated 501,669 people with AIDS in the United States had died.[5]
- The estimated annual number of AIDS-related deaths in the United States fell approximately 14 percent from 1998 to 2002, from 19,005 deaths in 1998 to 16,371 deaths in 2002.[5]
- Of the estimated 16,371 AIDS-related deaths in the United States in 2002, approximately 52 percent were among blacks, 28 percent among whites, 19 percent among Hispanics, and less than 1 percent among Asians/Pacific Islanders and American Indians/Alaska Natives.[5]

References

1. UNAIDS. *AIDS Epidemic Update*, December, 2003.
2. Fleming, P.L. et al. *HIV Prevalence in the United States, 2000*. 9th Conference on Retroviruses and Opportunistic Infections, Seattle, Wash., Feb. 24-28, 2002. Abstract 11.
3. Centers for Disease Control and Prevention (CDC). HIV and AIDS—United States, 1981-2001. *MMWR* 2001;50:430-434.

4. Centers for Disease Control and Prevention (CDC). *HIV Prevention Strategic Plan Through 2005*. January 2001.

5. Centers for Disease Control and Prevention (CDC). *HIV/AIDS Surveillance Report* 2002;14:1-40.

For More Information

AIDSinfo, located at www.AIDSinfo.nih.gov, is a comprehensive resource for up-to-date information on government and industry sponsored HIV/AIDS treatment and prevention clinical trials. AIDSinfo also maintains the most current, federally approved guidelines for the treatment and prevention of HIV/AIDS and AIDS-related illnesses in adults and children, for the management of occupational exposure to HIV, and for the prevention of HIV transmission from mother-to-child during pregnancy. AIDSinfo has a great deal of information available in Spanish, and provides links to other Spanish language resources, which can be accessed through the home page.

AIDSinfo is sponsored by the National Institutes of Health: Office of AIDS Research, National Institute of Allergy and Infectious Diseases (NIAID), National Library of Medicine; Centers for Disease Control and Prevention; Health Resources and Service Administration; and Centers for Medicare and Medicaid Services.

AIDSinfo
P.O. Box 6303
Rockville, MD 20849-6303
Toll-free: 1-800-HIV-0440 (1-800-448-0440)
Phone: 301-519-0459 (International)
Phone: 1-888-480-3739 (TTY/TDD)
Monday to Friday, 12:00 p.m. to 5:00 p.m. Eastern Time
Spanish-speaking health information specialists are available
Website: http://aidsinfo.nih.gov

For information specifically about clinical trials conducted by the NIAID Intramural AIDS Research Program, call 1-800-243-7644 (http://clinicaltrials.gov).

Chapter 40

Influenza (Flu)

The Influenza (Flu) Viruses

Influenza A, B, and C

Influenza types A or B viruses cause epidemics of disease almost every winter. In the United States, these winter influenza epidemics can cause illness in 10% to 20% of people and are associated with an average of 36,000 deaths and 114,000 hospitalizations per year. Getting a flu shot can prevent illness from types A and B influenza. Influenza type C infections cause a mild respiratory illness and are not thought to cause epidemics. The flu shot does not protect against type C influenza.

Influenza type A viruses are divided into subtypes based on two proteins on the surface of the virus. These proteins are called hemagglutinin (H) and neuraminidase (N). The current subtypes of influenza

---

This chapter includes text from "The Influenza (Flu) Viruses," January 15, 2002, "Influenza A (H1N2) Viruses," December 5, 2003, "Questions and Answers: The Disease," December 10, 2003, "Questions and Answers: Cold Versus Flu," January 8, 2004, "Preventing the Flu: Overview," December 12, 2004, "Questions and Answers: Flu Vaccine," December 10, 2003, "Questions and Answers: Flu Shot," December 10, 2003, "Questions and Answers: The Nasal-Spray Flu Vaccine (Live Attenuated Influenza Vaccine [LAIV])," December 15, 2003, "Questions and Answers: Treating the Flu," December 10, 2003, "When to Use Antiviral Drugs for the Flu," December 22, 2003, and "What to Do If You Get Sick: Overview (Interim Guidance)," January 15, 2004, Centers for Disease Control and Prevention (CDC).

A viruses found in people are A(H1N1) and A(H3N2). Influenza B virus is not divided into subtypes. Influenza A(H1N1), A(H3N2), and influenza B strains are included in each year's influenza vaccine.

On February 6, 2002, World Health Organization (WHO) and the Public Health Laboratory Service (PHLS) in the United Kingdom reported the recent identification of a new influenza virus strain, influenza A(H1N2), isolated from humans in England, Israel, and Egypt. In addition to the viruses reported by PHLS, the Centers for Disease Control and Prevention (CDC) has identified influenza A(H1N2) virus from patient specimens collected during the 2001–02 and 2002–03 seasons. Influenza A(H1N2) viruses have been identified in the past.

Transmission of Influenza Viruses from Animals to People

Influenza A viruses are found in many different animals, including ducks, chickens, pigs, whales, horses, and seals. Influenza B viruses circulate widely only among humans.

Influenza A viruses are divided into subtypes based on two proteins on the surface of the virus: the hemagglutinin (H) and the neuraminidase (N). There are 15 different hemagglutinin subtypes and 9 different neuraminidase subtypes, all of which have been found among influenza A viruses in wild birds. Wild birds are the primary natural reservoir for all subtypes of influenza A viruses and are thought to be the source of influenza A viruses in all other animals. Most influenza viruses cause asymptomatic or mild infection in birds; however, the range of symptoms in birds varies greatly depending on the strain of virus. Infection with certain avian influenza A viruses (for example, some strains of H5 and H7 viruses) can cause widespread disease and death among some species of wild and especially domestic birds such as chickens and turkeys.

Pigs can be infected with both human and avian influenza viruses in addition to swine influenza viruses. Infected pigs get symptoms similar to humans, such as cough, fever, and runny nose. Because pigs are susceptible to avian, human and swine influenza viruses, they potentially may be infected with influenza viruses from different species (e.g., ducks and humans) at the same time. If this happens, it is possible for the genes of these viruses to mix and create a new virus. For example, if a pig were infected with a human influenza virus and an avian influenza virus at the same time, the viruses could mix (reassort) and produce a new virus that had most of the genes from the human virus, but a hemagglutinin and/or neuraminidase from the avian virus. The resulting new virus would likely be able to infect humans and spread from person to person, but it would have surface proteins (hemagglutinin and/or neuraminidase) not previously seen in influenza viruses that infect humans. This type of major change in the influenza A viruses is known as antigenic shift. Antigenic shift results when a new influenza A subtype to which most people have little or no immune protection infects humans. If this new virus causes illness in people and can be transmitted easily from person to person, an influenza pandemic can occur.

While it is unusual for people to get influenza infections directly from animals, sporadic human infections and outbreaks caused by certain avian influenza A viruses have been reported.

How the Flu Virus Can Change—"Drift" and "Shift"

Influenza viruses can change in two different ways.

One is called "antigenic drift." These are small changes in the virus that happen continually over time. Antigenic drift produces new virus strains that may not be recognized by the body's immune system. This process works as follows: a person infected with a particular flu virus strain develops antibody against that virus. As newer virus strains appear, the antibodies against the older strains no longer recognize the "newer" virus, and reinfection can occur. This is one of the main reasons why people can get the flu more than one time. In most years, one or two of the three virus strains in the influenza vaccine are updated to keep up with the changes in the circulating flu viruses. So, people who want to be protected from flu need to get a flu shot every year.

The other type of change is called "antigenic shift." Antigenic shift is an abrupt, major change in the influenza A viruses, resulting in new hemagglutinin and/or new hemagglutinin and neuraminidase proteins in influenza viruses that infect humans. Shift results in a new influenza A subtype. When shift happens, most people have little or no protection against the new virus. While influenza viruses are changing by antigenic drift all the time, antigenic shift happens only occasionally. Type A viruses undergo both kinds of changes; influenza type B viruses change only by the more gradual process of antigenic drift.

Questions and Answers about Influenza

What is influenza (flu)?

Influenza, commonly called "the flu," is caused by the influenza virus, which infects the respiratory tract (nose, throat, lungs). Unlike many other viral respiratory infections, such as the common cold, the flu causes severe illness and life-threatening complications in many people.

What are the symptoms of the flu?

Influenza is a respiratory illness. Symptoms of flu include fever, headache, extreme tiredness, dry cough, sore throat, runny or stuffy nose, and muscle aches. Children can have additional gastrointestinal symptoms, such as nausea, vomiting, and diarrhea, but these symptoms are uncommon in adults. Although the term "stomach flu" is sometimes used to describe vomiting, nausea, or diarrhea, these illnesses are caused by certain other viruses, bacteria, or possibly parasites, and are rarely related to influenza.

When is the flu season in the United States?

In the United States, the peak of flu season can occur anywhere from late December through March. The overall health impact (e.g., infections, hospitalizations, and deaths) of a flu season varies from year to year. CDC monitors circulating flu viruses and their related disease activity and provides influenza reports each week from October through May.

How does the flu spread?

The main way that influenza viruses are spread is from person to person in respiratory droplets of coughs and sneezes. (This is called "droplet spread.") This can happen when droplets from a cough or sneeze of an infected person are propelled (generally up to 3 feet) through the air and deposited on the mouth or nose of people nearby. Though much less frequent, the viruses also can be spread when a person touches respiratory droplets on another person or an object and then touches their own mouth or nose (or someone else's mouth or nose) before washing their hands.

Does the flu have complications?

Yes. Some of the complications caused by flu include bacterial pneumonia, dehydration, and worsening of chronic medical conditions, such as congestive heart failure, asthma, or diabetes. Children may get sinus problems and ear infections as complications from the flu. Those aged 65 years and older and persons of any age with chronic medical conditions are at highest risk for serious complications of flu.

How do I find out if I have the flu?

It is very difficult to distinguish the flu from other viral or bacterial causes of respiratory illnesses on the basis of symptoms alone. A test can confirm that an illness is influenza if the patient is tested within the first two to three days after symptoms begin. In addition, a doctor's examination may be needed to determine whether a person has another infection that is a complication of influenza.

How soon will I get sick if I am exposed to the flu?

The time from when a person is exposed to flu virus to when symptoms begin is about one to four days, with an average of about two days.

How long is a person with flu virus contagious?

The period when an infected person is contagious depends on the age of the person. Adults may be contagious from one day prior to becoming sick and for three to seven days after they first develop symptoms. Some children may be contagious for longer than a week.

How many people get sick or die from the flu every year?

Each flu season is unique, but it is estimated that approximately 10% to 20% of U.S. residents get the flu, and an average of 114,000 persons are hospitalized for flu-related complications. About 36,000 Americans die on average per year from the complications of flu.

What is the difference between a cold and the flu?

The flu and the common cold are both respiratory illnesses but they are caused by different viruses. Because these two types of illnesses have similar flu-like symptoms, it can be difficult to tell the difference between them based on symptoms alone. In general, the flu is worse than the common cold, and symptoms such as fever, body aches, extreme tiredness, and dry cough are more common and intense. Colds are usually milder than the flu. People with colds are more likely to have a runny or stuffy nose. Colds generally do not result in serious health problems, such as pneumonia, bacterial infections, or hospitalizations.

How can you tell the difference between a cold and the flu?

Because colds and flu share many symptoms, it can be difficult (or even impossible) to tell the difference between them based on symptoms alone. Special tests that usually must be done within the first few days of illness can be carried out, when needed to tell if a person has the flu.

What are the symptoms of the flu versus the symptoms of a cold?

In general, the flu is worse than the common cold, and symptoms such as fever, body aches, extreme tiredness, and dry cough are more common and intense. Colds are usually milder than the flu. People with colds are more likely to have a runny or stuffy nose. Colds generally do not result in serious health problems, such as pneumonia, bacterial infections, or hospitalizations.

Preventing the Flu

The single best way to prevent the flu is to get vaccinated each fall. In the absence of vaccine, however, there are other ways to protect against flu. Antiviral medications can also be used to prevent the flu. Other good health habits include:

- **Avoid close contact:** Avoid close contact with people who are sick. When you are sick, keep your distance from others to protect them from getting sick too.
- **Stay home when you are sick:** If possible, stay home from work, school, and errands when you are sick. You will help prevent others from catching your illness.
- **Cover your mouth and nose:** Cover your mouth and nose with a tissue when coughing or sneezing. It may prevent those around you from getting sick.
- **Clean your hands:** Washing your hands often will help protect you from germs.
- **Avoid touching your eyes, nose, or mouth:** Germs are often spread when a person touches something that is contaminated with germs and then touches his or her eyes, nose, or mouth.

Flu Vaccine

What kind of flu vaccines are there?

There are two types of vaccines that protect against the flu. The "flu shot" is an inactivated vaccine (containing killed virus) that is given with a needle, usually in the arm. A different kind of vaccine, called the nasal-spray flu vaccine (sometimes referred to as LAIV for Live Attenuated Influenza Vaccine), was approved in 2003. The nasal-spray flu vaccine contains attenuated (weakened) live viruses, and is administered by nasal sprayer. It is approved for use only among healthy people between the ages of 5 and 49 years. The flu shot is approved for use among people over 6 months of age, including healthy people and those with chronic medical conditions.

Each of the two vaccines contains three influenza viruses, representing one of the three groups of viruses circulating among people in a given year. Each of the three vaccine strains in both vaccines—one A (H3N2) virus, one A (H1N1) virus, and one B virus—are representative of the influenza vaccine strains recommended for that year. Viruses for both vaccines are grown in eggs.

How do flu vaccines work?

Both flu vaccines (the flu shot and the nasal-spray flu vaccine (LAIV)) work in the same way; they cause antibodies to develop in the body, and these antibodies provide protection against influenza virus infection.

Why should people get vaccinated against the flu?

Influenza is a serious disease, and people of any age can get it. In an average year, the flu causes 36,000 deaths (mostly among those aged 65 years or older) and 114,000 hospitalizations in the United States. The "flu season" in the United States is usually from November through April each year. During this time, flu viruses are circulating in the population. An annual flu vaccine (either the flu shot or the nasal-spray flu vaccine) is the best way to reduce the chances that you will get the flu.

When should I get a flu vaccination?

Beginning each September, the flu shot should be offered to people at high risk when they are seen by health-care providers for routine care or as a result of hospitalization.

The best time to get vaccinated is from October through November. Flu activity in the United States generally peaks between late December and early March.

You can still benefit from getting vaccinated after November, even if flu is present in your community. Vaccine should continue to be offered to unvaccinated people throughout the flu season as long as vaccine is still available. Once you get vaccinated, your body makes protective antibodies in about two weeks.

Does flu vaccine work right away?

No. It takes about two weeks after vaccination for antibodies to develop in the body and provide protection against influenza virus infection. In the meantime, you are still at risk for getting the flu. That's why it's better to get vaccinated early in the fall, before the flu season really gets under way.

Can I get the flu even though I got a flu vaccine this year?

Yes. The ability of flu vaccine to protect a person depends on two things: 1) the age and health status of the person getting the vaccine, and 2) the similarity or "match" between the virus strains in the vaccine and those in circulation.

How effective is the flu vaccine?

The flu vaccine is the most effective way to prevent the flu. However, in limited studies, the flu shot and the nasal-spray flu vaccine (LAIV) have different rates of effectiveness.

Why do I need to get vaccinated against the flu every year?

Flu viruses change from year to year, which means two things. First, you can get the flu more than once during your lifetime. The immunity (natural protection that develops against a disease after a person has had that disease) that is built up from having the flu caused by one virus strain doesn't always provide protection when a new strain is circulating. Second, a vaccine made against flu viruses circulating last year may not protect against the newer viruses. That is why the influenza vaccine is updated to include current viruses every year.

Another reason to get flu vaccine every year is that after you get vaccinated, your immunity to the disease declines over time and may be too low to provide protection after one year.

How are the viruses for flu vaccine selected?

Each year, many laboratories throughout the world, including in the United States, collect flu viruses. Some of these flu viruses are sent to one of four World Health Organization (WHO) reference laboratories, one of which is at the Centers for Disease Control and Prevention (CDC) in Atlanta, for detailed testing. These laboratories also test how well antibodies made to the current vaccine react to the circulating virus and new flu viruses. This information, along with information about flu activity, is summarized and presented to an advisory committee of the U.S. Food and Drug Administration (FDA) and at a WHO meeting. These meetings result in the selection of three viruses (two subtypes of influenza A viruses and one influenza B virus) to go into flu vaccines for the following fall and winter. Usually, one or two of the three virus strains in the vaccine are changed each year.

Questions and Answers about Flu Shots

What is the flu shot?

The flu shot is an inactivated vaccine (containing killed virus) that is given with a needle, usually in the arm. It contains three influenza viruses. The three vaccine strains—one A (H3N2) virus, one A (H1N1) virus, and one B virus—are representative of the influenza vaccine strains recommended for that year. Viruses for the flu shot are grown in eggs.

Who should get a flu shot?

People at high risk for complications of the flu and people in close contact with them (including household members) should get a flu shot.

Who should not get a flu shot?

Talk with a doctor before getting a flu shot if you:

1. Have ever had a severe allergic reaction to eggs or to a previous flu shot or
2. Have a history of Guillain-Barré syndrome (GBS).

If you are sick with a fever when you go to get your flu shot, you should talk to your doctor or nurse about getting your shot at a later date. However, you can get a flu shot at the same time you have a respiratory illness without fever or if you have another mild illness.

How effective is the flu shot?

With the flu shot, when the "match" between vaccine and circulating strains is close, the vaccine prevents influenza in about 70%–90% of healthy persons younger than age 65 years. Among elderly persons living outside chronic-care facilities (such as nursing homes) and those persons with long-term (chronic) medical conditions, the flu shot is 30%–70% effective in preventing hospitalization for pneumonia and influenza. Among elderly nursing home residents, the flu shot is most effective in preventing severe illness, secondary complications, and deaths related to the flu. In this population, the shot can be 50%–60% effective in preventing hospitalization or pneumonia and 80% effective in preventing death from the flu.

What are the risks from getting a flu shot?

The viruses in the flu shot are killed (inactivated), so you cannot get the flu from a flu shot. The risk of a flu shot causing serious harm, or death, is extremely small. However, a vaccine, like any medicine, may rarely cause serious problems, such as severe allergic reactions. Almost all people who get influenza vaccine have no serious problems from it.

What are the side effects that could occur?

- Soreness, redness, or swelling where the shot was given
- Fever (low grade)
- Aches

If these problems occur, they begin soon after the shot and usually last one to two days.

Can severe problems occur?

- Life-threatening allergic reactions are very rare. Signs of serious allergic reaction can include breathing problems, hoarseness or wheezing, hives, paleness, weakness, a fast heartbeat, or dizziness. If they do occur, it is within a few minutes to a few hours after the shot. These reactions are more likely to occur among persons with a severe allergy to eggs, because the viruses used in the influenza vaccine are grown in hens' eggs. People who have had a severe reaction to eggs or to a flu shot in the past should not get a flu shot before seeing a physician.

- Guillain-Barré syndrome: Normally, about one person per 100,000 people per year will develop Guillain-Barré syndrome (GBS), an illness characterized by fever, nerve damage, and muscle weakness. In 1976, vaccination with the swine flu vaccine was associated with getting GBS. Several studies have been done to evaluate if other flu vaccines since 1976 were associated with GBS. Only one of the studies showed an association. That study suggested that one person out of 1 million vaccinated persons may be at risk of GBS associated with the vaccine.

What should I do if I have had a serious reaction to influenza vaccine?

- Call a doctor, or get to a doctor right away.
- Tell your doctor what happened, the date and time it happened, and when you got the flu shot.
- Ask your doctor, nurse, or health department to file a Vaccine Adverse Event Reporting System (VAERS) form, or call VAERS at 1-800-822-7967.

The Nasal-Spray Flu Vaccine (Live Attenuated Influenza Vaccine [LAIV])

What is the nasal-spray flu vaccine (or LAIV)?

The nasal-spray flu vaccine (sometimes called LAIV for Live Attenuated Influenza Vaccine) is a new flu vaccine that was licensed in 2003. It is different from the other licensed influenza vaccine (also called the "flu shot") because it contains weakened live influenza viruses instead of killed viruses and is administered by nasal spray instead of injection.

How does the nasal-spray flu vaccine (LAIV) work?

The nasal-spray flu vaccine contains three different live (but weakened) influenza viruses. When the viruses are sprayed into the nose, they stimulate the body's immune system to develop protective antibodies that will prevent infection by naturally occurring influenza viruses.

The live viruses in the nasal-spray flu vaccine (LAIV) are attenuated, cold-adapted, and temperature sensitive. What does this mean?

Attenuated means the viruses are weakened and will not cause severe symptoms often associated with influenza illness. Cold-adapted and temperature sensitive mean the viruses can grow in the nose and throat, but not in the lower respiratory tract where the temperature is higher.

How effective is the nasal-spray flu vaccine (LAIV)?

In one large study among children aged 15–85 months, the nasal-spray flu vaccine (LAIV) reduced the chance of influenza illness by 92% compared with placebo. In a study among adults, the participants were not specifically tested for influenza. However, the study found 19% fewer severe febrile respiratory tract illnesses, 24% fewer respiratory tract illnesses with fever, 23–27% fewer days of illness, 13–28% fewer lost work days, 15–41% fewer health care provider visits, and 43–47% less use of antibiotics compared with placebo.

Who can be vaccinated with the nasal-spray flu vaccine (LAIV)?

LAIV is approved for use in healthy people between the ages of 5 and 49 years.

Who should not be vaccinated with the nasal-spray flu vaccine (LAIV)?

- People less than 5 years of age
- People 50 years of age and over
- People with a medical condition that places them at high risk for complications from influenza, including those with chronic heart or lung disease, such as asthma or reactive airways disease; people with medical conditions such as diabetes or kidney failure; or people with illnesses that weaken the immune system, or who take medications that can weaken the immune system.
- Children or adolescents receiving aspirin
- People with a history of Guillain-Barré syndrome, a rare disorder of the nervous system

- Pregnant women
- People with a history of allergy to any of the components of LAIV or to eggs

Should the nasal-spray flu vaccine (LAIV) be given to patients with chronic diseases other than those specifically listed above?

No. The nasal-spray flu vaccine is approved for use only in healthy people between the ages of 5 and 49 years.

Can people receiving the nasal-spray flu vaccine (LAIV) pass the vaccine viruses to others?

In clinical studies, transmission of vaccine viruses to close contacts has occurred only rarely. The current estimated risk of getting infected with vaccine virus after close contact with a person vaccinated with the nasal-spray flu vaccine is low (0.6%–2.4%). Because the viruses are attenuated and cold-adapted, infection is unlikely to result in influenza illness symptoms since the vaccine viruses have not been shown to mutate into typical or naturally occurring influenza viruses.

Can contacts of people with weakened immune systems get the nasal-spray flu vaccine (LAIV)?

Use of inactivated influenza vaccine (the flu shot) is preferred for vaccinating household members, health-care workers, and others who have close contact with people who have weakened immune systems because of the theoretical risk that a vaccine virus could be transmitted and cause illness. Otherwise, either inactivated vaccine or the nasal-spray flu vaccine can be used for healthy people between the ages of 5 and 49 years who are in close contact with other people at high risk for flu-related complication (for example, people with heart disease who are not on medications that could weaken the immune system).

What side effects are associated with the nasal-spray flu vaccine (LAIV)?

In children, side effects can include runny nose, headache, vomiting, muscle aches, and fever. In adults, side effects can include runny nose, headache, sore throat, and cough. Fever is not a common side effect in adults receiving the nasal-spray flu vaccine.

When should the nasal-spray flu vaccine (LAIV) be given?

The optimal time to receive influenza vaccine is usually in October or November. Children between the ages of 5 and 8 years who have never received influenza vaccine should receive the nasal-spray flu vaccine for the first time in October or earlier because they need a second dose 6 to 10 weeks after the first dose.

How often should the nasal-spray flu vaccine (LAIV) be given?

LAIV should be given each year before the influenza season.

Can people who received inactivated influenza vaccine (the flu shot) last year get the nasal-spray flu vaccine (LAIV) this year?

Yes, people who got inactivated influenza vaccine (the flu shot) last year can get the nasal-spray flu vaccine (LAIV) this year.

Can the nasal-spray flu vaccine (LAIV) be given at the same time as other vaccines?

An inactivated vaccine may be given either at the same time or at any time before or after the nasal-spray flu vaccine. A live vaccine may be given together with the nasal-spray flu vaccine. If the two live vaccines are not given at the same visit, they should be given more than 4 weeks apart.

Can the nasal-spray flu vaccine (LAIV) be given to patients when they are ill?

The nasal-spray flu vaccine (LAIV) can be given to people with minor illnesses (e.g., diarrhea or mild upper respiratory tract infection with or without fever). However, if nasal congestion is present that might limit delivery of the vaccine to the nasal lining, then delaying of vaccination until the nasal congestion is reduced should be considered.

Can the nasal-spray flu vaccine (LAIV) be used together with influenza antiviral medications?

If a person is taking an influenza antiviral drug (including Symmetrel [amantadine] for Parkinson's disease), then the nasal-spray flu vaccine should not be given until 48 hours after the last dose of the influenza antiviral medication was given. If a person has received the nasal-spray flu vaccine, an influenza antiviral medication should not be given until 2 weeks after the flu mist was administered.

If a child under the age of 9 years is getting influenza vaccine for the first time and requires 2 doses, does the same type of vaccine have to be used for both doses?

No, the first and second doses do not have to match; live or inactivated vaccine can be used for either dose. If inactivated influenza vaccine (the flu shot) is used first, then the nasal-spray flu vaccine (LAIV) should be given at least 4 weeks later. If the nasal-spray flu vaccine is used first, the second vaccine should be given 6 to 10 weeks later.

How is the nasal-spray flu vaccine (LAIV) stored?

The nasal-spray flu vaccine (LAIV) must be stored frozen at -15° C or colder. It may not be stored in a frost-free freezer (because temperature cycling in these freezers may reach more than -15° C) unless a storage box provided by the manufacturer is used. After thawing, the vaccine may be stored for up to 24 hours in a refrigerator at 2–8°C, and it should not be refrozen. Vaccine thawed for more than 24 hours should be discarded.

What personal protective equipment is recommended for health-care workers who are giving the vaccine?

Disposable gloves should be worn by health-care workers administering the nasal-spray flu vaccine (LAIV).

Does the nasal-spray flu vaccine (LAIV) contain thimerosal?

No, the nasal-spray flu vaccine (LAIV) does not contain thimerosal or any other preservative.

Treating the Flu

How should the flu be treated?

- Rest
- Drink plenty of liquids

- Avoid using alcohol and tobacco
- Take medication to relieve the symptoms of flu (but never give aspirin to children or teenagers who have flu-like symptoms—and particularly fever—without first speaking to your doctor.)

In some cases, your doctors may choose to use certain antiviral drugs to treat the flu. (Influenza is caused by a virus, so antibiotics [like penicillin] don't work to cure it.)

Can antiviral drugs cure the flu?

Not exactly. When started within the first two days of illness, they can reduce the duration of the disease but cannot cure it outright.

Four different antiviral drugs (amantadine, rimantadine, zanamivir, and oseltamivir) have been approved for treating the flu. All four drugs can reduce the duration of flu by about one day if taken within 2 days of when symptoms begin. The four drugs differ in terms of side effects. In some patients, amantadine (Symmetrel®, others) can cause symptoms such as nervousness, difficulty concentrating, or lightheadedness. Rimantadine (Flumadine®) can also cause similar types of side effects, but less often. Caution is advised if zanamivir (Relenza®) is used by people who have asthma or chronic obstructive pulmonary disease, because the airways of these people may suddenly grow smaller after using zanamivir, leading to difficulty breathing. Oseltamivir (Tamiflu®) can cause nausea and vomiting in some people.

All of these drugs must be prescribed by a doctor. These drugs are effective against flu viruses, but they are not effective against other viruses or bacteria that can cause symptoms similar to influenza. These drugs are not effective for treating bacterial infections that can occur as complications of influenza.

When to Use Antiviral Drugs for the Flu

What antiviral drugs are used for the flu?

Three antiviral drugs (amantadine, rimantadine, and oseltamivir) are approved and commercially available for use in preventing flu. All of these medications are prescription drugs, and a doctor should be consulted before the drugs are used. When used for prevention, they are about 70% to 90% effective for preventing illness in healthy adults.

Four antiviral drugs (amantadine, rimantadine, zanamivir and oseltamivir) have been approved for treatment of the flu. If taken within 2 days of getting sick, these drugs can reduce the symptoms of the flu and shorten the time you are sick by 1 or 2 days. They also can make you less contagious to others. All of these drugs must be prescribed by a doctor and taken for 5 days. Antiviral drugs are effective only against influenza viruses. They will not help the symptoms associated with the common cold or many other flu-like illnesses caused by viruses that circulate in the winter.

All of the antiviral drugs are different in terms of who can take them, how they are given, any dosing changes based on age or medical conditions, and side effects. Your doctors will help decide whether you should get antivirals and which one you should get.

When are antivirals effective?

Antiviral drugs are most often used to control flu outbreaks in institutions, for example in nursing homes, or in hospital wards, where people at high risk (see below) for complications from flu are in close contact with each other. Antivirals also have been used on cruise ships or similar settings to control outbreaks of the flu.

In the event of an outbreak, public health practice is to combine the use of flu vaccine and antivirals. In a nursing home during an outbreak, for example, residents and staff are given the flu vaccine and antivirals to prevent flu until the vaccine takes effect (about 2 weeks). This practice continues as long as influenza is occurring in that setting.

Doctors also can prescribe antivirals for flu to people not living in institutional settings, but treatment must begin within 2 days of the onset of symptoms for it to be effective. Also, while all antivirals lessen the symptoms of illness and shorten the duration of illness, only 1 (oseltamivir) has been shown in a study to reduce some complications requiring antibiotics.

When considering antivirals, it's important to remember that most healthy people recover from the flu without complications.

Should antivirals be used for people at high risk for complications?

Some people are considered to be at high risk from complications of flu. This includes

- People 65 years of age and older
- Children 6–23 months of age*

- People of any age with chronic medical conditions (for example, heart or lung disease, diabetes)
- Pregnant women

Note that none of the antivirals are approved for use in children less than 1 year of age.

*Children 6–23 months of age are at increased risk for influenza-related hospitalization.

Who should get antiviral drugs?

For Treatment: If you get sick with flu-like symptoms this season, your doctor first may give you a test to find out whether you have influenza. (Symptoms of flu include: fever (usually high), headache, tiredness, a sore throat and dry cough, nasal congestion, and body aches.) Your doctor also will consider a number of things before making a treatment decision, such as your risk for complications from flu.

For Prevention: In the event of a flu outbreak in a home, institution, or community, your doctor may choose to give antivirals to you as a preventive measure, especially if you are at high risk for complications from the flu. Also, if you are in close contact with someone who is considered at high risk for complications from flu, you may be given antiviral drugs to prevent passing flu to the high-risk person.

What to Do If You Get Sick

What should you do if you get the flu?

If you develop flu-like symptoms, and you are not at high risk for complications from the flu:

- Get plenty of rest
- Drink a lot of liquids
- Avoid using alcohol and tobacco
- Consider taking over-the-counter medications to relieve the symptoms of flu (but never give aspirin to children or teenagers who have flu-like symptoms)
- Stay home and avoid contact with other people to protect them from catching your illness

- Cover your nose and mouth with a tissue when you cough or sneeze to protect others from your germs.

Most healthy people recover from the flu without complications.

What are the signs that medical attention is needed?

There are some "emergency warning signs" that require urgent medical attention.

In children, some emergency warning signs that need urgent medical attention include:

- High or prolonged fever
- Fast breathing or trouble breathing
- Bluish skin color
- Not drinking enough fluids
- Changes in mental status, such as not waking up or not interacting; being so irritable that the child does not want to be held; or seizures
- Flu-like symptoms improve but then return with fever and worse cough
- Worsening of underlying chronic medical conditions (for example, heart or lung disease, diabetes)

In adults, some emergency warning signs that need urgent medical attention include:

- High or prolonged fever
- Difficulty breathing or shortness of breath
- Pain or pressure in the chest
- Near-fainting or fainting
- Confusion
- Severe or persistent vomiting

Seek medical care immediately, either by calling your doctor or going to an emergency room, if you or someone you know is experiencing any of the signs described above or other unusually severe symptoms. When you arrive, tell the receptionist or nurse about your symptoms. You may be asked to wear a mask and/or sit in a separate area to protect others from getting sick.

What are special concerns for people at high risk for complications from the flu?

Some people are at increased risk to develop complications of flu. This group includes:

- People 65 years of age and older
- Children 6–23 months of age (children 6–23 months of age are at increased risk for influenza-related hospitalization)
- People of any age with chronic medical conditions (for example, heart or lung disease, asthma, diabetes, or HIV infection)
- Pregnant women

If you are in a group that is considered to be at high risk for complications from the flu and you get flu-like symptoms, you should consult your health-care provider when your symptoms begin.

Some of the complications caused by flu include bacterial pneumonia, dehydration, and worsening of chronic medical conditions, such as congestive heart failure, asthma, or diabetes. Children also may get sinus and ear infections.

What secondary infections may develop?

Persons infected with influenza are sometimes at higher risk for developing secondary infections, such as pneumonia. During the 2003–2004 U.S. influenza season, several cases of community-acquired MRSA (methicillin resistant *Staphylococcus aureus*) infections, including pneumonias, have occurred in association with influenza infection. This has not been reported previously.

Chapter 41

Measles (Rubeola)

Signs and Symptoms

Measles, also called rubeola, is best known for its typical skin rash. It is, however, primarily a respiratory infection. The first symptoms are irritability, runny nose, eyes that are red and sensitive to light, hacking cough, and a fever as high as 105 degrees Fahrenheit (40.6 degrees Celsius).

Fever peaks with the appearance of the rash, which typically begins on the forehead, then spreads downward over the face, neck, and body. The child is particularly ill-looking during the first days of the rash. It usually takes about 3 days for the rash to make its way down to the feet. Once the rash appears on the legs and feet, symptoms usually subside within 2 days.

The rash itself looks like large flat red to brown blotches that often flow into one another to completely cover the skin, especially on the face and shoulders. The rash fades in the same order that it appeared, forehead first and feet last. The total time for the rash, from beginning to end, head to toe, is usually about 6 days. As the rash disappears, the healing skin may look brown temporarily, before it sheds in a finely textured peel.

"Rubeola (Measles)," The Nemours Foundation, updated and reviewed by Kim Rutherford, MD., reprinted with permission. This information was provided by KidsHealth, one of the largest resources online for medically reviewed health information written for parents, kids, and teens. For more articles like this one, visit www.KidsHealth.org, or www.TeensHealth.org.

One special identifying sign of measles is Koplik's spots. These are small, red, irregularly-shaped spots with blue-white centers found inside the mouth. Koplik's spots usually appear 1 to 2 days before the measles rash and may be noticed by a doctor looking for the cause of a child's fever and cough.

Measles can lead to many different complications: croup, bronchitis, bronchiolitis, pneumonia, conjunctivitis, myocarditis, hepatitis, and encephalitis. Measles can also make the body more susceptible to ear infections or pneumonias caused by bacteria. Symptoms and complications of measles are usually most severe in adults.

Description

Measles is a respiratory infection caused by the measles virus. Before immunization was available, measles occurred in springtime epidemics, usually in cycles of 2 or 3 years.

Infants are generally protected from measles for 6 to 8 months after birth, due to immunity that was passed on from their mothers. Older children are usually immunized against measles according to state and school health regulations. Currently, outbreaks of measles are occurring most often on college campuses, among young persons who have either not been adequately immunized against measles, or whose immunity has decreased since childhood.

Prevention

Measles is prevented by a vaccine that can be given before, or within 3 days after, exposure to the disease. In most children, measles vaccine is given as part of the mumps-measles-rubella immunizations (MMR)—one given at age 15 months, and the second at 11 to 12 years. Measles vaccine is not usually given to infants younger than 13 months old, except in times of measles outbreaks. In this case, a dose of measles vaccine alone may be given at 9 months, followed by the usual MMR immunization at 15 months.

Measles vaccine made before 1979 may not have been as effective as vaccine made today. Because of this, doctors often recommend that persons vaccinated before 1980 receive another measles vaccination if a measles outbreak occurs in their area, especially if they are in school. A blood test can be performed to determine a person's immunity and whether they need another immunization.

Measles vaccine should not be given to pregnant women, or to persons with active tuberculosis, leukemia, lymphoma, or depressed immune systems. Also, persons with severe allergies to eggs, or to the antibiotic neomycin, may risk life-threatening reactions to measles vaccine.

Measles vaccine occasionally causes side effects in persons with no underlying health problems. In about 10% of cases there is a fever between 5 and 12 days after vaccination, and in about 5% of cases there is a rash.

In special situations (pregnant women, infants, persons with cancer, tuberculosis, or depressed immune systems), persons exposed to measles can also be protected from infection by an injection of antibodies called gamma globulin. Gamma globulin is given within 6 days of exposure, and it either prevents measles or makes symptoms less severe.

As is the case with all immunization schedules, there are important exceptions and special circumstances. Your doctor should have the most current information regarding recommendations about the measles immunization.

Incubation

The incubation period for measles is about 9 to 11 days between exposure and prodromal symptoms, or about 2 weeks between exposure and the appearance of a rash.

Duration

Measles usually lasts about 10 to 14 days, measured from the beginning of the prodromal symptoms to the fading of the rash. Most prodromal symptoms disappear 1 or 2 days after the rash begins, except for the cough, which may last as long as the rash.

Contagiousness

Measles is a highly contagious disease, and about 90% of nonimmunized persons will develop measles if they live in the same house as someone who has the disease. The measles virus spreads in fluid from the nose or mouth, and in airborne droplets. Persons with measles are contagious from 5 days after exposure to 5 days after the rash appears.

Home Treatment

Call your child's doctor if you suspect that your child has measles. Close contact with your doctor will let you both monitor your child's progress and will help you to spot any complications. Take your child's temperature at least once each morning and each evening, and keep a record. If fever goes above 103 degrees Fahrenheit (39.4 degrees Celsius) bring it down using nonaspirin fever medications such as acetaminophen. Unless instructed by your child's doctor, don't give aspirin to a child who has a viral illness since the use of aspirin in such cases has been associated with the development of Reye syndrome.

Encourage your child to drink clear fluids: water, fruit juice, tea, and lemonade. Fluids will help replace body water lost in the heat and sweating of fever episodes. Fluids will also help reduce the chance of lung infections (pneumonia) because they prevent lung secretions from becoming thick and clogging the breathing passages.

Use a cool-mist vaporizer to relieve cough and to soothe breathing passages. Clean the vaporizer each day to prevent mold from growing. Avoid hot-water or steam vaporizers that can cause accidental burns and scalds in children.

Children with measles should not read or watch television while their eyes are sensitive to light. They should rest and avoid busy activities. It is usually safe for them to return to school about 7 to 10 days after the fever and rash are gone.

Professional Treatment

If you think that your child may have measles, it's important to tell your doctor immediately. Your doctor can confirm that the illness is measles and can guide you in watching for complications. He or she can also notify those health authorities who keep track of childhood immunization programs and measles outbreaks.

After symptoms have begun, gamma globulin is not effective against measles, and antibiotics do not work against the measles virus.

Children who are weakened by measles are more susceptible to infections caused by bacteria, especially bacterial infections of the ear and lungs. When this happens, antibiotics are given to treat the bacterial infection.

When to Call Your Child's Doctor

Call your child's doctor immediately if you suspect that your child has measles. Also, call your doctor if your child has been exposed to measles and your child is an infant; is taking medicines that depress the immune system; has tuberculosis, cancer, or a disease that affects the immune system.

If your child has measles, ask your doctor what to watch for. Keep track of your child's temperature and call your doctor if it goes above 103 degrees Fahrenheit (39.4 degrees Celsius). Let your doctor know if your child has an earache, since this may be a sign of a bacterial infection.

Call your doctor if a child with measles has signs that a lung infection (pneumonia) may be starting. These signs may include: breathing that is difficult or very fast; a cough that lasts for more than four or five days or that brings up discolored mucus; lips or nails that are bluish or gray. Your doctor will give you more details.

Immediately call your doctor if your child has any of the following: severe headache; stiff neck; convulsion (seizure); severe drowsiness; difficulty waking up; or loss of consciousness.

Chapter 42

Mumps

Signs and Symptoms

Mumps is a disease caused by a virus that can infect many parts of the body, especially the parotid salivary glands. The parotid salivary glands, which produce saliva for the mouth, are found toward the back of each cheek, in the area between the ear and jaw. In mumps, the parotid glands become increasingly swollen and painful over a period of one to three days. Pain gets worse when the child swallows, talks, chews, or drinks juices that are acidic (like orange juice). As the glands swell, there is often a fever of up to 103 degrees Fahrenheit (39.4 degrees Celsius), with headache and loss of appetite.

In two out of three cases, both left and right parotid glands are affected, one side swelling a few days before the other. In rare cases, mumps will attack other groups of salivary glands instead of the parotids. If this happens, the swelling and pain may be under the tongue, under the jaw, or all the way down to the front of the chest. Mumps less commonly can also involve inflammation (swelling) of the brain, pancreas and other organs.

"Mumps," The Nemours Foundation, updated and reviewed by Kim Rutherford, MD., reprinted with permission. This information was provided by KidsHealth, one of the largest resources online for medically reviewed health information written for parents, kids, and teens. For more articles like this one, visit www.KidsHealth.org, or www.TeensHealth.org. © 2003 The Nemours Center for Children's Health Media, a division of The Nemours Foundation.

Mumps in young adult males (and older) may result in the development of orchitis, an inflammation of the testicles—a condition that ultimately can lead to a decreased sperm count. Usually one testicle becomes swollen and painful about 7 to 10 days after the parotids swell. There is a high fever (often to 106 degrees Fahrenheit or 41.1 degrees Celsius), with shaking chills, headache, nausea, and vomiting. After 3 to 7 days, testicular pain and swelling subside, usually about the same time as the fever passes. In some cases, both testicles are involved.

Mumps may also lead to encephalitis or meningitis (inflammation of the brain or the lining of the central nervous system). Symptoms appear 3 to 7 days after parotid swelling begins and may include: high fever, stiff neck, headache, nausea and vomiting, drowsiness, convulsions, and other signs of brain involvement.

Mumps may also affect the pancreas or, in females, the ovaries, causing pain and tenderness in the parts of the abdomen.

In some cases, signs and symptoms of mumps are so mild that no one suspects a mumps infection. Doctors believe that about one in four persons may have a mumps infection without symptoms.

Description

Mumps is an illness that affects the entire body, but especially the salivary glands. It is caused by a virus that usually spreads through an infected person's saliva, and possibly through the urine. Outbreaks of mumps are most common in the spring, especially in April and May. Mumps epidemics are fairly rare and happen most often where people live in close quarters, like army camps and schools.

Mumps infections are rare in children younger than two years, but become more common as children grow. Children ages 10 to 19 are most likely to get mumps.

It is very unusual to have a second mumps infection, since one attack of mumps almost always gives lifelong protection against another.

Prevention

Mumps can be prevented by vaccine. This vaccine can be given alone, or as part of the mumps-measles-rubella (MMR) immunizations given at age 15 months, and again at 11 to 12 years. As is the case with all immunization schedules, there are important exceptions and special circumstances. Your child's doctor will have the most current information. Mumps vaccine is effective in 75% to 95% of persons who receive it, but it should not be given to a child who has a fever, or to an infant younger than 1 year old. It should also not be given to pregnant women; persons who have certain types of cancer; those who are having radiation or chemotherapy treatment for cancer; persons with depressed immune systems or who are taking medicines that affect the immune system.

An antimumps globulin is available and can be given to children who have been exposed to mumps, but it doesn't always prevent the disease.

Incubation

The incubation period for mumps can be 12 to 25 days, but the average is 18 days.

Duration

Children usually recover from mumps in about 10 to 12 days. It takes about 1 week for the swelling to disappear in each parotid gland, but both glands don't usually swell at the same time.

Contagiousness

Experts disagree about how long someone with mumps is contagious. Some say that the contagious period lasts from 2 days before symptoms begin, to 6 days after symptoms end. Others say that persons with mumps can spread the virus in their saliva from 6 days before their glands begin swelling, to 2 weeks after. Mumps virus may also live in the urine of infected persons for 2 to 3 weeks.

Home Treatment

Call your child's doctor if you suspect that your child has mumps. Close contact with your child's doctor will let you both monitor your child's progress and will help you spot any complications. Take your child's temperature at least once each morning and each evening, and keep a record. If fever goes above 103 degrees Fahrenheit (39.4 Celsius), bring it down using nonaspirin fever medications such as acetaminophen. These medicines will also help relieve pain in the swollen parotid glands. Unless instructed by your child's doctor, aspirin should NOT be used in children with viral illnesses since the use of aspirin in such cases has been associated with the development of Reye syndrome.

In addition to giving pain medication, soothe your child's swollen parotid glands with either warm or cold packs—whichever feels better. Serve a soft, bland diet, and encourage your child to drink plenty of fluids. Avoid serving tart or acidic fruit juices (like orange juice, grapefruit juice or lemonade) that make parotid pain worse. Water, decaffeinated soft drinks and tea are better tolerated.

When mumps involves the testicles, your doctor may prescribe stronger medications for pain and swelling. He or she may also give you instructions about how to apply warm or cool packs to soothe the area.

A child with mumps doesn't need to stay in bed, but may play quietly. Ask your doctor about the best time for your child to return to school.

Professional Treatment

If you think that your child has mumps, call your child's doctor immediately. The doctor can confirm that your child's illness is mumps and can guide you in watching for complications. He or she can also notify those health authorities who keep track of childhood immunization programs and measles outbreaks.

Because mumps is caused by a virus, it cannot be treated with antibiotics. Although an antimumps globulin is available, it does not always stop mumps infection.

When to Call Your Child's Doctor

Call your child's doctor immediately if you suspect that your child has mumps. If your child has mumps, ask your doctor about signs that complications may be developing. Keep track of your child's temperature and call your doctor if it goes above 101 degrees Fahrenheit (38.3 degrees Celsius).

In boys, watch for high fever, with pain and swelling of the testicles. Watch for abdominal pain that can mean involvement of the pancreas in either sex, or involvement of the ovaries in girls. Call the doctor if your child has any of these symptoms.

Since mumps can also involve the brain and its membranes, call your doctor if your child shows any of the following: severe headache; stiff neck; convulsions (seizures); extreme drowsiness; twitching face muscles; headache; loss of consciousness.

Chapter 43

Polio

Polio (short for poliomyelitis, once called infantile paralysis), used to strike thousands of children each year. In 1955, it was announced that the Salk vaccine, which was developed with March of Dimes funding, was safe and effective against this disabling, sometimes fatal infection.

Questions and Answers about Polio

What is polio?

Polio is a disease that causes lasting disabilities in a minority of infected individuals. It is caused by any of three types of polio viruses. It attacks mainly infants and children, but young adults and some older people get it, too.

Polio often causes no more than a sore throat, headache, malaise, intestinal upset and fever. About 90 percent of infected persons have no more than these mild symptoms and recover completely. However, from the digestive tract (stomach and intestines), the virus also can get into the blood stream and be carried to the nervous system (brain and spinal cord). About 10 percent of infected individuals develop a

---

This chapter begins with "Polio," For additional information, contact the March of Dimes at their website, www.marchofdimes.com. To purchase a copy of this article from the March of Dimes, call 800-367-6630. "Questions and Answers about the Polio Vaccine" is from the National Immunization Program, Centers for Disease Control and Prevention, January 2002.

high fever, meningitis (inflammation of membranes surrounding the brain and spinal cord), and severe neck and back pain.

In about one of every hundred infected persons, the virus attacks nerves inside the spine that send messages to muscles in arms, legs, and other areas. This can result in partial or complete paralysis. If the virus gets into the brainstem (bulbar polio), muscles needed for breathing, swallowing, and other vital functions become paralyzed, and the patient may die.

How does polio spread?

The virus is spread from person-to-person contact, by contact with infected secretions from the nose or mouth or by contact with infected feces. It usually enters the body when the person ingests contaminated food or water, or touches the mouth with contaminated hands.

How is polio treated?

There is no drug that can cure polio once a person is infected. Patients are made as comfortable as possible, with bed rest, pain-relieving medications, and hot packs to help relieve the pain of extreme muscle tightness. Some need assistance with breathing, such as supplemental oxygen or a ventilator. During the epidemics of the 1930s, 1940s and 1950s, some patients with serious breathing problems were placed in an "iron lung," a cylindrical chamber that surrounded a patient's body from the neck down, and which used rhythmic alterations in air pressure to force air in and out of the patient's lungs.

After the active stage of the disease is over, surviving nerve cells gradually send out new nerve connections to orphaned muscle cells, in an attempt to take over the function of nerve cells that were destroyed. This often allows the patient to regain use of muscles and recover, partially or completely.

Patients with permanent, partial paralysis are taught to use remaining healthy muscles. They generally go on to lead active lives, although some require braces and wheelchairs.

How is polio prevented?

Polio is best prevented by vaccination. There are two types of polio vaccine; one is injected and one is given by mouth. The Salk vaccine—the first to be approved, in 1955—is made from completely inactivated polio viruses and injected into the body. The oral vaccine—known as the Sabin vaccine—is made from weakened polio viruses.

It was introduced in 1962. Both vaccines cause the body to produce antibodies—specialized proteins, formed by white blood cells and lymphoid tissue, that fight the polio viruses. The vaccines make a person immune to polio, almost as though he or she had the disease and recovered from it. (Immune means that once you've been infected by any of the three types of polio virus, it's nearly impossible to contract that same type again.) The vaccines immunize against all three virus types. Both vaccines were developed with funding by the March of Dimes.

Children in the United States now are routinely vaccinated against polio, along with other preventable diseases. They receive 4 doses of the vaccine at 2, 4, 6–18 months and 4–6 years. As a result of vaccination programs, natural polio infections have been eliminated from the Americas for the past two decades.

Until recently, the polio vaccine usually was given by mouth. Very rarely, paralytic polio occurs in children who have been vaccinated with the oral vaccine or in others with whom they've had contact. As of January 2000, the federal Centers for Disease Control and Prevention (CDC) and the American Academy of Pediatrics recommend that babies in the United States be vaccinated against polio with the shot, which cannot cause polio.

Adults or children who are traveling to less developed countries where polio is still common should check with their doctor or local health department to see if they need a "booster" dose.

Are there late effects of polio?

Yes. Some patients who had polio when young experience progressive new muscle weakness decades afterward. This weakness can affect muscles previously weakened by polio as well as muscles believed to have been unaffected. These people also sometimes report intense fatigue and pain in muscles and joints. This finding of new weakness, fatigue and pain many years after having polio is called post-polio syndrome (PPS). However, not all polio survivors with such symptoms have PPS. Some, when examined by doctors, are found to have arthritis or other common joint and muscle disorders.

What is the cause of PPS?

Many experts believe that the overburdened nerve cells that sent out new connections to take over for destroyed nerve cells eventually begin to fail, resulting in new muscle weakness. Other factors, including normal aging, probably also play a role.

What can be done about PPS?

Polio survivors who believe they are having the symptoms of PPS should be thoroughly evaluated by experts at a center for rehabilitation medicine. Before such evaluation, they should not increase exercise or activity in the hope that this will give their muscles more strength. This actually might do more damage. The best thing to do is seek expert medical help.

Sometimes, a change in braces, a decrease in activity, or treatment of conditions like arthritis will lessen symptoms. Specially designed exercise programs also can help improve strength and functioning.

What is the March of Dimes role?

Many people remember the March of Dimes for conquering epidemic polio and the Foundation continues to receive many questions about the disorder. The March of Dimes responds to these inquiries, and often refers people to sources of help.

In May 2000, funded by a special donation for the purpose, the March of Dimes sponsored an international conference on best practices in diagnosis and management of PPS. Findings from the conference have been widely disseminated to patients and health care professionals.

Historians have called the conquest of polio one of the great achievements of the 20th century. Thanks to the March of Dimes, and the millions of people who supported it, we no longer have to fear another devastating polio epidemic like those that terrorized previous generations.

References

American Academy of Pediatrics. Poliovirus infections, in: Pickering L.K. (ed.) *2000 Red Book: Report of the Committee on Infectious Diseases 25th edition*, Elk Grove Village, IL, American Academy of Pediatrics, 2000, pages 465-470.

Halstead, L.S. Post-polio syndrome. *Scientific American*, April, 1998, pages 42-47.

Jubelt, B., Agre, J.C. Characteristics and management of postpolio syndrome. *Journal of the American Medical Association*, volume 284, number 4, pages 412-414.

March of Dimes. *Guidelines for People Who Have Had Polio*. White Plains, N.Y., 2002.

March of Dimes Steering Committee on Post-Polio Syndrome. *March of Dimes International Conference on Post-Polio Syndrome: Identifying Best Practices in Diagnosis and Care*. White Plains, N.Y., 2002.

Questions and Answers about the Polio Vaccine

Why did Centers for Disease Control and Prevention (CDC) and Advisory Committee on Immunization Practices (ACIP) change the polio vaccination schedule to an all-IPV (inactivated poliovirus vaccine) series?

The CDC and ACIP changed the polio schedule in 2000 because the only indigenously acquired polio in the U.S. since 1980 had been due to the vaccine, while there had been no polio cases due to the wild poliovirus. The ACIP determined that the risk-benefit ratio associated with the exclusive use of the OPV for routine immunization had changed because of the rapid progress in global polio eradication efforts. In particular, the benefits of OPV had diminished in importance due to the elimination of wild virus associated poliomyelitis in the Western Hemisphere since 1991 and the reduced threat of poliovirus importation into the U.S.

Conversely, the risk of vaccine-associated poliomyelitis due to OPV, which caused an average of 8–9 reported cases of paralytic polio each year, was judged less acceptable due to the absence of indigenous disease and reduced risk of imported infection.

Consequently, in 1996 the ACIP and CDC recommended a transition policy to increase use of IPV and decrease use of OPV, and in 2000 recommended exclusive use of IPV.

Isn't IPV less effective than OPV?

No. The IPV that has been used in the U.S. since 1987 is as effective as OPV for preventing polio in the recipient. After two doses of IPV, 90% or more of recipients have protective antibody levels to all types of poliovirus, and after three doses more than 99% have protective antibodies.

Previously, IPV was recommended to be administered subcutaneously only. Now I've read that it may also be given intramuscularly. Is this correct?

IPV is approved for either subcutaneous or intramuscular administration.

After what age is routine polio vaccine no longer recommended?

Routine polio vaccination is not recommended for persons 18 years of age and older who reside in the United States.

What is the IPV schedule for unvaccinated children 4–18 years of age?

The schedule for routine polio vaccination of children 4–17 years of age is 2 doses of IPV separated by 4–8 weeks, and a third dose 6–12 months after the second dose. If an accelerated schedule is needed, three doses separated by at least 4 weeks may be given. Polio vaccine is not routinely administered to persons 18 years of age and older.

If a child received 4 doses of IPV before the 2nd birthday, with at least 4 weeks between doses, is a 5th dose necessary?

ACIP recommends that the fourth dose in the polio series be given at school entry (4–6 years of age), mainly to assure long-term protection. But a child who has received a total of four doses of polio vaccine at least 4 weeks apart does not need a fifth dose at school entry.

However, some states mandate a dose of polio vaccine to be administered on or after 4 years of age as a requirement for school entry. In this situation just give a fifth dose at school entry. There is no harm in giving an additional dose.

What is the risk of serious reactions following IPV?

There are no serious reactions known to occur following IPV.

Chapter 44

Respiratory Syncytial Virus (RSV)

Clinical Features

Respiratory syncytial virus (RSV) is the most common cause of bronchiolitis and pneumonia among infants and children under 1 year of age. Illness begins most frequently with fever, runny nose, cough, and sometimes wheezing. During their first RSV infection, between 25% and 40% of infants and young children have signs or symptoms of bronchiolitis or pneumonia, and 0.5% to 2% require hospitalization. Most children recover from illness in 8 to 15 days. The majority of children hospitalized for RSV infection are under 6 months of age. RSV also causes repeated infections throughout life, usually associated with moderate-to-severe cold-like symptoms; however, severe lower respiratory tract disease may occur at any age, especially among the elderly or among those with compromised cardiac, pulmonary, or immune systems.

The Virus

RSV is a negative-sense, enveloped RNA virus. The virion is variable in shape and size (average diameter of between 120 and 300 nanometers), is unstable in the environment (surviving only a few hours on environmental surfaces), and is readily inactivated with soap and water and disinfectants.

"Respiratory Syncytial Virus," National Center for Infectious Diseases, Centers for Disease Control and Prevention (CDC), reviewed November 2003.

Epidemiologic Features

RSV is spread from respiratory secretions through close contact with infected persons or contact with contaminated surfaces or objects. Infection can occur when infectious material contacts mucous membranes of the eyes, mouth, or nose, and possibly through the inhalation of droplets generated by a sneeze or cough. In temperate climates, RSV infections usually occur during annual community outbreaks, often lasting 4 to 6 months, during the late fall, winter, or early spring months. The timing and severity of outbreaks in a community vary from year to year. RSV spreads efficiently among children during the annual outbreaks, and most children will have serologic evidence of RSV infection by 2 years of age.

Diagnosis

Diagnosis of RSV infection can be made by virus isolation, detection of viral antigens, detection of viral RNA, demonstration of a rise in serum antibodies, or a combination of these approaches. Most clinical laboratories use antigen detection assays to diagnose infection.

Treatment

For children with mild disease, no specific treatment is necessary other than the treatment of symptoms (e.g., acetaminophen to reduce fever). Children with severe disease may require oxygen therapy and sometimes mechanical ventilation. Ribavirin aerosol may be used in the treatment of some patients with severe disease. Some investigators have used a combination of immune globulin intravenous (IGIV) with high titers of neutralizing RSV antibody (RSV-IGIV) and ribavirin to treat patients with compromised immune systems.

Prevention

Development of an RSV vaccine is a high research priority, but none is yet available. Current prevention options include good infection-control practices, RSV-IGIV, and an anti-RSV humanized murine monoclonal antibody. RSV-IGIV or the anti-RSV humanized murine monoclonal antibody can be given during the RSV outbreak season to prevent serious complications of infection in some infants and children at high risk for serious RSV disease (for example, those with chronic lung disease and prematurely born infants with or without chronic lung disease). Frequent handwashing and not sharing items such as cups, glasses, and utensils with persons who have RSV illness should decrease the spread of virus to others. Excluding children with colds or other respiratory illnesses (without fever) who are well enough to attend child care or school settings will probably not decrease the transmission of RSV, since it is often spread in the early stages of illness. In a hospital setting, RSV transmission can and should be prevented by strict attention to contact precautions, such as handwashing and wearing gowns and gloves.

References

American Academy of Pediatrics. Respiratory Syncytial Virus. In: Peter G, ed. *1997 Red Book: Report of the Committee on Infectious Diseases. 24th ed.* Elk Grove Village, IL: American Academy of Pediatrics; 1997: 443.

Collins PL, McIntosh K, Chanock RM. Respiratory Syncytial Virus. In: Fields BN, Knipe DM, Howley PM, eds. *Fields Virology. 3rd ed.* Philadelphia: Lippincott-Raven; 1995: 1313-51.

McIntosh K. Respiratory Syncytial Virus. In: Evans A, Kaslow R, eds. *Viral Infections in Humans: epidemiology and control. 4th ed.* New York: Plenum; 1997:691-705.

Chapter 45

Rubella

Rubella (German Measles)

Signs and Symptoms

Rubella infection is commonly known as "German measles" or "3-day measles." It may begin with 1 or 2 days of mild fever (99 degrees F to 100 degrees F) and swollen glands that are usually found either in the neck or behind the ears. On the second or third day, a rash appears that begins at the hairline and spreads downward on the rest of the body. As the rash spreads downward on the body, it usually clears on the face. The rubella rash appears as either pink or light red spots, about 0.1 inches (2 to 3 mm) in diameter, which may merge to form evenly colored patches. The rash doesn't itch, and lasts up to 5 days (the average is 3 days). As the rash passes, the affected skin may be shed in flakes.

Other symptoms of rubella may include: mild conjunctivitis (inflammation of the lining of the eyelids and eyeballs); stuffy or runny

---

"Rubella (German Measles)" was provided by KidsHealth, one of the largest resources online for medically reviewed health information written for parents, kids, and teens. For more articles like this one, visit www.KidsHealth.org, or www.TeensHealth.org. © 2003 The Nemours Center for Children's Health Media, a division of The Nemours Foundation. "Facts about Rubella for Adults," is reprinted with permission from the National Foundation for Infectious Diseases—National Coalition for Adult Immunization. © July 2002. For additional information visit the National Foundation for Infectious Diseases website at http://www.nfid.org, or the National Coalition for Adult Immunization at http://www.nfid.org/ncai/

nose; swollen lymph glands in other regions of the body; pain and swelling in the joints (especially in young women); and in males, pain in the testicles.

When rubella occurs in a pregnant woman, it may cause congenital rubella syndrome with serious malformations of her developing fetus. Children infected with rubella before birth (a condition known as congenital rubella) are at risk for the following: growth retardation; malformations of the heart, eyes, or brain; deafness; and liver, spleen, and bone marrow problems.

Description

Rubella is an infection that primarily affects the skin and lymph glands. It is caused by the rubella virus, which can be found in the throat, blood, and stool of an infected person. The virus usually enters the body through the nose or throat, but it can also pass through a pregnant woman's bloodstream to infect her unborn child. Since this is a generally mild disease in children, the primary medical danger of rubella is the infection of pregnant women, which may potentially cause congenital rubella syndrome in the developing infant.

Before a vaccine against rubella became available in 1969, there were rubella epidemics every 6 to 9 years. Those primarily affected by rubella were children ages 5 to 9 and adults, but there were also many cases of congenital rubella. Now, due to immunization of younger children and teens, fewer cases of congenital rubella occur. Estimates are that 10% of young women of childbearing age are currently susceptible to rubella; obstetricians usually will check for immunity.

The term “German” has nothing to do with the country, but probably came from the Old French term “germain” and the Latin term “germanus,” meaning “akin to” or “similar.”

Duration

The rubella rash may last from 1 to 5 days, but 3 days is the most common duration. Children with rubella usually recover in 1 week, but adults may take longer.

Contagiousness

The rubella virus passes from person to person through droplets and fluids from the nose and throat. Persons with rubella are contagious from 1 week before the rash appears until 1 week after it fades.

Incubation

The incubation period for rubella is 14 to 21 days; 18 days is the average incubation period.

Prevention

Rubella can be prevented by a rubella vaccine, which is usually given to children at 12 to 15 months as part of the scheduled measles-mumps-rubella (MMR) immunization. A second dose of MMR is generally given at 4 to 6 years of age, but should be given no later than 11 to 12 years of age. The rubella vaccine should not be given to pregnant women or to a woman who may become pregnant within 3 months of receiving the vaccine.

When to Call Your Child's Doctor

Call your child's doctor if your child develops a fever over 101 degrees F or if he appears to be getting sicker than the mild course of symptoms described above.

If you are contemplating getting pregnant, make sure that you are immune to rubella through a blood test or proof of immunization. If you are pregnant and you are exposed to rubella, call your obstetrician immediately.

Professional Treatment

Rubella cannot be treated with antibiotics, since antibiotics do not work against viral infections.

Any pregnant woman who has been exposed to rubella should contact her obstetrician immediately.

Home Treatment

Rubella is usually a mild illness, especially in children. To relieve minor discomfort, give acetaminophen. Record the child's temperature once each morning and each evening. Call your child's doctor for fever above 102 degrees F, or above 100.4 degrees F if your child is younger than 6 months.

Avoid giving aspirin to a child who has a viral illness since the use of aspirin in such cases has been associated with the development of Reye syndrome.

Facts about Rubella for Adults

- Rubella can be prevented with a safe, effective vaccine.
- You cannot get rubella from the rubella vaccine.
- Rubella is contagious from 7 days before to 5–7 days after the rash appears.
- In most cases of rubella, symptoms appear within 12–23 days, and 20% to 50% of cases may be asymptomatic.
- If a pregnant woman gets rubella during the first 3 months of pregnancy, her baby has a good chance of having serious birth defects such as deafness, cataracts, heart defects, liver and spleen damage, and mental retardation.
- During 2000, 87% of all reported cases of rubella occurred among people 15–39 years of age.
- As many as 8 million women of childbearing age are susceptible to rubella.
- Up to 10% of young adults are susceptible to the rubella virus.

Prevention

There is a safe and effective vaccine to protect against rubella. The vaccine is frequently given to adults as part of a combination vaccine, called the MMR vaccine, that protects against measles, mumps and rubella. There is also a vaccine that protects against rubella only.

Symptoms

Symptoms of rubella may include a rash, slight fever, aching joints, headaches, discomfort, runny nose and reddened eyes. The rash first appears on the face and spreads from head to toe. The lymph nodes just behind the ears and at the back of the neck may swell, causing soreness and pain. Many people with rubella have few or no symptoms, and only about half of the people who have the disease get a rash. In most cases of rubella, symptoms appear within 16–18 days after exposure.

Who Should Get MMR Vaccine?

- Adults born in 1957 or later who do not have a medical contraindication should receive at least one dose of MMR vaccine, unless they have documentation of vaccination with at least one dose of measles-, rubella-, and mumps-containing vaccine or other acceptable evidence of immunity to these three diseases.

- College and university students, healthcare personnel, non-pregnant women of childbearing age, child care workers such as teachers and day care personnel, and international travelers are at increased risk for measles, and these persons should receive two doses of MMR vaccine to ensure adequate protection.

Vaccine Safety

The rubella vaccine and the combined MMR vaccine are very safe. You cannot get rubella from either vaccine. The most common side effect is burning or stinging at the injection site. Other common side effects include fever, rash, headache, and general weakness. As with any medicine, there are very small risks that serious problems could occur after getting a vaccine. However, the potential risks associated with rubella are much greater than the potential risks associated with the rubella vaccine.

Chapter 46

Severe Acute Respiratory Syndrome (SARS)

What is SARS?

Severe acute respiratory syndrome (SARS) is a viral respiratory illness that was recognized as a global threat in March 2003, after first appearing in Southern China in November 2002.

What are the symptoms and signs of SARS?

The illness usually begins with a high fever (measured temperature greater than 100.4°F [>38.0°C]). The fever is sometimes associated with chills or other symptoms, including headache, general feeling of discomfort, and body aches. Some people also experience mild respiratory symptoms at the outset. Diarrhea is seen in approximately 10 percent to 20 percent of patients. After 2 to 7 days, SARS patients may develop a dry, nonproductive cough that might be accompanied by or progress to a condition in which the oxygen levels in the blood are low (hypoxia). In 10 percent to 20 percent of cases, patients require mechanical ventilation. Most patients develop pneumonia.

What is the cause of SARS?

SARS is caused by a previously unrecognized coronavirus, called SARS-associated coronavirus (SARS-CoV). It is possible that other infectious agents might have a role in some cases of SARS.

"Frequently Asked Questions about SARS," Centers for Disease Control and Prevention (CDC), February 13, 2004.

How is SARS spread?

The primary way that SARS appears to spread is by close person-to-person contact. SARS-CoV is thought to be transmitted most readily by respiratory droplets (droplet spread) produced when an infected person coughs or sneezes. Droplet spread can happen when droplets from the cough or sneeze of an infected person are propelled a short distance (generally up to 3 feet) through the air and deposited on the mucous membranes of the mouth, nose, or eyes of persons who are nearby. The virus also can spread when a person touches a surface or object contaminated with infectious droplets and then touches his or her mouth, nose, or eye(s). In addition, it is possible that SARS-CoV might be spread more broadly through the air (airborne spread) or by other ways that are not now known.

What does "close contact" mean?

Close contact is defined as having cared for or lived with a person known to have SARS or having a high likelihood of direct contact with respiratory secretions and/or body fluids of a patient known to have SARS. Examples include kissing or embracing, sharing eating or drinking utensils, close conversation (within 3 feet), physical examination, and any other direct physical contact between people. Close contact does not include activities such as walking by a person or briefly sitting across a waiting room or office.

If I were exposed to SARS-CoV, how long would it take for me to become sick?

The time between exposure to SARS-CoV and the onset of symptoms is called the "incubation period." The incubation period for SARS is typically 2 to 7 days, although in some cases it may be as long as 10 days. In a very small proportion of cases, incubation periods of up to 14 days have been reported.

How long is a person with SARS infectious to others?

Available information suggests that persons with SARS are most likely to be contagious only when they have symptoms, such as fever or cough. Patients are most contagious during the second week of illness. However, as a precaution against spreading the disease, CDC recommends that persons with SARS limit their interactions outside the home (for example, by not going to work or to school) until 10 days after their fever has gone away and their respiratory (breathing) symptoms have gotten better.

Is a person with SARS contagious before symptoms appear?

To date, no cases of SARS have been reported among persons who were exposed to a SARS patient before the onset of the patient's symptoms.

What medical treatment is recommended for patients with SARS?

CDC recommends that patients with SARS receive the same treatment that would be used for a patient with any serious community-acquired atypical pneumonia. SARS-CoV is being tested against various antiviral drugs to see if an effective treatment can be found.

If there is another outbreak of SARS, how can I protect myself?

If transmission of SARS-CoV recurs, there are some common-sense precautions that you can take that apply to many infectious diseases. The most important is frequent hand washing with soap and water or use of an alcohol-based hand rub. You should also avoid touching your eyes, nose, and mouth with unclean hands and encourage people around you to cover their nose and mouth with a tissue when coughing or sneezing.

Global SARS Outbreak, 2003

How many people contracted SARS worldwide during the 2003 outbreak? How many people died of SARS worldwide?

During November 2002 through July 2003, a total of 8,098 people worldwide became sick with severe acute respiratory syndrome that was accompanied by either pneumonia or respiratory distress syndrome (probable cases), according to the World Health Organization (WHO). Of these, 774 died. By late July 2003, no new cases were being reported, and WHO declared the global outbreak to be over.

How many people contracted SARS in the United States during the 2003 outbreak? How many people died of SARS in the United States?

In the United States, only eight persons were laboratory-confirmed as SARS cases. There were no SARS-related deaths in the United States. All of the eight persons with laboratory-confirmed SARS had traveled to areas where SARS-CoV transmission was occurring.

SARS Situation: 2004

What is the current SARS situation in the world?

There is currently no evidence of person-to-person transmission of SARS in the world. Since the end of the global outbreak in July 2003, two cases of SARS associated with laboratory exposures have been reported—one case in Singapore in September 2003 and one in Taiwan in December 2003. In addition, since December 16, 2003, a few sporadic cases of SARS have been reported in China. However, none of the contacts of these cases has developed a SARS-like illness, and there is no evidence of any association among the cases.

SARS-Associated Coronavirus

What are coronaviruses?

Coronaviruses are a group of viruses that have a halo or crown-like (corona) appearance when viewed under a microscope. These viruses are a common cause of mild to moderate upper-respiratory illness in humans and are associated with respiratory, gastrointestinal, liver and neurologic disease in animals.

If coronaviruses usually cause mild illness in humans, how could this new coronavirus be responsible for a potentially life-threatening disease such as SARS?

There is not enough information about the new virus to determine the full range of illness that it might cause. Coronaviruses have occasionally been linked to pneumonia in humans, especially people with weakened immune systems. The viruses also can cause severe disease in animals, including cats, dogs, pigs, mice, and birds.

How long can SARS-CoV survive in the environment?

Preliminary studies in some research laboratories suggest that the virus may survive in the environment for several days. The length of time that the virus survives likely depends on a number of factors. These factors could include the type of material or body fluid containing the virus and various environmental conditions such as temperature or humidity. Researchers at CDC and other institutions are designing standardized experiments to measure how long SARS-CoV can survive in situations that simulate natural environmental conditions.

Laboratory Testing

Is there a laboratory test for SARS?

Yes, several laboratory tests can be used to detect SARS-CoV. A reverse transcription polymerase chain reaction (RT-PCR) test can detect SARS-CoV in clinical specimens such as blood, stool, and nasal secretions. Serologic testing also can be performed to detect SARS-CoV antibodies produced after infection. Finally, viral culture has been used to detect SARS-CoV.

What is a PCR test?

PCR (or polymerase chain reaction) is a laboratory method for detecting the genetic material of an infectious disease agent in specimens from patients. This type of testing has become an essential tool for detecting infectious disease agents.

What does serologic testing involve?

A serologic test is a laboratory method for detecting the presence and/or level of antibodies to an infectious agent in serum from a person. Antibodies are substances made by the body's immune system to fight a specific infection.

What does viral culture and isolation involve?

For a viral culture, a small sample of tissue or fluid that may be infected is placed in a container along with cells in which the virus can grow. If the virus grows in the culture, it will cause changes in the cells that can be seen under a microscope.

Chapter 47

Smallpox

Smallpox Overview

The Disease

Smallpox is a serious, contagious, and sometimes fatal infectious disease. There is no specific treatment for smallpox disease, and the only prevention is vaccination. The name smallpox is derived from the Latin word for "spotted" and refers to the raised bumps that appear on the face and body of an infected person.

There are two clinical forms of smallpox. Variola major is the severe and most common form of smallpox, with a more extensive rash and higher fever. There are four types of variola major smallpox: ordinary (the most frequent type, accounting for 90% or more of cases); modified (mild and occurring in previously vaccinated persons); flat; and hemorrhagic (both rare and very severe). Historically, variola major has an overall fatality rate of about 30%; however, flat and

---

This chapter contains information from the following documents: "Smallpox Overview," Public Health Emergency Preparedness and Response, Centers for Disease Control and Prevention, December 2002; "Frequently Asked Questions and Answers On Smallpox," Communicable Disease Surveillance and Response, World Health Organization (WHO), © 2001 WHO, reprinted with permission; and "Vaccine Overview," April 2003, "Protecting Americans: Smallpox Vaccination Program," December 2002, "Reactions after Smallpox Vaccination," December 2002, "People Who Should Not Get the Smallpox Vaccine," April 2003, and "Smallpox Vaccine and Heart Problems," April 2003, U.S. Department of Health and Human Services (www.smallpox.gov).

hemorrhagic smallpox usually are fatal. Variola minor is a less common presentation of smallpox, and a much less severe disease, with death rates historically of 1% or less.

Smallpox outbreaks have occurred from time to time for thousands of years, but the disease is now eradicated after a successful worldwide vaccination program. The last case of smallpox in the United States was in 1949. The last naturally occurring case in the world was in Somalia in 1977. After the disease was eliminated from the world, routine vaccination against smallpox among the general public was stopped because it was no longer necessary for prevention.

Where Smallpox Comes From

Smallpox is caused by the variola virus that emerged in human populations thousands of years ago. Except for laboratory stockpiles, the variola virus has been eliminated. However, in the aftermath of the events of September and October, 2001, there is heightened concern that the variola virus might be used as an agent of bioterrorism. For this reason, the U.S. government is taking precautions for dealing with a smallpox outbreak.

Transmission

Generally, direct and fairly prolonged face-to-face contact is required to spread smallpox from one person to another. Smallpox also can be spread through direct contact with infected bodily fluids or contaminated objects such as bedding or clothing. Rarely, smallpox has been spread by virus carried in the air in enclosed settings such as buildings, buses, and trains. Humans are the only natural hosts of variola. Smallpox is not known to be transmitted by insects or animals.

A person with smallpox is sometimes contagious with onset of fever (prodrome phase), but the person becomes most contagious with the onset of rash. At this stage the infected person is usually very sick and not able to move around in the community. The infected person is contagious until the last smallpox scab falls off.

Smallpox Disease

Exposure to the virus is followed by an incubation period during which people do not have any symptoms and may feel fine. This incubation period averages about 12 to 14 days but can range from 7 to 17 days. During this time, people are not contagious.

The first symptoms of smallpox include fever, malaise, head and body aches, and sometimes vomiting. The fever is usually high, in the range of 101 to 104 degrees Fahrenheit. At this time, people are usually too sick to carry on their normal activities. This is called the prodrome phase and may last for 2 to 4 days. Smallpox may be contagious during the prodrome phase, but is most infectious during the first 7 to 10 days following rash onset.

A rash emerges first as small red spots on the tongue and in the mouth.

These spots develop into sores that break open and spread large amounts of the virus into the mouth and throat. At this time, the person becomes most contagious.

Around the time the sores in the mouth break down, a rash appears on the skin, starting on the face and spreading to the arms and legs and then to the hands and feet. Usually the rash spreads to all parts of the body within 24 hours. As the rash appears, the fever usually falls and the person may start to feel better.

By the third day of the rash, the rash becomes raised bumps.

By the fourth day, the bumps fill with a thick, opaque fluid and often have a depression in the center that looks like a bellybutton. (This is a major distinguishing characteristic of smallpox.)

Fever often will rise again at this time and remain high until scabs form over the bumps.

The bumps become pustules—sharply raised, usually round and firm to the touch as if there's a small round object under the skin. People often say the bumps feel like BB pellets embedded in the skin.

The pustules begin to form a crust and then scab.

By the end of the second week after the rash appears, most of the sores have scabbed over.

The scabs begin to fall off, leaving marks on the skin that eventually become pitted scars. Most scabs will have fallen off three weeks after the rash appears.

The person is contagious to others until all of the scabs have fallen off.

Scabs have fallen off. Person is no longer contagious.

Frequently Asked Questions about Smallpox

What is smallpox?

Smallpox is an ancient disease caused by the variola virus. Early symptoms include high fever and fatigue. The virus then produces a characteristic rash, particularly on the face, arms and legs. The resulting spots become filled with clear fluid and later, pus, and then form a crust, which eventually dries up and falls off. Smallpox was fatal in up to 30% of cases. Smallpox has existed for at least 3,000 years and was one of the world's most feared diseases until it was eradicated by a collaborative global vaccination program led by the World Health Organization (WHO). The last known natural case was in Somalia in 1977. Since then, the only known cases were caused by a laboratory accident in 1978 in Birmingham, England, which killed one person and caused a limited outbreak. Smallpox was officially declared eradicated in 1979.

Does it occur naturally?

Smallpox no longer occurs naturally since it was totally eradicated by a lengthy and painstaking process, which identified all cases and their contacts and ensured that they were all vaccinated. Until then, smallpox killed many millions of people.

How can I catch it and is it contagious?

The virus which causes smallpox is contagious and spreads through person-to-person contact and saliva droplets in an infected person's breath. It has an incubation period of between 7 and 17 days after exposure and only becomes infectious once the fever develops. A distinctive rash appears two to three days later. The most infectious period is during the first week of illness, although a person with smallpox is still infectious until the last scabs fall off.

How fast does smallpox spread?

The speed of smallpox transmission is generally slower than for such diseases as measles or chickenpox. Patients spread smallpox primarily to household members and friends because by the time patients are contagious, they are usually sick and stay in bed; large outbreaks in schools were uncommon.

Weren't the remaining stocks of the smallpox virus destroyed after smallpox was eradicated?

When smallpox was officially certified as eradicated, in December 1979, an agreement was reached under which all remaining stocks of the virus would either be destroyed or passed to one of two secure laboratories—one in the United States and one in the Russian Federation. That process was completed in the early 1980s and since then no other laboratory has officially had access to the virus which causes smallpox.

Then why is smallpox being talked about now?

Some governments believe there is a risk that the virus which causes smallpox exists in places other than these laboratories and could be deliberately released to cause harm. It is impossible to assess the risk that this might happen, but at their request, WHO is making efforts to help governments prepare for this possibility.

Can it be treated?

There is no cure for smallpox, but vaccination can be used very effectively to prevent infection from developing if given during a period of up to four days after a person has been exposed to the virus. This is the strategy that was used to eradicate the disease during the 20th century. New antiviral drugs, that have been developed for other diseases since smallpox was eradicated, may have a role. No studies of their usefulness, or safety, have been conducted on humans exposed to smallpox.

Is a vaccine currently available?

There is a vaccine against smallpox and it was a key tool in the eradication of the disease. The vaccine does not contain the variola virus which causes smallpox, but a closely related virus called vaccinia. When this vaccine is given to humans, it protects them against smallpox. However, it can have very serious side effects, which in extreme cases can be fatal. It has therefore not been recommended for the general public since smallpox was eradicated. It is used to protect researchers who work on the variola virus that causes smallpox and other viruses in the same virus family (known as orthopox viruses). It could also be used to protect anyone else judged to have a high risk of exposure to smallpox. The vaccine cannot be used in people whose immune systems are not functioning properly.

Should the smallpox vaccine be widely used to protect people?

Vaccination with the vaccinia virus as a protection against smallpox is not recommended for widespread use. No government gives or recommends the vaccine routinely since it can cause serious complications, and even death. It should be given only to those persons who have a high risk of coming into contact with the virus which causes smallpox, or who have been exposed.

What can be done to protect people from smallpox?

Doctors, health workers, and hospital personnel around the world have been trained to identify infectious diseases, verify their diagnosis and then respond accordingly. The same system would identify any possible outbreak of smallpox even if the virus is deliberately spread to cause harm. The public health system would then be mobilized to trace all known contacts of the infected person and vaccinate them to prevent more cases of smallpox from developing. If this is done rapidly and effectively, the number of cases could be kept to a minimum and the outbreak would be contained. This was the approach which successfully eradicated the disease. The key is a good disease detection system and a rapid response to infectious diseases, no matter what their cause. At this time, several governments have started to examine the potency and levels of their smallpox vaccine stocks, and to consider whether, and under what circumstances, to obtain additional supplies.

I had the vaccination when I was a child. Am I still protected?

Anyone who has been vaccinated against smallpox (in most countries, this means anyone aged 25–30 or over) will have some level of protection. The vaccination may not still be fully effective, but it is likely to protect you from the worst effects of the disease. However, if you were directly exposed to the virus which causes smallpox, a repeat vaccination would be recommended.

What is WHO doing now?

WHO receives information from governments and other sources on suspected occurrences of unusual outbreaks, including smallpox. It provides technical guidance to help them respond to these events. WHO has displayed practical information on smallpox diagnosis, surveillance, and outbreak response on its website. It can help countries identify potential sources of vaccine, should such a need arise.

Vaccine Overview

The Smallpox Vaccine

The smallpox vaccine helps the body develop immunity to smallpox. The vaccine is made from a virus called vaccinia which is a "pox"-type virus related to smallpox. The smallpox vaccine contains the "live" vaccinia virus—not dead virus like many other vaccines. For that reason, the vaccination site must be cared for carefully to prevent the virus from spreading. Also, the vaccine can have side effects (see the section "Smallpox Vaccine Safety" in this chapter). The vaccine does not contain the smallpox virus and cannot give you smallpox.

Currently, the United States has a big enough stockpile of smallpox vaccine to vaccinate everyone in the country who might need it in the event of an emergency. Production of new vaccine is underway.

Length of Protection

Smallpox vaccination provides high level immunity for 3 to 5 years and decreasing immunity thereafter. If a person is vaccinated again later, immunity lasts even longer. Historically, the vaccine has been effective in preventing smallpox infection in 95% of those vaccinated. In addition, the vaccine was proven to prevent or substantially lessen infection when given within a few days of exposure. It is important to note, however, that at the time when the smallpox vaccine was used to eradicate the disease, testing was not as advanced or precise as it is today, so there may still be things to learn about the vaccine and its effectiveness and length of protection.

Receiving the Vaccine

The smallpox vaccine is not given with a hypodermic needle. It is not a shot as most people have experienced. The vaccine is given using a bifurcated (two-pronged) needle that is dipped into the vaccine solution. When removed, the needle retains a droplet of the vaccine. The needle is used to prick the skin a number of times in a few seconds. The pricking is not deep, but it will cause a sore spot and one or two droplets of blood to form. The vaccine usually is given in the upper arm.

If the vaccination is successful, a red and itchy bump develops at the vaccine site in three or four days. In the first week, the bump becomes a large blister, fills with pus, and begins to drain. During the second week, the blister begins to dry up and a scab forms. The scab falls off in the third week, leaving a small scar. People who are being vaccinated for the first time have a stronger reaction than those who are being revaccinated.

Post-Vaccination Care

After vaccination, it is important to follow care instructions for the site of the vaccine. Because the virus is live, it can spread to other parts of the body, or to other people. The vaccinia virus (the live virus in the smallpox vaccine) may cause rash, fever, and head and body aches. In certain groups of people (see the section "Smallpox Vaccine Safety" in this chapter), complications from the vaccinia virus can be severe.

Benefit of Vaccine Following Exposure

Vaccination within 3 days of exposure will prevent or significantly lessen the severity of smallpox symptoms in the vast majority of people. Vaccination 4 to 7 days after exposure likely offers some protection from disease or may modify the severity of disease.

Smallpox Vaccine Safety

The smallpox vaccine is the best protection you can get if you are exposed to the smallpox virus. Anyone directly exposed to smallpox, regardless of health status, would be offered the smallpox vaccine because the risks associated with smallpox disease are far greater than those posed by the vaccine.

There are side effects and risks associated with the smallpox vaccine. Most people experience normal, usually mild reactions that include a sore arm, fever, and body aches. However, other people experience reactions ranging from serious to life-threatening. People most likely to have serious side effects are: people who have had, even once, skin conditions (especially eczema or atopic dermatitis) and people with weakened immune systems, such as those who have received a transplant, are HIV positive, are receiving treatment for cancer, or are currently taking medications (like steroids) that suppress the immune system. In addition, pregnant women should not get the vaccine because of the risk it poses to the fetus. Women who are breastfeeding should not get the vaccine. Children younger than 12 months of age should not get the vaccine. Also, the Advisory Committee on Immunization Practices (ACIP) advises against non-emergency use of smallpox vaccine in children younger than 18 years of age. In addition, those allergic to the vaccine or any of its components should not receive the vaccine. Also, people who have been diagnosed by a doctor as having a heart condition with or without symptoms, including conditions such as previous myocardial infarction (heart attack), angina (chest pain caused by lack of blood flow to the heart), congestive heart failure, cardiomyopathy, stroke or transient ischemic attack (a "mini-stroke" that produces stroke-like symptoms but no lasting damage), chest pain or shortness of breath with activity (such as walking up stairs), or other heart conditions being treated by a doctor should not get the vaccine at this time. (Heart disease may be a temporary exclusion and may change as more information is gathered.) Also, individuals who have 3 or more of the following risk factors should not get the vaccine at this time: high blood pressure diagnosed by a doctor; high blood cholesterol diagnosed by a doctor; diabetes or high blood sugar diagnosed by a doctor; a first degree relative (for example, mother, father, brother or sister) with a heart condition before the age of 50; and/or, currently a cigarette smoker. (These may be temporary exclusions and may change as more information is gathered.)

In the past, about 1,000 people for every 1 million people vaccinated for the first time experienced reactions that, while not life-threatening, were serious. These reactions included a toxic or allergic reaction at the site of the vaccination (erythema multiforme), spread of the vaccinia virus to other parts of the body and to other individuals (inadvertent inoculation), and spread of the vaccinia virus to other parts of the body through the blood (generalized vaccinia). These types of reactions may require medical attention. In the past, between 14 and 52 people out of every 1 million people vaccinated for the first time experienced potentially life-threatening reactions to the vaccine. Based on past experience, it is estimated that 1 or 2 people in 1 million who receive the vaccine may die as a result. Careful screening of potential vaccine recipients is essential to ensure that those at increased risk do not receive the vaccine.

Smallpox Vaccine Availability

Routine smallpox vaccination among the American public stopped in 1972 after the disease was eradicated in the United States. Until recently, the U.S. government provided the vaccine only to a few hundred scientists and medical professionals working with smallpox and similar viruses in a research setting.

After the events of September and October, 2001, however, the U.S. government took further actions to improve its level of preparedness against terrorism. One of many such measures—designed specifically to prepare for an intentional release of the smallpox virus—included updating and releasing a smallpox response plan. In addition, the U.S. government ordered production of enough smallpox vaccine to immunize the American public in the event of a smallpox outbreak. Right now, the U.S. government has access to enough smallpox vaccine to effectively respond to a smallpox outbreak in the United States.

Smallpox Vaccination Information for the General Public Regarding Bioterrorist Threat

What is the current threat assessment? Who are likely countries to obtain and use the virus?

Terrorists or governments hostile to the United States may have, or could obtain, some of the variola virus that causes smallpox disease. If so, these adversaries could use it as a biological weapon. This potential along with an appreciation for the potentially devastating consequences of a smallpox attack, suggests that we should take prudent steps to prepare our critical responders to protect the American public should an attack occur. People exposed to variola virus, or those at risk of being exposed, can be protected by vaccinia (smallpox) vaccine. The United States is taking precautions to deal with this possibility.

If a person wants to sign up to receive the vaccine as soon as possible, what should they do?

The federal government is not recommending that members of the general public be vaccinated at this point. The U.S. government has no information that a biological attack is imminent, and there are significant side effects and risks associated with the vaccine. The U.S. Department of Health and Human Services (HHS) is in the process of establishing an orderly process to make vaccines available to those adult members of the general public without medical contraindications who insist on being vaccinated. (A member of the general public may also be eligible to volunteer for an on-going clinical trial for next generation vaccines).

How long will it take before HHS begins administering vaccines to the general public?

Again, HHS does not recommend at this point that the general public be vaccinated. The immediate task for state and federal government will remain the implementation of our program to vaccinate our emergency responders. This is necessary to best protect Americans in the event of a release.

Of course, in the event of an actual attack, HHS will immediately make vaccine available to those at risk from disease.

Who will administer the vaccines?

State health departments, with guidance from CDC, will set up vaccination clinics and determine who will be staffing clinics and administering smallpox vaccine. The number of vaccination sites will be determined in the state plans, and depends in large part on the demand for the vaccines. CDC is assisting states with planning, technical assistance, and education.

How will the government monitor and report side effects?

The CDC will enlist an outside group to constitute an external data monitoring and safety review board. This external review board will review vaccine adverse event reports and data, interpret findings, and provide guidance and advice for strengthening the overall safety of the program.

Reactions after Smallpox Vaccination

The smallpox vaccine prevents smallpox. For most people, it is safe and effective. Most people experience normal, typically mild reactions to the vaccine, which indicate that it is beginning to work. Some people may experience reactions that may require medical attention.

Normal, Typically Mild Reactions

These reactions usually go away without treatment:

- The arm receiving the vaccination may be sore and red where the vaccine was given.
- The glands in the armpits may become large and sore.
- The vaccinated person may run a low fever.

- One out of 3 people may feel bad enough to miss work, school, or recreational activity or have trouble sleeping.

Serious Reactions

In the past, about 1,000 people for every 1 million people vaccinated for the first time experienced reactions that, while not life-threatening, were serious. These reactions may require medical attention:

- A vaccinia rash or outbreak of sores limited to one area. This is an accidental spreading of the vaccinia virus caused by touching the vaccination site and then touching another part of the body or another person. It usually occurs on the genitals or face, including the eyes, where it can damage sight or lead to blindness. Washing hands with soap and water after touching the vaccine site will help prevent this (inadvertent inoculation).
- A widespread vaccinia rash. The virus spreads from the vaccination site through the blood. Sores break out on parts of the body away from the vaccination site (generalized vaccinia).
- A toxic or allergic rash in response to the vaccine that can take various forms (erythema multiforme).

Life-Threatening Reactions

Rarely, people have had very bad reactions to the vaccine. In the past, between 14 and 52 people per 1 million people vaccinated for the first time experienced potentially life-threatening reactions. These reactions require immediate medical attention:

- Eczema vaccinatum. Serious skin rashes caused by widespread infection of the skin in people with skin conditions such as eczema or atopic dermatitis.
- Progressive vaccinia (or vaccinia necrosum). Ongoing infection of skin with tissue destruction frequently leading to death.
- Postvaccinal encephalitis. Inflammation of the brain.

People with certain medical conditions—including people with weakened immune systems or certain skin conditions—are more likely to have these reactions and should not get the smallpox vaccine unless they have been exposed to smallpox.

Based on past experience, it is estimated that between 1 and 2 people out of every 1 million people vaccinated may die as a result of life-threatening reactions to the vaccine.

Important Note: Statistical information about smallpox vaccine adverse reactions is based on data from two studies conducted in 1968. Adverse event rates in the United States today may be higher because there may be more people at risk from immune suppression (from cancer, cancer therapy, organ transplants, and illnesses such as HIV/AIDS) and eczema or atopic dermatitis. The outcome associated with adverse events may be less severe than previously reported because of advances in medical care. Rates may be lower for persons previously vaccinated.

People Who Should NOT Get the Smallpox Vaccine

Some people are at greater risk for serious side effects from the smallpox vaccine. Individuals who have any of the following conditions, or live with someone who does, should NOT get the smallpox vaccine unless they have been exposed to the smallpox virus:

- Eczema or atopic dermatitis. (This is true even if the condition is not currently active, mild, or experienced as a child.)
- Skin conditions such as burns, chickenpox, shingles, impetigo, herpes, severe acne, or psoriasis. (People with any of these conditions should not get the vaccine until they have completely healed.)
- Weakened immune system. (Cancer treatment, an organ transplant, HIV, Primary Immune Deficiency disorders, some severe autoimmune disorders and medications to treat autoimmune disorders, and other illnesses can weaken the immune system.)
- Pregnancy or plans to become pregnant within one month of vaccination.

In addition, individuals should not get the smallpox vaccine if they:

- Are allergic to the vaccine or any of its ingredients (polymyxin B, streptomycin, chlortetracycline, neomycin).
- Are younger than 12 months of age. However, the Advisory Committee on Immunization Practices (ACIP) advises against non-emergency use of smallpox vaccine in children younger

than 18 years of age. In addition, the vaccine manufacturer's package insert states that the vaccine is not recommended for use in geriatric populations in non-emergency situations. The term geriatric generally applies to people age 65 and above.

- Have a moderate or severe short-term illness. (These people should wait until they are completely recovered to get the vaccine.)
- Are currently breastfeeding.
- Are using steroid drops in their eyes. (These people should wait until they are no longer using the medication to get the vaccine).
- Have been diagnosed by a doctor as having a heart condition with or without symptoms, including conditions such as previous myocardial infarction (heart attack), angina (chest pain caused by lack of blood flow to the heart), congestive heart failure, cardiomyopathy (heart muscle becomes inflamed and doesn't work as well as it should), stroke or transient ischemic attack (a "mini-stroke" that produces stroke-like symptoms but not lasting damage), chest pain or shortness of breath with activity (such as walking up stairs), or other heart conditions being treated by a doctor. (While this may be a temporary exclusion, these people should not get the vaccine at this time.)
- Have 3 or more of the following risk factors: high blood pressure diagnosed by a doctor; high blood cholesterol diagnosed by a doctor; diabetes or high blood sugar diagnosed by a doctor; a first degree relative (for example, mother, father, brother, sister) who had a heart condition before the age of 50; and, you smoke cigarettes now. (While this may be a temporary exclusion, these people should not get the vaccine at this time.)

Again, people who have been directly exposed to the smallpox virus should get the vaccine, regardless of their health status.

If offered the smallpox vaccine, individuals should tell their immunization provider if they have any of the above conditions, or even if they suspect they might.

Smallpox Vaccine and Heart Problems

Careful monitoring of smallpox vaccinations has suggested that the vaccine may cause heart inflammation (myocarditis), inflammation of the membrane covering the heart (pericarditis), and/or a combination of these two problems (myopericarditis). Experts are exploring this more in depth.

Heart pain (angina) and heart attack also have been reported following smallpox vaccination. However, it is not known at this time if smallpox vaccination caused these problems or if they occurred by chance alone (heart problems are very common). Experts are investigating this question also.

Reported events are not necessarily caused by the vaccine, and some or all of these events might be coincidental.

What has been reported?

- **Past Experience:** Rare cases of heart inflammation following smallpox vaccination were reported in the 1960s and 1970s. Most of these did not occur in the United States and involved a different smallpox vaccine than is being used in the U.S. now.
- **Civilian Vaccinations:** Of the 25,645 civilians who had received the smallpox vaccine as of March 21, 2003, 7 reported heart problems. These included problems like angina (chest pain caused by lack of blood flow to the heart) and heart attacks. Two people who had heart attacks died. It is not known at this time if smallpox vaccination caused these events.
- **Military Vaccinations:** Between December 13, 2002 and March 31, 2003, approximately 325,000 troops received the smallpox vaccine. Eleven cases of heart inflammation have been reported among approximately 225,000 members of the military who received the vaccine for the first time (a rate of about 1 in 20,000). No such cases occurred in people who had been vaccinated before. According to the Department of Defense, one of the cases became severely ill with heart failure on March 27, 2003 and remains hospitalized as of March 31, 2003. The other 10 individuals had mild to moderate disease and have recovered.

As a precautionary step, if you have been diagnosed by a doctor as having a heart condition with or without symptoms you should NOT get the smallpox vaccine at this time while experts continue their investigations. These include conditions such as:

- known coronary disease including:
  - previous myocardial infarction (heart attack)

- angina (chest pain caused by lack of blood flow to the heart)
- congestive heart failure
- cardiomyopathy (heart muscle becomes inflamed and doesn't work as well as it should)
- stroke or transient ischemic attack (a "mini-stroke" that produces stroke-like symptoms but no lasting damage)
- chest pain or shortness of breath with activity (such as walking up stairs)
- other heart conditions under the care of a doctor

In addition, you should NOT get the smallpox vaccine if you have 3 or more of the following risk factors:

- You have been told by a doctor that you have high blood pressure.
- You have been told by a doctor that you have high blood cholesterol.
- You have been told by a doctor that you have diabetes or high blood sugar.
- You have a first degree relative (for example mother, father, brother, or sister) who had a heart condition before the age of 50.
- You smoke cigarettes now.

These may be temporary exclusions and may change as more information is gathered.

If you have received the smallpox vaccine, you should see a health care provider right away if you develop chest pain, shortness of breath, or other symptoms of cardiac disease after vaccination.

If you have been diagnosed by a doctor as having heart disease and you have already received the smallpox vaccine, you should contact your heart disease specialist or your regular health care provider if you have questions.

For more information, the visit the HHS smallpox website at www.smallpox.gov, visit the CDC smallpox website at www.cdc.gov/smallpox, or call the CDC public response hotline at (888) 246-2675 (English), (888) 246-2857 (Español), or (866) 874-2646 (TTY).

Chapter 48

Viral (Aseptic) Meningitis

What is meningitis?

Meningitis is an illness in which there is inflammation of the tissues that cover the brain and spinal cord. Viral or aseptic meningitis, which is the most common type, is caused by an infection with one of several types of viruses. Meningitis can also be caused by infections with several types of bacteria or fungi.

What are the symptoms of meningitis?

The symptoms of meningitis may not be the same for every person. The more common symptoms are fever, severe headache, stiff neck, bright lights hurt the eyes, drowsiness or confusion, and nausea and vomiting. In babies, the symptoms are more difficult to identify. They may include fever, fretfulness or irritability, difficulty in awakening the baby, or the baby refuses to eat.

Is viral meningitis a serious disease?

Viral (aseptic) meningitis is serious but rarely fatal in persons with normal immune systems. Usually, the symptoms last from 7 to 10 days and the person recovers completely. Bacterial meningitis, on the other hand, can be very serious and result in disability or death if not

---

"Viral (Aseptic) Meningitis," National Center for Infectious Diseases, Centers for Disease Control and Prevention (CDC), reviewed August 20, 2001

treated promptly. Often, the symptoms of viral meningitis and bacterial meningitis are the same. For this reason, if you think you or your child has meningitis, see your doctor as soon as possible.

What causes viral meningitis?

Many different viruses can cause meningitis. About 90% of cases of viral meningitis are caused by members of a group of viruses known as enteroviruses, such as coxsackieviruses and echoviruses. Herpesviruses and the mumps virus can also cause viral meningitis.

How is viral meningitis diagnosed?

Viral meningitis is usually diagnosed by laboratory tests of spinal fluid obtained with a spinal tap. It can also be diagnosed by tests that identify the virus in specimens collected from the patient, but these tests are not usually done.

How is viral meningitis treated?

No specific treatment for viral meningitis exists at this time. Most patients recover completely on their own, and doctors often will recommend bed rest, plenty of fluids, and medicine to relieve fever and headache.

Can I get viral meningitis if I'm around someone who has it?

The viruses that cause viral meningitis are contagious. Enteroviruses, for example, are very common during the summer and early fall, and many people are exposed to them. However, most infected persons either have no symptoms or develop only a cold or rash with low-grade fever. Typically, fewer than 1 of every 1,000 persons infected actually develop meningitis. Therefore, if you are around someone who has viral meningitis, you have a moderate chance of becoming infected, but a very small chance of developing meningitis.

How is the virus spread?

Enteroviruses, the most common cause of viral meningitis, are most often spread through direct contact with respiratory secretions (e.g., saliva, sputum, or nasal mucus) of an infected person. This usually happens by shaking hands with an infected person or touching something they have handled, and then rubbing your own nose, mouth, or eyes. The virus can also be found in the stool of persons who are infected. The virus is spread through this route mainly among small children who are not yet toilet trained. It can also be spread this way to adults changing the diapers of an infected infant. The incubation period for enteroviruses is usually between 3 and 7 days from the time you are infected until you develop symptoms. You can usually spread the virus to someone else beginning about 3 days after you are infected until about 10 days after you develop symptoms.

How can I reduce my chances of becoming infected?

Because most persons who are infected with enteroviruses do not become sick, it can be difficult to prevent the spread of the virus. If you are in contact with someone who has viral meningitis, however, the most effective method of prevention is to wash your hands thoroughly and often. In institutional settings such as child care centers, washing objects and surfaces with a dilute bleach solution (made by mixing 1 capful of chlorine-containing household bleach with 1 gallon water) can be a very effective way to inactivate the virus.

Part Four

Parasitic, Fungal, and Other Diseases

Chapter 49

Amebiasis

What is amebiasis?

Amebiasis is a disease caused by a one-celled parasite called *Entamoeba histolytica* (ent-a-ME-ba his-to-LI-ti-ka).

Who is at risk for amebiasis?

Although anyone can have this disease, it is most common in people who live in developing countries that have poor sanitary conditions. In the United States, amebiasis is most often found in immigrants from developing countries. It also is found in people who have traveled to developing countries and in people who live in institutions that have poor sanitary conditions. Men who have sex with men can become infected and can get sick from the infection, but they often do not have symptoms.

How can I become infected with E. histolytica*?*

- By putting anything into your mouth that has touched the stool of a person who is infected with *E. histolytica*.
- By swallowing something, such as water or food, that is contaminated with *E. histolytica*.

"Amebiasis," Division of Parasitic Diseases, Centers for Disease Control and Prevention (CDC), reviewed January 2004.

- By touching and bringing to your mouth cysts (eggs) picked up from surfaces that are contaminated with *E. histolytica*.

What are the symptoms of amebiasis?

On average, about one in 10 people who are infected with *E. histolytica* becomes sick from the infection. The symptoms often are quite mild and can include loose stools, stomach pain, and stomach cramping. Amebic dysentery is a severe form of amebiasis associated with stomach pain, bloody stools, and fever. Rarely, *E. histolytica* invades the liver and forms an abscess. Even less commonly, it spreads to other parts of the body, such as the lungs or brain.

If I swallowed E. histolytica, *how quickly would I become sick?*

Usually 1 to 4 weeks later but sometimes more quickly or more slowly.

What should I do if I think I have amebiasis?

See your health care provider.

How is amebiasis diagnosed?

Your health care provider will ask you to submit stool samples. Because *E. histolytica* is not always found in every stool sample, you may be asked to submit several stool samples from several different days.

Diagnosis of amebiasis can be very difficult. One problem is that other parasites and cells can look very similar to *E. histolytica* when seen under a microscope. Therefore, sometimes people are told that they are infected with *E. histolytica* even though they are not. *Entamoeba histolytica* and another amoeba, *Entamoeba dispar*, which is about 10 times more common, look the same when seen under a microscope. Unlike infection with *E. histolytica*, which sometimes makes people sick, infection with *E. dispar* never makes people sick and therefore does not need to be treated.

If you have been told that you are infected with *E. histolytica* but you are feeling fine, you might be infected with *E. dispar* instead. Unfortunately, most laboratories do not yet have the tests that can tell whether a person is infected with *E. histolytica* or with *E. dispar*. Until these tests become more widely available, it usually is best to assume that the parasite is *E. histolytica*.

A blood test is also available. However, the test is recommended only when your health care provider thinks that your infection has invaded the wall of the intestine (gut) or some other organ of your body, such as the liver. One problem is that the blood test may still be positive if you had amebiasis in the past, even if you are no longer infected now.

How is amebiasis treated?

Several antibiotics are available to treat amebiasis. Treatment must be prescribed by a physician. You will be treated with only one antibiotic if your *E. histolytica* infection has not made you sick. You probably will be treated with two antibiotics (first one and then the other) if your infection has made you sick.

I am going to travel to a country that has poor sanitary conditions. What should I eat and drink there so I will NOT become infected with **E. histolytica** *or other such germs?*

- Drink only bottled or boiled (for 1 minute) water or carbonated (bubbly) drinks in cans or bottles. Do not drink fountain drinks or any drinks with ice cubes. Another way to make water safe is by filtering it through an "absolute 1 micron or less" filter and dissolving iodine tablets in the filtered water. "Absolute 1 micron" filters can be found in camping/outdoor supply stores.
- Do not eat fresh fruit or vegetables that you did not peel yourself.
- Do not eat or drink milk, cheese, or dairy products that may not have been pasteurized.
- Do not eat or drink anything sold by street vendors.

Should I be concerned about spreading infection to the rest of my household?

Yes. However, the risk of spreading infection is low if the infected person is treated with antibiotics and practices good personal hygiene. This includes thorough hand washing with soap and water after using the toilet, after changing diapers, and before handling food.

Chapter 50

Cryptosporidiosis

What is cryptosporidiosis?

Cryptosporidiosis (krip-toe-spo-rid-e-o-sis), is a diarrheal disease caused by a microscopic parasite, *Cryptosporidium parvum.* It can live in the intestine of humans and animals and is passed in the stool of an infected person or animal. Both the disease and the parasite are also known as "crypto." The parasite is protected by an outer shell that allows it to survive outside the body for long periods of time and makes it very resistant to chlorine disinfection. During the past two decades, crypto has become recognized as one of the most common causes of waterborne disease (drinking and recreational) in humans in the United States. The parasite is found in every region of the United States and throughout the world.

What are the symptoms of crypto?

Symptoms include diarrhea, loose or watery stool, stomach cramps, upset stomach, and a slight fever. Some people have no symptoms.

How long after infection do symptoms appear?

Symptoms generally begin 2–10 days after being infected.

"Cryptosporidiosis," National Center for Infectious Diseases, Division of Parasitic Diseases, Centers for Disease Control and Prevention (CDC), reviewed November 2003.

How long will symptoms last?

In persons with average immune systems, symptoms usually last about 2 weeks; the symptoms may go in cycles in which you may seem to get better for a few days, then feel worse, before the illness ends.

How is crypto spread?

Crypto lives in the intestine of infected humans or animals. Millions of crypto can be released in a bowel movement from an infected human or animal. You can become infected after accidentally swallowing the parasite. Crypto may be found in soil, food, water, or surfaces that have been contaminated with the feces from infected humans or animals. Crypto is not spread by contact with blood. Crypto can be spread:

- By putting something in your mouth or accidentally swallowing something that has come in contact with the stool of a person or animal infected with crypto.
- By swallowing recreational water contaminated with crypto. Recreational water is water in swimming pools, hot tubs, Jacuzzis, fountains, lakes, rivers, springs, ponds, or streams that can be contaminated with sewage or feces from humans or animals. Note: Crypto is chlorine resistant and can live for days in pools.
- By eating uncooked food contaminated with crypto. Thoroughly wash with uncontaminated water all vegetables and fruits you plan to eat raw.
- By accidentally swallowing crypto picked up from surfaces (such as toys, bathroom fixtures, changing tables, diaper pails) contaminated with stool from an infected person.

I have been diagnosed with crypto. Should I worry about spreading infection to others?

Yes, crypto can be very contagious. Follow these guidelines to avoid spreading crypto to others.

- Wash your hands with soap and water after using the toilet, changing diapers, and before eating or preparing food.
- Avoid swimming in recreational water (pools, hot tubs, lakes or rivers, the ocean, etc.) if you have crypto and for at least 2

weeks after diarrhea stops. You can pass crypto in your stool and contaminate water for several weeks after your symptoms have ended. This has resulted in many outbreaks of crypto among recreational water users. Note: you are not protected in a chlorinated pool because crypto is chlorine resistant and can live for days in pools.

- Avoid fecal exposure during sex.

Am I at risk for severe disease?

Although crypto can infect all people, some groups are more likely to develop more serious illness. Young children and pregnant women may be more susceptible to the dehydration resulting from diarrhea and should drink plenty of fluids while ill.

If you have a severely weakened immune system, you are at risk for more serious disease. Your symptoms may be more severe and could lead to serious or life-threatening illness. Examples of persons with weakened immune systems include those with HIV/AIDS; cancer and transplant patients who are taking certain immunosuppressive drugs; and those with inherited diseases that affect the immune system. If you have a severely weakened immune system, consult with your health care provider for additional guidance. You can also call the CDC AIDS HOTLINE toll-free at 1-800-342-2437. Ask for more information on cryptosporidiosis.

What should I do if I think I have crypto?

See your health care provider.

How is a crypto infection diagnosed?

Your health care provider will ask you to submit stool samples to see if you are infected. Because testing for crypto can be difficult, you may be asked to submit several stool specimens over several days. Because tests for crypto are not routinely done in most laboratories, your health care provider should specifically request testing for the parasite.

What is the treatment for crypto?

There is no effective treatment. Most people with a healthy immune system will recover on their own. If you have diarrhea, drink plenty of fluids to prevent dehydration. Rapid loss of fluids because of diarrhea can be life threatening in babies; parents should consult their health care provider about fluid replacement therapy options for babies. Antidiarrheal medicine may help slow down diarrhea, but consult with your health care provider before taking it.

People who are in poor health or who have a weakened immune system are at higher risk for more severe and more prolonged illness. For persons with AIDS, antiretroviral therapy that improves immune status will also decrease or eliminate symptoms of crypto. However, crypto is usually not cured and may come back if the immune status worsens. See your health care provider to discuss anti-retroviral therapy used to improve immune status.

How can I prevent crypto?

Practice Good Hygiene

- Wash hands thoroughly with soap and water
  - Wash hands after using the toilet and before handling or eating food (especially for persons with diarrhea)
  - Wash hands after every diaper change, especially if you work with diaper-aged children, even if you are wearing gloves.
- Protect others by not swimming if experiencing diarrhea (essential for children in diapers).

Avoid Water that Might be Contaminated

- Avoid swallowing recreational water.
- Avoid drinking untreated water from shallow wells, lakes, rivers, springs, ponds, and streams.
- Avoid drinking untreated water during community-wide outbreaks of disease caused by contaminated drinking water. In the United States, nationally distributed brands of bottled or canned carbonated soft drinks are safe to drink. Commercially packaged noncarbonated soft drinks and fruit juices that do not require refrigeration until after they are opened (for example, those that can be stored unrefrigerated on grocery shelves) also are safe.
- Avoid using ice or drinking untreated water when traveling in countries where the water supply might be unsafe.

- If you are unable to avoid drinking or using water that might be contaminated, then treat the water yourself by:
- Heating the water to a rolling boil for at least 1 minute.

OR

- Using a filter that has an absolute pore size of at least 1 micron or one that has been NSF-rated for "cyst removal."
- Do not rely on chemical disinfection of crypto because it is highly resistant to inactivation by chlorine or iodine.

Avoid Food that Might be Contaminated

- Wash and/or peel all raw vegetables and fruits before eating.
- Use uncontaminated water to wash all food that is to be eaten raw.
- Avoid eating uncooked foods when traveling in countries with minimal water treatment and sanitation systems.

Avoid Fecal Exposure during Sex

Chapter 51

Lice

Body Lice (Pediculosis)

What are body lice?

Body lice are parasitic insects that live on the body and in the clothing or bedding of infested humans. Infestation is common, found worldwide, and affects people of all races. Body lice infestations spread rapidly under crowded conditions where hygiene is poor and there is frequent contact among people. Are body lice infestations common in the United States? Body lice are found only in homeless, transient populations who don't have access to changes of clothes or bath. Infestation is unlikely in anyone who bathes regularly.

Where are body lice found?

Body lice are found on the body and on clothing or bedding used by infested people; lice eggs are lain in the seams of clothing or on bedding. Occasionally eggs are attached to body hair.

Lice found on the hair and head are not body lice; they are head lice.

"Body Lice," June 2000, "Head Lice Infestation," November 2003, "Treating Head Lice," May 2001, "Treating Head Lice with Malathion," December 2003, and "Pubic Lice or 'Crabs,'" June 2000. Division of Parasitic Diseases, Centers for Disease Control and Prevention (CDC).

Can body lice transmit disease?

Yes. Epidemics of typhus and louse-borne relapsing fever have been caused by body lice. Though typhus is no longer widespread, epidemics still occur during times of war, civil unrest, natural disasters, in refugee camps, and prisons where people live crowded together in unsanitary conditions. Typhus still exists in places where climate, chronic poverty, and social customs prevent regular changes and laundering of clothing.

What are the signs and symptoms of body lice?

Itching and rash are common; both are your body's allergic reaction to the lice bite. Long-term body lice infestations may lead to thickening and discoloration of the skin, particularly around the waist, groin, and upper thighs. Sores on the body may be caused by scratching. These sores can sometimes become infected with bacteria or fungi.

How are body lice spread?

Body lice are spread directly through contact with a person who has body lice, or indirectly through shared clothing, beds, bed linens, or towels.

What do body lice look like?

There are three forms of body lice: the egg (sometimes called a nit), the nymph, and the adult.

Nit: Nits are body lice eggs. They are generally easy to see in the seams of clothing, particularly around the waistline and under armpits. They are about 1/16 of an inch long. Nits may also be attached to body hair. They are oval and usually yellow to white. Nits may take 30 days to hatch.

Nymph: The egg hatches into a baby louse called a nymph. It looks like an adult body louse, but is smaller. Nymphs mature into adults about 7 days after hatching. To live, the nymph must feed on blood.

Adult: The adult body louse is about the size of a sesame seed, has 6 legs, and is tan to grayish-white. Females lay eggs. To live, adult lice need to feed on blood. If the louse falls off a person, it dies within 10 days.

How is a body lice infestation diagnosed?

By looking closely in the seams of clothing and on the body for eggs and for crawling lice. Diagnosis should be made by a health care provider if you are unsure about infestation. How are body lice treated? Lice infestations are generally treated by giving the infested person a clean change of clothes, a shower, and by laundering all worn clothing, bed linens, and towels. When laundering items, use the hot cycle (130° F) of the washing machine. Set the dryer to the hot cycle to dry items. Additionally, a 1% permethrin or pyrethrin lice shampoo, (also called pediculicide, pronounced "peh-DICK-you-luh-side"), may be applied to the body. Medication should be applied exactly as directed on the bottle or by your physician.

Head Lice Infestation

What are head lice?

Also called *Pediculus humanus capitis* (peh-DICK-you-lus HUE-man-us CAP-ih-TUS), head lice are parasitic insects found on the heads of people. Having head lice is very common. However, there are no reliable data on how many people get head lice in the United States each year.

Who is at risk for getting head lice?

Anyone who comes in close contact with someone who already has head lice, contaminated clothing, and other belongings. Preschool and elementary-age children, 3–10, and their families are infested most often. Girls get head lice more often than boys, women more than men. In the United States, African-Americans rarely get head lice.

What do head lice look like?

There are three forms of lice: the nit, the nymph, and the adult.

Nit: Nits are head lice eggs. They are hard to see and are often confused for dandruff or hair spray droplets. Nits are found firmly attached to the hair shaft. They are oval and usually yellow to white. Nits take about 1 week to hatch.

Nymph: The nit hatches into a baby louse called a nymph. It looks like an adult head louse, but is smaller. Nymphs mature into adults about 7 days after hatching. To live, the nymph must feed on blood.

Adult: The adult louse is about the size of a sesame seed, has six legs, and is tan to grayish-white. In persons with dark hair, the adult louse will look darker. Females lay nits; they are usually larger than males. Adult lice can live up to 30 days on a person's head. To live, adult lice need to feed on blood. If the louse falls off a person, it dies within 2 days.

Where are head lice most commonly found?

On the scalp behind the ears and near the neckline at the back of the neck. Head lice hold on to hair with hook-like claws found at the end of each of their six legs. Head lice are rarely found on the body, eyelashes, or eyebrows.

What are the signs and symptoms of head lice infestation?

- Tickling feeling of something moving in the hair.
- Itching, caused by the an allergic reaction to the bites.
- Irritability.
- Sores on the head caused by scratching. These sores can sometimes become infected.

How did my child get head lice?

- By contact with an already infested person. Contact is common during play at school and at home (slumber parties, sports activities, at camp, on a playground).
- By wearing infested clothing, such as hats, scarves, coats, sports uniforms, or hair ribbons.
- By using infested combs, brushes, or towels.
- By lying on a bed, couch, pillow, carpet, or stuffed animal that has recently been in contact with an infested person.

How is head lice infestation diagnosed?

By looking closely through the hair and scalp for nits, nymphs, or adults. Finding a nymph or adult may be difficult; there are usually few of them and they can move quickly from searching fingers. If crawling lice are not seen, finding nits within a 1/4 inch of the scalp confirms that a person is infested and should be treated. If you only find nits more than 1/4 inch from the scalp, the infestation is probably an old one and does not need to be treated. If you are not sure if a person has head lice, the diagnosis should be made by a health care provider, school nurse, or a professional from the local health department or agricultural extension service.

Treating Head Lice

I have heard that head lice medications do not work, or that head lice are resistant to medication. Is this true?

A recent study done by Harvard University did show that SOME, but NOT ALL (or even most) head lice are resistant to common prescription and over-the-counter medications (OTC). There is no information on how widespread resistance may be in the United States. Resistance (medication not working) is more likely in people who have been treated many times for head lice. There are many reasons why medications may seem not to work. Below are some of those reasons:

1. **Misdiagnosis of a head lice infestation.** A person has head lice if they have crawling bugs on their head or many lice eggs (also called nits) within a quarter inch (approximately the width of your pinky finger) of the scalp. Nits found on the hair shaft further than 1/4 inch from the scalp have already hatched out. Treatment is not recommended for people who only have nits further than one-quarter inch away from the scalp.

2. **Not following treatment instructions fully.** See instructions below for how to treat a head lice infestation. Using medication alone is not likely to cure a head lice infestation.

3. **Medication not working at all (resistance).** If head lice medication does not kill any crawling bugs, then resistance is likely. If the medication kills some of the bugs, then resistance to medication is probably not the reason for treatment failure (see item #2 and #4).

4. **Medication kills crawling bugs, but is not able to penetrate the nits.** It is very difficult for head lice medication to penetrate the nit shell. Medication may effectively kill crawling bugs, but may not treat the nits. This is why follow-up treatment is recommended. See instructions below for a detailed summary.

5. **New infection.** You can get infested more than once with head lice. Teach family members how to prevent re-infection.

How can I treat a head lice infestation?

By treating the infested person, any other infested family members, and by cleaning clothing and bedding.

Step 1: Treat the Infested Person/Any Infested Family Members

Requires using an OTC or prescription medication. Follow these treatment steps:

1. Before applying treatment, remove all clothing from the waist up.
2. Apply lice medicine, also called pediculicide, according to label instructions. If your child has extra long hair, you may need to use a second bottle.

   WARNING: Do not use a creme rinse or combination shampoo/conditioner before using lice medicine. Do not re-wash hair for 1–2 days after treatment.
3. Have the infested person put on clean clothing after treatment.
4. If some live lice are still found 8–12 hours after treatment, but are moving more slowly than before, do not retreat. Comb dead and remaining live lice out of the hair. The medicine sometimes takes longer to kill the lice.
5. If no dead lice are found 8–12 hours after treatment and lice seem as active as before, the medicine may not be working. See your health care provider for a different medication and follow their treatment instructions.
6. A nit comb should be used to remove nits and lice from the hair shaft. Many flea combs made for cats and dogs are also effective. Finer-toothed nit combs, available through Wal-Med* and the National Pediculosis Association*, may also be helpful.
7. After treatment, check hair every 2–3 days and use a nit comb to remove any nits or lice you see.
8. Retreat in 7–10 days.

9. Check all treated persons for 2–3 weeks after you think that all lice and nits are gone.

Step 2: Treat the Household

1. To kill lice and nits, machine wash all washable clothing and bed linens that the infested person touched during the 2 days before treatment. Use the hot water cycle (130° F) to wash clothes. Dry laundry using the hot cycle for at least 20 minutes.
2. Dry clean clothing that is not washable, (coats, hats, scarves, etc.) OR
3. Store all clothing, stuffed animals, comforters, etc., that cannot be washed or dry cleaned into a plastic bag and seal for 2 weeks.
4. Soak combs and brushes for 1 hour in rubbing alcohol, Lysol*, or wash with soap and hot (130° F) water.
5. Vacuum the floor and furniture. Do not use fumigant sprays; they can be toxic if inhaled.

My child has head lice. I don't. Should I treat myself to prevent being infested?

No, although anyone living with an infested person can get head lice. Have another person check the back and sides of your head for lice and nits. Check family members for lice and nits every 2–3 days. Treat only if crawling lice or nits are found within a 1/4 inch of the scalp.

Is there a product I can use to prevent getting head lice?

No.

Should my pets be treated for head lice?

No. Head lice do not live on pets.

My child is under 2 years old and has been diagnosed with head lice. Can I treat him or her with prescription or OTC drugs?

No. For children under 2 years old, remove crawling bugs and nits by hand. If the problem persists, consult your pediatrician.

What OTC medications are available to treat head lice?

Many head lice medications are available at your local drug store. Each OTC product contains one of the following active ingredients.

1. Pyrethrins (pie-WREATH-rins): often combined with piperonyl butoxide (pie-PER-a-nil beu-TOX-side): Brand name products: A-200*, Pronto*, R&C*, Rid*, Triple X* Pyrethrins are natural extracts from the chrysanthemum flower. Though safe and effective, pyrethrins only kill crawling lice, not unhatched nits. A second treatment is recommended in 7–10 days to kill any newly hatched lice. Sometimes the treatment does not work.

2. Permethrin (per-meth-rin): Brand name product: Nix* Permethrins are similar to natural pyrethrins. Permethrins are safe and effective and may continue to kill newly hatched eggs for several days after treatment. A second treatment may be necessary in 7–10 days to kill any newly hatched lice. Sometimes the treatment does not work.

Note: If OTC permethrin (1%) does not effectively kill crawling bugs, prescription-strength (5%) permethrin will not be any more effective. If lice are resistant to 1%, they will also be resistant to 5% permethrin.

What are the prescription drugs used to treat head lice?

Malathion (Ovide*): Malathion has just been reapproved for the treatment of head lice infestations. When used as directed, malathion is very effective in treating lice and nits. Few side-effects have been reported. Malathion may sting if applied to open sores on the scalp caused by scratching. Therefore, do not use if excessive scratching has caused a large number of open sores on the head.

Lindane (Kwell*): Lindane is one of the most common treatments used to treat head lice. When used as directed, the drug is usually safe. Overuse, misuse, or accidentally swallowing of Lindane can be toxic to the brain and nervous system. Lindane should not be used if excessive scratching has caused open sores on the head.

Which head lice medicine is best for me?

If you aren't sure, ask your pharmacist or health care provider. When using medicine, always follow the instructions.

When Treating Head Lice

1. Do not use extra amounts of the lice medication unless instructed. Drugs are insecticides and can be dangerous when misused or overused.
2. Do not treat the infested person more than 3 times with the same medication if it does not seem to work. See your health care provider for alternative medication.
3. Do not mix head lice medications.

Should household sprays be used to kill adult lice?

No. Spraying the house is NOT recommended. Fumigants and room sprays can be toxic if inhaled.

Should I have a pest control company spray my house?

No. Vacuuming floors and furniture is enough to treat the household.

Treating Head Lice with Malathion

Malathion (Ovide* lotion) was re-approved Food and Drug Administration (FDA) as a prescription drug for the treatment of head lice infestation in the United States. Follow the directions below to treat a head lice-infestation in your home.

Step 1: Treat the Person Infested with Head Lice

1. Before applying malathion lotion, remove all clothing.
2. Apply malathion according to label directions, to dry hair until the scalp and hair are wet and thoroughly coated. Leave the medication on the hair for 8–12 hours; allow the hair to dry naturally. Have the person put on clean clothing once medication has been applied.

   (Consider treating just before bedtime. Once malathion has been applied to the hair and scalp, cover any pillow(s) with a towel to keep medication from staining the pillow.)
3. After 8–12 hours, thoroughly wash hair.
4. A nit (head lice egg) comb should be used to remove lice and nits from the hair. Many flea combs made for cats and dogs are also effective.

5. After treatment, check hair and comb with a nit comb to remove nits and lice every 2–3 days. Continue checking for 2–3 weeks until you are sure all lice and nits are gone.
6. If crawling bugs are found 7–10 days after treatment, retreat with the same or different louse medication.

Warnings and Precautions

1. Malathion may cause stinging, especially if the scalp has open sores from scratching.
2. Malathion is flammable. Keep medication out of the eyes and away from heat sources such as hair dryers, electric curlers, cigarettes, or open flames.
3. Pregnant and nursing mothers should only use malathion after consulting their physician.

Step 2: Treat the Household

Head lice do not live long if they fall off a person. You do not need to spend a lot of time or money on house cleaning activities. Follow these steps to help avoid re-infestation by lice that have recently fallen off the hair or crawled onto clothing or furniture.

1. To kill lice and nits, machine wash all washable clothing and bed linens that the infested person has worn or slept on during the 2 days before treatment. Use the hot water (130° F) cycle. Dry laundry using high heat for at least 20 minutes.
2. Dry clean clothing worn 2 days before treatment if it is not washable, (coats, hats, scarves, etc.) OR store all clothing, stuffed animals, comforters, etc., that cannot be washed or dry cleaned into a plastic bag and seal for 2 weeks.
3. Soak combs and brushes for 1 hour in rubbing alcohol, Lysol*, or wash with soap and hot (130° F) water.
4. Vacuum the floor and furniture. Do not use fumigant sprays; they can be toxic if inhaled or absorbed through the skin.

Step 3: Prevent Reinfestation

Lice are most commonly spread directly by head-to-head contact and indirectly though sharing contaminated clothing or belongings.

Teach your child to avoid playtime and other activities that are likely to spread lice.

- Avoid head-to-head contact common during play at school and at home (slumber parties, sports activities, at camp, on a playground).
- Do not share clothing, such as hats, scarves, coats, sports uniforms, hair ribbons, or barrettes.
- Do not share infested combs, brushes, or towels.
- Do not lie on beds, couches, pillows, carpets, or stuffed animals that have recently been in contact with an infested person.

Are treatment failures common?

No, however reinfestation is common.

Is a second treatment needed?

Maybe. If crawling lice are still found, a second treatment may be given in 7–9 days. Other family members should be checked for signs of infestation.

Does malathion kill head lice eggs?

Yes. Some medication remains on the hair for several days to kill any eggs that may hatch.

Pubic Lice or "Crabs" (Pthirus pubis)

What are pubic lice?

Also called "crabs," pubic lice are parasitic insects found in the genital area of humans. Infection is common and found worldwide.

How did I get pubic lice?

Pubic lice are usually spread through sexual contact. Rarely, infestation can be spread through contact with an infested person's bed linens, towels, or clothes. A common misbelief is that infestation can be spread by sitting on a toilet seat. This isn't likely, since lice cannot live long away from a warm human body. Also, lice do not have feet designed to walk or hold onto smooth surfaces such as toilet seats.

Infection in a young child or teenager may indicate sexual activity or sexual abuse.

Where are pubic lice found?

Pubic lice are generally found in the genital area on pubic hair; but may occasionally be found on other coarse body hair, such as hair on the legs, armpit, mustache, beard, eyebrows, and eyelashes. Infestations of young children are usually on the eyebrows or eyelashes. Lice found on the head are not pubic lice; they are head lice.

Animals do not get or spread pubic lice.

What are the signs and symptoms of pubic lice?

Itching in the genital area. Nits (lice eggs) or crawling lice may be seen.

What do pubic lice look like?

There are three stages in the life of a pubic louse: the nit, the nymph, and the adult.

Nit: Nits are pubic lice eggs. They are hard to see and are found firmly attached to the hair shaft. They are small (about 1/16"), oval, and usually yellow to white. Nits take about 1 week to hatch.

Nymph: The nit hatches into a baby louse called a nymph. It looks like an adult pubic louse, but is smaller. Nymphs mature into adults about 7 days after hatching. To live, the nymph must feed on blood.

Adult: The adult pubic louse resembles a miniature crab when viewed through a strong magnifying glass. Pubic lice have six legs, but their two front legs are very large and look like the pincher claws of a crab; this how they got the nickname "crabs." Pubic lice are tan to grayish-white in color. Females lay nits; they are usually larger than males. To live, adult lice need to feed on blood. If the louse falls off a person, it dies within 1–2 days.

How is a pubic lice infestation diagnosed?

By looking closely through pubic hair for nits, nymphs, or adults. Finding a nymph or adult may be difficult; there are usually few of them and they can move quickly away from light. If crawling lice are not seen, finding nits confirms that a person is infested and should be treated. Diagnosis should be made by a health care provider if you are unsure about infestation or if treatment is not successful.

How are pubic lice treated?

A 1% permethrin or pyrethrin lice shampoo, also called pediculicide, is recommended to treat pubic lice. These products are available with out a prescription at your local drug store. Medication is generally very effective; apply the medication exactly as directed on the bottle. A prescription medication, called Lindane (1%) is available through your health care provider. Lindane is not recommended for pregnant or nursing women or for children less than 2 years old.

How to treat pubic lice infestations: (Note: see section below for treatment of eyelashes or eyebrows. The lice medications described in this section should not be used near the eyes.)

1. Wash the infested area; towel dry.
2. Thoroughly saturate hair with lice medication. If using permethrin or pyrethrins, leave medication on for 10 minutes; if using Lindane, shampoo should only be left on for 4 minutes. Thoroughly rinse off medication with water. Dry off with a clean towel.
3. Following treatment, most nits will still be attached to hair shafts. Nits may be removed with fingernails.
4. Put on clean underwear and clothing after treatment.
5. To kill any lice and nits that may be left on clothing or bedding, machine wash those washable items that the infested person used during the 2–3 days before treatment. Use the hot water cycle (130° F) of the washing machine to wash clothes. Use the hot cycle of the dryer for at least 20 minutes to dry clothes.
6. Dry clean clothing that is not washable.
7. Inform any sexual partners that they are at risk for infestation.
8. Avoid any sexual partners until partners have been treated and infestation has been cured.
9. Retreat in 7–10 days if lice are still found.

To treat nits and lice found on eyebrows or eyelashes:

If only a few nits are found, it may be possible to remove live lice and nits with your fingernails or a nit comb.

If additional treatment is needed for pubic lice nits found on the eyelashes, applying an ophthalmic-grade petrolatum ointment (only available by prescription) to the eyelids twice a day for 10 days is effective. Vaseline* is a kind of petrolatum, but is likely to irritate the eyes if applied.

Note

* Use of trade names is for identification only and does not imply endorsement by the Public Health Service or by the U.S. Department of Health and Human Services.

Chapter 52

Pinworm

What is pinworm infection?

This infection is caused by a small, white intestinal worm called *Enterobius vermicularis* (EN-ter-O-be-us ver-MIK-u-lar-is). Pinworms are about the length of a staple and live in the rectum of humans. While an infected person sleeps, female pinworms leave the intestines through the anus and deposit eggs on the surrounding skin.

What are the symptoms of a pinworm infection?

Itching around the anus, disturbed sleep, and irritability are common symptoms. If the infection is heavy, symptoms may also include loss of appetite, restlessness, and difficulty sleeping. Symptoms are caused by the female pinworm laying her eggs. Most symptoms of pinworm infection are mild; many infected people have no symptoms.

Who is at risk for pinworm infection?

Pinworm is the most common worm infection in the United States. School-age children, followed by preschoolers, have the highest rates of infection. In some groups nearly 50% of children are infected. Infection often occurs in more than one family member. Adults are less likely to have pinworm infection, except mothers of infected children.

"Pinworm Infection," Division of Parasitic Diseases, Centers for Disease Control and Prevention (CDC), reviewed August 15, 1999. Despite the older date of this document, the information is still accurate.

Child care centers, and other institutional settings often have cases of pinworm infection.

How is pinworm infection spread?

Pinworm eggs are infective within a few hours after being deposited on the skin. They can survive up to 2 weeks on clothing, bedding, or other objects. You or your children can become infected after accidentally ingesting (swallowing) infective pinworm eggs from contaminated surfaces or fingers.

How is pinworm infection diagnosed?

If pinworms are suspected, transparent adhesive tape (often called the "scotch tape test") or a pinworm paddle (supplied by your health care provider) are applied to the anal region. The eggs become glued to the sticky tape or paddle and are identified by examination under a microscope. Because bathing or having a bowel movement may remove eggs, the test should be done as soon as you wake up in the morning. You may have to provide several samples to your health care provider for examination. Since scratching of the anal area is common, samples taken from under the fingernails may also contain eggs. Eggs are rarely found during lab examinations of stool or urine. At night, the adult worms can sometimes be seen directly in bedclothes or around the anal area.

How is pinworm infection treated?

With either prescription or over-the-counter drugs. You should consult your health care provider before treating a suspected case of pinworm. Treatment involves a two-dose course. The second dose should be given 2 weeks after the first.

What if the pinworm infection occurs again?

The infected person should be treated with the same two-dose treatment. Close family contacts should also be treated. If the infection occurs again, you should search for the source of the infection. Playmates, schoolmates, close contacts outside the house, and household members should be considered. Each infected person should receive the usual two-dose treatment. In some cases it may be necessary to treat with more than two doses. One option is four to six treatments spaced 2 weeks apart.

How can I prevent the spread of infection and reinfection?

- Bathe when you wake up to help reduce the egg contamination.
- Change and wash your underwear each day. Frequent changing of night clothes are recommended.
- Change underwear, night clothes, and sheets after each treatment. Because the eggs are sensitive to sunlight, open blinds or curtains in bedrooms during the day.
- Personal hygiene should include washing hands after going to the toilet, before eating and after changing diapers.
- Trim fingernails short.
- Discourage nail-biting and scratching bare anal areas. These practices help reduce the risk of continuous self reinfection.

Cleaning and vacuuming the entire house or washing sheets every day are probably not necessary or effective. Screening for pinworm infection in schools or institutions is rarely recommended. Children may return to day care after the first treatment dose, after bathing, and after trimming and scrubbing nails.

Chapter 53

Scabies

What is scabies?

Scabies (SKAY-bees) is an infestation of the skin with the microscopic mite *Sarcoptes scabei*. Infestation is common, found worldwide, and affects people of all races and social classes. Scabies spreads rapidly under crowded conditions where there is frequent skin-to-skin contact between people, such as in hospitals, institutions, child-care facilities, and nursing homes.

What are the signs and symptoms of scabies infestation?

- Pimple-like irritations, burrows or rash of the skin, especially the webbing between the fingers; the skin folds on the wrist, elbow, or knee; the penis, the breast, or shoulder blades.
- Intense itching, especially at night and over most of the body.
- Sores on the body caused by scratching. These sores can sometimes become infected with bacteria.

How did I get scabies?

By direct, prolonged, skin-to-skin contact with a person already infested with scabies. Contact must be prolonged (a quick handshake

---

"Scabies," Division of Parasitic Diseases, Centers for Disease Control and Prevention (CDC), reviewed August 15, 1999. Despite the older date of this document, the information is still accurate.

or hug will usually not spread infestation). Infestation is easily spread to sexual partners and household members. Infestation may also occur by sharing clothing, towels, and bedding.

Who is at risk for severe infestation?

People with weakened immune systems and the elderly are at risk for a more severe form of scabies, called Norwegian or crusted scabies.

How long will mites live?

Once away from the human body, mites do not survive more than 48–72 hours. When living on a person, an adult female mite can live up to a month.

Did my pet spread scabies to me?

No. Pets become infested with a different kind of scabies mite. If your pet is infested with scabies, (also called mange) and they have close contact with you, the mite can get under your skin and cause itching and skin irritation. However, the mite dies in a couple of days and does not reproduce. The mites may cause you to itch for several days, but you do not need to be treated with special medication to kill the mites. Until your pet is successfully treated, mites can continue to burrow into your skin and cause you to have symptoms.

How soon after infestation will symptoms begin?

For a person who has never been infested with scabies, symptoms may take 4–6 weeks to begin. For a person who has had scabies, symptoms appear within several days. You do not become immune to an infestation.

How is scabies infestation diagnosed?

Diagnosis is most commonly made by looking at the burrows or rash. A skin scraping may be taken to look for mites, eggs, or mite fecal matter to confirm the diagnosis. If a skin scraping or biopsy is taken and returns negative, it is possible that you may still be infested. Typically, there are fewer than 10 mites on the entire body of an infested person; this makes it easy for an infestation to be missed.

Can scabies be treated?

Yes. Several lotions are available to treat scabies. Always follow the directions provided by your physician or the directions on the package insert. Apply lotion to a clean body from the neck down to the toes and left overnight (8 hours). After 8 hours, take a bath or shower to wash off the lotion. Put on clean clothes. All clothes, bedding, and towels used by the infested person 2 days before treatment should be washed in hot water; dry in a hot dryer. A second treatment of the body with the same lotion may be necessary 7–10 days later. Pregnant women and children are often treated with milder scabies medications.

Who should be treated for scabies?

Anyone who is diagnosed with scabies, as well as his or her sexual partners and persons who have close, prolonged contact to the infested person should also be treated. If your health care provider has instructed family members to be treated, everyone should receive treatment at the same time to prevent reinfestation.

How soon after treatment will I feel better?

Itching may continue for 2–3 weeks, and does not mean that you are still infested. Your health care provider my prescribe additional medication to relieve itching if it is severe. No new burrows or rashes should appear 24–48 hours after effective treatment.

Chapter 54

Tinea Infections

Fungus Infections: Tinea

Tinea is the name given to a fungal skin infection. Most people will develop some resistance to skin fungus after being infected. Others appear to have a susceptibility to fungal infections. Sometime the susceptibility will run in the family.

Tinea Pedis (Athlete's Foot)

This is the commonest type of fungal infection and only affects humans. It is spread by direct contact, most often through bare feet in bathrooms and health clubs. Leather or plastic footwear that doesn't "breathe" encourages tinea pedis. It is rare in children.

In most cases, the skin becomes white, soft and peels away between the toes (especially between the fourth and little toes). It may infect the sole of the foot resulting in peeling, scaling, itching, and sometimes blistering. Only one, or both feet may be involved.

This chapter includes "Fungus Infections: Tinea," and "Fungus Infections: Preventing Recurrence" which are reprinted with permission from the American Osteopathic College of Dermatology (AOCD). For additional information, visit the AOCD website at www.aocd.org. Also included is "Tinea Versicolor," reprinted with permission from the American Academy of Dermatology.

Onychomycosis (Tinea Unguium; Nail Fungus)

Toenail infection is usually associated with tinea pedis. It is very difficult to eradicate. Often the great toenail is the first to show signs, especially if it has been injured. The nail yellows, and after years thickens and breaks easily. Fingernail infections are similar, but less common.

Tinea Cruris (Jock Itch)

Some subjects with tinea pedis also develop a rash in the groin (tinea cruris), especially if they tend to sweat a lot. It is common and affects men more often than women. It has an itchy spreading red border.

Tinea Corporis (Ringworm)

Tinea corporis may be spread from person to person, from contact with an infected animal, most often a cat, or from exposure to fungus in the soil. Itchy red scaly patches come up anywhere the animal has rubbed. They often develop into a ring. This kind of tinea usually clears up with appropriate creams. If due to an animal, even if it has no signs of a skin problem it will need treatment too.

Tinea Capitis (Scalp Ringworm)

Tinea capitis usually occurs mostly in children and results in scaling and patchy hair loss. It is epidemic in many African American communities. The scalp can look quite moth-eaten but with the right treatment the hair will grow back normally and will not result in permanent hair loss.

An exception may be a kerion; this is a very inflammatory tinea of the scalp and looks like a boil or abscess. It is hard to immediately confirm that the symptoms are due to tinea infection and to establish the identity of the infecting organism. This may be treated with prednisone to prevent permanent hair loss.

Treatment

Tinea infections can be treated by a variety of different medications. For tinea pedis, cruris, and corporis, creams such as Lamisil-AT and Micatin AF can be bought over the counter at a pharmacy. Prescription creams are stronger, faster, and require fewer applications. Sometimes oral medications are necessary. These are very effective, and include griseofulvin (Gris-PEG, Fulvicin), Lamisil (terbinafine), Sporanox (itraconazole), and Diflucan (fluconazole). Tinea capitis, tinea unguium, and chronic tinea pedis are difficult to eradicate completely and require oral treatment.

Prevention

People with tinea pedis should discourage further growth of the fungus by keeping their feet as dry as possible. Wear open-toed sandals whenever possible, avoid boots, dry carefully after washing, and use an antifungal foot powder (Zeasorb-AF) daily.

Tinea Versicolor

Tinea versicolor is a common skin condition due to overgrowth of a skin surface yeast. This overgrowth results in uneven skin color and scaling that can be unsightly and sometimes itch. The yeast normally lives in the pores of the skin and thrives in oily areas such as the neck, upper chest, and back.

What does tinea versicolor look like and how do you recognize it?

Tinea versicolor has small, scaly white-to-pink or tan-to-dark spots which can be scattered over the upper arms, chest and back. They may sometimes appear on the neck and the face. On light skin, tinea versicolor may be faint or can appear as tan-to-pink spots, while on dark skin tinea versicolor may be light or dark. The fungus grows slowly and prevents the skin from tanning normally. As the rest of the skin tans in the sun, the pale spots, which are affected by the yeast, become more noticeable, especially on dark skin.

What are the symptoms?

Tinea versicolor usually produces few symptoms. Occasionally, there is some slight itching that is more intense when a person gets hot.

Who may get this rash?

Most people get tinea versicolor when they are teenagers or young adults. It is rare in the elderly and children, except in tropical climates where it can occur at any age. Both dark and light skinned people are equally prone to its development. People with oily skin may be more susceptible than those with naturally dry skin.

The yeast is normally present in small numbers on everyone's skin. Anyone can develop an overgrowth of yeast. During the summer months

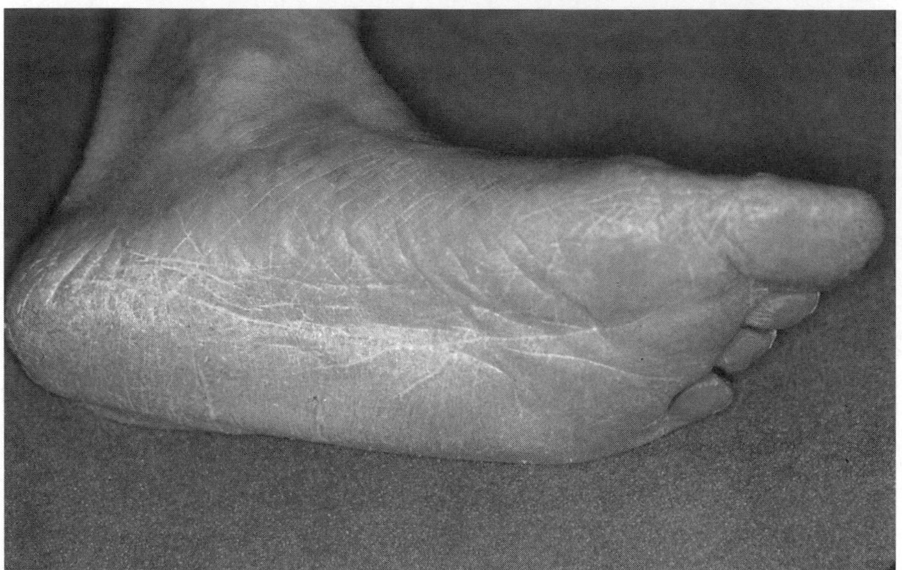

Figure 54.1. *Athlete's foot (tinea pedis). Photograph © Jere Mammino, D.O.; reprinted with permission.*

when the temperature and humidity are high, the yeast can increase. The excess yeast on the skin prevents the normal pigmentation process, resulting in light and dark spots. In tropical countries with continuous high heat and high humidity, people can have these spots year round. In other climates, the spots generally fade in the cooler and drier months of the year. Why some people get tinea versicolor and others do not is unclear.

In tropical countries with continuous high heat and high humidity, people can have these spots year round. In other climates, the spots generally fade in the cooler and drier months of the year.

How is tinea versicolor diagnosed?

Although the light or dark colored spots can resemble other skin conditions, tinea versicolor can be easily recognized by a dermatologist. In most cases, the appearance of the skin is diagnostic, but a simple examination of the fine scales scraped from the skin can confirm the diagnosis. Scales are lightly scraped onto a slide and examined under a microscope for the presence of the yeast. A special light may help to make the diagnosis by showing a yellow green color where the skin is affected.

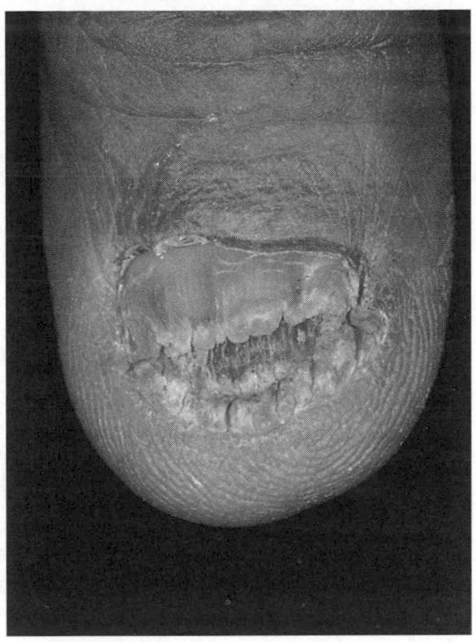

Figure 54.2. *Nail fungus (onychomycosis). Photograph © Jere Mammino, D.O.; reprinted with permission.*

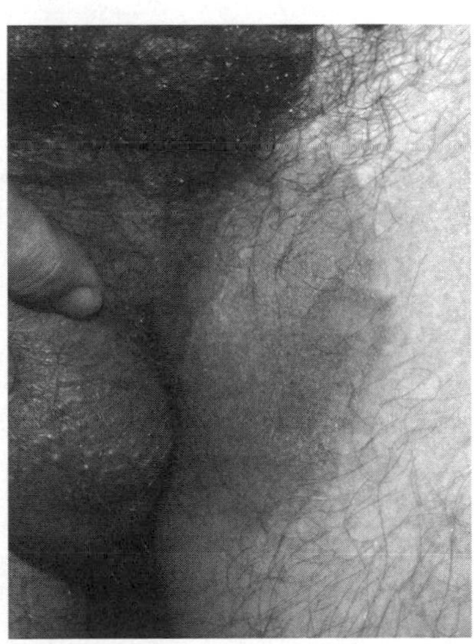

Figure 54.3. *Jock itch (tinea cruris). Photograph © Jere Mammino, D.O.; reprinted with permission.*

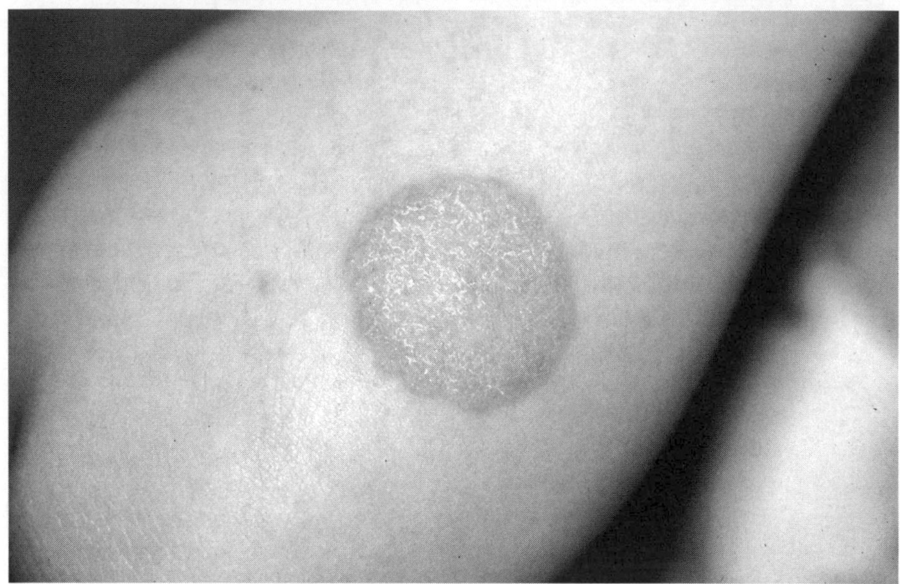

Figure 54.4. *Ringworm (tinea corporis). Photograph © Jere Mammino, D.O.; reprinted with permission.*

Figure 54.5. *Scalp ringworm (tinea capitis). Photograph © Jere Mammino, D.O.; reprinted with permission.*

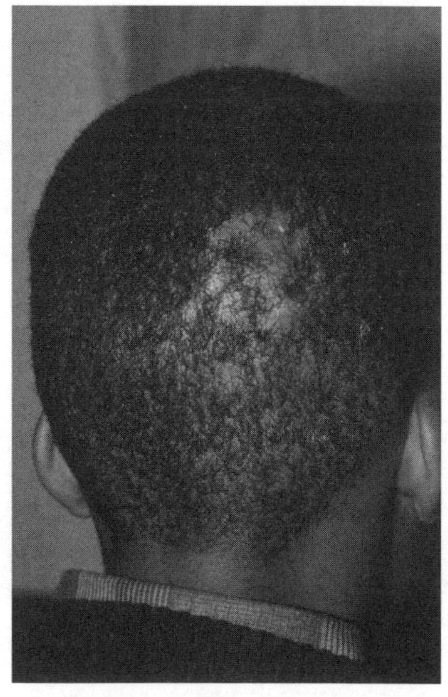

How is it treated?

Tinea versicolor is treated with topical or oral medications. Topical treatment includes special cleansers including some shampoos, creams, or lotions applied directly to the skin.

Several oral medications have been used successfully to treat tinea versicolor. Because of possible side effects, or interactions with other medications, the use of these prescription medicines should be supervised by your dermatologist. After any form of treatment, the uneven color of the skin may remain several months after the yeast has been eliminated until the skin repigments normally.

Tinea versicolor may recur. Special cleansers may decrease episodes when used once or twice a month, especially during warm humid months of the year.

Each patient is treated by the dermatologist according to the severity and location of the disease, the climate, and the desire of the patient. It's important to remember that the yeast is easy to kill, but it can take weeks or months for the skin to regain its normal color.

Fungus Infections: Preventing Recurrence

Doctors have excellent treatments for skin fungus infections that occur on the feet, nails, groin, hands, and other locations. Unfortunately, there is a strong tendency for fungal infections to recur in many people even after effective clearing with medication. This is because we all have our strengths and weaknesses. Some people are prone to allergies. Others get lots of colds. Others get stomach ulcers. And some people are prone to recurrent skin fungus infections.

The tendency for fungus to recur in many adults, especially on the feet and toenails, is a genetic condition. Their skin cannot recognize the fungus as foreign and get rid of it. After having a fungus there for a while the body's immune system learns to live with the fungus and no longer tries to get rid of it.

Children only rarely get fungal infections of the feet, especially before the age of five. Their bodies still react vigorously to the fungus. For some reason, they are more likely to get it on the scalp than adults are.

Fungus is all around us, on floors, in dirt, and on other people. It is hard to avoid forever. It likes warmth and moisture, making certain parts of the skin more vulnerable. A fungus is a superficial skin problem, not an internal one. It does not spread by going inside the body. Cortisone creams, tried by many patients, help fungus grow! The rash may get less red and itchy at first, but spreads out and recurs, itchier than ever, when the cortisone is stopped.

A fungus sheds "spores", like tiny seeds, which wait for the right moment to grow into new fungus. The most common place for these spores to collect is in shoes. Therefore, after effective treatment, a fungus may recur quickly where spores are present. Fungus doesn't care what color the socks are. White socks offer no advantage. Absorbent cotton or wool socks are best.

Some Rules for Prevention: Remember, nothing works one hundred per cent. Try combinations of these ideas.

1. Use the medicine completely and as recommended. The fungus may till be present long after it is no longer visible as a rash.
2. Keep feet clean, cool and dry. Change socks. Wear shoes that "breathe" like leather, rather than plastic.
3. Make sure shoes fit correctly and are not too tight.
4. Apply an anti-fungal cream, like Lotrimin or Lamisil, or a prescription antifungal cream to the bottom of the feet, and on the nails, about twice a week. This may help prevent early regrowth of the fungus. In some cases, an oral medication may be prescribed.
5. Avoid walking barefoot, especially in bathrooms, locker rooms, gyms, on carpeting, and in public bathing areas. Wear slippers or stand on a towel or piece of paper.
6. Keep toenails short, cut straight across and avoid ingrown nails. Do not use the same clippers on abnormal nails and normal nails.
7. Family members and close personal contacts should treat any fungus infections they may have to avoid trading back and forth.
8. Apply an anti-fungal powder, like Zeasorb-AF to the shoes every day, to keep spores from growing.
9. Discard old shoes, boots, slippers and sneakers. Do not share footwear with others.
10. If one has had a body fungus, in the groin or elsewhere on the skin, consider using an anti-dandruff shampoo, like Selsun Blue on this area twice a month. Lather up and leave it on the skin for about five minutes, then wash off completely. In some cases a preventive medication may be prescribed.

Chapter 55

Transmissible Spongiform Encephalopathies

What are transmissible spongiform encephalopathies?

Transmissible spongiform encephalopathies (TSEs), also known as prion diseases, are a group of rare degenerative brain disorders characterized by tiny holes that give the brain a "spongy" appearance. These holes can be seen when brain tissue is viewed under a microscope.

Creutzfeldt-Jakob disease (CJD) is the most well-known of the human TSEs. It is a rare type of dementia that affects about one in every one million people each year. Other human TSEs include kuru, fatal familial insomnia (FFI), and Gerstmann-Straussler-Scheinker disease (GSS). Kuru was identified in people of an isolated tribe in Papua New Guinea and has now almost disappeared. FFI and GSS are extremely rare hereditary diseases, found in just a few families around the world. A new type of CJD, called variant CJD (vCJD), was first described in 1996 and has been found in Great Britain and several other European countries. The initial symptoms of vCJD are different from those of classic CJD and the disorder typically occurs in younger patients. Research suggests that vCJD may have resulted from human consumption of beef from cattle with a TSE disease called bovine spongiform encephalopathy (BSE), also known as "mad cow disease." Other TSEs found in animals include scrapie, which affects

---

This chapter contains information from "Transmissible Spongiform Encephalopathies," December 2001, and "Creutzfeldt-Jakob Disease Fact Sheet," reviewed August 2003, National Institute of Neurological Disorders and Stroke (NINDS), National Institutes of Health (NIH).

sheep and goats; chronic wasting disease, which affects elk and deer; and transmissible mink encephalopathy. In a few rare cases, TSEs have occurred in other mammals such as zoo animals. These cases are probably caused by contaminated feed. CJD and other TSEs also can be transmitted experimentally to mice and other animals in the laboratory.

Research suggests that TSEs are caused by an abnormal version of a protein called a prion (prion is short for proteinaceous infectious particle). Prion proteins occur in both a normal form, which is a harmless protein found in the body's cells, and in an infectious form, which causes disease. The harmless and infectious forms of the prion protein are nearly identical, but the infectious form takes on a different folded shape from the normal protein.

Human TSEs can occur three ways: sporadically; as hereditary diseases; or through transmission from infected individuals. Sporadic TSEs may develop because some of a person's normal prions spontaneously change into the infectious form of the protein and then alter the prions in other cells in a chain reaction. Inherited cases arise from a change, or mutation, in the prion protein gene that causes the prions to be shaped in an abnormal way. This genetic change may be transmitted to an individual's offspring. Transmission of TSEs from infected individuals is relatively rare. TSEs cannot be transmitted through the air or through touching or most other forms of casual contact. However, they may be transmitted through contact with infected tissue, body fluids, or contaminated medical instruments. Normal sterilization procedures such as boiling or irradiating materials do not prevent transmission of TSEs.

Symptoms of TSEs vary, but they commonly include personality changes, psychiatric problems such as depression, lack of coordination, and/or an unsteady gait. Patients also may experience involuntary jerking movements called myoclonus, unusual sensations, insomnia, confusion, or memory problems. In the later stages of the disease, patients have severe mental impairment and lose the ability to move or speak.

Questions and Answers about Creutzfeldt-Jakob Disease

What is Creutzfeldt-Jakob disease?

Creutzfeldt-Jakob disease (CJD) is a rare, degenerative, invariably fatal brain disorder. It affects about one person in every one million people per year worldwide; in the United States there are about 200 cases per year. CJD usually appears in later life and runs a rapid course. Typically, onset of symptoms occurs about age 60, and about 90 percent of patients die within 1 year. In the early stages of disease, patients may have failing memory, behavioral changes, lack of coordination, and visual disturbances. As the illness progresses, mental deterioration becomes pronounced and involuntary movements, blindness, weakness of extremities, and coma may occur.

There are three major categories of CJD:

- In sporadic CJD, the disease appears even though the person has no known risk factors for the disease. This is by far the most common type of CJD and accounts for at least 85 percent of cases.
- In hereditary CJD, the person has a family history of the disease and/or tests positive for a genetic mutation associated with CJD. About 5 to 10 percent of cases of CJD in the United States are hereditary.
- In acquired CJD, the disease is transmitted by exposure to brain or nervous system tissue, usually through certain medical procedures. There is no evidence that CJD is contagious through casual contact with a CJD patient. Since CJD was first described in 1920, fewer than 1 percent of cases have been acquired CJD.

CJD belongs to a family of human and animal diseases known as the transmissible spongiform encephalopathies (TSEs). Spongiform refers to the characteristic appearance of infected brains, which become filled with holes until they resemble sponges under a microscope. CJD is the most common of the known human TSEs. Other human TSEs include kuru, fatal familial insomnia (FFI), and Gerstmann-Straussler-Scheinker disease (GSS). Kuru was identified in people of an isolated tribe in Papua New Guinea and has now almost disappeared. Fatal familial insomnia and GSS are extremely rare hereditary diseases, found in just a few families around the world. Other TSEs are found in specific kinds of animals. These include bovine spongiform encephalopathy (BSE), which is found in cows and often referred to as "mad cow" disease, scrapie, which affects sheep and goats, mink encephalopathy, and feline encephalopathy. Similar diseases have occurred in elk, deer, and exotic zoo animals.

What are the symptoms of the disease?

CJD is characterized as a rapidly progressive dementia. Initially, patients experience problems with muscular coordination; personality changes, including impaired memory, judgment, and thinking; and impaired vision. People with the disease also may experience insomnia, depression, or unusual sensations. CJD does not cause a fever or other flu-like symptoms. As the illness progresses, the patients' mental impairment becomes severe. They often develop involuntary muscle jerks called myoclonus, and they may go blind. They eventually lose the ability to move and speak and enter a coma. Pneumonia and other infections often occur in these patients and can lead to death.

There are several known variants of CJD. These variants differ somewhat in the symptoms and course of the disease. For example, a variant form of the disease—called new variant or variant (nv-CJD, v-CJD), described in Great Britain and France—begins primarily with psychiatric symptoms, affects younger patients than other types of CJD, and has a longer than usual duration from onset of symptoms to death. Another variant, called the panencephalopathic form, occurs primarily in Japan and has a relatively long course, with symptoms often progressing for several years. Scientists are trying to learn what causes these variations in symptoms and course of the disease. Some symptoms of CJD can be similar to symptoms of other progressive neurological disorders, such as Alzheimer's or Huntington's disease. However, CJD causes unique changes in brain tissue which can be seen at autopsy. It also tends to cause more rapid deterioration of a person's abilities than Alzheimer's disease or most other types of dementia.

How is CJD diagnosed?

There is currently no single diagnostic test for CJD. When a doctor suspects CJD, the first concern is to rule out treatable forms of dementia such as encephalitis (inflammation of the brain) or chronic meningitis. A neurological examination will be performed and the doctor may seek consultation with other physicians. Standard diagnostic tests will include a spinal tap to rule out more common causes of dementia and an electroencephalogram (EEG) to record the brain's electrical pattern, which can be particularly valuable because it shows a specific type of abnormality in CJD. Computerized tomography of the brain can help rule out the possibility that the symptoms result from other problems such as stroke or a brain tumor. Magnetic resonance imaging (MRI) brain scans also can reveal characteristic patterns of brain degeneration that can help diagnose CJD.

The only way to confirm a diagnosis of CJD is by brain biopsy or autopsy. In a brain biopsy, a neurosurgeon removes a small piece of tissue from the patient's brain so that it can be examined by a neuropathologist. This procedure may be dangerous for the patient, and the operation does not always obtain tissue from the affected part of the brain. Because a correct diagnosis of CJD does not help the patient, a brain biopsy is discouraged unless it is needed to rule out a treatable disorder. In an autopsy, the whole brain is examined after death. Both brain biopsy and autopsy pose a small, but definite, risk that the surgeon or others who handle the brain tissue may become accidentally infected by self-inoculation. Special surgical and disinfection procedures can minimize this risk. A fact sheet with guidance on these procedures is available from the National Institute of Neurological Disorders and Stroke (NINDS) and the World Health Organization.

Scientists are working to develop laboratory tests for CJD. One such test, developed at NINDS, is performed on a person's cerebrospinal fluid and detects a protein marker that indicates neuronal degeneration. This can help diagnose CJD in people who already show the clinical symptoms of the disease. This test is much easier and safer than a brain biopsy. The false positive rate is about 5 to 10 percent. Scientists are working to develop this test for use in commercial laboratories. There have been reports of other ways of diagnosing the disease, including tonsil biopsies, which may lead to other tests.

How is the disease treated?

There is no treatment that can cure or control CJD. Researchers have tested many drugs, including amantadine, steroids, interferon, acyclovir, antiviral agents, and antibiotics. However, none of these treatments has shown any consistent benefit.

Current treatment for CJD is aimed at alleviating symptoms and making the patient as comfortable as possible. Opiate drugs can help relieve pain if it occurs, and the drugs clonazepam and sodium valproate may help relieve myoclonus. During later stages of the disease, changing the person's position frequently can keep him or her comfortable and helps prevent bedsores. A catheter can be used to drain urine if the patient cannot control bladder function, and intravenous fluids and artificial feeding also may be used.

What causes Creutzfeldt-Jakob disease?

Some researchers believe an unusual "slow virus" or another organism causes CJD. However, they have never been able to isolate a virus or other organism in people with the disease. Furthermore, the agent that causes CJD has several characteristics that are unusual for known organisms such as viruses and bacteria. It is difficult to kill, it does not appear to contain any genetic information in the form of nucleic acids (DNA or RNA), and it usually has a long incubation period before symptoms appear. In some cases, the incubation period may be as long as 40 years. The leading scientific theory at this time maintains that CJD and the other TSEs are caused not by an organism but by a type of protein called a prion.

Prions occur in both a normal form, which is a harmless protein found in the body's cells; and in an infectious form, which causes disease. The harmless and infectious forms of the prion protein are nearly identical, but the infectious form takes a different folded shape than the normal protein. Sporadic CJD may develop because some of a person's normal prions spontaneously change into the infectious form of the protein and then alter the prions in other cells in a chain reaction.

Once they appear, abnormal prion proteins stick together and form fibers and/or clumps called plaques that can be seen with powerful microscopes. Fibers and plaques may start to accumulate years before symptoms of CJD begin to appear. It is still unclear what role these abnormalities play in the disease or how they might affect symptoms.

About 5 to 10 percent of all CJD cases are inherited. These cases arise from a mutation, or change, in the gene that controls formation of the normal prion protein. While prions themselves do not contain genetic information and do not require genes to reproduce themselves, infectious prions can arise if a mutation occurs in the gene for the body's normal prions. If the prion gene is altered in a person's sperm or egg cells, the mutation can be transmitted to the person's offspring. Several different mutations in the prion gene have been identified. The particular mutation found in each family affects how frequently the disease appears and what symptoms are most noticeable. However, not all people with mutations in the prion gene develop CJD. This suggests that the mutations merely increase susceptibility to CJD and that other, still-unknown factors also play a role in the disease.

How is CJD transmitted?

CJD is not a contagious disease. Although it can be transmitted to other people, the risk of this happening is extremely small. CJD cannot be transmitted through the air or through touching or most other forms of casual contact. Spouses and other household members of sporadic CJD patients have no higher risk of contracting the disease than the general population. However, direct or indirect contact with brain tissue and spinal cord fluid from infected patients should be avoided to prevent transmission of the disease through these materials.

In a few very rare cases, CJD has spread to other people from grafts of dura mater (a tissue that covers the brain), transplanted corneas, implantation of inadequately sterilized electrodes in the brain, and injections of contaminated pituitary growth hormone derived from human pituitary glands taken from cadavers. Doctors call these cases that are linked to medical procedures iatrogenic cases. Since 1985, all human growth hormone used in the United States has been synthesized by recombinant DNA procedures, which eliminates the risk of transmitting CJD by this route.

The appearance of the new variant of CJD (nv-CJD or v-CJD) in several younger than average people in Great Britain and France has led to concern that BSE may be transmitted to humans through consumption of contaminated beef. Although laboratory tests have shown a strong similarity between the prions causing BSE and v-CJD, there is no direct proof to support this theory. Furthermore, BSE has never been found in the United States, and importation of cattle and beef from countries with BSE has been banned in the United States since 1989 to reduce the risk that it will occur in this country.

Many people are concerned that it may be possible to transmit CJD through blood and related blood products such as plasma. Some animal studies suggest that contaminated blood and related products may transmit the disease, although this has never been shown in humans. If there are infectious agents in these fluids, they are probably in very low concentrations. Scientists do not know how many abnormal prions a person must receive before he or she develops CJD, so they do not know whether these fluids are potentially infectious or not. They do know that, even though millions of people receive blood transfusions each year, there are no reported cases of someone contracting CJD from a transfusion. Even among hemophiliacs, who sometimes receive blood plasma concentrated from thousands of people, there are no reported cases of CJD. This suggests that, if there is a risk of transmitting CJD through blood or plasma, it is extremely small.

How can people avoid spreading the disease?

To reduce the already very low risk of CJD transmission from one person to another, people should never donate blood, tissues, or organs if they have suspected or confirmed CJD, or if they are at increased risk because of a family history of the disease, a dura mater graft, or other factor.

Normal sterilization procedures such as cooking, washing, and boiling do not destroy prions. Caregivers, health care workers, and undertakers should take the following precautions when they are working with a person with CJD:

- Wash hands and exposed skin before eating, drinking, or smoking.
- Cover cuts and abrasions with waterproof dressings.
- Wear surgical gloves when handling a patient's tissues and fluids or dressing the patient's wounds.
- Avoid cutting or sticking themselves with instruments contaminated by the patient's blood or other tissues.
- Use disposable bedclothes and other cloth for contact with the patient. If disposable materials are not available, regular cloth should be soaked in undiluted chlorine bleach for an hour or more, then washed in a normal fashion after each use.
- Use face protection if there is a risk of splashing contaminated material such as blood or cerebrospinal fluid.
- Soak instruments that have come in contact with the patient in undiluted chlorine bleach for an hour or more, then use an autoclave (pressure cooker) to sterilize them in distilled water for at least one hour at 132–134 degrees Centigrade.

A fact sheet listing additional precautions for healthcare workers and morticians is available from the NINDS and the World Health Organization.

What research is taking place?

Many researchers are studying CJD. They are examining whether the transmissible agent is, in fact, a prion or a product of the infection, and are trying to discover factors that influence prion infectivity and how the disorder damages the brain. Using rodent models of the disease and brain tissue from autopsies, they are also trying to identify factors that influence susceptibility to the disease and that govern when in life the disease appears. They hope to use this knowledge to develop improved tests for CJD and to learn what changes ultimately kill the neurons so that effective treatments can be developed.

Chapter 56

Trichomoniasis

What is Trichomonas *infection?*

Trichomonas vaginalis is a microscopic parasite found worldwide. Infection with *Trichomonas* is called trichomoniasis (trick-oh-moe-nye-uh-sis). Trichomoniasis is one of the most common sexually transmitted diseases, mainly affecting 16–35 year old women. In the United States, it is estimated that 2 million women become infected each year.

How is trichomoniasis spread?

Trichomoniasis is spread through sexual activity. Infection is more common in women who have had multiple sexual partners.

A common misbelief is that infection can be spread by a toilet seat; this isn't likely, since the parasite cannot live long in the environment or on objects.

What are the signs and symptoms of infection?

Women: Signs and symptoms of infection range from having no symptoms (asymptomatic) to very symptomatic. Typical symptoms include foul smelling or frothy green discharge from the vagina, vaginal itching, or redness. Other symptoms can include painful sexual intercourse, lower abdominal discomfort, and the urge to urinate.

"Trichomonas Infection," Division of Parasitic Diseases, Centers for Disease Control and Prevention (CDC), reviewed January 2004.

Men: Most men with this infection do not have symptoms. When symptoms are present, they most commonly are discharge from the urethra, the urge to urinate, and a burning sensation with urination.

How long after infection do symptoms occur?

Most women who develop symptoms do so within 6 months of being infected.

What should I do if I think I have trichomoniasis?

See your health care provider who can test you for infection.

How is infection diagnosed?

Women: Your health care provider will perform a pelvic exam to collect vaginal samples for examination. Diagnosis is most commonly made by viewing the parasite under a microscope. Culturing for the parasite is the best way to diagnose infection; results may take 3–7 days.

Men: Diagnosis is made by collecting specimens from the urethra.

Remember: No diagnostic test is 100% accurate; mistakes can be made. Your health care provider may order additional testing to confirm the diagnosis.

I have trichomoniasis and am pregnant; can I spread infection to my baby?

Yes, but this is rare. Babies born to infected mothers may contract infection during delivery. Infants may develop fever; girls may develop vaginal discharge. Children should be treated if diagnosed. See your health care provider about treatment of trichomoniasis during pregnancy.

How can a child get trichomoniasis?

Infants: If an infant is infected, it is possible that the mother spread infection during childbirth. The mother should be checked for infection.

Young children: Because trichomoniasis is an STD, infection in a young child may indicate sexual abuse. If sexual abuse is suspected, an evaluation for other STDs is recommended.

Teenagers: Because trichomoniasis is a STD, infection in a teenager may indicate sexual activity or sexual abuse. An evaluation for other STDs is recommended.

Is infection treatable?

Yes. Your doctor will prescribe an antibiotic for you and all sexual partners you have had since becoming infected. If all current sexual partners are not treated, it is possible to become reinfected. Infants and children who are infected should be treated.

Treatment failed, is there another recommendation?

Yes. However, you may be treated with the same drug, for a longer time and at a higher dose. Your doctor may prescribe more than one drug to treat you. All sexual partners should be treated at the same time. Use a latex condom or avoid having sexual intercourse to prevent reinfection during treatment.

Can infection be prevented?

Yes. Follow these guidelines:

- Abstain from sexual intercourse; or,
- Use a latex condom properly, every time you have sexual intercourse, with every partner.
- Limit your sexual partners. The more sex partners you have, the greater your risk of encountering someone who has this or other STDs.
- If you are infected, your sexual partner(s) should be treated. This will prevent you from getting reinfected.

Once I am infected, am I immune?

No. You can get infected again.

Part Five

Vaccination Information

Chapter 57

Immunization Remains Our Best Defense Against Deadly Disease

Smallpox and polio have been wiped out in the United States. Cases of measles, mumps, tetanus, whooping cough (pertussis), and other life-threatening illnesses have been reduced by more that 95 percent. Immunization against influenza and pneumonia prevent tens of thousands of deaths annually among elderly persons and those who are chronically ill. As a result, millions of lives have been saved. But don't let the success of vaccines fool you into thinking we no longer need them. Most vaccine-preventable diseases aren't gone.

Steve Berman, M.D., president of the American Academy of Pediatrics and a pediatrician in Denver, says he and his colleagues were devastated to recently see an infant die of whooping cough. "This was a case where the family thought the risks of vaccination outweighed the benefits," Dr. Berman says. The baby was exposed to the disease by two older brothers who hadn't been vaccinated.

Vaccines contain a weakened (attenuated) or killed (inactivated) form of disease-causing bacteria or viruses, or components of these microorganisms, that trigger a response by our body's immune system. For example, vaccines stimulate our bodies to make antibodies—proteins that specifically recognize and target the bacteria and viruses against which the vaccines are designed, and that help eliminate them from the body when we encounter them.

"Understanding Vaccine Safety: Immunization Remains Our Best Defense Against Deadly Disease," by Michelle Meadows, *FDA Consumer*, Food and Drug Administration (FDA), July-August 2001.

Without vaccine protection, we can easily contract and transmit infectious diseases. It may only take one person, whether it's a family member, a neighbor, or a visitor from another country, to start the spread of a disease. And even immunized individuals can be at risk because no vaccine is ever 100 percent effective for everyone.

Most parents believe in the benefits of vaccination, as evidenced by record high childhood vaccination rates, and more and more adults are getting vaccinated against influenza, pneumococcal disease, and tetanus. But some people who need vaccines don't get them for a variety of reasons, including fear of side effects. Lately, a surge of negative publicity focusing on the risks of vaccines—some of which are unproven or inaccurate—has some wondering whether they do more harm than good. But vaccine experts and the overwhelming majority of healthcare providers caution consumers against skipping important vaccinations because of an evening news report or a posting on the Internet.

Sometimes such reports contain unsubstantiated or inaccurate information and don't reflect a balanced view of the risks and benefits of a particular vaccine.

The Food and Drug Administration recommends that consumers arm themselves with the facts about the benefits and risks of vaccines, along with the potential consequences of not vaccinating against certain diseases. According to a Washington state-based organization called Parents of Kids with Infectious Diseases (PKIDS), some parents are shocked to learn that children can die of chickenpox and other vaccine-preventable diseases they hadn't considered a threat.

The FDA's Center for Biologics Evaluation and Research (CBER) regulates vaccines in the United States, and works with several other agencies, including the Centers for Disease Control and Prevention (CDC) and the National Institutes of Health (NIH), to study and monitor vaccine safety and effectiveness. New vaccines are licensed only after the FDA thoroughly reviews the results of extensive laboratory studies and clinical trials performed by scientists, physicians, and manufacturers.

For vaccines intended for wide use in healthy populations such as children, clinical testing with careful safety monitoring typically involves thousands of patients before a vaccine is ever licensed. And after a vaccine hits the market, the safety monitoring continues, as does FDA oversight to assure the highest levels of quality control in the vaccine production process.

"We are always monitoring for evidence that might suggest possible problems with vaccines," says Karen Midthun, M.D., director of CBER's office of vaccine research and review. CBER scientists also conduct research to better ensure vaccine safety and to better understand vaccine-related side effects.

A Commitment to Safety

On the surface, it may seem that approaching vaccine safety as a continuous process—always looking into problems and potential problems—implies that vaccines are unsafe. "But it's actually a reflection of our ongoing commitment to safety, and to assuring the prevention of potentially lethal infectious diseases," says Jesse Goodman, M.D., M.P.H., deputy director for medicine at CBER. "It's also the nature of science to seek and implement improvements which make for safer and more effective medical products."

Since 1996, for example, CBER has licensed several acellular pertussis vaccines. Acellular pertussis vaccines use only parts of the disease-causing bacteria and are associated with fewer side effects than the whole cell pertussis vaccines that had been in use. In 1997, the CDC's Advisory Committee on Immunization Practices (ACIP) recommended a switch from using the whole cell pertussis component of the diphtheria, tetanus, pertussis (DTP) vaccine to using acellular pertussis vaccines for all five doses in the childhood schedule.

The National Institute of Allergy and Infectious Diseases (NIAID) sponsored clinical trials for some of the experimental acellular vaccines. "We set out to develop an improved vaccine that would be as effective as the standard whole cell vaccine but cause less extended crying, fevers, and other side effects," says Carole Heilman, Ph.D., director of NIAID's division of microbiology and infectious diseases. CBER scientists also played a critical role by developing methods to evaluate the acellular vaccines, which helped them get to clinical trials faster.

There have been other recent policy changes to improve vaccine safety, including ACIP's 1999 recommendation to change from the use of oral polio vaccine (OPV) to the inactivated polio virus (IPV). OPV had been highly effective in controlling naturally occurring polio outbreaks, preventing thousands of cases of paralysis a year. But as a live virus, it mutated in extremely rare cases to cause polio itself. Continued use of OPV resulted in about 10 cases of paralytic polio each year among millions vaccinated and their contacts, according to William Egan, Ph.D., deputy director of CBER's office of vaccine research and review. Switching to the use of IPV eliminated this risk and was appropriate once epidemic polio was controlled.

"There are times when we also take action even when there is just the theoretical potential for harm," Goodman says. Thimerosal, a mercury-containing compound, had been the most widely used preservative in vaccines. Its use in minute amounts helped to prevent bacteria from contaminating multi-dose vials of vaccines and other medicines, protecting against potentially serious infections. But thimerosal has been nearly eliminated from vaccines because of legitimate and growing scientific concerns about the possible effects of mercury on the nervous system, Goodman says.

"In addition, as the numbers of vaccines used in children have increased, small infants who received every recommended vaccine could be exposed to cumulative doses of mercury that exceeded some, but not all, federal guidelines," Goodman explains.

Even though there are no convincing data that show harm because of thimerosal in vaccines, the U.S. Public Health Service recommended moving rapidly to vaccines that are thimerosal-free. The FDA encouraged manufacturers to comply and set the highest priority for its reviews of such products, Goodman says. As a result, all recommended pediatric vaccines available are now thimerosal free or have greatly reduced thimerosal contents. In March 2001, the FDA approved a newly formulated version of Tripedia, a diphtheria and tetanus toxoids and acellular pertussis (DTAP) vaccine with only a trace amount of thimerosal.

A Thorough Process

The most common components of vaccines are weakened microbes (disease-causing microorganisms), killed microbes, and inactivated toxins. In addition, subunit vaccines, which only use a part of the bacterium or virus, are increasingly being used.

Manufacturers conduct stringent tests to make sure that cell lines used for producing viral vaccines do not contain adventitious agents (unwanted viruses) such as simian virus 40 (SV40), which was found in some early polio vaccines. These vaccines had been manufactured in kidney cells from simians (monkeys) that harbored SV40. Following its discovery, SV40 was removed from vaccines, and vaccines have been free of the virus since the early 1960s. CBER scientists are developing potentially better methods to detect such infectious agents.

Developing vaccines is a thorough and rigorous process, Egan says. Vaccines are tested for safety on animals first, and then in humans during several phases of clinical trials. The most important clinical trial for the recently licensed vaccine Prevnar involved nearly 40,000 people, equally divided between those who received the vaccine and those who did not. Prevnar was approved to prevent invasive pneumococcal diseases such as meningitis.

A group of FDA scientists reviews data and the proposed labeling of the vaccine, which includes directions for use and information about potential side effects. The committee also reviews manufacturing protocols, conducts its own tests, and inspects the manufacturing facility. The FDA's Vaccines and Related Biological Products Advisory Committee, which includes scientific experts and consumer representatives, can be consulted at any time to review data and recommend action to the agency.

After a vaccine is licensed, the FDA generally requires that manufacturers use validated methods to test samples from each vaccine lot for safety, potency, and purity prior to its release for public use. The FDA also tests selected lots and products to help assure the accuracy of tests conducted by the manufacturers.

Common Concerns

"Most vaccines cause some side effects, but they are usually minor and short-lived like low-grade fever and soreness at the injection site," Midthun says. Serious vaccine reactions—causing disability, hospitalization, or death—are extremely rare but they can happen.

Like any medicine, vaccines carry a small risk of serious harm such as severe allergic reaction. But experts point out that the risk of being harmed by a vaccine is much lower than the risk that comes with infectious diseases.

For example, in 1976, the swine influenza (flu) vaccine was associated with a severe paralytic illness called Guillain-Barré Syndrome (GBS). According to the CDC's vaccine information sheet on the influenza vaccine, "if there is a risk of GBS from current influenza vaccines, it is estimated at 1 or 2 cases per million persons vaccinated, much less than the risk of severe influenza, which can be prevented by vaccination." Each year, flu causes tens of thousands of deaths, mostly among older people. Most people who get the influenza vaccine have no serious problem from it.

And though some people worry about it, you can't get the flu from the flu vaccine, Midthun says. "Just as there are no vaccines that are 100 percent safe, there are also none that are 100 percent effective," she says. "So you may get the flu soon after you received the vaccine, before it could be expected to protect you. It does not mean the shot gave you the flu," she says.

Some live virus vaccines, such as the chickenpox vaccine, can cause mild versions of the disease they protect against, says Goodman. "But this is usually only a serious problem if the patient has a severely compromised immune system." And vaccines are generally not advised for such people. It's important to talk with your doctor about the benefits and risks of vaccines, and any concerns you may have, specifically as it relates to you and your family. If you or your child has previously had a significant reaction to a vaccine, that may affect the risk/benefit ratio for the individual and whether that vaccine should be recommended again.

How Reactions Are Evaluated

Before a vaccine is put into standard medical practice, it must be studied in clinical trials of thousands of people, which allows for evaluation of relatively common side effects. For example, a common side effect might occur in one or more of several hundred vaccine recipients. But rare events (fewer than one case in several thousand recipients) aren't usually evident in clinical trials. "Unless you've studied something in a million or more people, you might never see the very rare event or be able to know whether it occurred due to vaccination or simply by chance," Goodman says.

Through the Vaccine Adverse Event Reporting System (VAERS), jointly operated by the FDA and the CDC to monitor the safety of licensed vaccines, experts look for patterns and any unusual trends that may raise questions about a vaccine's safety once it is used more widely in the population. The FDA continuously reviews and evaluates individual reports, in addition to monitoring overall reporting patterns. The FDA also monitors reporting trends for individual vaccine lots. Most reports come from health-care providers, but anyone can report an unexpected event after vaccination to VAERS.

VAERS receives 800 to 1,000 reports each month. Because it often can't be determined whether an adverse event occurring after vaccination was actually caused by the vaccination, health-care providers and consumers are encouraged to report any event that might be attributable to a vaccine.

"You don't have to be sure," says Susan Ellenberg, Ph.D., director of CBER's office of biostatistics and epidemiology. "Reporting possible reactions will help identify adverse events that might be truly associated with vaccinations and need further study." But this approach to reporting means that one can't assume that all VAERS reports describe true vaccination reactions.

VAERS is a passive, voluntary reporting system, which means not all adverse events get reported. It also means that many reports are incomplete or even contain inaccurate information because the forms are not filled out by trained personnel. Another problem with interpreting

VAERS data is the lack of information on the total number of individuals who received a particular vaccine, making it impossible to estimate the incidence of reported adverse events. It's also often the case that multiple vaccines are given at the same time, further complicating the interpretation of what might have caused the event, Ellenberg says.

Despite these problems, VAERS does contribute in important ways to understanding vaccine safety. VAERS data may suggest the need for more research on certain vaccines. "In this sense, VAERS is a signal generator," Egan says. Recently, VAERS data were instrumental in evaluating RotaShield, a vaccine licensed to protect against rotavirus infection. Rotavirus is the most common cause of gastroenteritis in children younger than five and can result in severe diarrhea, dehydration, and death. This virus is an especially serious problem in developing nations, where it kills hundreds of thousands of children every year.

Following the vaccine's licensure, VAERS started to receive reports of bowel obstruction in a number of infants who had received RotaShield. Careful review of these reports revealed that the bowel obstruction occurred most often in the first two weeks after RotaShield was administered. As a result, the CDC recommended postponing any further distribution or administration of RotaShield until more data could be collected and evaluated.

The FDA discussed the concerns with the manufacturer, which decided to voluntarily withdraw the product from use. In November 1999, ACIP withdrew its previous recommendation for universal use of the vaccine. At this time, the FDA, NIH, and CDC are still studying the bowel obstruction and RotaShield-associated cases, Egan says. "We continue to look into mechanisms for any serious adverse events. We want to understand why they happen so that we can prevent them from occurring in the future."

The CDC's Vaccine Safety DataLink, which links computerized histories of vaccination to hospitalization records and other medical information for members of eight large managed care organizations, supplements the information in VAERS and permits more rigorous evaluation of possible safety concerns. For example, the system allows researchers to compare how often an adverse event occurs in people recently vaccinated with those not recently vaccinated, to evaluate the likelihood that the vaccine caused the adverse event.

Alleged Associations

Some have looked to vaccines to explain a host of serious conditions that we don't fully understand, including sudden infant death syndrome (SIDS), multiple sclerosis, diabetes, and autism. There have been a number of epidemiological studies of these possible associations, and experts say there is no good scientific evidence at this time showing that vaccines cause these diseases or conditions.

"Physicians give vaccines to children at multiple time points during their development and a lot can happen during that time," says Midthun. She stresses that both the FDA and the CDC take concerns of parents seriously. After careful review of all available information, neither agency has found that existing data support any link between the measles, mumps, and rubella (MMR) vaccines and autism, a hypothesis that has received considerable publicity over the last year.

The CDC and the NIH recently contracted with the Institute of Medicine, part of the National Academy of Sciences, to establish the Immunization Safety Review Committee. The independent committee is charged with evaluating nine vaccine safety topics over a three-year span. The possible association of the MMR vaccine and autism was the first topic.

On April 23, 2001, the Immunization Safety Review Committee reported its finding that the current evidence does not favor the hypothesis that there is a link between MMR and autism, and that no changes should be made in the current policy of administering the MMR vaccine. The committee could not rule out the possibility that the MMR vaccine might be linked to autism in some sub-population, and recommended that targeted research in this area be conducted. To date, there is no indication as to whether there is any such subpopulation, or what the genetic makeup or other characteristics of such a subpopulation would be, Egan says.

"It's important that policy decisions about vaccine safety be based on science," says Martin G. Myers, M.D., director of the U.S. Department of Health and Human Service's National Vaccine Program Office. As vaccine safety research continues, Myers says, we can't afford to lose sight of what life was like before immunization. Vaccination is the reason we don't see the suffering, disability, and death from whooping cough, measles, polio, and other infectious diseases like we used to.

"Vaccines are very safe," Myers adds, "but nothing is without risk." Not vaccinating against certain diseases means choosing another type of risk, he says. Myers recalls treating an infant with seizures from tetanus so strong they shook the baby's whole body. These types of seizures and many deaths are preventable by vaccination. And Myers still has an audiotape from the early eighties of a child hacking and gasping for air because of whooping cough. "The child's mother asked me to play it for parents who might be undecided about getting vaccinated."

Chapter 58

What Would Happen If We Stopped Vaccinations?

In the U.S., vaccines have reduced or eliminated many infectious diseases that once routinely killed or harmed many infants, children, and adults. However, the viruses and bacteria that cause vaccine-preventable disease and death still exist and can be passed on to people who are not protected by vaccines. Vaccine-preventable diseases have many social and economic costs: sick children miss school and can cause parents to lose time from work. These diseases also result in doctor's visits, hospitalizations, and even premature deaths.

Polio

Polio virus causes acute paralysis that can lead to permanent physical disability and even death. Before polio vaccine was available, 13,000 to 20,000 cases of paralytic polio were reported each year in the United States. These annual epidemics of polio often left thousands of victims—mostly children—in braces, crutches, wheelchairs, and iron lungs. The effects were life-long.

Development of polio vaccines and implementation of polio immunization programs have eliminated paralytic polio caused by wild polio viruses in the U.S. and the entire Western hemisphere.

In 1999, as a result of global immunization efforts to eradicate the disease, there were about 2,883 documented cases of polio in the world.

"What Would Happen If We Stopped Vaccinations?" National Immunization Program (NIP), Centers for Disease Control and Prevention (CDC), November 2003.

In 1994, wild polio virus was imported to Canada from India, but high vaccination levels prevented it from spreading in the population.

Measles

Before measles immunization was available, nearly everyone in the U.S. got measles. An average of 450 measles-associated deaths were reported each year between 1953 and 1963.

In the U.S., up to 20 percent of persons with measles are hospitalized. Seventeen percent of measles cases have had one or more complications, such as ear infections, pneumonia, or diarrhea. Pneumonia is present in about six percent of cases and accounts for most of the measles deaths. Although less common, some persons with measles develop encephalitis (swelling of the lining of the brain), resulting in brain damage.

As many as three of every 1,000 persons with measles will die in the U.S. In the developing world, the rate is much higher, with death occurring in about one of every 100 persons with measles.

Measles is one of the most infectious diseases in the world and is frequently imported into the U.S. In the period 1997–2000, most cases were associated with international visitors or U.S. residents who were exposed to the measles virus while traveling abroad. More than 90 percent of people who are not immune will get measles if they are exposed to the virus.

According to the World Health Organization (WHO), nearly 900,000 measles-related deaths occurred among persons in developing countries in 1999. In populations that are not immune to measles, measles spreads rapidly. If vaccinations were stopped, each year about 2.7 million measles deaths worldwide could be expected.

In the U.S., widespread use of measles vaccine has led to a greater than 99 percent reduction in measles compared with the pre-vaccine era. If we stopped immunization, measles would increase to pre-vaccine levels.

Haemophilus Influenzae Type b (Hib) Meningitis

Before Hib vaccine became available, Hib was the most common cause of bacterial meningitis in U.S. infants and children. Before the vaccine was developed, there were approximately 20,000 invasive Hib cases annually. Approximately two-thirds of the 20,000 cases were meningitis, and one-third were other life-threatening invasive Hib diseases such as bacteria in the blood, pneumonia, or inflammation of the epiglottis. About one of every 200 U.S. children under 5 years of age got an invasive Hib disease. Hib meningitis once killed 600 children each year and left many survivors with deafness, seizures, or mental retardation.

Since introduction of conjugate Hib vaccine in December 1987, the incidence of Hib has declined by 98 percent. From 1994–1998, fewer than 10 fatal cases of invasive Hib disease were reported each year.

This preventable disease was a common, devastating illness as recently as 1990; now, most pediatricians just finishing training have never seen a case. If we were to stop immunization, we would likely soon return to the pre-vaccine numbers of invasive Hib disease cases and deaths.

Pertussis (Whooping Cough)

Since the early 1980s, reported pertussis cases have been increasing, with peaks every 3–4 years; however, the number of reported cases remains much lower than levels seen in the pre-vaccine era. Compared with pertussis cases in other age groups, infants who are 6 months old or younger with pertussis experience the highest rate of hospitalization, pneumonia, seizures, Encephalopathy (a degenerative disease of the brain), and death. From 1990 to 1996, 57 persons died from pertussis; 49 of these were less than six months old.

Before pertussis immunizations were available, nearly all children developed whooping cough. In the U.S., prior to pertussis immunization, between 150,000 and 260,000 cases of pertussis were reported each year, with up to 9,000 pertussis-related deaths.

Pertussis can be a severe illness, resulting in prolonged coughing spells that can last for many weeks. These spells can make it difficult for a child to eat, drink, and breathe. Because vomiting often occurs after a coughing spell, infants may lose weight and become dehydrated. In infants, it can also cause pneumonia and lead to brain damage, seizures, and mental retardation.

The newer pertussis vaccine (acellular or DTaP) that has been available for use in the United States since 1991 and has been recommended for exclusive use since 1998. These vaccines are effective and associated with fewer mild and moderate adverse reactions when compared with the older (whole-cell DTP) vaccines.

During the 1970s, widespread concerns about the safety of the older pertussis vaccine led to a rapid fall in immunization levels in the United Kingdom. More than 100,000 cases and 36 deaths due to pertussis were reported during an epidemic in the mid 1970s. In Japan, pertussis vaccination coverage fell from 80 percent in 1974 to 20 percent in 1979. An epidemic occurred in 1979, resulted in more than 13,000 cases and 41 deaths.

Pertussis cases occur throughout the world. If we stopped pertussis immunizations in the U.S., we would experience a massive resurgence of pertussis disease. A recent study* found that, in eight countries where immunization coverage was reduced, incidence rates of pertussis surged to 10 to 100 times the rates in countries where vaccination rates were sustained.

*Reference for study: Gangarosa EJ, et al. Impact of anti-vaccine movements on pertussis control: the untold story. *Lancet* 1998;351: 356-61.

Rubella (German Measles)

While rubella is usually mild in children and adults, up to 90 percent of infants born to mothers infected with rubella during the first trimester of pregnancy will develop congenital rubella syndrome (CRS), resulting in heart defects, cataracts, mental retardation, and deafness.

In 1964–1965, before rubella immunization was used routinely in the U.S., there was an epidemic of rubella that resulted in an estimated 20,000 infants born with CRS, with 2,100 neonatal deaths and 11,250 miscarriages. Of the 20,000 infants born with CRS, 11,600 were deaf, 3,580 were blind, and 1,800 were mentally retarded.

Due to the widespread use of rubella vaccine, only six CRS cases were provisionally reported in the U.S. in 2000. Because many developing countries do not include rubella in the childhood immunization schedule, many of these cases occurred in foreign-born adults. Since 1996, greater than 50 percent of the reported rubella cases have been among adults. Since 1999, there have been 40 pregnant women infected with rubella.

If we stopped rubella immunization, immunity to rubella would decline and rubella would once again return, resulting in pregnant women becoming infected with rubella and then giving birth to infants with CRS.

Varicella (Chickenpox)

Chickenpox is always present in the community and is highly contagious. Prior to the licensing of chickenpox vaccine in 1995, almost all persons in the U.S. had suffered from chickenpox by adulthood. An estimated 4 million cases of chickenpox occurred annually, resulting in 11,000 hospitalizations and 100 deaths.

Chickenpox is usually mild, but may be severe in some infants, adolescents, and adults. Some people who get chickenpox have also suffered from complications such as secondary bacterial infections, loss of fluids (dehydration), pneumonia, and central nervous system involvement. In addition, only persons who have had chickenpox in the past can get shingles, a painful inflammation of the nerves. About 500,000 cases of shingles occur each year when inactivated chickenpox virus is activated in people who have had chickenpox in the past.

Vaccine coverage among children 19–35 months was 80 percent in 2002.

Hepatitis B

More than 2 billion persons worldwide have been infected with the hepatitis B virus at some time in their lives. Of these, 350 million are life-long carriers of the disease and can transmit the virus to others. One million of these people die each year from liver disease and liver cancer.

National studies have shown that about 12.5 million Americans have been infected with hepatitis B virus at some point in their lifetime. One and one quarter million Americans are estimated to have chronic (long-lasting) infection, of whom 20 percent to 30 percent acquired their infection in childhood. Chronic hepatitis B virus infection increases a person's risk for chronic liver disease, cirrhosis, and liver cancer. About 5,000 persons will die each year from hepatitis B-related liver disease resulting in over $700 million medical and work loss costs.

The number of new infections per year has declined from an average of 450,000 in the 1980s to about 80,000 in 1999. The greatest decline has occurred among children and adolescents due to routine hepatitis B vaccination.

Infants and children who become infected with hepatitis B virus are at highest risk of developing lifelong infection, which often leads to death from liver disease (cirrhosis) and liver cancer. Approximately 25 percent of children who become infected with life-long hepatitis B virus would be expected to die of related liver disease as adults.

CDC estimates that one-third of the life-long hepatitis B virus infections in the United States resulted from infections occurring in infants and young children. About 16,000–20,000 hepatitis B antigen infected women give birth each year in the United States. It is estimated that

12,000 children born to hepatitis B virus infected mothers were infected each year before implementation of infant immunization programs. In addition, approximately 33,000 children (10 years of age and younger) of mothers who are not infected with hepatitis B virus were infected each year before routine recommendation of childhood hepatitis B vaccination.

Diphtheria

Diphtheria is a serious disease caused by a bacteria. This germ produces a poisonous substance or toxin which frequently causes heart and nerve problems. The death rate is 5 percent to 10 percent, with higher death rates (up to 20 percent) in the very young and the elderly.

In the 1920's, diphtheria was a major cause of illness and death for children in the U.S. In 1921, a total of 206,000 cases and 15,520 deaths were reported. With vaccine development in 1923, new cases of diphtheria began to fall in the U.S., until in 2001 only two cases were reported.

Although diphtheria is rare in the U.S., it appears that the bacteria continues to get passed among people. In 1996, 10 isolates of the bacteria were obtained from persons in an American Indian community in South Dakota, none of whom had classic diphtheria disease. There has been one death reported in 2000 from clinical diphtheria caused by a related bacteria.

There are high rates of susceptibility among adults. Screening tests conducted since 1977 have shown that 41 percent to 84 percent of adults 60 and over lack protective levels of circulating antitoxin against diphtheria.

Although diphtheria is rare in the U.S., it is still a threat. Diphtheria is common in other parts of the world and with the increase in international travel, diphtheria and other infectious diseases are only a plane ride away. If we stopped immunization, the U.S. might experience a situation similar to the Newly Independent States of the former Soviet Union. With the breakdown of the public health services in this area, diphtheria epidemics began in 1990, fueled primarily by persons who were not properly vaccinated. From 1990–1999, more than 150,000 cases and 5,000 deaths were reported.

Tetanus (Lockjaw)

Tetanus is a severe, often fatal disease. The bacteria that cause tetanus are widely distributed in soil and street dust, are found in the waste of many animals, and are very resistant to heat and germ-killing cleaners. From 1922–1926, there were an estimated 1,314 cases of tetanus per year in the U.S. In the late 1940's, the tetanus vaccine was introduced, and tetanus became a disease that was officially counted and tracked by public health officials. In 2000, only 41 cases of tetanus were reported in the U.S.

People who get tetanus suffer from stiffness and spasms of the muscles. The larynx (throat) can close causing breathing and eating difficulties, muscles spasms can cause fractures (breaks) of the spine and long bones, and some people go into a coma, and die. Approximately 20 percent of reported cases end in death.

Tetanus in the U.S. is primarily a disease of adults, but unvaccinated children and infants of unvaccinated mothers are also at risk for tetanus and neonatal tetanus, respectively. From 1995–1997, 33 percent of reported cases of tetanus occurred among persons 60 years of age or older and 60 percent occurred in patients greater than 40 years of age. The National Health Interview Survey found that in 1995, only 36 percent of adults 65 or older had received a tetanus vaccination during the preceding 10 years.

Worldwide, tetanus in newborn infants continues to be a huge problem. Every year tetanus kills 300,000 newborns and 30,000 birth mothers who were not properly vaccinated. Even though the number of reported cases is low, an increased number of tetanus cases in younger persons has been observed recently in the U.S. among intravenous drug users, particularly heroin users.

Tetanus is infectious, but not contagious, so unlike other vaccine-preventable diseases, immunization by members of the community will not protect others from the disease. Because tetanus bacteria are widespread in the environment, tetanus can only be prevented by immunization. If vaccination against tetanus were stopped, persons of all ages in the U.S. would be susceptible to this serious disease.

Mumps

Before the mumps vaccine was introduced, mumps was a major cause of deafness in children, occurring in approximately 1 in 20,000 reported cases. Mumps is usually a mild viral disease. However, rare conditions such as swelling of the brain, nerves, and spinal cord can lead to serious side effects such as paralysis, seizures, and fluid in the brain.

Serious side effects of mumps are more common among adults than children. Swelling of the testes is the most common side effect in males past the age of puberty, occurring in up to 20 percent to 50 percent of men who contract mumps. An increase in miscarriages has been found among women who develop mumps during the first trimester of pregnancy.

An estimated 212,000 cases of mumps occurred in the U.S. in 1964. After vaccine licensure in 1967, reports of mumps decreased rapidly. In 1986 and 1987, there was a resurgence of mumps with 12,848 cases reported in 1987. Since 1989, the incidence of mumps has declined, with 266 reported cases in 2001. This recent decrease is probably due to the fact that children have received a second dose of mumps vaccine (part of the two-dose schedule for measles, mumps, rubella or MMR) and the eventual development of immunity in those who did not gain protection after the first mumps vaccination.

If we were to stop vaccination against mumps, we could expect the number of cases to climb back to pre-vaccine levels, since mumps is easily spread among unvaccinated persons.

Chapter 59

Making Sure Kids Get All Their Shots

The Food and Drug Administration (FDA) is part of the U.S. government's Department of Health and Human Services. One of the FDA's jobs is to make sure that vaccines are safe and effective.

Vaccinations Are Important

It's important that children get vaccinated—get their "shots"—so they don't get childhood diseases. Your child can be vaccinated at the doctor's office or your local health department. Ask the doctor to give you a list of the shots your child has received. Keep this list so that you have records for school, and so you'll know if your child needs more shots.

Vaccines are available today to protect your child against:

- diphtheria
- whooping cough (pertussis)
- tetanus
- polio
- measles

"Protecting Your Child Against Serious Diseases: Making Sure Kids Get All Their 'Shots'," Food and Drug Administration (FDA), Department of Health and Human Services, January 2002; and "The Advisory Committee on Immunization Practices Vote to Recommend Influenza Vaccination for Children Aged 6 to 23 Months," Office of Communication, Centers for Disease Control and Prevention (CDC), October 16, 2003.

- mumps
- German measles (rubella)
- chickenpox (varicella)
- hepatitis B
- HIB (haemophilus influenzae type B)
- pneumococcal diseases

In most of the United States, many of these vaccinations are required for school or day care. The first shots for most of these illnesses should be given when the child is still a baby. This is important because most of the diseases these vaccines protect your child against can be serious or even deadly.

Like any medicine, vaccines carry a small risk of serious harm such as a severe allergic reaction. But side effects from shots are usually mild and last only a short time. Some children have no side effects at all. None of the possible side effects should keep your child from getting shots unless your doctor says so.

Be sure to tell your doctor if anyone in your immediate family has ever had a bad reaction to a vaccine, and ask if there are certain conditions under which vaccination is not recommended. Also talk to your doctor about whether certain reactions to vaccines can be controlled, such as by giving your child acetaminophen before or after vaccination.

Here are common vaccinations your child needs, the recommended age to get them, and possible side effects:

DTaP (Diphtheria, Tetanus, Pertussis)

Protects against: diphtheria, whooping cough (pertussis), and tetanus. The vaccines against these three diseases are combined in a single shot.

Diphtheria is a serious infection of the throat, mouth, and nose, which can lead to suffocation, pneumonia, heart failure, and paralysis.

A child who catches whooping cough develops a bad cough that sounds like a "whoop." The severe coughing can interfere with eating, drinking, and breathing. Whooping cough can be life-threatening, especially in children younger than 1.

Tetanus is caused by germs in dirt and rusty metal that get into the body through a cut. Tetanus attacks the jaw muscles first, often causing lockjaw. It can also affect the muscles used to breathe. It causes death in 3 out of 10 people who get it.

Ages to get vaccine: Shot is given at 2 months, 4 months, 6 months, and 15–18 months, with a booster given between the ages of 4 and 6 years. After that, everyone should get a tetanus booster every 10 years throughout life.

Possible side effects include: Fever, soreness where shot is given, irritability. In rare cases, the shot can cause very high fever and convulsions.

Polio

Protects against: polio, a virus that can cause paralysis and death.

There are two kinds of polio vaccines: the inactivated polio virus (IPV), which is the shot recommended in the United States today, and a live, oral polio virus (OPV). OPV causes polio in a few people and experts believe that using OPV is no longer worth the slight risk, except in limited cases. IPV does not cause polio.

Ages to get vaccine: Shot is usually given at 2 months, 4 months, 6–18 months, and at 4–6 years.

Possible side effects include: The main side effect of IPV is soreness where the shot is given.

MMR (Measles, Mumps, and Rubella)

Protects against: measles, mumps, and German measles (rubella). The vaccines against these three diseases are combined in a single shot.

Measles is easy to catch and causes a rash, high fever, and cough. Measles can also cause hearing loss, convulsions, brain damage, and death.

Mumps makes the saliva glands under the jaws swell and hurt. It also usually causes fever and headache, and can have serious complications. It is even more painful for teen-age boys, whose testicles may swell.

German measles is mild in children but can damage the unborn baby if a woman gets it while she is pregnant.

Ages to get vaccine: One shot is given at 12–15 months and another is usually given at 4–6 years. Women who do not know if they are immune to rubella can be tested to see if they are. If they have no immunity they should get the rubella vaccine more than three months before they plan to get pregnant.

Possible side effects include: Pain where the shot is given and a rash. The shot can also cause swollen glands or mild joint pain, but these are rare.

Chickenpox

Protects against: chickenpox, which is usually a mild disease that causes an itchy rash and fever. But some children experience serious complications.

Ages to get vaccine: One shot is given for children between the ages of 12 months and 12 years. It is recommended that children receive the shot at 12 to 18 months of age. Adults and adolescents older than 13 who have not had chickenpox get two shots, at least 4–8 weeks apart.

Possible side effects include: Pain where the shot is given, rash, fever.

Hepatitis B

Protects against: hepatitis B, a disease of the liver caused by the hepatitis B virus. It can cause lifelong liver problems or death.

Ages to get vaccine: For babies, three shots are given before 18 months of age. Older children, adolescents, and adults who didn't get the shot when they were babies can get the first shot any time, a second shot 1–2 months later, and a third shot 4–6 months after the first shot.

Possible side effects include: Soreness where the shot is given and fever.

*HIB (*Haemophilus Influenzae *Type B)*

Protects against: *Haemophilus influenzae* type b, an infection that can seriously harm a child's brain, blood, bones, throat, and the area around the heart.

Ages to get vaccine: Shot is given at 2 months, 4 months, 6 months, and 12–15 months.

Possible side effects include: Soreness where the shot is given and fever.

Pneumococcal Conjugate

Protects against: Invasive pneumococcal diseases, which can cause brain damage and death.

Table 59.1. Recommended Childhood Immunization Schedule (*continued on next page*)

Hepatitis B	
1st dose	Birth–2 months
2nd dose	1 month–4 months
3rd dose	6 months–18 months
catch up	11–12 years
Diphtheria, Tetanus, Pertussis	
1st dose	2 months
2nd dose	4 months
3rd dose	6 months
4th dose	15 months–18 months
5th dose	4–6 years
Td	11–12 years-14–16 years
H. influenzae type b	
1st dose	2 months
2nd dose	4 months
3rd dose	6 months
4th dose	12 months–15 months
Inactivated Polio	
1st dose	2 months
2nd dose	4 months
3rd dose	6 months–18 months
4th dose	4–6 years

Ages to get vaccine: Shot is given at 2 months, 4 months, 6 months, and 12 to 15 months.

Possible side effects include: Soreness where the shot is given and mild fever.

Reporting Injuries Caused by Vaccines

When there are side effects from childhood vaccinations, they are usually mild. But because there have been rare reports of more serious

Table 59.1. Recommended Childhood Immunization Schedule (*continued from previous page*)

Pneumococcal Conjugate	
1st dose	2 months
2nd dose	4 months
3rd dose	6 months
4th dose	12 months–15 months
Measles, Mumps, Rubella	
1st dose	12 months–15 months
2nd dose	4–6 years
catch up	11–12 years
Varicella (chickenpox)	
1st dose	12 months–18 months
catch up	11–12 years
Hepatitis A	
1 dose (in selected areas)	24 months-14–18 years

These are recommended ages for shots. Any dose not given at the recommended age should be given as a 'catch up" shot at the following visit. For the complete details, visit the Web site www.cdc.gov/nip.

Source: The Advisory Committee on Immunization Practices (ACIP), the American Academy of Pediatrics (AAP) and the American Academy of Family Physicians (AAFP).

side effects, Congress passed the National Childhood Vaccine Injury Act in 1986. This law set up a way for people to report side effects that they believe are associated with the vaccine, and a way for families to be compensated for injuries related to vaccines.

The FDA encourages you to report unexpected problems after vaccines to your doctor and the FDA's Vaccine Adverse Event Reporting System (VAERS) at 1-800-822-7967. Also visit www.fda.gov/cber/vaers/vaers.htm.

For more information about The National Vaccine Injury Compensation Program, call 1-800-338-2382, or visit www.bhpr.hrsa.gov/vicp.

The FDA may have an office near you. Look for the number in the blue pages of the phone book. You can also contact the FDA through its toll-free number, 1-888-INFO-FDA (1-888-463-6332). Or, visit the FDA's website at http://www.fda.gov.

Update Regarding Influenza Vaccination for Children Aged 6 to 23 Months

The Advisory Committee on Immunization Practices (ACIP) voted to recommend that children 6 to 23 months of age be vaccinated annually against influenza. The ACIP recommended this change be implemented in the fall of 2004.

The ACIP had previously encouraged physicians to vaccinate 6 to 23 month old children when feasible; that is, when they had resources and capacity to educate parents about influenza, to administer the needed doses, and to monitor vaccine adverse events.

The current inactivated influenza vaccine is not approved by FDA for use among children less than six months of age.

Two doses of inactivated influenza vaccine administered more than one month apart are recommended for previously unvaccinated children less than nine years of age. If possible, the second dose should be administered before December. All subsequent annual influenza vaccinations require only one dose of vaccine.

Annual vaccination with the current vaccine is recommended because immunity declines during the year after vaccination and because the vaccine composition usually changes each year. Vaccine prepared for a previous influenza season should not be administered to provide protection for the current season.

The recommendations of the ACIP are forwarded to the Director of the CDC and the Secretary of Health and Human Services (HHS) for review. If the ACIP recommendations are accepted by the Director of CDC and the Secretary of HHS, they are published in the *Morbidity and Mortality Weekly Report* and become recommendations of CDC.

The ACIP consists of 15 experts in fields associated with immunization who have been selected for the Secretary of HHS to provide guidance to the Secretary, the Assistant Secretary for Health, and the CDC on the most effective means to prevent vaccine-preventable diseases. The Committee reviews and reports on immunization practices and recommends improvements in the national immunization efforts.

Chapter 60

Adolescent and Adult Immunization

Facts about Adolescent Immunization

- Vaccines are among the safest medicines available.
- Approximately 340,000 children and adolescents aged 2–18 years have chronic illnesses, placing them at risk for influenza and pneumococcal diseases and their complications.
- More than 8 million children and adolescents aged 2–18 years have at least one medical condition placing them at high risk for complications of the flu.
- Although no longer a very common disease in the United States, diphtheria remains a large problem in other countries and can pose a serious threat to United States citizens who may not be fully immunized and who travel to other countries or have contact with immigrants or international travelers coming to the U.S.
- Forty to fifty cases of tetanus (lockjaw) occur each year, resulting in approximately 5 deaths annually in the United States.

"Facts about Adolescent Immunization," "Prematriculation Immunization Requirement (PIR)," "Adult Immunization Questions and Answers," and "Facts about Adult Immunization," are reprinted with permission from the National Foundation for Infectious Diseases - National Coalition for Adult Immunization. "Prematriculation Immunization Requirement (PIR)" is © 2000, other documents are © 2002. For additional information visit the National Foundation for Infectious Diseases website at www.nfid.org or the National Coalition for Adult Immunization at http://www.nfid.org/ncai.

- The majority of the estimated 80,000 new cases of hepatitis B reported each year strike adolescents and young adults. The hepatitis B virus is 100 times more infectious than HIV, the virus that causes AIDS.
- The hepatitis B vaccine is recognized as the first anti-cancer vaccine because it can prevent primary liver cancer caused by hepatitis B infection.
- The highest rates of hepatitis A occur among children and adolescents 5–14 years old, and most cases can be attributed to person-to-person transmission.
- Of the 575 measles cases in 1996 for whom age was known, one-third were 10–19 years old.
- About one-fifth of people infected with the mumps virus do not have any symptoms.

Are there vaccines that protect against communicable diseases?

Yes. Immunizations against hepatitis B, measles, mumps, rubella (German measles), tetanus (lockjaw), diphtheria, and varicella (chickenpox) are available for all adolescents. In addition, vaccinations against hepatitis A, influenza (flu) and pneumococcal disease are needed by some adolescents.

Should all adolescents be immunized?

Yes. All adolescents require measles, mumps, rubella, tetanus and diphtheria immunizations. All adolescents with diabetes or chronic heart, lung, liver, or kidney disorders need protection against influenza and pneumococcal disease, and should consult their healthcare providers regarding their need for these shots. Varicella (chickenpox) vaccine is recommended for those not previously vaccinated and who have no reliable history of the disease. Hepatitis B vaccine is indicated for all adolescents aged 8–18 who have not been vaccinated previously. Hepatitis A vaccine is recommended for adolescents traveling to or working in countries where the disease is common, and for those living in communities with outbreaks of the disease, and those living in states that have hepatitis A rates that exceed the national average. It is also recommended for adolescents who have chronic liver disease or clotting-factor disorders, use illegal injection drugs, or are male and have sex with other males.

How often do I need to be immunized?

Hepatitis B vaccine is generally administered in 3 doses. Adolescents not previously vaccinated with 2 doses of MMR vaccine require these. Immunization against tetanus and diphtheria (Td vaccine) should be supplemented with a booster shot at 11–12 years of age and every 10 years thereafter. Those who deferred Td boosters during 2001 and early 2002 because of vaccine shortages should get back on track—the supply problems have been resolved. One dose of chickenpox vaccine is recommended for adolescents 11–12 years of age, or 2 doses for those 13 or older, if there is no proof of prior chickenpox disease or immunization. The flu shot should be administered yearly to adolescents who have any medical condition that places them at high risk for complications associated with influenza, such as diabetes, asthma, or chronic heart, lung, or other diseases. Immunization against pneumococcal disease is recommended for adolescents with certain chronic diseases who are at increased risk for this disease or its complications, and a booster dose is recommended 5 years after the initial dose for this group. Hepatitis A vaccine is administered in 2 doses.

Are there side effects to these shots?

Vaccines are among the safest medicines available. Some common side effects are a sore arm or low fever. As with any medicine, there are very small risks that serious problems could occur after getting a vaccine. However, the potential risks associated with the diseases that these vaccines prevent are much greater than the potential risks associated with the vaccines themselves.

Should I carry a personal immunization record?

Yes. This record will help you and your healthcare provider ensure that you are protected against vaccine-preventable diseases. Ask your provider for this record, and be sure to take it with you every time you visit so it can be reviewed by your provider and updated each time you are immunized.

Prematriculation Immunization Requirement (PIR)

The following section provides data to support college and university health professionals in their efforts to implement Prematriculation Immunization Requirements (PIRs). A PIR requires incoming students to provide documentation of immunization against, or immunity to, vaccine-preventable diseases, and is a cornerstone of disease prevention for colleges and universities.

Recent Centers for Disease Control and Prevention (CDC) epidemiological data indicate that as occurrences of measles, mumps, and rubella have been decreasing among the entire population, the proportion of cases among young adults has been increasing. For example, people age 20 and older accounted for:

- 36 percent of all measles cases in 1995.
- About one-third of rubella cases in 1994.
- Almost 20 percent of all cases of mumps in 1993.

In addition to including large populations of young adults, universities and colleges are susceptible to outbreaks because:

- Students usually live and work in a closed environment which can facilitate the spread of disease.
- The increasing enrollment of international students means that more students are likely to need vaccinations not provided in their native countries. The CDC found that 11 percent of all measles cases were imported in 1994.

The costs of containing outbreaks of vaccine-preventable disease on campus include an enormous outlay of school and public health resources, which strain the public health system and disrupt college life. For example, a 1995 measles outbreak at a university in the state of Washington resulted in:

- A total cost of more than a $300,000 to the university and to the state and county health departments, not including 850+ volunteer hours donated by students, faculty and staff.
- A public health logistics challenge—between days 2 and 10 of the outbreak, the state and county health departments had to mobilize personnel and administer more than 8,200 doses of vaccine.

The following examples demonstrate the effectiveness of PIRs.

- A study published in the *Journal of the American Medical Association* (Oct. 12, 1994, p. 1127) concluded that campuses in states with mandated PIRs had significantly reduced risks of measles outbreaks.

- All states have PIRs for grades K–12; this has substantially reduced outbreaks of vaccine-preventable diseases among students.
- After requiring immunization or proof of immunity upon enlistment, the U.S. Armed Forces experienced a marked decrease in outbreaks of vaccine-preventable diseases, including measles.

Adult Immunization Questions and Answers

Are there vaccines that protect against communicable diseases for adults?

Yes. Immunizations are readily available for such common adult illnesses as influenza (flu), pneumococcal disease, and hepatitis B. Vaccinations against measles, mumps, rubella (German measles), hepatitis A, tetanus (lockjaw), diphtheria, and varicella (chickenpox) are also needed by some adults. U.S. Public Health Service recommendations clearly identify people who are at risk for these diseases and who should be immunized to prevent these diseases and their complications. Consult your healthcare provider or local health department regarding your own immunization status and recommendations for immunizations.

Why immunize?

Some of these illnesses, once contracted, do not have a cure, and all may cause tremendous health problems or even death. Vaccines are some of the safest medicines available, are very effective, and can relieve suffering costs related to these preventable diseases for us all.

Should all adults be immunized?

Yes. All adults require tetanus and diphtheria (Td) immunizations at 10 year intervals throughout the life. Adults who deferred Td boosters during 2001 and early 2002 because of vaccine shortages should get back on track—the supply problems have been resolved. Adults born after 1956 need to be immunized against measles, mumps and rubella. All adults aged 65 or older, as well as persons aged 2–64 years who have diabetes or chronic heart, lung, liver, or kidney disorders need protection against pneumococcal disease, and should consult their healthcare providers regarding their need for this shot. Influenza vaccination is recommended for adults 50 years of age or older, pregnant women and residents of long-term care facilities, as well as for persons older than 6 months of age who have chronic illness and persons 6 months–18 years of age who receive chronic aspirin therapy. High-risk individuals such as these should be immunized before non-high risk individuals under the age of 65. Hepatitis B vaccine is recommended for adults in certain high-risk groups, such as healthcare workers and persons with multiple sex partners. Hepatitis B vaccine is also recommended for all adolescents who may not have not received it during infancy or childhood. Hepatitis A vaccine is recommended for all susceptible travelers to, for persons working in, countries with intermediate or high rates of hepatitis A virus (HAV) infection, and for those residing in states where the hepatitis A rate exceeds the national average. Many adults, including teachers of young children and day care workers, residents and staff in institutional settings, military personnel, nonpregnant women of childbearing age, international travelers, healthcare workers, and family members of immunocompromised persons, who have not had chickenpox and have not been immunized previously against chickenpox should receive varicella vaccine.

Where can I obtain my immunizations?

Immunizations should be available from family doctors and internists. Additionally, your city or county health department or local hospital may hold clinics to administer these vaccines, and many pharmacies offer vaccinations as well.

How often do I need to be immunized?

Immunizations for pneumococcal disease (except for patients at particular risk for pneumococcal complications), measles, mumps, and rubella are usually administered once, and offer protection for life. Some persons born after 1956 may require a second measles vaccination. Influenza vaccine must be administered yearly due to the appearance of new strains of virus which are not addressed by previous vaccines. Additional booster doses of tetanus and diphtheria vaccines (usually given as a combination Td vaccine) are required every 10 years to maintain immunity against these diseases. Hepatitis B vaccine is administered in 3 doses given over a 6-month period. Two doses of chickenpox vaccine are recommended for people 13 years or older who have not had the disease. Two doses of hepatitis A are needed 6 to 12 months apart to ensure long-term protection.

What do these shots cost?

The cost may vary depending on insurance coverage. Check with your healthcare provider or clinic, and your health insurance for exact rates. Remember, both influenza and pneumococcal vaccinations are fully paid for by Medicare Part B if your healthcare provider accepts the Medicare-approved payment amount. Medicare Part B also will pay up to 80% of the costs of hepatitis B vaccinations for qualifying individuals.

Are there side effects to these immunizations?

Vaccines are among the safest medicines available. Some common side effects are a sore arm or low fever. As with any medicine, there are very small risks that serious problems could occur after getting a vaccine. However, the potential risks associated with the diseases these vaccines prevent are much greater than the potential risks associated with the vaccines themselves.

What shots do I need if I'm traveling abroad?

Contact your healthcare provider or the public health department as early as possible to check on the immunizations you may need. Vaccines against certain diseases such as hepatitis A, yellow fever and typhoid fever are recommended for different countries. The time required to receive all immunizations will depend on whether you need one dose or a vaccine series. There are several books available which provide information on specific vaccines required by different countries and general health measures for travelers. You may also call the Centers for Disease Control and Prevention (CDC) information line for international travelers toll-free at (877) 394-8747 or visit the CDC Travel Web site at http://www.cdc.gov/travel.

Should I carry a personal immunization record?

Definitely yes. A permanent immunization record should be kept by every adult. It will help you and your healthcare provider ensure that you are fully protected against vaccine-preventable diseases. It can also prevent needless revaccination during a health emergency or when you change providers. Ask your provider for an immunization record, and be sure to take it with you to every time you visit so it can be reviewed by your provider and updated each time you are immunized.

Facts about Adult Immunization

- Each year in the United States, up to 60,000 adults die from vaccine-preventable diseases or their complications.
- Pneumonia and influenza together are the seventh leading cause of death in the U.S., and the fifth leading cause of death among older adults.
- Medicare Part B fully reimburses healthcare providers who accept the Medicare-approved payment amount for both influenza and pneumococcal immunizations.
- During most influenza seasons, 10% to 20% of the Nation's population is infected with influenza with an annual estimated cost to society of up to $12 billion during severe epidemics.
- The 1918 Spanish influenza pandemic killed more than 500,000 people in the U.S. and over 21 million worldwide. The 1957–58 "Asian flu" and the 1968–69 "Hong Kong flu" epidemics led to 68,000 and 34,000 deaths in the United States, respectively.
- Each year in the United States, pneumococcal disease accounts for an estimated 500,000 cases of pneumonia (infection of the lungs), 6,000 cases of bacteremia (bloodstream infection), and 3,300 cases of meningitis (inflammation of the tissues and fluids surrounding the brain and spinal cord).
- Pneumococcal pneumonia accounts for up to 175,000 hospitalizations each year and is the most common cause of pneumonia.
- The hepatitis B virus is found in blood and other body fluids such as semen and vaginal secretions. It is 100 times more infectious than HIV, the virus that causes AIDS.
- The hepatitis B vaccine is recognized as the first anti-cancer vaccine because it can prevent primary liver cancer caused by hepatitis B infection.
- In the United States there are 1–1 1/4 million people with chronic hepatitis B infections who can infect other household members and sexual partners.
- An estimated 80,000 people in the United States are infected with hepatitis B each year, the majority are adolescents and young adults.
- Vaccines are among the safest medicines available.

- An estimated 180,000 Americans are infected with hepatitis A each year.
- Hepatitis A is the most common vaccine-preventable disease in travelers to other countries.
- Fifty or fewer cases of tetanus occur each year, but result in about 5 deaths annually in the United States. Most deaths occur in those 60 years of age or older.
- Almost all reported cases of tetanus occur in persons who have either never been vaccinated, or who completed their primary series but have not had a booster vaccination in the past 10 years.
- Nearly one out of every 10 people who get diphtheria will die from it.
- Unimmunized persons of any age can get measles, but those born after 1956 who do not have proof of immunity are particularly at risk and should be immunized.
- If rubella (German measles) occurs during pregnancy, it can result in severe birth defects, miscarriages, and stillbirths.
- Approximately one-fifth of infected people do not exhibit symptoms of mumps.
- Serious complications of mumps are more common among adults than among children.
- Adolescents and adults are more likely than children to develop severe complications when infected with the chickenpox virus.
- Less than 5% of adults are susceptible to infection with the chickenpox virus, but adults are much more likely to die from chickenpox than are children.

Chapter 61

Vaccine and Treatment Evaluation Units

For more than 40 years, vaccine research and development has been a vital component of the National Institute of Allergy and Infectious Diseases (NIAID) research agenda. Established in 1962, the NIAID Vaccine and Treatment Evaluation Units (VTEUs) have played a key role in this effort.

The VTEUs are a network of university research hospitals across the United States that conduct Phase I and II clinical trials to test and evaluate candidate vaccines for infectious diseases. Through these sites, researchers can quickly carry out safety and efficacy studies of promising vaccines in children, adults, and specific high-risk populations, such as premature infants and the elderly. The results of these trials may have a profound effect on public health here and abroad.

The VTEU network is a critical player in the success of NIAID vaccine research and development. Through numerous studies at the VTEUs, researchers have tested and advanced vaccines for malaria, tuberculosis, pneumonia, cholera, and whooping cough. In the last six years alone, NIAID has supported more than 110 clinical studies through the VTEU network.

One of the many strengths of the VTEUs is their ability to conduct studies to address important public health questions. The VTEUs have the flexibility to focus on developing orphan vaccines for rare conditions. They also allow researchers to compare products from different

---

"NIAID's Vaccine and Treatment Evaluation Units," National Institute of Allergy and Infectious Diseases (NIAID), National Institutes of Health (NIH), August 2002.

manufacturers and to test the additive effects of products from different manufacturers in a prime-boost strategy.

Highlights and Accomplishments

NIAID-supported research led to the development of several group A streptococcal (GAS) vaccine candidates, which are in various stages of testing. Major disorders associated with GAS infection include scarlet fever, strep throat, impetigo, pneumonia, bacteremia, acute kidney inflammation, toxic shock syndrome, necrotizing fasciitis (caused by so-called flesh-eating bacteria), and rheumatic fever. Rheumatic fever occurs in all parts of the world and is the leading cause of acquired heart disease in children in developing countries.

Researchers are conducting clinical trials to evaluate the safety of a recombinant protein vaccine against GAS. In addition, the VTEU is evaluating the safety of a novel bacterial delivery system in which commensal bacteria (so-called "good" bacteria) may be engineered to produce a GAS protective antigen. In recent years, there have been few clinical trials testing GAS vaccines, adding to the importance of these studies.

NIAID has invested more than 30 years of research into developing pneumococcal vaccines. Early product development support as well as Phase I and II studies conducted by VTEU sites in infants were helpful in developing Prevnar, a vaccine to prevent pneumococcal diseases in children younger than 2 years of age.

By delivering more than one vaccine at a time, combination vaccines minimize needlesticks and trips to the doctor. A five-site VTEU trial evaluated the impact of inactivated (killed) poliovirus vaccine versus oral poliovirus vaccines when given with a combined vaccine against Haemophilus influenzae type b, pertussis, diphtheria, and tetanus. As a result of the study, health experts now recommend that children get the inactivated poliovirus vaccine as part of their routine immunizations.

Novel Delivery Systems

VTEU research has also helped usher in a new era of ways to deliver vaccines, such as a nasal spray. Six VTEUs enrolled young children in a Phase III trial of FluMist, an influenza vaccine administered by nasal spray. The vaccine proved to be 93 percent effective against the predominant flu strains of the 1996 to 1997 flu season. In 1998, researchers again inoculated the children against three flu strains thought to be circulating that season. They found the nasal spray vaccine to be 86 percent effective against not only the flu strains covered in the vaccine but also against a circulating strain not included in the vaccine.

Issues such as lack of refrigeration can make immunizing people using traditional vaccines very difficult in developing countries. To help address this issue, scientists have developed plants genetically engineered to contain an antigen for the *Escherichia coli* bacteria and the Norwalk virus. This development shows that safe and effective edible vaccines can be made.

The first clinical study of an edible vaccine was conducted at the University of Maryland VTEU in 1998. In it, potatoes were genetically engineered to produce an immune response to *E. coli* when eaten raw. This novel technology may be an inexpensive and effective way to safely immunize people in developing countries against vaccine-preventable illnesses.

Vaccine Safety

The evaluation of vaccine safety is an important part of every vaccine clinical trial sponsored by the National Institutes of Health, including the VTEUs. Study participants are closely monitored for any adverse effects of the vaccinations they receive. All trials include safety as a primary study objective. In addition to the rigorous evaluation of vaccine safety that takes place during every trial, VTEU research explores emerging hypotheses regarding possible vaccine-related adverse events.

Recent Federal efforts to improve the safety of vaccination have found that it is prudent to remove thimerosal, a possible source of organic mercury, from vaccines routinely given to infants. The University of Rochester VTEU has conducted a study to assess mercury levels in blood, hair, and stool samples from infants who received routine vaccines containing thimerosal. Mercury levels were compared with similar samples from infants who received vaccines without thimerosal.

Several important results have been obtained from this study. Mercury levels in blood were low in all infants studied and uniformly below the Environmental Protection Agency safety guidelines for methyl mercury. Mercury levels in the stool of infants receiving vaccines containing thimerosal were relatively high compared to mercury levels in the stool of infants who were not exposed to thimerosal. These results indicate that thimerosal appears to be removed from the blood and body more rapidly than methyl mercury. Thus, exposure to thimerosal is likely less dangerous than exposure to methyl mercury—and the guidelines for methyl mercury offer an even greater margin of safety.

Biodefense

Responding to the concern that the smallpox virus could be used as a bioterrorist weapon against the United States, NIAID is exploring the best way to use existing smallpox vaccine supplies to protect military and civilian populations. Approximately 15 million doses of Dryvax smallpox vaccine have been stored since production stopped in 1983.

Because the estimated amount needed to control a U.S. outbreak is 40 million doses, NIAID began a study to determine whether Dryvax vaccine could be diluted effectively to make more doses of this smallpox vaccine available. This clinical trial showed that the existing U.S. supply of smallpox vaccine could successfully be diluted up to five times and retain its potency, effectively expanding the number of individuals it could protect from the contagious disease to 75 million. Dryvax, the vaccine used in this study, was made by Wyeth Laboratories (Marietta, Pa.). The vaccine is freeze-dried, live vaccinia virus, a poxvirus related to smallpox virus.

A report describing these findings appears in the April 2002 issue of *The New England Journal of Medicine*. The Dryvax vaccine will soon be studied in previously vaccinated populations to determine whether any residual immunity exists from earlier vaccination.

In addition to Dryvax, NIAID is sponsoring clinical trials of another vaccine against smallpox. Eighty million doses of Wetvax or APSV, a different formulation of the vaccinia smallpox vaccine produced by Aventis Pasteur (Paris, France) has been in storage for 40 years. The VTEU studies will determine the safety and preliminary efficacy of various concentrations of Aventis Pasteur's Smallpox Vaccine, USP (APSV) in adults who have never received vaccinia.

Researchers are also working on new, improved anthrax vaccines that may be more easily given to a diverse population. NIAID is collaborating with the U.S. Department of Defense to develop a next-generation vaccine. This new vaccine is based on a laboratory-produced recombinant version of PA protein, the major component of the existing vaccine that protects against infection. The Institute will supervise phase I and phase II trials of the recombinant PA vaccine in different formulations at VTEU sites.

VTEU Sites

The VTEUs are set up to respond to changing health needs. The sites are listed below.

Baylor College of Medicine
Department of Microbiology and Immunology
One Baylor Plaza, M929
Houston, TX 77030
Phone: 713-798-6054
Fax: 713-798-3700
Website: http://www.bcm.tmc.edu/departments/immunology.htm
E-mail: immunology@bcm.tmc.edu

Cincinnati University Children's Hospital
Medical Center
Gamble Program for Clinical Studies
3333 Burnet Avenue
Cincinnati, Ohio 45229-3039
Toll-Free: 800-344-2462
Phone: 513-636-7699
Website: http://www.cincinnatichildrens.org/svc/prog/gamble/default.htm
E-mail: gambleprogram@chmcc.org

University of California at Los Angeles
Center for Vaccine Research
1124 West Carson Street
Building E6
Torrance, CA 90502
Phone: 310-781-3636
Fax: 310-972-2962
Website: http://www.rei.edu

Saint Louis University School of Medicine
Division of Infectious Diseases and Immunology
3635 Vista Avenue
7th Floor, Desloge Towers
St. Louis, Missouri 63110-0250
Phone: 314-577-8648
Fax: 314-771-3816
Website: http://internalmed.slu.edu/infectiousdis

University of Maryland School of Medicine
Center for Vaccine Development
HSF Room 480
685 West Baltimore Street
Baltimore, MD 21201
Phone: 410-706-5328
Fax: 410-706-6205
Website: http://medschool.umaryland.edu/CVD/about.asp
E-mail: cvd@medicine.umaryland.edu

University of Rochester
School of Medicine and Dentistry
601 Elmwood Avenue, Box 706
Rochester, NY 14642
Phone: 585-275-3409
Fax: 585-256-1131
Website: http://www.umc.rochester.edu/smd

Vanderbilt University Medical Center
Department of Pediatrics
2200 Children's Way
Nashville, TN 37232
Phone: 615-322-2250
Fax: 615-343-9723
Website: http://www.vanderbiltchildrens.com

Chapter 62

Vaccine Safety

Importance of Vaccine Safety

Perhaps the greatest success story in public health is the reduction of infectious diseases resulting from the use of vaccines. Routine immunization has eradicated smallpox from the globe and led to the near elimination of wild polio virus. Vaccines have reduced preventable infectious diseases to an all-time low and now few people experience the devastating effects of measles, pertussis and other illnesses. Prior to approval by the U.S. Food and Drug Administration (FDA), vaccines are extensively tested by scientists to ensure that they are effective and safe. Vaccines are the best defense we have against infectious diseases. However, no vaccine is 100% safe or effective. Differences in the way individual immune systems react to a vaccine account for rare occasions when people are not protected following immunization or when they experience side effects.[1,2,3]

As infectious diseases continue to decline, some people have become less interested in the consequences of preventable illnesses like diphtheria and tetanus. Instead, they have become increasingly concerned about the risks associated with vaccines. After all, vaccines are given to healthy individuals, many of whom are children, and therefore a high standard of safety is required. Since vaccination is such a common and memorable event, any illness following immunization may be attributed to the vaccine. While some of these reactions may be

---

"Overview of Vaccine Safety," National Immunization Program, Centers for Disease Control and Prevention (CDC), March 12, 2003.

caused by the vaccine, many of them are unrelated events that occur after vaccination by coincidence. Therefore, the scientific research that attempts to distinguish true vaccine side effects from unrelated, chance occurrences is crucial. This knowledge is necessary in order to maintain public confidence in immunization programs. As science continues to advance, we are constantly striving to develop safer vaccines and improve delivery in order to better protect ourselves against disease. This overview will focus on vaccine research, how vaccines are licensed, how safety is monitored, and how risks are communicated to the public.[1,2,3]

National Childhood Vaccine Injury Act (NCVIA)

The topic of vaccine safety became prominent during the mid 1970's with increases in lawsuits filed on behalf of those presumably injured by the diphtheria, pertussis, tetanus (DPT) vaccine.[4] Legal decisions were made and damages awarded despite the lack of scientific evidence to support vaccine injury claims.[4] As a result of the liability, prices soared and several manufacturers halted production. A vaccine shortage resulted and public health officials became concerned about the return of epidemic disease. In order to reduce liability and respond to public health concerns, Congress passed the National Childhood Vaccine Injury Act (NCVIA) in 1986. This act was influential in many ways.

1. As a result of the NCVIA, the National Vaccine Program Office (NVPO) was established within the Department of Health and Human Services (DHHS). The responsibility of NVPO is to coordinate immunization-related activities between all DHHS agencies including the Centers for Disease Control and Prevention (CDC), Food and Drug Administration (FDA), National Institutes of Health (NIH) and the Health Resources and Services Administration (HRSA).

2. The NCVIA requires that all health care providers who administer vaccines containing diphtheria, tetanus, pertussis, polio, measles, mumps, rubella, hepatitis B, *Haemophilus influenzae* type b, and varicella must provide a Vaccine Information Statement (VIS) to the vaccine recipient, their parent or legal guardian prior to each dose. A VIS must be given with every vaccination including each dose in a multi-dose series. Each VIS contains a brief description of the disease as well as the risks and benefits of the vaccine. VISs are developed by

the CDC and distributed to state and local health departments as well as individual providers.

3. The NCVIA also mandates that all health care providers must report certain adverse events following vaccination to the Vaccine Adverse Event Reporting System (VAERS). This system will be described in detail later in the chapter.

4. Under the NCVIA, the National Vaccine Injury Compensation Program (NVICP) was created to compensate those injured by vaccines on a "no fault" basis. This program will be described in detail later in the chapter.

5. The NCVIA established a committee from the Institute of Medicine (IOM) to review the existing literature on vaccine adverse events (health effects occurring after immunization that may or may not be related to the vaccine). This group concluded that there are limitations in our knowledge of the risks associated with vaccines. Of the 76 adverse events they reviewed for a causal relationship, 50 (66%) had no or inadequate research.[1] Specifically, IOM identified the following problems:

   - limited understanding of biological processes that underlie adverse events
   - incomplete and inconsistent information from individual reports
   - poorly constructed research studies (not enough people enrolled for a long enough period of time)
   - inadequate systems to track vaccine adverse events
   - few experimental studies published in the medical literature.[1] Significant progress has been made over the past few years to better monitor adverse events and conduct research relevant to vaccine safety.[4,5]

Monitoring Vaccine Safety: Pre-Licensure

Before vaccines are licensed by the FDA, they are extensively tested in the laboratory and in human beings to ensure their safety. First, computers are used to predict how the vaccine will interact with the immune system. Then researchers test the vaccine on animals including mice, guinea pigs, rabbits, and monkeys. Once the vaccine successfully completes these laboratory tests, it is approved for use in clinical studies by the FDA. During clinical trials, the vaccine is tested on human beings. Participation in these studies is completely voluntary. Many individuals choose to contribute their time and energy for the advancement of science. Informed consent must be obtained from all participants before they become involved in research. This ensures that they understand the purpose of the study and potential risks and that they are willing to participate. Volunteers agree to receive the vaccine and undergo any medical testing necessary to assess its safety and efficacy.[6]

Vaccine licensure is a lengthy process that may take ten years or longer. The FDA requires that vaccines undergo three phases of clinical trials in human beings before they can be licensed for use in the general public. Phase one trials are small, involving only 20–100 volunteers, and last only a few months. The purpose of phase one trials is to evaluate basic safety and identify very common adverse events. Phase two trials are larger and involve several hundred participants. These studies last anywhere from several months to two years and collect additional information on safety and efficacy. Data gained from phase two trials can be used to determine the composition of the vaccine, how many doses are necessary and a profile of common adverse events. Unless the vaccine is completely ineffective or causes serious side effects, the trials are expanded to phase three which involve several hundred to several thousand volunteers. Typically these trials last several years. Because the vaccinated group can be compared to those who have not received the vaccine, researchers are able to identify true side effects.[1,3,6,7,8]

If the clinical trials demonstrate that the vaccine is safe and effective, the manufacturer applies to the FDA for two licenses, one for the vaccine (product license) and one for the production plant (establishment license). During the application process, the FDA reviews the clinical trial data and proposed product labeling. In addition, the FDA inspects the plant and goes over manufacturing protocols to ensure that vaccines are produced in a safe and consistent manner. Only after the FDA is satisfied that the vaccine is safe is it licensed for use in the general population.[7]

Monitoring Vaccine Safety: Post-Licensure

After a vaccine is licensed for public use, its safety is continually monitored. The FDA requires all manufacturers to submit samples from each vaccine lot prior to its release. In addition, the manufacturers must provide the FDA with their test results for vaccine safety, potency, and purity. Each lot must be tested because vaccines are sensitive to environmental factors (like temperature) and can be contaminated during production. During the last ten years, only three vaccine lots have been recalled by the FDA. One lot was mislabeled and another was contaminated with particles during production. A third lot was recalled after the FDA discovered potential problems with the manufacturing process at a production plant.[7]

While clinical trials provide important information on vaccine safety, the data are somewhat limited because of the small number (hundreds to thousands) of study participants. Rare side effects and delayed reactions may not be evident until the vaccine is administered to millions of people. Therefore, the Federal Government has established a surveillance system to monitor adverse events that occur following vaccination. This project is known as the Vaccine Adverse Events Reporting System (VAERS). More recently, large-linked databases (LLDBs) containing information on millions of individuals have been created in order to study rare vaccine side effects.[1,3]

Vaccine Adverse Event Reporting System (VAERS)

The National Childhood Vaccine Injury Act of 1986 mandated that all health care providers report certain adverse events that occur following vaccination. As a result, the Vaccine Adverse Events Reporting System (VAERS) was established by the FDA and the Centers for Disease Control and Prevention (CDC) in 1990. VAERS provides a mechanism for the collection and analysis of adverse events associated with vaccines currently licensed in the United States. Adverse events are defined as health effects that occur after immunization that may or may not be related to the vaccine. VAERS data are continually monitored in order to detect previously unknown adverse events or increases in known adverse events.[1,9]

Approximately 10,000–12,000 VAERS reports are filed annually, with 20% classified as serious (causing disability, hospitalization, life threatening illness, or death).[1] Anyone can file a VAERS report including health care providers, manufacturers, vaccine recipients or, when appropriate, parents/guardians. Those who have experienced an adverse reaction following immunization are encouraged to seek help from a health care professional when filling out the form. VAERS forms can be obtained in several ways. Each year the form is mailed to more than 200,000 physicians specializing in pediatrics, family practice, internal medicine, infectious diseases, emergency medicine, obstetrics, and gynecology. In addition, copies are sent to health departments and clinics that administer vaccines. The VAERS form requests the following information: the type of vaccine received, the timing of vaccination, the onset of the adverse event, current illnesses or medication, past history of adverse events following vaccination, and demographic information about the recipient (age, gender, etc.). The form is pre-addressed and stamped so it can be mailed directly to VAERS. To request a VAERS form or assistance in filling in out, call 1-800-822-7967.[1,9]

A contractor, under the supervision of FDA and CDC, collects the information and enters it into a database. Those reporting an adverse event to VAERS receive a confirmation letter by mail indicating that the form was received. This letter will contain a VAERS identification number. Additional information may be submitted to VAERS using the assigned identification number. Selected cases of serious adverse reactions are followed up at 60 days and one year post-vaccination to check the recovery status of the patient. The FDA and CDC have access to VAERS data and use this information to monitor vaccine safety and conduct appropriate research studies. VAERS data (minus any personal information) is also available to the public.[1,9]

While VAERS provides useful information on vaccine safety, the data are somewhat limited. Specifically, judgments about causality (whether the vaccine was truly responsible for an adverse event) cannot be made from VAERS reports because of incomplete information. VAERS reports often lack important information such as laboratory results. As a result, researchers have turned more recently to large-linked databases (LLDBs) in order to study vaccine safety. LLDBs provide scientists with access to the complete medical records of millions of individuals receiving vaccines (all identifying information is deleted to protect the confidentiality of the patient). One example of a LLDB is the Vaccine Safety Datalink (VSD) project described below, which is coordinated by the CDC. Studies conducted using LLDBs, like the VSD, are also known as post-marketing research or phase four clinical trials.[1]

Vaccine Safety Datalink (VSD) Project

The gaps that exist in the scientific knowledge of rare vaccine side effects prompted the CDC to develop the Vaccine Safety Datalink (VSD) project in 1990. This project involves partnerships with seven large health maintenance organizations (HMOs) to continually monitor vaccine safety. VSD is an example of a large-linked database (LLDB) and includes information on more than six million people. All vaccines administered within the study population are recorded. Available data include vaccine type, date of vaccination, concurrent vaccinations (those given during the same visit), the manufacturer, lot number, and injection site. Medical records are then monitored for potential adverse events resulting from immunization. The VSD project allows for planned vaccine safety studies as well as timely investigations of hypotheses. At present, the VSD project is examining potential associations between vaccines and a number of serious conditions. The database is also being used to test new vaccine safety hypotheses that result from the medical literature, VAERS, changes in the immunization schedule or from the introduction of new vaccines. This project is a powerful and cost-effective tool for the on-going evaluation of vaccine safety.[1,10]

Vaccine Injury Compensation Program

In order to reduce the liability of manufacturers and health care providers, the National Childhood Vaccine Injury Act of 1986 established the National Vaccine Injury Compensation Program (NVICP). This program is intended to compensate those individuals who have been injured by vaccines on a "no-fault" basis. No fault means that people filing claims are not required to prove negligence on the part of either the health care provider or manufacturer to receive compensation. The program covers all routinely recommended childhood vaccinations. Settlements are based on the Vaccine Injury Table which summarizes the adverse events caused by vaccines. This table was developed by a panel of experts who reviewed the medical literature and identified the serious adverse events that are reasonably certain to be caused by vaccines. Examples of table injuries include anaphylaxis (severe allergic reaction), paralytic polio, and encephalopathy (general brain disorder). The Vaccine Injury Table was created to justly compensate those injured by vaccines while separating out unrelated claims. As more information becomes available from research on vaccine side effects, the Vaccine Injury Table is updated.[11,12]

Individuals and their families can qualify for compensation in three ways. First, is to show that an injury found on the Vaccine Injury Table occurred in the appropriate time interval following immunization. The other two ways to qualify include proving that the vaccine caused the condition or demonstrating that the vaccine worsened or aggravated a pre-existing condition.[11,12]

The vaccine injury compensation process begins when an individual files a petition with the United States Court of Federal Claims.

At that point, a physician from the program reviews the petition to determine whether it meets the criteria for compensation. This recommendation is not binding. A Court attorney then reviews the case and makes an initial decision for or against entitlement to compensation. Decisions may be appealed to the Court of Federal Claims, and then to the Federal Circuit Court of Appeals. This process occurs at no cost to the individual filing the claim. NVICP is coordinated by the Department of Health and Human Services and the Department of Justice. For more information on the program or for assistance in making a claim, call 1-800-338-2382.[11,12]

Improvements in Vaccine Safety

In the last decade, numerous changes in vaccine production and administration have reduced the number of adverse events and resulted in safer vaccines. A more purified acellular pertussis (aP) vaccine has been licensed for use and has replaced the whole-cell pertussis vaccine used in DTP (diphtheria, tetanus, pertussis vaccine). Several studies have evaluated the safety and efficacy of DTaP as compared to DTP and have concluded that DTaP is effective in preventing disease and that mild side effects and serious adverse events occurred less frequently when the DTaP vaccine was given.[3] Recent changes in the schedule of polio vaccines have also resulted in fewer reports of serious side effects. In 1997, the Advisory Committee on Immunization Practice recommended a change in the vaccination schedule to include sequential administration of inactivated polio vaccine (IPV) and oral polio vaccine (OPV).[13] This sequential schedule was expected to produce a high level of individual protection against the disease caused by wild polio virus, while reducing by 50 to 70% vaccine-associated paralytic polio (VAPP) that occurs in 8–10 people a year who receive OPV.[14] Today, only IPV is on the recommended childhood immunization schedule.

Risk Communication

At some point, almost every person in the United States is vaccinated. Therefore, many individuals question how vaccines are made, if they are effective, and whether they are safe.[15] People seek answers to these questions from a wide variety of sources including family, friends, health care providers, the internet, television, and medical literature. The information they receive is complex and, at times, inaccurate or misleading. Therefore, health professionals have a responsibility to provide accurate, understandable information and to handle vaccine safety concerns appropriately. As mentioned previously, the NCVIA requires all health care providers who administer vaccines to discuss the potential risks and benefits of immunization. In these situations, risk communication is a necessary skill.[1]

Risk communication involves a dynamic exchange of information between individuals, groups, and institutions. This information must acknowledge and define the risks associated with vaccination in a way the public can understand. This is difficult given the current environment where few people experience the devastation of vaccine-preventable diseases. It is further complicated by the fact that immunization is associated with some degree of personal discomfort when needles are used to administer vaccines.[1]

In 1996, the Institute of Medicine's Vaccine Safety Forum held a workshop on risk communication and vaccination. Three key concepts emerged:

"First, risk communication is a dynamic process in which many participate, and these individuals are influenced by a wide variety of circumstances, interests, and information needs. Effective risk communication depends on the providers' and recipients' understanding more than simply the risks and benefits; background experiences and values also influence the process."[18] Good risk communication recognizes a diversity of form and context needs in the general population.

Second, the goal that all parties share regarding vaccine risk communication should be informed decision making. Consent for vaccination is truly 'informed' when the members of the public know the risks and benefits and make voluntary decisions.

Finally, there is often uncertainty about estimates of the risk associated with vaccination. Risk communication is more effective when this uncertainty is stated and when the risks are quantified as much as science permits. Trust is a key component of the exchange of information at every level, and overconfidence about risk estimates that are later shown to be incorrect contributes to a breakdown of trust among public health officials, vaccine manufacturers, and the public. "Continued research to improve the understanding of vaccine risks is critical to maximizing mutual understanding and trust."[19]

Several resources are available to address the risks and benefits of vaccination. Federal law requires all health care providers who administer vaccines in the United States to provide Vaccine Information Statements (VISs) to vaccine recipients (or their parent/guardian) prior to each dose being administered. VISs are developed by CDC and contain information on the disease as well as the risks and benefits associated with immunization. These documents, and others, can be obtained from the National Immunization Hotline 1-800-232-2522.

Conclusion: The Future of Vaccine Safety

The importance of vaccine safety will continue to grow throughout the twenty-first century. The development and licensure of new vaccines will add to the already complicated immunization schedule. Scientists may also perfect new ways of administering immunizations including edible vaccines and needleless injections. However they are formulated or delivered, vaccines will remain the most effective tool we possess for preventing disease and improving public health in the future.

References

1. Chen RT, Hibbs B. Vaccine safety: Current and future challenges. *Pediatric Annals*. July 1998; 27(7): 445-455.

2. Ellenberg SS, Chen RT. The complicated task of monitoring vaccine safety. *Public Health Reports*. Jan/Feb 1997; 112: 10-19.

3. Centers for Disease Control and Prevention. (1997) *Epidemiology and prevention of vaccine-preventable diseases, vaccine safety* (chapter 15). Washington DC: Government Printing Office.

4. Freed GL, Katz SL, Clark SJ. Safety of vaccinations: Miss America, the media, and public health. *JAMA*. 1996; 276(23): 1869-1872.

5. Brink EW, Hinman AR. The vaccine injury compensation act: The new law and you. *Contemporary Pediatrics*. July 1989; 6(3): 28-32, 35-36, 39, 42.

6. National Institutes of Health. (1998) *Understanding vaccines*. Bethesda, MD: NIH.

7. Food and Drug Administration (FDA) web site (http://www.fda.gov/fdac/features/095_vacc.html)

8. Chen RT, Orenstein WA. Epidemiologic methods in immunization programs. *Epidemiologic Reviews*. 1996; 18(2): 99-117.

9. Chen RT, Rastogi SC, Mullen JR, Hayes SW, Cochi SL, Donlon JA, Wassilak SG. The Vaccine Adverse Event Reporting System (VAERS). *Vaccine*. 1994; 12(6): 542-550.

10. Chen RT, Glasser JW, Phodes PH, Davis RL, Barlow WE, Thompson RS, Mullooly JP, Black SB, Shinefield HR, Badheim CM, Marcy SM, Ward JI, Wise RP, Wassilak SG, Hadler SC. Vaccine safety datalink project: A new tool for improving vaccine safety monitoring in the United States. *Pediatrics*. June 1997; 99(6): 765-773.

11. Vaccine Injury Compensation Program web site (http://www.hrsa.gov/osp/vicp)

12. National Immunization Program, Satellite Course on Vaccine Safety and Risk Communication. February 26, 1998.

13. Advisory Committee on Immunization Practice (ACIP). Poliomyelitis prevention in the United States: Introduction of a sequential vaccination schedule of inactivated poliovirus vaccine followed by oral poliovirus vaccine. *MMWR*. 1997; 46 (RR-3); 1-25.

14. Advisory Committee on Immunization Practice (ACIP). Poliomyelitis prevention in the United States: Introduction of a sequential vaccination schedule of inactivated poliovirus vaccine followed by oral poliovirus vaccine. *MMWR*. 1997; 46 (RR-3); 1-25.

15. Offit PM, Bell LM. *What every parent should know about vaccines*. New York: Simon & Schuster Macmillan Company, 1998:1.

16. Hance BJ, Chess C, Sandman P. *Industry risk communication manual*. Chelsea, MI: Lewis Publishers, 1990.

17. Meszaros JR, Asch, DA, Baron J, Hershey JC, Kunreuther H, Schwartz-Buzaglo J. Cognitive processes and the decisions of some parents to forego pertussis vaccination for their children. *J Clin Epidemiol*. 1996; 49: 697-703.

18. Zeckhauser R. Coverage for catastrophic illness. *Public Policy* 1973; 21:149-72.

19. Institute of Medicine, Vaccine Safety Forum. (1997). *Risk communication and vaccination: summary of a workshop*. Washington, DC: National Academy Press.

Chapter 63

Additives in Vaccines

Millions of doses of vaccines are administered to children in this country each year. Ensuring that those vaccines are potent, sterile, and safe requires the addition of minute amounts of chemical additives.

Chemicals are added to vaccines to inactivate a virus or bacteria and stabilize the vaccine, helping to preserve the vaccine and prevent it from losing its potency over time. The amount of chemical additives found in vaccines is very small and may not be enough to cause a serious allergic response.

In July 1999, the Federal government asked vaccine manufacturers to work towards eliminating or reducing the use of thimerosal, a preservative which contains small amounts of mercury, in any products currently available on the market. Today, all routinely recommended pediatric vaccines manufactured for the U.S. market contain no thimerosal or only trace amounts.

Facts

Additives used in the production of vaccines may include:

- suspending fluid (for example, sterile water, saline, or fluids containing protein)
- preservatives and stabilizers to help the vaccine remain unchanged (for example, albumin, phenols, and glycine); and

---

"Additives in Vaccines," National Immunization Program, Centers for Disease Control and Prevention (CDC), December 2003.

- adjuvants or enhancers that help the vaccine improve its work.

Common substances found in vaccines include:

- Aluminum gels or salts of aluminum which are added as adjuvants to help the vaccine stimulate production of antibodies to fight off diseases and aid other substances in their action. In vaccines, adjuvants may be added to help promote an earlier response, more potent response, or more persistent immune response to disease.
- Antibiotics which are added to vaccines to prevent the growth of germs (bacteria) in vaccine cultures.
- Egg protein which is found in vaccines prepared using chick embryos. Ordinarily, persons who are able to eat eggs or egg products safely can receive these vaccines.
- Formaldehyde which is used to inactivate bacterial products for toxoid vaccines. It is also used to kill unwanted viruses and bacteria that might be found in cultures used to produce vaccines.
- Monosodium glutamate (MSG) and 2-phenoxy-ethanol which are used as stabilizers in a few vaccines to help the vaccine remain unchanged even in the presence of forces such as heat, light, acidity, humidity, etc. MSG is also found in many foods, especially Asian foods and flavor enhancers.
- Thimerosal which is a preservative that might be added to prevent the vaccine from spoiling. Thimerosal is also found in some contact lens solutions and throat sprays.

For children with a prior history of allergic reactions to any of these substances in vaccines, parents should consult their child's health care provider before vaccination.

What You Should Know

- To find out what chemical additives are in specific vaccines, ask your health care provider or pharmacist for a copy of the vaccine package insert, which lists all ingredients in the vaccine and discusses any known adverse reactions.
- To assure the safety of vaccines, the Centers for Disease Control and Prevention (CDC), the Food and Drug Administration (FDA), the National Institutes of Health (NIH), and other Federal

agencies routinely monitor and conduct research to examine any new evidence that would suggest possible problems with the safety of vaccines.

- To report a health problem that followed vaccination you or your provider should call the Vaccine Adverse Event Reporting System (VAERS) at 1-800-822-7967.

For more information call the National Immunization Hotline: English (800) 232-2522; Spanish (800) 232-0233; or visit the National Immunization Program web site at http://www.cdc.gov/nip.

Additional information may also be found in the following journal article: "Addressing Parents' Concerns: Do Vaccines Contain Harmful Preservatives, Adjuvants, Additives, or Residuals?" *Pediatrics*, Vol. 112, No. 6, December 2003, pp. 1394-1397.

Chapter 64

Studies Regarding the Safety of Mercury and Thimerosal in Vaccines

National Institute of Allergy and Infectious Diseases (NIAID) Research on Thimerosal

Mercury is a naturally occurring chemical element found throughout the environment. Mercury is found in three forms: as a pure metal (as found in thermometers), as inorganic salts, and as an organic derivative. Humans and wildlife are exposed to all three forms. Most environmental mercury consists of the metallic and inorganic forms. Because mercury is everywhere, it is not possible to prevent all exposure to it. High levels of mercury are toxic.

Methyl mercury, the most common organic derivative of mercury, is mainly produced by microorganisms in water and soil. Methyl mercury is of particular concern because it can accumulate in certain edible freshwater and saltwater fish, especially in larger and older fish, to levels that are much greater than levels in the surrounding water. Methyl mercury can also accumulate in humans who eat these fish. Exposure to high levels of methyl mercury is toxic and can cause mental retardation, cerebral palsy, and seizures. The fetus is especially sensitive to methyl mercury exposure, and may suffer brain damage or even death if exposed to high levels.

"NIAID Research on Thimerosal," National Institute of Allergy and Infectious Diseases (NIAID), National Institutes of Health (NIH), December 2003; "Thimerosal and Vaccines," May 20, 2003, and "Availability of Thimerosal-Free Vaccines," July 7, 2001, National Immunization Program, Centers for Disease Control and Prevention (CDC).

Since the 1930s, thimerosal has been added to some vaccines and other products because it is effective in killing bacteria and in preventing bacterial contamination, particularly in multi-dose containers. When thimerosal is degraded or metabolized, one product is ethyl mercury, another organic derivative of mercury. Not much is known about the effects of thimerosal exposure on humans and how this compares to methyl mercury exposure. The only known side-effects of receiving low doses of thimerosal in vaccines have been minor reactions such as redness and swelling at the injection site.

In July 1999, the Public Health Service (PHS) agencies, the American Academy of Pediatrics (AAP), and vaccine manufacturers agreed that thimerosal should be reduced or eliminated in vaccines as a precautionary measure and to reduce exposure to mercury from all sources. Today, all routinely recommended licensed pediatric vaccines that are currently being manufactured for the U.S. market are either thimerosal-free or contain markedly reduced amounts of thimerosal. However, thimerosal remains in some vaccines given to adults and adolescents, as well as some pediatric vaccines not on the Recommended Childhood Immunization Schedule. Thimerosal is a common preservative found in vaccines used outside the United States.

The decision to move toward reduced/eliminated thimerosal in vaccines was based on the various federal guidelines for methyl mercury exposure and the assumption that the health risks from methyl- and ethyl mercury were the same. Methyl mercury exposure is primarily through fish consumption. People who regularly eat mercury-contaminated fish can accumulate methyl mercury in their body over time. Some of this methyl mercury may be passed from the mother to the fetus before birth and to infants through breast milk. The fetus is most sensitive to damage by this exposure. Prior to the removal of thimerosal from childhood recommended vaccines, during vaccination, infants were exposed to ethyl mercury by intramuscular injection, not by ingestion. Furthermore, infants received thimerosal from childhood vaccines that were administered days or months apart. In contrast, methyl mercury exposure, primarily from foods, tends to occur over a longer sustained period of time. More research is needed to determine if the guidelines for methyl mercury exposure are also appropriate guidelines for thimerosal. Additionally, guidelines for maximal levels for short-term exposure (days, weeks, months) need to be established.

NIAID funds thimerosal research that focuses on better understanding what happens to thimerosal once it is introduced in the body and how this compares to current knowledge of methyl mercury pathways. At the University of Rochester, NIAID sponsored researchers are performing an assessment of mercury levels in infants receiving routine immunizations. In addition, NIAID and the National Institutes of Environmental Health Sciences (NIEHS) are funding studies comparing the pharmacokinetics and tissue distribution of thimerosal, ethyl mercury, and methyl mercury in non-human primates.

Assessment of Mercury Levels in Infants Receiving Routine Immunizations

NIAID has supported studies at the University of Rochester (one of NIAID's Vaccine Treatment and Evaluation Units) and Bethesda Naval Hospital to assess levels of mercury in the blood, hair, urine, and stool of forty infants who received vaccines containing thimerosal and twenty infants who received vaccines without thimerosal, as controls. The infants studied were six months of age or younger. Several important results have been obtained from this study. Mercury levels in blood and urine were low in all infants studied and in many cases too small to measure. There was no observed dose-dependent relationship between the level of thimerosal received through vaccination and the level of mercury in the body. Mercury levels in blood did not exceed, at any time, the blood levels that correspond to the Environmental Protection Agency's (EPA) guidelines for exposure. Mercury levels in the stool of infants receiving vaccines containing thimerosal were relatively high compared to mercury levels in the stool of infants who were not exposed to thimerosal, providing evidence that mercury from thimerosal is eliminated in the stool of infants. These results were recently published in the *Lancet*.

Questions and Answers about Mercury, Thimerosal, and Vaccine Safety

Why is thimerosal used as a preservative in vaccines?

Thimerosal is used as a preservative in some multi-dose vials of vaccines to prevent contamination. Preservatives are not required for vaccines in single-dose vials. As a preservative, thimerosal is added at the end of the production process to the bulk or final container to prevent contamination after multi-dose vials are opened. Today, all routinely recommended licensed pediatric vaccines that are currently being manufactured for the U.S. market are free of thimerosal as a preservative. Thimerosal still may be used in the early stages of manufacturing of certain vaccines, but is removed through a purification process, with only trace, or insignificant, amounts remaining.

If thimerosal was used in vaccines for many years, why is it of concern now?

The Food and Drug Administration (FDA) Modernization Act of 1997 called for the FDA to review and assess the risk of all mercury containing food and drugs. As part of this effort, the FDA conducted a review of mercury content in vaccines.

What recommendations did the Federal government make with respect to thimerosal in vaccines?

A review conducted by the Food and Drug Administration (FDA) concluded that the use of thimerosal as a preservative in vaccines might result in the intake of mercury during the first 6 months of life that exceeds the Environmental Protection Agency (EPA), but not the FDA, the Agency for Toxic Substances and Disease Registry (ATSDR), or the World Health Organization (WHO) guidelines for methyl mercury intake (Ball et al., 2001). Thimerosal contains ethyl mercury. Methyl mercury is a related compound and has been more thoroughly researched than ethyl mercury. Thus, federal safety standards are based on information we have about methyl mercury.

FDA's review found no evidence of harm caused by doses of thimerosal in vaccines, except for minor local reactions (Ball et al., 2001). Nevertheless, in July 1999 the Public Health Service agencies (PHS), the American Academy of Pediatrics (AAP), and vaccine manufacturers agreed that thimerosal levels in vaccines should be reduced or eliminated as a precautionary measure, and the Food and Drug Administration (FDA) committed to expediting the review of new vaccines that do not contain thimerosal.

What progress has been made since July 1999 in removing thimerosal from vaccines routinely recommended for infants?

Substantial progress has been made in the effort to reduce thimerosal exposure from vaccines. At this time, all routinely recommended licensed pediatric vaccines that are currently being manufactured for the U.S. market, contain no thimerosal or contain only trace amounts of thimerosal. The vaccines with trace amount of thimerosal licensed to date contain less than 0.5 micrograms of mercury per dose, that is, a given dose of vaccine contains less than 1 part per million.

Events that contributed to accomplishing this goal include the licensure of a thimerosal free Hepatitis B Vaccine (Recombinant) manufactured by Merck and Company in August 1999. FDA licensed another hepatitis B vaccine with trace amounts of thimerosal, manufactured by GlaxoSmithKline in March 2000. A supplement for a new formulation of Aventis Pasteur's DTaP Vaccine with only a trace amount of thimerosal was approved in March 2001. Additionally, Wyeth-Lederle Vaccines and Pediatrics now only markets a single-dose, thimerosal-free formulation of its Haemophilus b (Hib) Conjugate Vaccine in the U.S. Thus, two hepatitis B vaccines are thimerosal free, four Hib vaccines are thimerosal free, and two DTaP vaccines are thimerosal free.

Prior to the recent initiative to reduce or eliminate thimerosal from childhood vaccines, the maximum cumulative exposure to mercury via routine childhood vaccinations during the first six months of life was 187.5 micrograms. With the newly formulated vaccines, the maximum cumulative exposure during the first six months of life will now be less than three micrograms of mercury; this represents a greater than 98 percent reduction in the amount of mercury a child would receive from vaccines in the first six months of life.

I've heard that children may be getting toxic levels of mercury from vaccines. Is that true?

No. There is no evidence of harm caused by the minute doses of thimerosal in vaccines, except for minor effects like swelling and redness at the injection site due to sensitivity to thimerosal.

Most importantly, since 1999, newly formulated thimerosal preservative-free vaccines have been licensed. With the newly formulated vaccines, the maximum cumulative exposure during the first six months of life will now be less than three micrograms of mercury. No children are receiving toxic levels of mercury from vaccines.

What research is being conducted by the Federal Government regarding the safety of vaccines containing thimerosal?

There is no evidence to suggest that thimerosal in vaccines causes any health problems in children and adults beyond local hypersensitivity reactions (like redness and swelling at the injection site). However, efforts to remove thimerosal from the U.S. vaccine supply have been accompanied by research investigations to better assess the potential health effects of exposure to thimerosal containing vaccines:

- The National Institute of Allergy and Infectious Diseases (NIAID) at the National Institutes of Health (NIH) funds thimerosal research that focuses on better understanding of what happens to thimerosal once it is introduced into the body and how this compares to current knowledge of methyl mercury pathways.

- A recent study sponsored by the NIAID and conducted at the University of Rochester assessed mercury levels in 40 infants who received vaccines containing thimerosal and 21 infants who received thimerosal-free vaccines. The scientists measured the level of mercury in the infants' blood, urine and stool up to 28 days after vaccination. They found that 1) infants who were given vaccines with thimerosal had levels of mercury well below the safe level of 29 nmol/L (this level is set ten times lower than the level at which mercury begins to cause neurological problems) and 2) the body seems to be able to get rid of thimerosal (ethyl mercury) via the gastrointestinal tract (stools) much quicker than it gets rid of methyl mercury. For more information about the different types of mercury visit http://www.cdc.gov/nip/vacsafe/concerns/thimerosal/faqs-mercury.htm.
- NIAID and the National Institutes of Environmental Health Sciences (NIEHS) are also funding studies comparing the pharmacokinetics and tissue distribution of thimerosal, ethyl mercury, and methyl mercury in non-human primates. Pharmacokinetics is the study of how an agent is absorbed, distributed, metabolized (broken down), and excreted. For more information visit http://www.niaid.nih.gov/factsheets/thimerosal.htm.

- The Food and Drug Administration (FDA) has been actively addressing the issue of thimerosal as a preservative in vaccines. For information on FDA activities related to thimerosal and vaccines visit http://www.fda.gov/cber/vaccine/thimerosal.htm
- The CDC used large automated databases that link vaccination and International Classification of Disease codes (ICD-9) stored in the medical records in three managed care organizations (i.e., the Vaccine Safety Datalink project, or VSD) to screen for any possible associations between exposure to thimerosal-containing vaccines and a variety of neurologic, developmental, and renal outcomes. In phase I of this investigation, using data from 2 of the managed care organizations, CDC and VSD researchers found statistically significant associations between thimerosal

and several neurodevelopmental disorders, including language delays, speech delays, attention deficit hyperactivity disorder (ADHD), unspecified developmental delays, stammering, sleep disorders, emotional disorders, and tics. However, the associations were not consistent between the two VSD sites. Reviews of these preliminary observations by expert consultants, first at CDC and then from outside CDC, identified many important limitations and potential biases in the data set, including weak and inconsistent statistical associations, potential inaccuracies in the diagnostic codes, and inadequate control for socio-economic factors. In phase II of the investigation, CDC investigators obtained and examined data from a third managed care organization. Analyses of these data using the same methods and having similar limitations as in the above study, did not confirm results for speech or language delay and attention deficit disorder. The number of events was too small to examine the association with tics and the category of unspecified developmental delays was not defined clearly enough to permit reanalysis. CDC has developed a research protocol for a follow-up to this study. The Thimerosal Follow-Up study will include 1,200 children who are 7 to 9 years of age and who are current members of one of seven managed care organizations that participate in the VSD. Data collection is expected to begin during the spring of 2003 and be completed during the spring of 2004.

- The CDC's Center for Environmental Health and the National Center for Health Statistics are doing a study looking at all mercury exposures and working with the National Health and Nutrition Examination Survey (NHANES). NHANES 4 will collect samples of blood, hair, and urine from all women of reproductive age and children under 5 in order to assess mercury levels in the body from all sources of mercury a person can be exposed to in the environment. Findings of a study conducted using NHANES 3 data to check blood and hair mercury levels suggest that the mercury levels in young children and in women of childbearing age are generally below the level considered hazardous (MMWR;50, 140-143).

Does thimerosal cause autism?

There is no evidence that any vaccine or vaccine additive increases the risk of developing autism or any other behavior disorder. Nonetheless, given the level of concern among parents and others regarding vaccines and autism, the CDC is committed to investigating this issue to the fullest extent possible, using the best scientific methods available.

What about the recent study that claimed to find a relationship between thimerosal in vaccines and autism, speech disorders, and heart disease?

In 2003, Geier and Geier reported conducting two analyses to test whether thimerosal in vaccines is associated with autism, speech disorders, and heart disease. The researchers inadequately described the methods they used, making it impossible to determine exactly what was done and how the results should be interpreted. In the first analysis, the researchers reviewed Vaccine Adverse Event Reporting System (VAERS) reports involving autism, speech disorders, and heart disease. They state that they compared VAERS reports involving thimerosal-containing DTP and DTaP vaccines with those involving thimerosal-free DTaP vaccines. There are a number of weaknesses in this analysis, including an apparent misunderstanding among the authors regarding VAERS reporting requirements. VAERS is a passive surveillance system for reporting possible vaccine adverse events that depends on health care providers, patients, and/or others to file reports. Health effects reported to VAERS as following vaccination may be true adverse events, coincidental occurrences, or mistakes in filing. Because of this, VAERS has certain weaknesses that limit the system, including incomplete reporting, lack of verification of diagnoses, and lack of data on those who were vaccinated and did not report problems. VAERS data are useful for "hypothesis generation" (raising questions), but should not be used for research aimed at determining whether vaccines cause certain health problems as done by Geier and Geier. Moreover, children who could have received thimerosal-free DTaP vaccine were less likely to have autism or speech disorders diagnosed because they were younger than the children in the thimerosal-containing vaccines group. In the heart disease evaluation, the authors examined reports coded as "heart arrest," these cases in VAERS are completely different from the coronary heart disease cases in the studies that the authors cite to support a possible association between mercury and heart disease. It is also unclear how the researchers calculated levels of mercury exposure, because their calculations are inconsistent with the known levels of mercury that were in thimerosal-containing DTP or DTaP vaccines.

In the second analysis, the authors looked at the estimated amount of mercury exposure from vaccines over time and the number of children enrolled in U.S. special education programs for selected disabilities. The authors present figures with very high correlations, but from the limited description provided, it does not seem that the appropriate data were available to perform the analyses and derive the conclusions that the authors report. Although enrollment in special education of children with autism did increase during the 1990s, it has not been determined whether this represents a real increase in the incidence of autism as opposed to increased awareness and acceptance of the diagnosis, better recognition, changing diagnostic criteria, or educational and service incentives to make the diagnosis.

The American Academy of Pediatrics has more information on this study at http://www.aap.org/profed/thimaut-may03.htm.

Did the preliminary Vaccine Safety Datalink (VSD) study described above find that exposure to thimerosal within the first three months of life increases a child's risk of developing autism?

No. A statistically significant relationship between autism and thimerosal was not found in either the preliminary study or the later, larger analysis. While a graph in the preliminary report does show an apparent elevation in risk for autism among children exposed to a certain level of thimerosal (> 62.5µg) by the third month of life, this risk was not statistically significant and was likely a chance fluctuation. In fact, later analyses of additional cases showed that a child's exposure to thimerosal, either by three months of life or by seven months of life, did not increase his or her risk for developing autism. There was no suggestion of an increased risk for autism even among those children who were exposed to the highest levels of thimerosal by seven months of age (i.e., those receiving 162.5 µg, 175 µg, or more than 175 µg thimerosal by 7 months of age). These preliminary negative results from the VSD project, however, cannot be considered definitive since the study was not specifically designed to evaluate a complex condition such as autism. CDC is planning a more thorough investigation of thimerosal exposure through infant vaccines and risk of autism.

Researchers must study as many people as possible in order to detect rare vaccine side effects and to reduce the chance fluctuations that often occur when studies are done with smaller groups of people. The Vaccine Safety Datalink (VSD) project is a partnership between CDC and several large health maintenance organizations (HMO's). Children who are born into the HMO's are added to the study on an ongoing basis. Information is continually accumulated on children in the study and each HMO compiles and sends this data to the CDC on a yearly basis. Therefore, a major difference between the preliminary study and the later analyses (presented to the Institute of Medicine's Immunization Safety Review Committee on July 16, 2001) is one of size and duration of follow-up. The preliminary study included over 75,000 children (67 with autism) who were followed up no further than December of 1997, whereas the study that was presented to the Institute of Medicine (IOM) included over 130,000 children (169 with autism) followed up until May of 1998.

Great Britain experienced a rapid rise in autism among children born in the 1980s and early 1990s. Could this be due to thimerosal in vaccines?

It is unlikely that the rapid increase in autism cases in the UK was due to thimerosal. The only vaccine in the UK's childhood immunization program that contains thimerosal is DTP. All other vaccines (OPV, BCG, MMR, Hib, menC) added to the program since the 1950s are and have always been thimerosal free. In addition, if thimerosal in vaccines were causing autism, we would expect to see a simultaneous increase in both thimerosal exposure and autism cases. However, from the 1950s on, there was no increase in the amount of thimerosal UK children were receiving from vaccines, yet there was a jump in autism cases in the 1980s.

A significant change in the UK's program did occur in 1990 when they accelerated their immunization schedule so vaccines would be given earlier (changed from 3, 5, and 8 months to 2, 3 and 4 months). However, the rate of autism was rising long before this change occurred (see Fombonne, 2001).

I understand some people are sensitive to mercury and must avoid it. Do they have problems with thimerosal-containing vaccines?

Some individuals experience local skin reactions such as redness and swelling that may suggest a delayed-type of minor allergic reaction following injection with products containing thimerosal. Research suggests that most people who have a contact or skin allergy to thimerosal will not have the reaction when thimerosal is injected under the skin (Forstrom, 1980; Jacobs 1982). A prior history of a minor reaction to thimerosal in a vaccine is not considered a contraindication to further vaccination with thimerosal-containing vaccines. Severe anaphylactic (allergic) reaction to any vaccine is a contraindication to further vaccination with the vaccine.

Do measles, mumps, and rubella (MMR) vaccines contain thimerosal?

No, MMR vaccine does not and never did contain thimerosal. Varicella (chickenpox), inactivated polio (IPV), and pneumococcal conjugate vaccines have also never contained thimerosal.

Why are chemicals and other substances added to vaccines?

Many foods and medicines, including vaccines, have chemicals added to them to prevent the growth of germs, reduce spoilage, and prevent it from losing its potency over time.

Some additives are used in the production of vaccines. Vaccines may include suspending fluid (e.g., sterile water, saline, or fluids containing protein); preservatives and stabilizers (e.g., albumin, phenols, and glycine); and adjuvants, or enhancers, that help the vaccine improve its immunogenicity (ability to protect against disease).

For more information on additives, visit: http://www.cdc.gov/nip/vacsafe/concerns/gen/additives.htm.

How can I find out what chemical additives are in specific vaccines?

Ask your healthcare provider or pharmacist for a copy of the vaccine package insert. The package insert lists ingredients in the vaccine and discusses any known adverse reactions.

Availability of Thimerosal-Free Vaccines

Which vaccines do not contain thimerosal?

Today, all vaccines in the recommended childhood immunization schedule that are for use in the U.S. market contain no thimerosal or only trace amounts. (Those with a concentration of less than 0.0002% contain what is considered "trace," or insignificant, amounts.) Influenza (flu) vaccines and tetanus and diphtheria vaccines (Td and DT) are not available without thimerosal. For more information on thimerosal content in some currently manufactured U.S. licensed vaccines, visit http://www.fda.gov/cber/vaccine/thimerosal.htm.

Why weren't thimerosal-containing vaccines taken off the market?

Scientific data have not established that vaccines containing thimerosal, used as a preservative, create an imminent or substantial hazard to public health or are in violation of FDA laws or regulations, and therefore do not justify such a recall. A mandatory recall requires that the product present "an imminent or substantial hazard to the public health."

The U.S. Food and Drug Administration (FDA) is responsible for voluntary and mandatory recalls of drug and vaccine products. The FDA continuously monitors the safety of these products.

Should immunization providers stop using licensed pediatric vaccines that contain thimerosal?

No. Immunization providers should use the vaccines available in their stock. The use of vaccines should continue according to the currently recommended schedule. The risks of not vaccinating children on time are significant, whereas the risks of thimerosal-containing vaccines have not been proven scientifically. Furthermore, availability of any vaccine containing thimerosal preservative is rare.

What is the availability of the thimerosal-free hepatitis B vaccine?

All hepatitis B vaccines intended for use in infants and children are free of thimerosal as a preservative, and an adequate supply of these vaccines is available for all infant and childhood vaccinations. This vaccine should be administered to all newborn infants and is a major cornerstone in the prevention of a potentially fatal disease in children and adults.

Are there adequate supplies of thimerosal-free vaccines to meet national demand?

Yes, there are sufficient supplies of thimerosal-free vaccines to assure an uninterrupted supply to meet national demand. Because of the expiration date of current vaccines, it is believed that few, if any, of those containing thimerosal preservative are still being administered. Thus, only pediatric thimerosal preservative-free vaccines may be available for use in the immediate future.

Chapter 65

National Vaccine Injury Compensation Program

Background

In the early 1980s, reports of harmful side effects following the DTP (diphtheria, tetanus, pertussis) vaccine posed major liability concerns for vaccine companies and health care providers, and caused many to question the safety of the DTP vaccine. Parents began filing many more lawsuits against vaccine companies and health care providers. Vaccination rates among children began to fall and many companies that develop and produce vaccines decided to leave the marketplace, creating significant vaccine shortages and a real threat to the nation's health.

The dilemma facing the nation was so great that Congress decided to act. A coalition of physicians, public health organizations, leaders of industry, government representatives and private citizens developed the idea of a no-fault alternative to the tort system for resolving vaccine injury claims. Lawmakers passed the National Childhood Vaccine Injury Act of 1986 (P. L.99–660), which established the National Vaccine Injury Compensation Program (VICP).

The VICP is administered jointly by the U.S. Department of Health and Human Services (HHS), the U.S. Court of Federal Claims (the Court), and the U.S. Department of Justice (DOJ). The VICP is located

---

"National Vaccine Injury Compensation Program," November 2002, and "Commonly Asked Questions about the National Vaccine Injury Compensation Program," December 2002, Health Resources and Services Administration (HRSA), Department of Health and Human Services.

in the Division of Vaccine Injury Compensation, Health Resources and Services Administration, HHS.

Overview

Congress created the VICP to ensure an adequate supply of vaccines, stabilize vaccine costs, and establish and maintain an accessible and efficient forum for individuals thought to be injured by childhood vaccines. The VICP, which went into effect on October 1, 1988, is a no-fault alternative to the traditional tort system for resolving vaccine injury claims, whether the vaccine is administered in the public or private sector. Since its inception, the VICP has been a key component in stabilizing the U.S. vaccine market by providing liability protection to both vaccine companies and health care providers, by encouraging research and development of new and safer vaccines, and by providing for a more streamlined and "less adversarial" alternative to the traditional tort system for resolving claims. The VICP covers all vaccines recommended by the Centers for Disease Control and Prevention for routine administration to children. The vaccines currently covered include: diphtheria, tetanus, pertussis (DTP, DTaP, DT, TT or Td), measles, mumps, rubella (MMR or any components), polio (OPV or IPV), hepatitis B, haemophilus influenza type b (Hib), varicella, rotavirus, and pneumococcal conjugate.

The 9-member Advisory Commission on Childhood Vaccines (ACCV) provides oversight of the VICP. Members recommend ways to improve the VICP, including changing the Vaccine Injury Table, proposing legislation, covering new and safer childhood vaccines, gathering information about vaccine-related injuries from federal, state, and local immunization programs, and revising vaccine information statement and adverse reaction reporting requirements.

The Vaccine Injury Table

There are three means of qualifying for compensation: 1) a petitioner must show that an injury listed on the Vaccine Injury Table (the Table) occurred; 2) a petitioner must prove that the vaccine significantly aggravated a pre existing condition; or 3) a petitioner must prove that the vaccine caused the condition.

The Table lists specific injuries or conditions and the time frames in which they must occur after vaccine administration. The Table is a legal mechanism for defining complex medical conditions and allows a statutory "presumption of causation." The Table serves as the basis for presumptions of causation for vaccines covered under the VICP. It is much easier to demonstrate a Table injury than to prove that the vaccine caused the condition. However, if an adverse event is not listed on the Table, an individual may still file a claim but must prove that the vaccine did "in fact" cause the alleged injury. Compensation may not be awarded if the Court determines that the injury or death was due to an alternative cause unrelated to the vaccine, even if a Table injury is demonstrated.

Filing a Claim

An individual claiming a vaccine-related injury or death files a petition for compensation with the Court, and is often represented by an attorney (which is not a requirement). The Secretary of HHS is named as the Respondent. As of February 1, 1991, the time has expired for filing claims for injuries resulting from vaccines administered prior to October 1, 1988. Any claims filed for that time period are subject to dismissal by the Court. For injuries or deaths resulting from a vaccine administered on or after October 1, 1988, the following restrictions apply:

- In the case of an injury, the claim must be filed within 36 months after the first symptoms appeared. The effects of the injury must have lasted at least 6 months after the vaccine administration, or the injury must have resulted in inpatient hospitalization and surgical intervention.
- In the case of a death, the claim must be filed within 24 months of the death, and within 48 months after the onset of the vaccine-related injury from which the death occurred.

An HHS physician reviews each petition to determine whether it meets the medical criteria for compensation. This recommendation is provided to the Court through a Respondent's report filed by the DOJ. The HHS position is presented by an attorney from the DOJ in hearings before a "special master" who makes the decision for compensation under the VICP. A special master is an attorney appointed by the judges of the Court. Decisions may be appealed to the Court, then to the Federal Circuit Court of Appeals, and eventually to the U.S. Supreme Court.

If a case is found eligible for compensation, the amount of the award is usually negotiated between the DOJ and the petitioner's attorneys. If the attorneys can't agree, the case is scheduled for a hearing for the special master to assess the amount of compensation. Compensable

Table 65.1. Vaccine Injury Table (Effective August 26, 2002)

Vaccine	Adverse Event	Time Period
Tetanus-containing (DTaP, DTP, DT, Td, TT)	Anaphylaxis or anaphylactic shock	0–4 hours
	Brachial neuritis	2–28 days
Pertussis antigen-containing (DTaP, DTP, P, DTP-Hib)	Anaphylaxis or anaphylactic shock	0–4 hours
	Encephalopathy (or encephalitis)	0–72 hours
MMR or in any combination (MMR, MR, M, R)	Anaphylaxis or anaphylactic shock	0–4 hours
	Encephalopathy	5–15 days
Rubella-containing (MMR, MR, R)	Chronic Arthritis	7–42 days
Measles-containing (MMR, MR, M)	Thrombocytopenic purpura	7–30 days
	Vaccine-strain measles viral infection in an immunodeficient receipt	0–6 months
OPV	Paralytic polio (recipient and community contact cases)	0–30 days/0–6 months*
	Vaccine-strain polio viral infection	0–30 days/0–6 months*

IPV	Anaphylaxis or anaphylactic shock	0–4 hours
Hepatitis B	Anaphylaxis or anaphylactic shock	0–4 hours
Hib (conjugate)	No condition specified	Not applicable**
Varicella	No condition specified	Not applicable**
Rotavirus	No condition specified	Not applicable**
Live, oral, rhesus-based rotavirus vaccine	Intussusception	0–30 days
Pneumococcal conjugate vaccines	No condition specified	Not applicable**
New vaccines	No condition specified	Not applicable**

*Time intervals for immunocompetent/immunodeficient individuals who receive OPV. Contact cases have no time limit.

**No condition has been identified requiring inclusion on the Vaccine Injury Table; and therefore, compensation for alleged injuries must be pursued on a causation in fact basis.

claims, and even most claims found to be non-compensable, are awarded reimbursement for attorney's fees and costs. A petitioner may file a claim in civil court against the vaccine company and/or the vaccine administrator only after first filing a claim under the VICP and then rejecting the decision of the Court.

Commonly Asked Questions about the National Vaccine Injury Compensation Program

What is the National Vaccine Injury Compensation Program (VICP)?

The National Childhood Vaccine Injury Act of 1986, as amended, (the Act) established the VICP. The VICP went into effect on October 1, 1988 and is a Federal "no-fault" system designed to compensate individuals or families of individuals, who have been injured by covered childhood vaccines, whether administered in the private or public sector.

What vaccines are covered?

Diphtheria, tetanus, pertussis (DTP, DTaP, DT, TT, or Td), measles, mumps, rubella (MMR or any components), polio (OPV or IPV), hepatitis B, Haemophilus influenzae type b (Hib), varicella (chicken pox), rotavirus and pneumococcal conjugate vaccines. Eight years' retroactive coverage is provided for any vaccine or vaccine-related adverse event added for coverage under the VICP.

The only live, oral, rhesus-based rotavirus vaccine licensed in the U.S., which was routinely distributed beginning on October 1, 1998, was withdrawn from the market on October 15, 1999, and is no longer being administered in the U.S. Because the Secretary of Health and Human Services determined that a causal link existed between this vaccine and the injury of intussusception, the Secretary modified the Vaccine Injury Table (the Table) to add the injury of intussusception.

Specifically, effective as of August 26, 2002, the Secretary added vaccines containing live, oral, rhesus-based rotavirus as a separate category to the Table, with an associated injury of intussusception. Prior to this date, the Table already contained the general category of rotavirus vaccines, with no associated Table injury. The new Table injury of intussusception applies to all cases in which the injury occurred within 30 days of the administration of the vaccine, provided that the rotavirus vaccine was administered on or before August 26, 2002.

Under current law, petitioners may be eligible for compensation for vaccine-related intussusceptions if the condition: (i) had residual effects or complications lasting for more than 6 months; (ii) resulted in inpatient hospitalization and surgery; or (iii) resulted in death.

Petitioners wishing to file claims relating to injuries (or deaths) thought to be related to a rotavirus vaccine must generally comply with the statute of limitations contained at 42 U.S.C. 300aa-16 (which provides that injury claims must be filed within 36 months of the date of the first symptom or manifestation of the onset or significant aggravation of the injury). If the addition of the Table injury of intussusception will significantly increase a petitioner's likelihood of obtaining compensation with the VICP, a petitioner is also entitled to file a claim within 2 years of the effective date of the Table change (August 26, 2002), so long as the underlying vaccine-related injury or death occurred within an 8-year period before that date.

How are new vaccines added for coverage under the VICP?

On March 24, 1997, a final rule was published which, in part, provided for the "automatic" addition of future vaccines recommended by the Centers for Disease Control and Prevention (CDC) for routine administration to children. However, Congress will still need to set an appropriate excise tax on any new vaccines recommended by CDC before those vaccines are effectively covered under the Vaccine Injury Compensation Program. Under the current statutory language, 8 years' retroactive coverage will be provided for those claiming injury or death resulting from a vaccine or vaccine-related adverse event newly added to the VICP.

Who may file a claim?

Any injured individual or a parent, legal guardian, or trustee of an injured child or an incapacitated person may file a claim. A claim may be made for any injury or death thought to be a result of a covered vaccine. These injuries may include, but are not limited to: anaphylaxis, paralytic polio, and encephalopathy.

How does the VICP work?

The VICP is administered jointly by the U.S. Court of Federal Claims (the Court), the Department of Health and Human Services (HHS), and the Department of Justice (DOJ). The process is as follows:

- An individual claiming injury or death from a vaccine files a petition for compensation with the Court;

- A physician at the Division of Vaccine Injury Compensation, HHS, reviews each petition to determine whether it meets the criteria for compensation. This recommendation is provided to the Court through a report filed by the DOJ, although it is not binding.
- The HHS position is represented by an attorney from the DOJ in hearings before a "special master" who makes the initial decision for compensation under the VICP. A special master is an attorney appointed by the judges of the Court.
- Decisions may be appealed to the Court and then to the Federal Circuit Court of Appeals.

How is eligibility for compensation determined?

There are three means to qualify for compensation:

- A petitioner must show that an injury found on the Vaccine Injury Table (the Table) occurred; or
- A petitioner must prove that the vaccine caused the condition; or
- A petitioner must prove that the vaccine significantly aggravated a pre-existing condition.

The Table lists specific injuries or conditions and the time frames in which they must occur after vaccine administration. The Table is a legal mechanism for defining complex medical conditions and allows a statutory "presumption of causation." It is much easier to demonstrate a "Table Injury" than to prove that the vaccine caused the condition, and most claims allege that a Table Injury occurred. Compensation is not awarded, however, if the Court determines that the injury or death was due to a cause unrelated to the vaccine, even if it was a Table Injury.

In contrast to civil liability suits, hearings to determine eligibility under the VICP usually last only 1 or 2 days. A case found eligible for compensation is scheduled for a hearing to assess the amount of compensation. Most claims found to be noncompensable receive awards for attorney's fees and costs.

What is the amount of an award under the VICP?

Awards to the estate in a vaccine-related death are limited to $250,000 plus attorney's fees and costs. Awards to individuals with an injury judged to be vaccine-related have averaged $824,463. There is no limitation on the amount of an award in a vaccine-related injury; however, the law does contain certain restrictions.

How does the VICP protect vaccine administrators and vaccine manufacturers?

The Act requires that vaccine injury claims involving covered vaccines given on or after October 1, 1988 must first be filed with the VICP before civil litigation through the tort system can be pursued. If a petitioner accepts an award under the VICP, the claim cannot be brought subsequently to the tort system.

Under what circumstances may a vaccine administrator or manufacturer be sued?

- If the petition has been judged non-compensable or dismissed under the VICP; or
- If the award granted by the VICP is otherwise rejected by the petitioner; or
- If the vaccine is not covered under the VICP.

Have there been changes to the Vaccine Injury Table?

On March 10, 1995, a modified Table (and the accompanying Qualifications and Aids to Interpretation) became effective for all claims filed on or after that date. Significant changes include the addition of chronic arthritis under vaccines containing rubella (e.g., MMR, MR, R vaccines), and the removal of Residual Seizure Disorder and Hypotonic-Hyporesponsive Episode (HHE) under the DTP vaccine. The definition of Encephalopathy was clarified in the Qualifications and Aids to Interpretation.

On March 24, 1997, further modifications to the Table took effect that include the addition of brachial neuritis and removal of encephalopathy for tetanus-containing vaccines, addition of thrombocytopenia and vaccine-strain measles virus infection, removal of residual seizure disorder for measles-containing vaccines, and addition of vaccine-strain poliovirus infection for live polio virus vaccine. Modifications also included the addition of three new vaccines: hepatitis B, Haemophilus influenzae type b, and varicella. Coverage for these three new vaccines went into effect August 6, 1997. The Rule also provided for "automatic" addition of future vaccines recommended by the Centers for Disease Control and Prevention for routine administration to children, although injuries for such vaccines will be specified only after additional rulemaking. All other Table changes became effective for all claims filed on or after March 24.

On October 22, 1998, rotavirus vaccine was added to the Table for coverage.

On August 26, 2002, a modified Table (and the accompanying Qualifications and Aids to Interpretation) became effective for all claims filed on or after that date. A second category of rotavirus (live, oral, rhesus-based) vaccine was added to the Table with intussusception listed as an injury with a time interval of onset of 0–30 days. A separate category was added for pneumococcal conjugate vaccines with no condition specified. Haemophilus influenzae type b (Hib) polysaccharide vaccines was removed from the Table; however, Haemophilus influenzae type b (Hib) conjugate vaccines remains on the Table with no condition specified. Under the Table's Qualifications and Aids to Interpretation, early-onset Hib disease and residual seizure disorder were removed.

What documentation are vaccine administrators required to keep?

The National Childhood Vaccine Injury Act of 1986 (as amended) requires that the date of administration; vaccine manufacturer; lot number; and name, address, and title of the health care provider be recorded in the patient's permanent medical record.

What adverse events are health care providers required to report?

The Vaccine Adverse Event Reporting System (VAERS), operated by the Food and Drug Administration (FDA) and the CDC, should be notified of any adverse event by completing a VAERS reporting form. The following events are required to be reported:

- Any event set forth in the Vaccine Injury Table that occurs within the time period specified or within 7 days, if that is longer.
- Any contraindicating event listed in the manufacturer's package insert.

In addition, VAERS accepts all reports by any interested party of real or suspected adverse events occurring after the administration of any vaccine.

The VAERS form may be obtained by calling 1-800-822-7967 or from the FDA website at http://www.hrsa.gov/osp/vicp/www.fda.gov/cber/vaers/report.htm.

Please note: Submitting a reporting form to VAERS in not the same as filing a claim under the VICP as they are two separate programs.

How many petitions have been filed under the VICP? Of those petitions filed, how many have been awarded compensation? How much money has been spent on compensation awards?

To obtain a copy of the most recent VICP "Monthly Statistics Report" please visit the VICP Website at http://www.hrsa.gov/osp/vicp/www.hrsa.gov/osp/vicp/monthly.htm, telephone 1-800-338-2382, or write to the National Vaccine Injury Compensation Program, Parklawn Building, Room 16C-17, 5600 Fishers Lane, Rockville, Maryland 20857.

If I believe that the thimerosal (mercury) in a vaccine caused an injury or death, can I file a claim with the VICP?

For vaccines covered under the VICP, individuals alleging that the thimerosal in a vaccine caused an injury or death must first file a claim with the VICP before any civil litigation can be pursued. According to section 2133 of the Public Health Service Act (42 U.S.C. 300aa-33(5)), a "vaccine-related injury or death" eligible for compensation under the VICP does not include an injury or death associated with an adulterant or contaminant intentionally added to a vaccine. Components, such as thimerosal, that are added to microorganisms to create vaccines cannot and should not be considered adulterants or contaminants. Instead, preservatives and components, such as thimerosal, should be considered one of several elements that comprise vaccines.

Because thimerosal is not an adulterant to or a contaminant in vaccines, individuals who have claims relating to thimerosal in vaccines covered under the VICP are not statutorily barred from filing claims with the VICP. As such, the Department of Health and Human Services (HHS) believes individuals interested in filing such a claim must first file the claim with the VICP before pursuing any other civil litigation.

On October 11, the U.S. Court of Federal Claims (the Court) ruled that thimerosal-related injury claims are subject to the Court's jurisdiction pursuant to the National Childhood Vaccine Injury Act of 1986, as amended. Plaintiffs had filed a petition for compensation in the Court, but then filed a motion to challenge the jurisdiction of the Court for thimerosal-related injuries. The Court found the plaintiff's arguments to be without merit. As such, the Court's Chief Special Master accepted HHS's arguments and found that the Court's jurisdiction was mandated on all fronts. Leroy v. Secretary of HHS is the first definitive statement by the Court that thimerosal-related vaccine injury claims are subject to its jurisdiction. For further information on the "Omnibus Autism Proceeding, visit the Court's Website at http://www.uscfc.uscourts.gov/osmPage.htm.

Where can I get information about anthrax or smallpox vaccines?

Currently, the anthrax and smallpox vaccines are not covered under the VICP. To obtain information about these vaccines, contact the National Immunization Program, Centers for Disease Control and Prevention (CDC) at 1600 Clifton Road, N.E., Mail Stop E-61, Atlanta, Georgia 30333. You may also contact them at 1-800-232-2522 or visit their Internet Website at: http://www.hrsa.gov/osp/vicp/www.cdc.gov/nip.

Contact Information

For further information regarding the VICP:

National Vaccine Injury Compensation Program
Parklawn Building
5600 Fishers Lane
Room 16C-17
Rockville, Maryland 20857
Phone: 800-338-2382

For information on the Rules of the Court, including requirements for filing a petition visit the Court's Website at http://www.uscfc.uscourts.gov/osmPage.htm or contact:

Clerk, U.S. Court of Federal Claims
717 Madison Place, N.W.
Washington, D.C. 20005
Phone: 202-219-9657

Chapter 66

Vaccine Adverse Event Reporting System (VAERS)

Overview

The Vaccine Adverse Event Reporting System (VAERS) is a valuable tool for post-marketing safety surveillance (monitoring after a product has been approved and is on the market). Although extensive studies are required for licensure of new vaccines, post-marketing research and surveillance are necessary to identify safety issues that may only be detected following vaccination of a much larger and more diverse population. Rare events may not come to light before licensure. Sometimes an event is noted, but the evidence may not be adequate to conclude that a noted event is due to the vaccine.

VAERS is a program created as an outgrowth of the National Childhood Vaccine Injury Act of 1986 (NCVIA) and is administered by the Food and Drug Administration (FDA) and Centers for Disease Control and Prevention (CDC). VAERS accepts reports of adverse events that may be associated with U.S. licensed vaccines from health care providers, manufacturers, and the public. The FDA continually monitors VAERS reports for any unexpected patterns or changes in rates of adverse events.

The report of an adverse event to VAERS is not proof that a vaccine caused the event. More than ten million vaccinations per year are given to children less than one year old, usually between 2 months

---

This chapter includes "Vaccine Adverse Event Report System (VAERS) Overview," and "Vaccine Adverse Event Report System (VAERS) Frequently Asked Questions," U.S. Food and Drug Administration (FDA), April 2003.

and 6 months of age. At this stage of development infants are at risk for a variety of medical events and serious childhood illnesses. These naturally occurring events include fevers, seizures, sudden infant death syndrome (SIDS), cancer, congenital heart disease, asthma, and other conditions. Some infants coincidentally experience an adverse event shortly after a vaccination. In such situations an infection, congenital abnormality, injury, or some other provocation may cause the event. Because of such coincidences, it is usually not possible from VAERS data alone to determine whether a particular adverse event resulted from a concurrent condition or from a vaccination—even when the event occurs soon after vaccination. Doctors and other vaccine providers are encouraged to report adverse events, whether or not they believe that the vaccination was the cause. If the VAERS data suggest a possible link between an adverse event and vaccination, the relationship may be further studied in a controlled fashion.

Analyzing VAERS reports is a complex task. Children are often administered more than one vaccine at a time, making it difficult to know which vaccine, if any, may have contributed to any subsequent adverse events. While about 85% of adverse events reported to VAERS are minor (such as mild fevers or redness and swelling at the injection site), the remaining 15% describe more serious events. The more serious events include hospitalizations, life-threatening events, and deaths. As part of the VAERS program, FDA reviews the deaths and serious reports weekly, and conducts follow up. In some cases, certain vaccines and potentially associated symptoms will receive more intense follow up.

In addition to analyzing individual VAERS reports, the FDA also analyzes patterns of reporting associated with vaccine lots. Many complex factors must be considered in comparing reports between different vaccine lots. More reports may be received for a large lot than for a small one simply because more doses of vaccine from the large lot will be given to more children. Some lots contain as many as 700,000 doses, while others as few as 20,000 doses. Similarly, more reports will be received for a lot that has been in use for a long time than for a lot that has been in use for a short time. Even among lots of similar size and time in use, some lots will receive more reports than others will simply due to chance. The FDA continually looks for lots that have received more death reports than would be expected on the basis of such factors as time in use and chance variation as well as any unusual patterns in other serious reports within a lot. If such a lot is detected, further review is conducted to determine if the lot continues to be safe for use, or if additional FDA actions are needed.

Frequently Asked Questions

Who can report to VAERS?

Anyone can report to VAERS. VAERS reports are usually submitted by health care providers, vaccine manufacturers, vaccine recipients (or their parents/guardians) and state immunization programs. Patients, parents, and guardians are encouraged to seek the help of a health-care professional in reporting to VAERS.

Why should I report to VAERS?

VAERS is a valuable tool for post-marketing safety surveillance. Each report provides valuable information that is added to the VAERS database. Complete reporting of post-vaccination events supplies public health professionals with the information they need to ensure the safest strategies of vaccine administration.

What events should be reported to VAERS?

VAERS encourages the reporting of any significant adverse event occurring after the administration of any vaccine licensed in the United States. You should report any significant adverse event even if you are unsure whether a vaccine caused the event.

The National Childhood Vaccine Injury Act (NCVIA) requires health care providers to report:

- Any event listed by the vaccine manufacturer as a contraindication to subsequent doses of the vaccine.
- Any event listed in the Reportable Events Table that occurs within the specified time period after vaccination.

The Reportable Events Table specifically outlines the reportable post-vaccination events and the time frames in which they must occur in order to qualify as being reportable. To obtain a copy of the Reportable Events Table, call 1-800-822-7967 or go to http://www.vaers.org/reportable.htm.

How are VAERS reports analyzed?

Both the CDC and the FDA review data reported to VAERS. The FDA reviews reports to assess whether a reported event is adequately reflected in product labeling, and closely monitors reporting trends for individual vaccine lots. Approximately 85% of the reports describe mild events such as fever, local reactions, episodes of crying or mild irritability, and other less serious experiences. The remaining 15% of the reports reflect serious adverse events involving life-threatening conditions, hospitalization, permanent disability, or death, which may or may not have been truly caused by an immunization.

Can information reported to VAERS cause a recall of a vaccine?

The FDA has the authority to recall a vaccine from use in the United States if they feel it represents a risk to the American public. VAERS reports may signal that there is the potential for a safety risk, which would prompt a wider evaluation of the safety of the vaccine lot. If the evaluation confirms a risk, the batch can be recalled.

Are all events reported to VAERS caused by vaccinations?

No. Because VAERS accepts all reports of adverse events following vaccination, not all events reported to VAERS are caused by vaccines. Some events may occur coincidentally after the administration of a vaccine while others may in fact be caused by a vaccine. Studies help determine if there is more than a temporal (time) association between immunization and adverse events. An occurrence of an adverse event following the administration of a vaccine is not conclusive evidence that the event was caused by the vaccine. Various factors (e.g., medical history, other medications given near the time of the vaccination) must be examined to determine if they could have caused the adverse event. Many adverse events reported to VAERS may not be caused by vaccines.

What if I can't tell if a reaction was caused by a vaccine or another medication?

We encourage you to report any reaction following vaccination to VAERS, even if you cannot tell if the vaccine or another product caused it. Reports sent to the VAERS program that also make reference to non-vaccine pharmaceutical products are shared with MedWatch, the FDA's drug safety surveillance system.

How do I find out if a vaccine adverse event has been reported to VAERS?

The Freedom of Information Office can be contacted to obtain specific data from VAERS. The requester will be billed for the cost of retrieving and copying the data. You can request information about adverse events reported to VAERS by faxing requests to (301) 443-1726, or by sending requests to:

Food and Drug Administration
Freedom of Information Staff (HFI-35)
5600 Fishers Lane
Rockville, MD 20857
(301) 827-6500

Is VAERS involved in the Vaccine Injury Compensation Program?

No. The National Childhood Vaccine Injury Act created the Vaccine Injury Compensation Program (VICP) to compensate individuals whose injuries may have been caused by vaccines recommended by the CDC for routine use. VICP is separate from the VAERS program. Reporting an event to VAERS does not file a claim for compensation to the VICP. A petition must be filed with VICP to start a claim for compensation. For more information call (800) 338-2382, or go to http://www.hrsa.gov/osp/vicp.

Chapter 67

Autism and Vaccines

Frequently Asked Questions about MMR Vaccine and Autism

The weight of currently available scientific evidence does not support the hypothesis that MMR (measles, mumps, and rubella) vaccine causes autism. The Centers for Disease Control and Prevention (CDC) recognizes there is considerable public interest in this issue, and therefore supports additional research regarding this hypothesis. CDC is committed to maintaining the safest, most effective vaccine supply in history.

What is autism?

Autism is a term that refers to a collection of neurologically-based developmental disorders in which individuals have impairments in social interaction and communication skills, along with a tendency to have repetitive behaviors or interests. The severity of autism varies greatly, from individuals with little speech and poor daily living skills, to others who function well in most settings. Autism is typically diagnosed during the toddler or preschool years, although some children are diagnosed at older ages. It has been reported that approximately 20 percent of children with autism experience a "regression;" that is,

---

"FAQs (frequently asked questions) about MMR (Measles, Mumps, and Rubella) Vaccine and Autism," National Immunization Program, Centers for Disease Control and Prevention (CDC), February 12, 2003.

they have apparently normal development followed by a loss of communication and social skills. Boys are three-to-four times more likely to have autism than girls. Autism occurs in all racial, ethnic, and social groups. A variety of factors could be associated with some forms of autism, including infectious, metabolic, genetic, neurological, and environmental factors. Genetic factors and brain abnormalities at birth are considered to be some of the most recognized causes of autism.

Does the measles-mumps-rubella (MMR) vaccine cause autism?

Current scientific evidence does not support the hypothesis that measles-mumps-rubella (MMR) vaccine, or any combination of vaccines, causes the development of autism, including regressive forms of autism. The question about a possible link between MMR vaccine and autism has been extensively reviewed by independent groups of experts in the U.S. including the National Academy of Sciences, Institute of Medicine. These reviews have concluded that the available epidemiologic evidence does not support a causal link between MMR vaccine and autism.

What have studies found regarding MMR vaccine and autism?

Epidemiologic studies have shown no relationship between MMR vaccination in children and development of autism:

- In 1997, the National Childhood Encephalopathy Study (NCES) was examined to see if there was any link between measles vaccine and neurological events. The researchers found no indication that measles vaccine contributes to the development of long-term neurological damage, including educational and behavioral deficits (Miller et al., 1997).
- A study by Gillberg and Heijbel (1998) examined the prevalence of autism in children born in Sweden from 1975–1984. There was no difference in the prevalence of autism among children born before the introduction of the MMR vaccine in Sweden and those born after the vaccine was introduced.
- In 1999, the British Committee on Safety of Medicines convened a “Working Party on MMR Vaccine” to conduct a systematic review of reports of autism, gastrointestinal disease, and similar

disorders after receipt of MMR or measles/rubella vaccine. It was concluded that the available information did not support the posited associations between MMR and autism and other disorders.

- Taylor and colleagues (1999) studied 498 children with autism in the UK and found the age at which they were diagnosed was the same regardless of whether they received the MMR vaccine before or after 18 months of age or whether they were never vaccinated. Importantly, the first signs or diagnoses of autism were not more likely to occur within time periods following MMR vaccination than during other time periods. Also, there was no sudden increase in cases of autism after the introduction of MMR vaccine in the UK. Such a jump would have been expected if MMR vaccine was causing a substantial increase in autism.
- Kaye and colleagues (2001) assessed the relationship between the risk of autism among children in the UK and MMR vaccine. Among a subgroup of boys aged 2–5 years, the risk of autism increased almost 4 fold from 1988 to 1993, while MMR vaccination coverage remained constant at approximately 95% over these same years.
- Researchers in the U.S. found that among children born between 1980 and 1994 and enrolled in California kindergartens, there was a 373% relative increase in autism cases, though the relative increase in MMR vaccine coverage by the age of 24 months was only 14% (Dales et al., 2001). For more on this study, see California Data on Theory of Autism and MMR Immunization.
- Researchers in the UK (Frombonne & Chakrabarti, 2001) conducted a study to test the idea that a new form, or "new variant," of Inflammatory Bowel Disease (IBD) exists. This new variant IBD has been described as a combination of developmental regression and gastrointestinal symptoms occurring shortly after MMR immunization. Information on 96 children (95 immunized with MMR) who were born between 1992 and 1995 and were diagnosed with pervasive developmental disorder were compared with data from 2 groups of autistic patients (one group of 98 born before MMR was ever used and one group of 68 who were likely to have received MMR vaccine). No evidence was found to support a new syndrome of MMR-induced

IBD/autism. For instance, the researchers found that there were no differences between vaccinated and unvaccinated groups with regard to when their parents first became concerned about their child's development. Similarly, the rate of developmental regression reported in the vaccinated and unvaccinated groups was not different; therefore, there was no suggestion that developmental regression had increased in frequency since MMR was introduced. Of the 96 children in the first group, no inflammatory bowel disorder was reported. Furthermore, there was no association found between developmental regression and gastrointestinal symptoms.

- Another group of researchers in the UK (Taylor et al., 2002) also examined whether MMR vaccination is associated with bowel problems and developmental regression in children with autism, looking for evidence of a "new variant" form of IBD/autism. The study included 278 cases of children with autism and 195 with atypical autism (cases with many of the features of childhood autism but not quite meeting the required criteria for that diagnosis, or with atypical features such as onset of symptoms after the age of 3 years). The cases included in this study were born between 1979 and 1998. The proportion of children with developmental regression or bowel symptoms did not change significantly from 1979 to 1988, a period which included the introduction of MMR vaccination in the UK in 1988. No significant difference was found in rates of bowel problems or regression in children who received the MMR vaccine before their parents became concerned about their development, compared with those who received it only after such concern and those who had not received the MMR vaccine. The findings provide no support for an MMR associated "new variant" form of autism and further evidence against involvement of MMR vaccine in autism.
- Madsen et al. (2002) conducted a study of all children born in Denmark from January 1991 through December 1998. There were a total of 537,303 children in the study; 440,655 of the children were vaccinated with MMR and 96,648 were not. The researchers did not find a higher risk of autism in the vaccinated than in the unvaccinated group of children. Furthermore, there was no association between the age at time of vaccination, the amount of time that had passed since vaccination, or the date of vaccination and the development of any autistic disorder.

Though there were many more vaccinated than unvaccinated children in the study group, the sample was large enough to contain more statistical power than other MMR and autism studies. Therefore, this study provides strong evidence against the hypothesis that MMR vaccination causes autism.

Are there studies that suggest there might be a connection between autism and MMR vaccine?

The existing studies that suggest a causal relationship between MMR vaccine and autism have generated media attention. However, these studies have significant weaknesses and are far outweighed by the epidemiologic studies described above that have consistently failed to show a causal relationship between MMR vaccine and autism.

- The MMR-autism theory is based on the idea that intestinal problems, like Crohn's disease, are the result of viral infection and can contribute to the development of autism. The theory has its origins in research by Wakefield and colleagues (1989; 1990) which suggested that inflammatory bowel disease (IBD) is linked to persistent viral infection.
- In 1993, Wakefield and colleagues reported isolating measles virus in the intestinal tissue of persons with IBD. However, the validity of this finding was later called into question when it could not be reproduced by other researchers (Afzal, 1998; Iizuka et al., 2000).
- Thompson and colleagues (1995) suggested in a retrospective cohort study that MMR vaccine might be a risk factor for Crohn's disease. However, the selection and recall biases and the differences in data collection in this study were so substantial as to cast doubt on the validity of the findings.
- Two studies out of Sweden linked measles infection *in utero* to the development of IBD (Ekbom et al., 1994; Ekbom et al., 1996). However, these studies involved a very small number of cases and when researchers identified the persons to be included in the 1996 study, they had prior knowledge that cases of Crohn's disease had occurred in the offspring of two women who were infected with measles during pregnancy. This is called "selection bias" and limits the strength of the study.
- The MMR-autism theory came to the forefront when, in 1998, Wakefield and colleagues reviewed reports of children with

bowel disease and regressive developmental disorders, mostly autism. The researchers suggested that MMR vaccination led to intestinal abnormalities, resulting in impaired intestinal function and developmental regression within 24 hours to a few weeks of vaccination. This hypothesis was based on 12 children. In 9 of the cases, the child's parents or pediatrician speculated that the MMR vaccine had contributed to the behavioral problems of the children in the study. There are a number of limitations in the Wakefield et al. (1998) study:

1. The study used too few cases to make any generalizations about the causes of autism; only 12 children were included in the study. Further, the cases were referred to the researchers and may not be a representative sample of cases of autism.
2. There were no healthy control children for comparison. As a result, it is difficult to determine whether the bowel changes seen in the 12 children included in the study were similar to changes in normal children, or to determine if the rate of vaccination in autistic children was higher than in the general population.
3. The study did not identify the time period during which the cases were identified.
4. In at least 4 of the 12 cases, behavioral problems appeared before the onset of symptoms of bowel disease; that is, the effect preceded the proposed cause. It is unlikely, therefore, that bowel disease or the MMR vaccine triggered the autism.

- In another study that generated media attention and raised public concern in the UK (Uhlmann et al, 2002), researchers found measles virus fragments in the intestines of children with "new variant" IBD (children with both IBD and developmental disorder). Scientists looked for the presence of measles virus in the intestinal tissue of 91 children with new variant IBD and 70 "controls" (children without this type of IBD). The researchers found measles virus fragments in 75 out of the 91 children with "new variant" IBD, and in only 5 of the 70 controls. While this provides evidence for an association between the presence of measles virus and IBD in children with developmental disorder, it does not mean that the measles component of the MMR vaccine causes IBD or developmental disorder. As a commentary published with the article asserts, the data could just as easily be interpreted as indicating that the IBD or the developmental disorder cause the persistence of measles in the intestines (Morris & Aldulaimi, 2002). In addition, the researchers did not compare the virus found in the intestines of patients with the virus used in the MMR vaccine; nor did they provide information regarding whether or not the children in the study had been previously vaccinated with MMR or had previously contracted measles disease. The limitations of this study are further discussed in a letter written by the Director of CDC's National Immunization Program to the UK's Chief Medical Officer.

What about the claim that the number of children with autism has been increasing ever since the MMR vaccine has been in use?

Data from California (Department. of Developmental Services, 1999) have been used to illustrate an increase in cases of autism since the introduction of MMR vaccine. However, the data have been presented inaccurately (Fombonne, 2001). Fombonne (2001) lists several reasons why the data are misrepresented, for instance:

1. the figures presented are based on numbers, not rates and do not account for population growth and changes in the composition of the population,
2. changes in diagnostic definitions were not controlled in the report, and
3. as in other areas of the country, children with autism are currently being diagnosed at earlier ages meaning that there will be an increase in the number of reported cases.

A 2001 study (Dales et al.) used the autism case numbers provided by the California Department of Developmental Services and compared them with early childhood MMR immunization level estimates for California children. Results showed that for children born from 1980 through 1987, there was no major change in MMR immunization levels with the exception of a small increase in children born in 1988. This small increase was followed again by steady levels in children born through 1994. On the other hand, the cases of autism increased markedly, from 44 cases per 100,000 live births in 1980 to 208 cases per 100,000 live births in 1994. Even if one allows that a true increase in autism has occurred and the increase is not due to changes in diagnostic methods, diagnostic categorization, and improved identification of individuals with autism because of the level of services offered (Fombonne, 2001), this analysis shows that receipt of the MMR vaccine is not a factor. If it were a factor, one would expect the shape of the MMR level of immunization curve to be very similar to the autism case numbers. This is not the case, thus the analysis in this study argues against a link between MMR vaccination and autism.

Would it be safer to separate the MMR vaccine into its individual components—in other words, give children three separate shots, at different times (for example, six months or one year apart), instead of one combined shot?

There is no confirmed scientific research or data to indicate that there is any benefit to separating the MMR vaccine into its individual components. A publication by Wakefield and Montgomery (2001) suggests that there is an increased risk of immune-mediated disease when the MMR vaccine is administered as one vaccine versus when the 3 vaccines are administered separately. The specific issue of the safety of multiple vaccines given as one vaccine was addressed by the Institute of Medicine (IOM) (1994, p.63). They stated that the number of separate antigens in a vaccine would not likely result in a significant burden on the immune system that would result in immunosuppression. The issue of multiple vaccines and immune dysfunction was addressed again by the IOM in 2002. An IOM Immunization Safety Review Committee concluded that a review of the available scientific evidence does not support the suggestion that the infant immune system is inherently incapable of handling the number of antigens that children are exposed to during routine immunizations. The IOM committee also did not suggest any need to change the current U.S. vaccination schedule for MMR.

Splitting the MMR vaccine into three separate doses given at three different times would cause more discomfort from additional injections and would leave children exposed to potentially serious diseases. For instance, if rubella vaccine were delayed, 4 million children would be susceptible to rubella for an additional 6 to 12 months. This would potentially allow otherwise preventable cases of congenital rubella syndrome (CRS) to occur through transmission of rubella from infected children to pregnant women. Ironically, infection of pregnant woman with "wild" rubella virus is one of the few known causes of autism. Thus, by preventing rubella infection of pregnant women, MMR vaccine also prevents autism.

Should a younger sibling of an autistic child, or a child of someone who has autism be vaccinated with MMR or other vaccines?

Yes. Current scientific evidence does not show that MMR vaccine, or any combination of vaccines, causes the development of autism, including regressive forms of autism.

A younger sibling or the child of someone who suffered a vaccine side effect usually can, and should, safely receive the same vaccine. This is especially true since the large majority of side effects after vaccination are local reactions and fever, which do not represent a contraindication.

Should we delay vaccination until we know more about the negative effects of vaccines?

No. There is no convincing evidence that vaccines such as MMR cause long term health effects. On the other hand, we do know that people will become ill and some will die from the diseases this vaccine prevents. Measles outbreaks have recently occurred in the UK and Germany following an increase in the number of parents who chose not to have their children vaccinated with the MMR vaccine. Discontinuing a vaccine program based on unproven theories would not be in anyone's best interest. Isolated reports about these vaccines causing long term health problems may sound alarming at first. However, careful review of the science reveals that these reports are isolated and not confirmed by scientifically sound research. Detailed medical reviews of health effects reported after receipt of vaccines have often proven to be unrelated to vaccines, but rather have been related to other health factors. Because these vaccines are recommended widely to protect the health of the public, research on any serious hypotheses about their safety are important to pursue. Several studies are underway to investigate still unproven theories about vaccinations and severe side effects.

Chapter 68

Inflammatory Bowel Disease and Vaccines

Frequently Asked Questions about Measles Vaccine and Inflammatory Bowel Disease (IBD)

There is strong scientific evidence to show that measles vaccine does not cause inflammatory bowel disease (IBD). The Centers for Disease Control and Prevention (CDC) recognizes there is considerable public interest in this issue, and therefore supports additional research regarding this hypothesis. CDC is committed to maintaining the safest, most effective vaccine supply in history.

What is Inflammatory Bowel Disease (IBD)?

Inflammatory bowel disease, also known as IBD, is a general medical term used to refer to chronic inflammatory diseases of the intestine.

Two common inflammatory bowel diseases are ulcerative colitis and Crohn's disease. These chronic illnesses can inflame the gastrointestinal tract causing bloody diarrhea, abdominal pain, and weight loss. Ulcerative colitis can affect the entire large intestine or the rectum. Crohn's disease mainly affects short segments of both the small and large intestine. Although IBD can begin at any age, its usual onset is from age 15 to 30 years. IBD is a rare disease with 3–20 new cases recognized per 100,000 persons per year.

"FAQs (frequently asked questions) about Measles Vaccine and Inflammatory Bowel Disease (IBD)," National Immunization Program, Centers for Disease Control and Prevention (CDC), May 10, 2002.

What causes inflammatory bowel disease?

The cause(s) of inflammatory bowel disease is not known. There are several unproven theories as to the cause(s) of IBD:

1. IBD is known to "run in families" suggesting a possible inherited, or genetic cause.
2. A possible environmental cause is suggested because Crohn's disease most often occurs in people who smoke, are residents of Northern European countries and live in urban areas.
3. Another theory is that significant emotional events in a person's life may trigger the disease.
4. Other researchers speculate that the disease may be caused by an infection or virus.
5. Still others believe that the body's immune system is reacting to unidentified or unknown antigens. This antigen would cause the immune system to respond inappropriately against normal intestinal tissue, resulting in chronic inflammation.

Measles, mumps or rubella virus infection is not known cause IBD. The virus that causes measles disease infects the respiratory system and then spreads to lymphatic tissue (an important part of our immune system). During the acute infection, lymph cells in the gastrointestinal (GI) tract are infected but whether this causes chronic inflammation is highly questionable. One theory speculates that measles virus may persist in the intestine in certain individuals and later trigger a chronic inflammatory infection, however this has not been proven. Because MMR vaccine contains a very weak live measles virus it has been suggested that measles vaccine could cause an inflammatory process in the intestine. This theory has not been proven and is speculative. Two types of scientific data—epidemiological and pathological—can be studied to look at a possible link between measles infection and IBD. However, because conflicting results have been obtained for both types of data by different investigators, this link can not be established.

What about studies that suggest an association between measles vaccine and IBD?

The possibility of an association between measles virus and chronic inflammatory bowel disease was discussed in a 1998 study by Wakefield and colleagues. The researchers believed they discovered a new childhood illness that caused bowel disease and psychiatric problems including behavioral disorders and autism. MMR vaccine was suggested as a possible cause. The theory is that MMR vaccine could lead to intestinal inflammation resulting in decreased absorption by the intestinal tract of essential vitamins and nutrients which in turn could lead to developmental disorders. An editorial expressing concerns about the study was also published in the same issue (Chen 1998). That all patients in the study had bowel disease is not surprising since all were referred to a department of gastroenterology. Some of the concerns expressed were that in this small study (12 patients) there is no report of detection of vaccine viruses in intestinal or brain tissue for any of the patients. Multiple laboratories using more sensitive and specific tests, have failed to detect any findings to suggest this. In addition, the GI pathology should have existed prior to the behavioral symptoms to support their theory. The researchers reported the onset of GI symptoms was unknown in 5 patients and noted that GI problems occurred after the onset of behavioral symptoms in another 5 patients.

Two Swedish studies have also suggested a high risk of Crohn's Disease in those exposed to measles in utero. However, these studies involved very small numbers of cases, 2 cases in the first study and 4 in the second study, 2 of which were cases in the first study (Ekbom et al. 1994, Ekbom ct al. 1996).

In 1995, researchers (Thompson et al.) suggested in a retrospective cohort study that MMR vaccine might be a risk factor for Crohn's disease. However, the selection and recall biases and the differences in data collection in this study were so substantial as to cast doubt on the validity of the findings.

Another study has reported finding measles virus proteins and RNA in the intestinal tissue of cases of Crohn's disease using in situ hybridization and immunologic staining (Wakefield 1993). However, the validity of this finding was later called into question when it could not be reproduced by other researchers.

In 2002, researchers (Uhlmann et al., 2002) found measles virus fragments in the intestines of children with "new variant" IBD (children with both IBD and developmental disorder). Scientists looked for the presence of measles virus in the intestinal tissue of 91 children with new variant IBD and 70 "controls" (children without this type of IBD). The researchers found measles virus fragments in 75 out of the 91 children with IBD, and in only 5 of the 70 controls. While this provides evidence for an association between the presence of measles virus and IBD in children with developmental disorder, it does not mean that natural measles virus or the measles component of the MMR vaccine causes IBD or developmental disorder. A commentary published with the article asserts that the data could just as easily be interpreted as indicating that the IBD or the developmental disorder cause the persistence of measles in the intestines (Morris & Aldulaimi, 2002). In addition, the researchers did not compare the virus found in the intestines of patients with the virus used in the vaccine; nor did they provide information regarding whether or not the children in the study had been previously vaccinated with MMR or had previously contracted measles disease. The limitations of this study are further discussed in a letter written by the Director of CDC's National Immunization Program to the UK's Chief Medical Officer.

Is there scientific evidence to show there is no association between measles vaccine and IBD?

There is strong scientific evidence (both epidemiological and laboratory) to show there is no association between measles vaccine and inflammatory bowel disease.

A population-based study conducted by the CDC in collaboration with four large HMO's, part of the Vaccine Safety Datalink Project, concluded that there was no evidence that vaccination with MMR or other measles-containing vaccines, or the age of vaccination early in life, was associated with an increased risk for the development of IBD (Davis et al., 2001). Using a case-control design, the study compared patients diagnosed with IBD and those without IBD, and looked at the vaccination history of MMR vaccine and the timing of vaccinations. Vaccination with MMR or other measles-containing vaccines, or the timing of vaccination early in life, did not increase the risk for IBD.

Researchers in the UK (Frombonne & Chakrabarti, 2001) conducted a study to test the idea that a new form, or "new variant," of Inflammatory Bowel Disease (IBD) exists which is a combination of developmental regression and gastrointestinal symptoms occurring shortly after MMR immunization. Information on 96 children (95 immunized with MMR) who were born between 1992 and 1995 and were diagnosed with pervasive developmental disorder were compared with data from 2 groups of autistic patients (one group of 98 born before MMR was ever used and one group of 68 who were likely to have received MMR vaccine). No evidence was found to support a new syndrome of MMR-induced autism. For instance, the researchers found that there were no differences between vaccinated and unvaccinated groups with regard to when their parents first became concerned about their child's development. Similarly, the rate of developmental regression reported in the vaccinated and unvaccinated groups was not different; therefore, there was no suggestion that developmental regression had increased in frequency since MMR was introduced. Of the 96 children in the first group, no inflammatory bowel disorder was reported.

Another group of researchers in the UK (Taylor et al., 2002) also examined whether MMR vaccination is associated with bowel problems and developmental regression in children with autism, looking for evidence of a "new variant" form of IBD/autism. The study included 278 cases of children with autism and 195 with atypical autism (cases with many of the features of childhood autism but not quite meeting the required criteria for that diagnosis, or with atypical features such as onset of symptoms after the age of 3 years). The cases included in this study were born between 1979 and 1998. The proportion of children with developmental regression or bowel symptoms did not change significantly from 1979 to 1988, a period which included the introduction of MMR vaccination in the UK in 1988. No significant difference was found in rates of bowel problems or regression in children who received the MMR vaccine before their parents became concerned about their development, compared with those who received it only after such concern and those who had not received the MMR vaccine. The findings provide no support for an MMR associated "new variant" form of autism and further evidence against involvement of MMR vaccine in the initiation of autism.

Four other epidemiologic studies have failed to confirm the possible association between measles virus and inflammatory bowel disease. Nielsen et al. (1998) examined all possible cases of measles in pregnant women admitted to a Copenhagen hospital from 1915–1966. None of the offspring of the 25 identified women had developed Crohn's disease. In their case-control studies, Jones et al. (1997) and Feeney et al. (1997) found no association between IBD and measles infection or measles vaccine, respectively. In 1995, Hermon-Taylor compared the incidence of Crohn's disease in England and Wales with measles infection, including information after the introduction of measles vaccine. No association was found.

In another study, researchers used the same laboratory methodology as Wakefield et al. (1993), and could not identify any measles virus in patients with IBD, although they did find the presence of other viral and bacterial agents (Liu et al., 1995). Several other research groups using more sensitive and specific tests (polymerase chain reaction, PCR) have not found any evidence of measles virus RNA in the gastrointestinal tissues of patients with Crohn's Disease or ulcerative colitis (Haga 1996, Iizuka 1995, Afzal 1998).

What does CDC recommend for measles-mumps-rubella (MMR) vaccine?

The CDC continues to recommend two doses of MMR vaccine for all persons; for children, the first dose is recommended at 12–15 months of age and the second dose is recommended at 4–6 years of age. MMR vaccine protects children against dangerous, even deadly, diseases. For instance, one out of 30 children with measles gets pneumonia. For every 1,000 children who get the disease, one or two will die from it. Thanks to vaccines, we have few cases of measles in the U.S. today. However, the disease is extremely contagious and each year dozens of cases are imported from abroad into the U.S., threatening the health of people who have not been vaccinated and those for whom the vaccine was not effective.

Although the risk of Inflammatory Bowel Disease (IBD) is higher for those who have relatives with IBD, there are no data to suggest that measles vaccine will increase or decrease this risk. Measles vaccine is recommended for children with a family history of IBD unless there is another specific reason not to vaccinate (for example, in persons who are very ill and are not able to fight infections).

IBD References

Afzal MA, Minor PD, Begley J, Bentley ML, Armitage E, Gosh S, Ferguson A. Absence of measles virus genome in inflammatory bowel disease. *Lancet*. 1998; 351:646.

Chen RT, DeStefano F. Vaccine Adverse Events: Causal or Coincidental? *Lancet*. 1998; 351:611-612.

Davis RL, Kramarz P, Bohlke K, Benson P, Thompson RS, et al. Measles-mumps-rubella and other measles-containing vaccines do not increase the risk for inflammatory bowel disease. *Arch Pediatr Adolesc Med*. 2001;155:354-359.

Ekbom A, Adami HO, Helmick CG, Jonzon A, Zack MM. Perinatal risk factors for inflammatory bowel disease: a case control-study. *Am J Epidemiol* 1990;132:1111-1119.

Ekbom A, Wakefield AJ, Zack M, Adami HO. Perinatal measles infection and subsequent Crohn's disease. *Lancet*. 1994;344:508-510.

Ekbom A, Daszak P, Kraaz W, Wakefield AJ. Crohn's disease after in-utero measles virus exposure. *Lancet* 1996;348:515-517.

Feeney M, Clegg A, Winwood P, Snook J. A case-control study of measles vaccination and inflammatory bowel disease. *Lancet*. 1997;350: 764-766.

Fombonne E, FRCPsych, Chakrabarti S, FRCPCH, MRCP. No evidence for a new variant of measles-mumps-rubella-induced autism. *Pediatrics* 2001; 108:e58.

Haga Y, Funakoshi O, Kuroe K, et al. Absence of measles viral genomic sequence in intestinal tissues from Crohn's disease by nested polymerase chain reaction. *Gut* 1996;38:211-5.

Iizuka M, Nakagomi O, Chiba M, et al. Absence of measles virus in Crohn's disease. *Lancet* 1995;345:199.

Jones P, Fine P, Piracha S. Crohn's disease and measles. *Lancet*. 1997; 349:473.

Liu Y, Van Kruiningen HJ, West AB, Cartun RW, Cortot A, Colombel JF. Immunocytochemical evidence of Listeria, Escherichia coli, and Streptococcus antigens in Crohn's Disease. *Gastroenterology* 1995;108: 1396-1404.

Metcalf J. Is measles infection associated with Crohn's disease? The current evidence does not prove a causal link. *BMJ* 1998;316:166.

Morris A & Aldulaimi D. New evidence for a viral pathogenic mechanism for new variant inflammatory bowel disease and development disorder? *J Clin Pathol: Mol Pathol* 2002;55:0.

Nielsen LLW, Nielsen NM, Melbye M, Sodermann M, Jacobsen M, Aaby P. Exposure to measles in utero and Crohn's disease: Danish register study. *BMJ* 1998;316:196-7.

Taylor B, Miller E, Lingam R, Andrews N, Simmons A, Stove J. Measles, mumps, and rubella vaccination and bowel problems or developmental regression in children with autism: Population study. *BMJ* 2002;324(7334):393-396.

Thompson NP, Montgomery SM, Pounder RE, Wakefield AJ. Is measles vaccination a risk factor for inflammatory bowel disease? *Lancet* 1995;345:1071-1074.

Uhlmann V, Martin CM, Sheils O, Pilkington L, Silva I, Killalea A, Murch SB, Wakefield AJ, O'Leary JJ. Potential viral pathogenic mechanisms for new variant inflammatory bowel disease. *J Clin Pathol:Mol Pathol* 2002;55:0-6.

Wakefield AJ, Murch S, Anthony A, Linnell J, Casson DM, et al. Ileal lymphoid nodular hyperplasia, non-specific colitis, and regressive developmental disorder in children. *Lancet*. 1998; 351: 637-641.

Wakefield AJ, Pittilo RM, Sim R, Cosby SL, Stephenson JR, Dhillon AP, Pounder RE. Evidence of persistent measles virus infection in Crohn's disease. *J Med Virol* 1993;39:345-353.

Ward B, DeWals P. Association between measles infection and the occurrence of chronic inflammatory bowel disease. *CCDR* 1997;23:1-4.

Chapter 69

Diabetes and Vaccines

What is diabetes?

Most of the food we eat is turned into glucose, or sugar, for our bodies to use for energy. The pancreas, an organ that lies near the stomach, makes a hormone called insulin to help glucose get into the cells of our bodies. If a person has diabetes, their body can't make enough insulin or can't use its own insulin as well as it should. This causes sugar to build up in the blood. Diabetes is classified into two main types:

- **Type 1:** Previously known as insulin-dependent diabetes mellitus (IDDM) or juvenile diabetes. In Type 1 diabetes, which accounts for 5–10% of all diabetes cases, the body does not produce insulin. Risk factors are less well defined for type 1 diabetes than for type 2 diabetes, but genetic, environmental and autoimmune factors are involved in the development of this type of diabetes.
- **Type 2:** Previously known as non-insulin dependent diabetes mellitus (NIDDM) or adult-onset diabetes. In Type 2 diabetes, which accounts for 90–95% of all cases of diabetes, either the body does not produce enough insulin or the insulin does not work. Risk factors for type 2 diabetes include older age, obesity, family history, impaired glucose tolerance, physical inactivity and race/ethnicity (African Americans, Hispanic/Latino Americans,

---

"Diabetes and Vaccines," National Immunization Program, Centers for Disease Control and Prevention (CDC), September 2002.

Native Americans, and some Asian Americans and Pacific Islanders are at increased risk).

In following discussion, "diabetes" refers to type 1.

Do vaccines cause diabetes?

No. Carefully performed scientific studies show that vaccines do not cause diabetes or increase a person's risk of developing diabetes (DeStefano 2001, EURODIAB Substudy 2 Study Group 2000, Karvonen 1999, Heijbel 1997, Parent 1997, Dahlquist 1995, Hyoty 1993, Blom 1991). In 2002, the Institute of Medicine reviewed the existing studies and released a report concluding that the scientific evidence favors rejection of the theory that immunizations cause diabetes. Furthermore, DeStefano and colleagues (2001) recently conducted the first study looking at whether the timing of childhood vaccinations, particularly of Hepatitis B, is related to the risk of a child getting diabetes. This study, which examined data from 1,020 children in the U.S., did not show an association between any of the recommended childhood vaccines and diabetes, regardless of when the vaccines were given. Other studies also provide evidence that vaccination does not cause diabetes:

- A European study that examined 900 diabetic and 2,302 non-diabetic children found a slight relationship between infections during early infancy and risk of developing diabetes. However, the researchers did not find a relationship between any of the common childhood infections or childhood vaccines and diabetes in children. (EURODIAB Substudy 2 Study Group 2000)
- A study conducted in Sweden looked at 1,267 diabetic children in two groups: a group of children that were born during the time that pertussis vaccination was used and a group of children that were born after pertussis vaccine had been removed from the immunization schedule. The researchers found no difference in the incidence rate of diabetes between the children born before and the children born after 1979, when pertussis was excluded from routine immunizations in Sweden. (Heijbel 1997)
- The results from a study that examined 339 diabetic and 528 non-diabetic Swedish children showed that children that received measles vaccine were slightly protected against getting diabetes. The study showed no relationship, positive or negative, between tuberculosis, smallpox, tetanus, whooping cough, rubella, and mumps vaccines and diabetes in children. (Blom 1991)

What about evidence that suggests that vaccines cause diabetes?

The only evidence suggesting a relationship between vaccination and diabetes comes from Dr. John B. Classen (Classen 1996; Classen and Classen 1997; Classen and Classen 2002). He has suggested that certain vaccines if given at birth may decrease the occurrence of diabetes, whereas if initial vaccination is performed after 2 months of age the occurrence of diabetes increases. Dr. Classen's studies have a number of limitations and have not been verified by other researchers.

- This theory is based on results from experiments in laboratory animals, as well as comparisons of the rates of diabetes between countries with different immunization schedules (Classen, 1996; Classen & Classen 1997). Applying findings from laboratory animals to humans is fraught with uncertainty. Findings that are noted in animals cannot be directly applied to people because of the large biological differences. In addition, many of the animal experiments involved anthrax vaccine, which is not used in infants and children.
- Comparison of diabetes rates between countries provides weak evidence because many factors, including vaccination schedules, may differ by country. For instance, comparisons between countries included vaccines that are infrequently used in the U.S. (BCG) or are no longer used (smallpox). Furthermore, factors such as genetic predisposition and a number of possible environmental exposures unrelated to vaccines, may influence the development of diabetes in different countries.

Dr. Classen also performed an analysis of data from a large study conducted in Finland of *Haemophilus influenzae* type B (Hib) vaccine. Over 100,000 children were randomly assigned to receive either 4 doses of vaccine starting at 3 months of age or a single dose at 24 months. Over about a 10-year follow up period, 205 children in the multiple dose group developed diabetes compared with 185 in the single dose group.

- These results are inconclusive because the exact number of children in each group is not known and the noted differences may not be statistically significant (that is, they could be due to "chance").
- The results from a similar study using the same data from Finland were not the same as Dr. Classen's results (Karvonen et al.

1999). This study was similar to Dr. Classen's study except that it compared children in 3 (rather than 2) different groups: #1) children who were born before Hib vaccination was recommended (and therefore did not receive the shot as part of their routine immunizations), #2) children who began receiving Hib vaccine at 3 months of age, and #3) children who received a single dose of Hib at 24 months. This study did not find a difference in diabetes risk between any of the 3 groups of children.

Dr. Classen recently performed another analysis using the same data from the group of children in Finland (Classen and Classen 2002). In this study Dr. Classen suggests that by the age of 7 years old a greater number of diabetes cases occurred in Finnish children that had received the Hib vaccine than in children who had not received the vaccine.

- In order for an association between Hib vaccination and diabetes to be confirmed, the results would have to be replicated in several other scientific studies. No other studies, not even one using the exact same data from the children in Finland (Karvonen 1999), have found a relationship between Hib vaccine and an increase in diabetes (DeStefano 2001, EURODIAB Substudy 2 Study Group 2000).
- It appears that Dr. Classen may have conducted his statistical analysis after seeing the results and noting that the largest difference was apparent by 7 years. The validity of this type of 'post-hoc' statistical testing, however, is highly questionable. When the full 10 years of follow-up was evaluated the differences were not statistically significant, which is also what was found by Karvonen and colleagues.

What is being done to monitor the safety of vaccines?

To assure the safety of vaccines, The Centers for Disease Control and Prevention (CDC), the Food and Drug Administration (FDA), the National Institutes of Health (NIH), and other Federal agencies routinely monitor vaccine safety and conduct research to examine any new evidence that would suggest possible problems with the safety of vaccines. The CDC's Vaccine Safety Datalink (VSD) project links the immunization and medical records on members of seven HMOs, totaling 2.5% of the U.S. population for various vaccine safety studies. The VSD project is a powerful and cost-effective tool for the on-going evaluation of vaccine safety. The Vaccine Adverse Event Reporting System, or VAERS, was designed to give health care workers and others a place to report possible problems following vaccination. VAERS helps the FDA and CDC to continuously monitor vaccine safety. To request a VAERS form or to get more information about VAERS, please call 800-822-7967 or go to the VAERS website http://www.vaers .org.

For more information about vaccines and vaccinations, contact CDC's National Immunization Information Hotline:

English: 800-232-2522
Spanish: 800-232-0233

References

Blom L, Nystrom L, Dahlquist G. The Swedish childhood diabetes study: Vaccinations and infections as risk determinants for diabetes in childhood. *Diabetologia* 1991;34(3):176-81.

Classen DC, Classen JB. The timing of pediatric immunization and the risk of insulin-dependent diabetes mellitus. *Infectious Diseases in Clinical Practice* 1997;6:449-454.

Classen JB. The timing of immunization affects the development of diabetes in rodents. *Autoimmunity* 1996;24:137-145.

Classen JB, Classen DC. Clustering of cases of insulin dependent diabetes (IDDM) occurring three years after Haemophilus Influenza B (HiB) immunization support causal relationship between immunization and IDDM. *Autoimmunity* 2002; 35(4):247-353.

Dahlquist G, Gothefors L. The cumulative incidence of childhood diabetes mellitus in Sweden unaffected by BCG-vaccination. *Diabetologia* 1995;38:873-874.

DeStefano F, Mullooly JP, Okoro CA, Chen RT, Marcy SM, Ward JI, Vadheim CM, Black SB, Shinefield HR, Davis RL, Bohlke K. Childhood vaccinations, vaccination timing, and risk of type 1 diabetes mellitus. *Pediatrics* 2001;108(6):E112.

EURODIAB Substudy 2 Study Group. Infections and vaccinations as risk factors for childhood type 1 (insulin-dependent) diabetes mellitus: a multicentre case-control investigation. *Diabetologia* 2000;43(1): 47-53.

Heijbel H, Chen RT, Dahlquist G. Cumulative incidence of childhood-onset IDDM is unaffected by pertussis immunization. *Diabetes Care* 1997;20:173-175.

Hyoty H, Hiltunen M, Reunanen A, et al. Decline of mumps antibodies in Type 1 (insulin-dependent) diabetic children and a plateau in the rising incidence of type 1 diabetes after introduction of the mumps-measles-rubella vaccine in Finland. *Diabetologia* 1993;36:1303-1308.

Institute of Medicine. Stratton K, Wilson CB, McCormick MC, eds. *Multiple immunizations and immune dysfunction*. National Academy Press, Washington, DC. 2002. http://www.nap.edu/books/0309083281/html.

Karvonen M, Cepaitis Z, Tuomilehto J. Association between type 1 diabetes and Haemophilus influenzae type b vaccination: birth cohort study. *British Medical Journal* 1999;318(7192):1169-1172.

Parent M, Fritschi L, Siemiatycki J, Colle E, Menzies R. Bacille Calmette-Guerin vaccination and incidence of IDDM in Montreal, Canada. *Diabetes Care* 1997;20:767-772.

Chapter 70

Seizure Risks after Vaccination

Information in this chapter was drawn from a study published in the August 30, 2001 issue of the *New England Journal of Medicine* entitled "The Risk of Seizures after Receipt of Whole-Cell Pertussis or Measles, Mumps, and Rubella Vaccine" by William E. Barlow and colleagues.

Febrile Seizures after MMR and DTP Vaccinations

What are febrile seizures and what causes them?

Fever-related seizures are the most common type of seizure that occurs during childhood. These seizures generally develop when a child's temperature reaches 103.5 degrees or higher. Such seizures generally occur between 9 months and 5 years of age, and have a variety of causes. The most frequent causes of febrile seizures are viral infections of the upper respiratory tract (for example, ear infections) and conditions like roseola. However, fever-related seizures may happen with any condition that causes a high fever.

What are the health effects of fever-related seizures?

Children who have fever-related seizures uniformly have an excellent prognosis. This study found that febrile seizures following vaccination had no long-term effects.

"Febrile Seizures after MMR and DTP Vaccinations," National Immunization Program, Centers for Disease Control and Prevention (CDC), September 18, 2001.

How often do fever-related seizures happen after DTP and MMR vaccination?

Fever-related seizures following vaccination are very rare. In this study, the number of fever-related seizures following DTP vaccination was six to nine per 100,000 vaccinated children. The number after MMR vaccine was 25 to 34 per 100,000 vaccinated children.

When do fever-related seizures tend to happen?

According to this research, children vaccinated with DTP vaccine are at most risk for seizures on the day of the vaccination. Previously it was believed that the risk period was the same for three days following the vaccination. Fever-related seizures tended to occur 8 to 14 days after getting the MMR vaccine.

Given the risks of seizures, should parents have their children vaccinated?

Yes. Despite the small risk for seizures linked to fever following vaccination, MMR and DTaP immunizations are strongly recommended. These vaccines prevent serious diseases that pose a much greater risk to most children's health than the seizures associated with vaccination. Pertussis, for example, is a highly contagious respiratory disease ("whooping cough") that can lead to pneumonia, brain damage, and even death. Tetanus, diphtheria, measles, and mumps can also be life-threatening. Rubella can cause pregnant women to miscarry or have babies with serious birth defects.

What can be done to prevent fever-related seizures following vaccination?

Many pediatricians recommend giving children an aspirin-free pain reliever such as acetaminophen (Tylenol®) at the time the child receives DTP or DTaP. DTaP is a new vaccine with fewer side effects that has recently replaced DTP in the United States. Do not give aspirin to a child under 18. Aspirin can cause Reye's Syndrome, a rare but dangerous disease.

Seizures following DTP usually occur in the first three days following immunization, with the greatest frequency happening in the first 24 hours.

Preventing seizures following an MMR vaccination is more difficult because fever-related seizures typically occur eight to 14 days following the shot. Still, it may be helpful to start giving your child an aspirin-free pain reliever as soon as you notice a fever.

What should you do if your child has a seizure following a vaccination?

Contact a medical professional right away. Although fever-related seizures typically are not associated with long-term harmful effects, it's important that your child be evaluated to rule out other possible health problems.

Who conducted this study?

The study was conducted by researchers from Group Health Cooperative's Center for Health Studies, the University of Washington's departments of Pediatrics and Epidemiology, the U.S. Centers for Disease Control and Prevention, Northwest Kaiser Permanente, Kaiser Permanente of Northern California, UCLA Center for Vaccine Research, and Southern California Kaiser Permanente.

How was the study done?

Medical records at four large health maintenance organizations (HMOs) were reviewed. These HMOs are part of the Vaccine Safety Datalink Project, coordinated by the Centers for Disease Control and Prevention. In their review, the researchers looked at the immunization and medical information among 679,942 children after 340,386 vaccinations with DTP vaccine, 137,457 vaccinations with MMR vaccine, or no recent vaccination. Children who had febrile seizures after vaccination were followed to identify the risk of subsequent seizures and other neurological disabilities.

Part Six

Additional Help and Information

Chapter 71

Glossary of Terms Related to Contagious Diseases

AAP: American Academy of Pediatrics[4]

acellular vaccine: A vaccine containing partial cellular material as opposed to complete cells.[3]

ACIP: See Advisory Committee on Immunization Practices.[4]

active immunity: The production of antibodies against a specific disease by the immune system. Active immunity can be acquired in two ways, either by contracting the disease or through vaccination. Active immunity is usually permanent, meaning an individual is protected from the disease for the duration of their lives.[3]

adjuvant: A substance (for example, aluminum salt) that is added during production to increase the body's immune response to a vaccine.[3]

adverse events: Undesirable experiences occurring after immunization that may or may not be related to the vaccine.[3]

Advisory Committee on Immunization Practices (ACIP): A panel of 10 experts who make recommendations on the use of vaccines in

---

Terms in this glossary were excerpted from (1) "Microbes in Sickness and in Health," July 2002, and (2) "How HIV Causes AIDS," October 2001, publications of the National Institute of Allergy and Infectious Diseases (NIAID); and (3) "Glossary," February 2004, and (4) "Acronyms and Abbreviations," December 2003, publications of the National Immunization Program, Centers for Disease Control and Prevention (CDC).

the United States. The panel is advised on current issues by representatives from the Centers for Disease Control and Prevention, Food and Drug Administration, National Institutes of Health, American Academy of Pediatrics, American Academy of Family Physicians, American Medical Association and others. The recommendations of the ACIP guide immunization practice at the federal, state and local level.[3]

AIDS: Acquired Immune Deficiency Syndrome[4]

AIRA: American Immunization Registry Association[4]

antibiotic: A drug used to treat some bacterial diseases.[2]

antibody: A protein found in the blood that is produced in response to foreign substances (for example, bacteria or viruses) invading the body. Antibodies protect the body from disease by binding to these organisms and destroying them.[3]

antigen: A substance or molecule that is recognized by the immune system. The molecule can be from a foreign material such as bacteria or viruses.[2]

antitoxin: Antibodies capable of destroying microorganisms including viruses and bacteria.[3]

antiviral: Literally "against-virus"—any medicine capable of destroying or weakening a virus.[3]

association: The degree to which the occurrence of two variables or events is linked. Association describes a situation where the likelihood of one event occurring depends on the presence of another event or variable. However, an association between two variables does not necessarily imply a cause and effect relationship. The term association and relationship are often used interchangeably.[3]

asymptomatic infection: The presence of an infection without symptoms. Also known as inapparent or subclinical infection.[3]

ATSDR: Agency for Toxic Substances and Disease Registry[4]

attenuated vaccine: A vaccine in which live virus is weakened through chemical or physical processes in order to produce an immune response without causing the severe effects of the disease. Attenuated vaccines currently licensed in the United States include measles, mumps, rubella, polio, yellow fever and varicella. Also known as a live vaccine.[3]

B cells: Small white blood cells crucial to the immune defenses. Also known as B lymphocytes, they come from bone marrow and develop into blood cells called plasma cells, which are the source of antibodies.[2]

bacteria: Tiny one-celled organisms present throughout the environment that require a microscope to be seen. While not all bacteria are harmful, some cause disease. Examples of bacterial disease include diphtheria, pertussis, tetanus, *Haemophilus influenza* and pneumococcus (pneumonia).[3]

BCG: Bacillus of Calmette and Guérin (tuberculosis vaccine)[4]

booster shots: Additional doses of a vaccine needed periodically to "boost" the immune system. For example, the tetanus and diphtheria (Td) vaccine which is recommended for adults every ten years.[3]

breakthrough infection: Development of a disease despite a person's having responded to a vaccine.[3]

carriers: Apparently healthy people who harbor disease-causing microbes in the body and who can infect others by passing the microbes on to them.[2]

causal association: The presence or absence of a variable (for example, smoking) is responsible for an increase or decrease in another variable (for example, cancer). A change in exposure leads to a change in the outcome of interest.[3]

CBER: Center for Biologics Evaluation and Research (FDA)[4]

CD4+ T cells: White blood cells that orchestrate the immune response, signaling other cells in the immune system to perform their special functions. Also known as T helper cells.[1]

CD8+ T cells: White blood cells that kill cells infected with HIV or other viruses, or transformed by cancer.[1]

CDC: Centers for Disease Control and Prevention[4]

cell: The smallest unit of life; the basic living unit that makes up tissues.[2]

chronic health condition: A health related state that lasts for a long period of time (for example, cancer, asthma).[3]

COID: Committee on Infectious Diseases (AAP)[4]

combination vaccine: Two or more vaccines administered at once in order to reduce the number of shots given; for example, the MMR (measles, mumps, rubella) vaccine.[3]

communicable: That which can be transmitted from one person or animal to another.[3]

community immunity: Having a large percentage of the population vaccinated in order to prevent the spread of certain infectious diseases. Even individuals not vaccinated (such as newborns and those with chronic illnesses) are offered some protection because the disease has little opportunity to spread within the community. Also known as herd immunity.[3]

conjugate vaccine: The joining together of two compounds (usually a protein and polysaccharide) to increase a vaccine's effectiveness.[3]

CRS: Congenital rubella syndrome[4]

cytokines: Proteins used for communication by cells of the immune system. Central to the normal regulation of the immune response.[1]

cytoplasm: The living matter within a cell.[1]

DAT: Diphtheria antitoxin[4]

dendritic cells: Immune system cells with long, tentacle-like branches. Some of these are specialized cells at the mucosa that may bind to HIV following sexual exposure and carry the virus from the site of infection to the lymph nodes. See also follicular dendritic cells.[1]

DFA: Direct fluorescent antibody[4]

diphtheria: A bacterial disease marked by the formation of a false membrane, especially in the throat, which can cause death.[3]

disease: A state in which a function or part of the body is no longer in a healthy condition.[2]

DNA (deoxyribonucleic acid): A complex molecule found in the cell nucleus which contains an organism's genetic information.[2]

DRSP: Drug-resistant *Streptococcus pneumonia*[4]

DT: Diphtheria and tetanus toxoids[4]

DTaP: Diphtheria and tetanus toxoids and acellular pertussis vaccine[4]

DTP: Diphtheria and tetanus toxoids and whole-cell pertussis vaccine[4]

EBV: Epstein-Barr virus[4]

encephalitis: Inflammation of the brain caused by a virus. Encephalitis can result in permanent brain damage or death.[3]

endemic: The continual, low-level presence of disease in a community.[3]

enzyme: A protein that accelerates a specific chemical reaction without altering itself.[1]

epidemic: A disease outbreak that affects many people in a region at the same time.[2]

EPO: Epidemiology Program Office[4]

etiology: The cause of.[3]

exposure: Contact with infectious agents (bacteria or viruses) in a manner that promotes transmission and increases the likelihood of disease.[3]

FDA: U.S. Food and Drug Administration[4]

febrile: Relating to fever; feverish.[3]

follicular dendritic cells (FDCs): Cells found in the germinal centers (B cell areas) of lymphoid organs. FDCs have thread-like tentacles that form a web-like network to trap invaders and present them to B cells, which then make antibodies to attack the invaders.[1]

GBS: See Guillain-Barré syndrome.[4]

genes: Units of genetic material (DNA) that carry the directions a cell uses to perform a specific function.[2]

germinal centers: Structures within lymphoid tissues that contain FDCs and B cells, and in which immune responses are initiated.[1]

Guillain-Barré syndrome (GBS): A rare neurological disease characterized by loss of reflexes and temporary paralysis. Symptoms include weakness, numbness, tingling, and increased sensitivity that spreads over the body. Muscle paralysis starts in the feet and legs and moves upwards to the arms and hands. Sometimes paralysis can result in the respiratory muscles causing breathing difficulties. Symptoms usually appear over the course of one day and may continue to progress for 3 or 4 days up to 3 or 4 weeks. Recovery begins within

2–4 weeks after the progression stops. While most patients recover, approximately 15%–20% experience persistent symptoms. GBS is fatal in 5% of cases.[3]

***Haemophilus influenzae* type b (Hib):** A bacterial infection that may result in severe respiratory infections, including pneumonia, and other diseases such as meningitis.[3]

HAV: See hepatitis A.[4]

HBcAg: Hepatitis B core antigen[4]

HBeAg: Hepatitis B e antigen[4]

HBIG: Hepatitis B immune globulin[4]

HBsAg: Hepatitis B surface antigen[4]

HBV: See hepatitis B.[4]

HCV: See hepatitis C.[4]

HDV: See hepatitis D.[4]

hepatitis A: A minor viral disease, that usually does not persist in the blood; transmitted through ingestion of contaminated food or water.[3]

hepatitis B: A viral disease transmitted by infected blood or blood products, or through unprotected sex with someone who is infected.[3]

hepatitis C: A liver disease caused by the Hepatitis C virus (HCV), which is found in the blood of persons who have the disease. HCV is spread by contact with the blood of an infected person.[3]

hepatitis D: A defective virus that needs the hepatitis B virus to exist. Hepatitis D virus (HDV) is found in the blood of persons infected with the virus.[3]

hepatitis E: A virus (HEV) transmitted in much the same way as hepatitis A virus. Hepatitis E, however, does not often occur in the United States.[3]

herpes zoster: A disease characterized by painful skin lesions that occur mainly on the trunk (back and stomach) of the body but which can also develop on the face and in the mouth. Complications include headache, vomiting, fever and meningitis. Recovery may take up to 5 weeks. Herpes zoster is caused by the same virus that is responsible for chickenpox. Most people are exposed to this virus during childhood. After the primary infection (chickenpox), the virus becomes dormant, or inactivated. In some people the virus reactivates years, or even decades, later and causes herpes zoster (also known as the shingles).[3]

Hi: *Haemophilus influenzae*

Hib: See *Haemophilus influenzae* type b.[4]

HRSA: Health Resources and Services Administration[4]

IAC: Immunization Action Coalition[4]

IAVG: Interagency Vaccine Group[4]

IG: Immune globulin[4]

IgE: Immunoglobulin E[4]

immune globulin: A protein found in the blood that fights infection. Also known as gamma globulin.[3]

immune system: The complex system in the body responsible for fighting disease. Its primary function is to identify foreign substances in the body (bacteria, viruses, fungi or parasites) and develop a defense against them. This defense is known as the immune response. It involves production of protein molecules called antibodies to eliminate foreign organisms that invade the body.[3]

immunity: Protection against a disease. There are two types of immunity, passive and active. Immunity is indicated by the presence of antibodies in the blood and can usually be determined with a laboratory test.[3]

immunization: Vaccination or other process that induces protection (immunity) against infection or disease caused by a microbe.[2]

immunosuppression: When the immune system is unable to protect the body from disease. This condition can be caused by disease (like HIV infection or cancer) or by certain drugs (like those used in chemotherapy). Individuals whose immune systems are compromised should not receive live, attenuated vaccines.[3]

inactive vaccine: A vaccine made from viruses and bacteria that have been killed through physical or chemical processes. These killed organisms cannot cause disease.[3]

inapparent infection: The presence of infection without symptoms. Also known as subclinical or asymptomatic infection.[3]

incidence: The number of new disease cases reported in a population over a certain period of time.[3]

incubation period: The time from contact with infectious agents (bacteria or viruses) to onset of disease.[3]

infection: A state in which disease-causing microbes have invaded or multiplied in body tissues.[2]

infectious agents: Organisms capable of spreading disease (for example, bacteria or viruses).[3]

infectious diseases: Diseases caused by microbes that can be passed to or among humans by several methods. [2]

infectious: Capable of spreading disease. Also known as communicable.[3]

inflammation: An immune system process that stops the progression of disease-causing microbes, often seen at the site of an injury like a cut. Signs include redness, swelling, pain, and heat.[2]

influenza: A highly contagious viral infection characterized by sudden onset of fever, severe aches ad pains, and inflammation of the mucous membrane.[3]

investigational vaccine: A vaccine that has been approved by the Food and Drug Administration (FDA) for use in clinical trials on humans. However, investigational vaccines are still in the testing and evaluation phase and are not licensed for use in the general public.[3]

IOM: Institute of Medicine[4]

IPV: Inactivated poliovirus vaccine[4]

IRB: Institutional Review Board[4]

killer T cells: see CD8+ T cells.[1]

LAIV: Live, attenuated influenza vaccine[4]

latent: Present but not seen. A latent viral infection is one in which no virus can be found in the blood cells but in which those virus-infected cells can produce virus under certain circumstances.[2]

lentivirus: "Slow" virus characterized by a long interval between infection and the onset of symptoms.[1]

live vaccine: A vaccine in which live virus is weakened through chemical or physical processes in order to produce an immune response without causing the severe effects of the disease. Attenuated vaccines currently licensed in the United States include measles, mumps, rubella, polio, yellow fever and varicella. Also known as an attenuated vaccine.[3]

lymphocytes: Small white blood cells that help the body defend itself against infection. These cells are produced in bone marrow and develop into plasma cells which produce antibodies. Also known as B cells.[3]

lymphoid organs: These include tonsils, adenoids, lymph nodes, spleen and other tissues. Act as the body's filtering system, trapping invaders and presenting them to squadrons of immune cells that congregate there.[1]

macrophage: A large immune system cell that devours invading pathogens and other intruders. Stimulates other immune system cells by presenting them with small pieces of the invaders.[1]

MCV: Measles-containing vaccines[4]

measles: A contagious viral disease marked by the eruption of red circular spots on the skin.[3]

memory cell: A group of cells that help the body defend itself against disease by remembering prior exposure to specific organisms (for example, viruses or bacteria). Therefore these cells are able to respond quickly when these organisms repeatedly threaten the body.[3]

meningitis: Inflammation of the meninges, the membranes that surround the brain and spinal cord.[2]

microbes: Tiny organisms (including viruses and bacteria) that can only be seen with a microscope.[3]

microorganisms: Microscopic organisms, including bacteria, viruses, fungi, plants, and animals.[2]

MMR: measles-mumps-rubella vaccine[4]

MMWR: *Morbidity and Mortality Weekly Report*[4]

molecules: The smallest physical units of a substance that still retain the chemical properties of that chemical substance; molecules are the building blocks of a cell. Some examples are proteins, fats, carbohydrates, and nucleic acids.[2]

monocyte: A circulating white blood cell that develops into a macrophage when it enters tissues.[1]

MR: Measles-rubella vaccine[4]

mumps: Acute contagious viral illness marked by swelling, especially of the parotid glands.[3]

NCCLS: National Committee for Clinical Laboratory Standards[4]

NCHS: National Center for Health Statistics[4]

NCID: National Center for Infectious Diseases[4]

NCRSR: National Congenital Rubella Syndrome Registry[4]

NCVIA: National Childhood Vaccine Injury Act of 1986[4]

NIH: National Institutes of Health[4]

NIP: National Immunization Program[4]

NNDSS: National Notifiable Diseases Surveillance System[4]

NVAC: National Vaccine Advisory Committee[4]

NVICP: National Vaccine Injury Compensation Program[4]

NVPO: National Vaccine Program Office[4]

opportunistic infection: An illness caused by an organism that usually does not cause disease in a person with a normal immune system.[1]

OPV: Oral poliovirus vaccine[4]

orchitis: A complication of mumps infection occurring in males (who are beyond puberty). Symptoms begin 7–10 days after onset of mumps and include inflammation of the testicles, headache, nausea, vomiting, pain and fever. Most patients recover but in rare cases sterility occurs.[3]

otitis media: A viral or bacterial infection that leads to inflammation of the middle ear. This condition usually occurs along with an upper respiratory infection. Symptoms include earache, high fever, nausea, vomiting and diarrhea. In addition, hearing loss, facial paralysis and meningitis may result.[3]

outbreak: Sudden appearance of a disease in a specific geographic area (for example, neighborhood or community) or population (for example, adolescents).[3]

pandemic: An epidemic occurring over a very large area.[3]

parasites: Plants or animals that live, grow, and feed on or within another living organism.[2]

passive immunity: Protection against disease through antibodies produced by another human being or animal. Passive immunity is effective, but protection is generally limited and diminishes over time (usually a few weeks or months). For example, maternal antibodies are passed to the infant prior to birth. These antibodies temporarily protect the baby for the first 4–6 months of life.[3]

pathogenesis: The production or development of a disease. May be influenced by many factors, including the infecting microbe and the host's immune response.[1]

pathogens: Organisms (for example, bacteria, viruses, parasites and fungi) that cause disease in human beings.[3]

PCV7: Pneumococcal conjugate vaccine (7-valent)[4]

pertussis: Whooping cough; bacterial infectious disease marked by a convulsive spasmodic cough, sometimes followed by a crowing intake of breath.[3]

pneumonia: Inflammation of the lungs characterized by fever, chills, muscle stiffness, chest pain, cough, shortness of breath, rapid heart rate and difficulty breathing.[3]

poliomyelitis: Polio; an acute infectious viral disease characterized by fever, paralysis, and atrophy of skeletal muscles.[3]

polysaccharide vaccines: Vaccines that are composed of long chains of sugar molecules that resemble the surface of certain types of bacteria. Polysaccharide vaccines are available for pneumococcal disease, meningococcal disease and *Haemophilus influenzae* type b.[3]

potency: A measure of strength.[3]

PPD: Purified protein derivative[4]

PPV23: Pneumococcal polysaccharide vaccine (23-valent) [4]

prevalence: The number of disease cases (new and existing) within a population over a given time period.[3]

provirus: DNA of a virus, such as HIV, that has been integrated into the genes of a host cell.[1]

quarantine: The isolation of a person or animal who has a disease (or is suspected of having a disease) in order to prevent further spread of the disease.[3]

recombinant: Of or resulting from new combinations of genetic material or cells; the genetic material produced when segments of DNA from different sources are joined.[3]

retrovirus: HIV and other viruses that carry their genetic material in the form of RNA and that have the enzyme reverse transcriptase.[1]

reverse transcriptase: The enzyme produced by HIV and other retroviruses that allows them to synthesize DNA from their RNA.[1]

ribonucleic acid (RNA): A complex molecule that is found in the cell cytoplasm and nucleus. One function of RNA is to direct the building of proteins.[2]

risk: The likelihood that an individual will experience a certain event.[3]

RNA: See ribonucleic acid.[4]

rotavirus: A group of viruses that can cause digestive problems and diarrhea in young children.[2]

rubella: German measles; viral infection that is milder than normal measles but as damaging to the fetus when it occurs early in pregnancy.[3]

rubeola: See measles. [3]

serology: Measurement of antibodies, and other immunological properties, in the blood serum.[3]

smallpox: An acute, highly infectious, often fatal disease caused by a poxvirus and characterized by high fever and aches with subsequent widespread eruption of pimples that blister, produce pus, and form pockmarks. Also called variola.[3]

strain: A specific version of an organism. Many diseases, including HIV/AIDS and hepatitis, have multiple strains.[3]

subclinical infection: The presence of infection without symptoms. Also known as inapparent or asymptomatic infection.[3]

susceptible: Unprotected against disease.[3]

T cells: Small white blood cells (also known as T lymphocytes) that direct or directly participate in immune defenses.[2]

temporal association: Two or more events that occur around the same time but are unrelated, chance occurrences.[3]

thimerosal: Thimerosal is a mercury-containing preservative that has been used in some vaccines and other products since the 1930's. There is no evidence that the low concentrations of thimerosal in vaccines have caused any harm other than minor reactions like redness or swelling at the injection site. However, in July 1999 the U.S. Public Health Service, the American Academy of Pediatrics, and vaccine manufacturers agreed that thimerosal should be reduced or eliminated from vaccines as a precautionary measure. Today, all routinely recommended childhood vaccines manufactured for the U.S. market contain either no thimerosal or only trace amounts.[3]

vaccination: Injection of a killed or weakened infectious organism in order to prevent the disease.[3]

Vaccine Adverse Event Reporting System (VAERS): A database managed by the Centers for Disease Control and Prevention and the Food and Drug Administration. VAERS provides a mechanism for the collection and analysis of adverse events associated with vaccines currently licensed in the United States. Reports to VAERS can be made by the vaccine manufacturer, recipient, their parent/guardian or health care provider. For more information on VAERS call (800) 822-7967.[3]

Vaccine Safety Datalink Project (VSD): In order to increase knowledge about vaccine adverse events, the Centers for Disease Control and Prevention have formed partnerships with eight large health Management Organizations (HMOs) to continually evaluate vaccine safety. The project contains data on more than 6 million people. Medical records are monitored for potential adverse events following immunization. The VSD project allows for planned vaccine safety studies as well as timely investigations of hypothesis.[3]

vaccines: Substances that contain parts of antigens from an infectious organism. By stimulating an immune response (but not disease), they protect the body against subsequent infection by that organism.[2]

VAE: Vaccine adverse event[4]

VAERS: See Vaccine Adverse Event Reporting System.[4]

VAPP: Vaccine-associated paralytic poliomyelitis[4]

varicella: Chickenpox; an acute contagious disease characterized by papular and vesicular lesions.[3]

variola: See smallpox.[3]

VICP: Vaccine Injury Compensation Program[4]

VIG: Vaccinia immune globulin[4]

viremia: The presence of a virus in the blood.[3]

virulence: The relative capacity of a pathogen to overcome body defenses.[3]

virus: A tiny organism that multiples within cells and causes disease such as chickenpox, measles, mumps, rubella, pertussis and hepatitis. Viruses are not affected by antibiotics, the drugs used to kill bacteria.[3]

VIS: Vaccine Information Statement[4]

VPD: Vaccine-preventable disease[4]

VSD: See Vaccine Safety Datalink project.[4]

VZIG: Varicella-zoster immune globulin[4]

VZV: Varicella-zoster virus[4]

waning immunity: The loss of protective antibodies over time.[3]

WBC: White blood-cell count[4]

WHO: World Health Organization[4]

Chapter 72

Resources for More Information about Contagious Diseases and Antimicrobial Resistance

More Information

You can get more in-depth information on microbes and infectious diseases from a local library or a health care provider. Other sources of information include:

Alliance for the Prudent Use of Antibiotics (APUA)
75 Kneeland Street
Boston, MA 02111-1901
Phone: 617-636-0966
Fax: 617-636-3999
Website: www.tufts.edu/med/apua
E-mail: apua@tufts.edu

APUA is an organization dedicated educating medical consumers and physicians about the appropriate use of antibiotics so that the effectiveness of antibiotic medications can be maintained. Their website offers information for patients, physicians, and researchers.

American Academy of Dermatology (AAD)
P.O. Box 4014
Schaumburg, IL 60168-4014
Toll-Free: 888-462-DERM

Resources listed in this chapter were excerpted from "Microbes in Sickness and in Health," National Institute of Allergy and Infectious Diseases (NIAID), National Institutes of Health (NIH), July 2, 2002 and other sources deemed reliable. All contact information was updated and verified in March 2004.

Phone: 847-330-0230
Fax: 847-330-0050
Website: http://www.aad.org

Medical consumers can find information about contagious diseases that affect the skin and other dermatological concerns on the AAD website.

American Association of Blood Banks (AABB)
8101 Glenbrook Road
Bethesda, MD 20814-2749
Phone: 301-907-6977
Fax: 301-907-6895
Website: http://www.aabb.org
E-mail: aabb@aabb.org

AABB is an association of blood banks that together with its member facilities collect almost all of the blood supply in the United States. In addition, AABB members are located in 80 other countries around the world. Its mission is to promote a high standard of care regarding the use of blood products. Information about contagious disease risks associated with blood donation is available on the organization's website.

American Lung Association (ALA)
61 Broadway, 6th Floor
New York, NY 10006
Toll-Free: 800-LUNG-USA (1-800-586-4872)
Phone: 212-315-8700
Website: http://www.lungusa.org

The American Lung Association was founded in 1904 to fight tuberculosis. Today the organization also works to help eliminate many other forms of lung disease. Information about lung function and lung disease is available on the ALA website.

American Osteopathic College of Dermatology
1501 East Illinois Street
Kirksville, MO 63501
Toll-Free: 800-449-2623
Phone: 660-665-2184
Fax: 660-627-2623
Website: http://www.aocd.org
E-mail: info@aocd.org

The American Osteopathic College of Dermatology focuses on the treatment of skin, hair, and nail diseases. A directory of contagious and other dermatologic diseases can be found at http://www.aocd.org/skin/dermatologic_diseases/index.html

American Social Health Association (ASHA)

P.O. Box 13827
Research Triangle Park, NC 27709
Toll-free: 1-877-HPV-5868 (1-877-478-5868) (2:00 p.m. to 7:00 p.m. ET)
Phone: 919-361-8400
Fax: 919-361-8425
Website: http://www.ashastd.org

ASHA's mission is to provide medically accurate information about sexually transmitted diseases (STDs), including facts about how they are transmitted, how they can be prevented, and what is currently known and recommended regarding their treatment. A directory of STD information, including disease facts, statistics, a glossary, and condom use instructions, is available on their website at http://www.ashastd.org/stdfaqs/index.html.

Association for Professionals in Infection Control and Epidemiology

1275 K Street, NW
Suite 1000
Washington, DC 20005-4006
Phone: 202-789-1890
Fax: 202-789-1899
Website: http://www.apic.org
E-mail: APICinfo@apic.org

Infection control professionals work to control the spread of infections in hospitals and other health care settings such as long-term care and rehabilitation facilities. News items and other information resources regarding current concerns in nosocomial infection control are available on the organization's website.

Centers for Disease Control and Prevention (CDC)

1600 Clifton Road
Atlanta, GA 30333
Toll-Free: 800-311-3435
Phone: 404-639-3311
Website: http://www.cdc.gov

Among its other duties, CDC is the U.S. Government agency charged with tracking outbreaks of infectious disease in the United States and sometimes other countries. The agency also searches for disease causes and issues guidelines for preventing and treating many of them. In addition, CDC is the main U.S. Government agency that develops policy and recommendations for immunizations. Individual agencies within CDC of special interest to people with questions about contagious diseases include:

- Epidemiology Program Office
  http://www.cdc.gov/epo/index.htm
  E-mail: epo@cdc.gov
- National Center for HIV, STD, and TB Prevention
  http://www.cdc.gov/nchstp/od/nchstp.html
  E-mail: nchstp@cdc.gov
- National Center for Infectious Diseases
  Website: http://www.cdc.gov/ncidod
  E-mail: ncid@cdc.gov
- National Immunization Information Program
  Toll Free: 800-232-2522
  Website: http://www.cdc.gov/nip
  E-mail: NIPINFO@cdc.gov

Hepatitis Foundation International
504 Blick Drive
Silver Spring, MD 20904-2901
Toll-Free: 800-891-0707
Phone: 301-622-4200
Fax: 301-622-4702
Website: http://www.hepfi.org
E-mail: hfi@comcast.net

Hepatitis Foundation International (HFI) provides educational materials and training to the public, patients, health educators, and medical professionals about the prevention, diagnosis, and treatment of viral hepatitis, and also provides support to hepatitis patients and researchers. HFI has a variety of materials available through its Liver Wellness/Hepatitis Education program including: videos for lending libraries; brochures on liver wellness and hepatitis; posters on hepatitis prevention; workplace programs; teacher and parent information; and coloring books for children.

March of Dimes

1275 Mamaroneck Avenue
White Plains, NY 10605
Toll-Free: 800-996-2724
Fax: 914-997-4537
Website: http://www.modimes.org

The first March of Dimes chapter was founded in 1939 and the organization's original focus was to help in the fight against polio. Today the organization works to help prevent birth defects, prematurity, and low birth weight. As part of this effort, the organization provides information concerning infectious disease risks to pregnant women and infants.

National Foundation for Infectious Diseases (NFID)

4733 Bethesda Avenue
Suite 750
Bethesda, MD 20814
Phone: 301-656-0003
Fax: 301-907-0878
Website: http://www.nfid.org
E-mail: info@nfid.org

NFID works to educate the public and medical professionals about the prevention and treatment of infectious diseases. A directory of disease fact sheets is available on their website at http://www.nfid.org/factsheets.

National Hansen's Disease Programs

1770 Physicians Park Drive
Baton Rouge, LA 70816
Toll-Free: 800-642-2477
Phone: 225-756-3762
Website: http://www.bphc.hrsa.gov/nhdp

The National Hansen's Disease Programs (NHDP), based in Baton Rouge, Louisiana, is primarily responsible for inpatient and outpatient care and treatment of Hansen's disease (leprosy). In addition to the clinical programs in Baton Rouge, the NHDP also coordinates outpatient care for Hansen's disease patients throughout the U.S. at Bureau of Primary Health Care grant-funded clinics as well as private physician offices.

National Institute of Allergy and Infectious Diseases (NIAID)
Building 31, Room 7A50
31 Center Drive, MSC 2520
Bethesda, MD 20892-2520
Website: http://www.niaid.nih.gov

NIAID supports basic and applied research to prevent, diagnose, and treat infectious and immune-mediated illnesses, including HIV/AIDS and other sexually transmitted diseases, illness from potential agents of bioterrorism, tuberculosis, malaria, autoimmune disorders, asthma, and allergies. The website has information on many of these diseases as well as links to other sources of information.

National Institutes of Health
9000 Rockville Pike
Bethesda, MD 20892
Phone: 301-496-4000
Website: http://www.nih.gov
E-mail: nihinfo@od.nih.gov

NIH is the U.S. Government agency that, through its institutes and centers, conducts and supports a broad range of biomedical research. Links available on the website contain information on the causes, symptoms, prevention, and treatment of many diseases and conditions that affect the human body. National Institutes of Health (NIH) is an agency of the Department of Health and Human Services.

National Library of Medicine (NLM)
8600 Rockville Pike
Bethesda, MD 20894
Phone: 301-496-6308
Website: http://www.medlineplus.gov
E-mail: custserv@nlm.nih.gov

NLM is the largest medical library in the world. The MEDLINEplus Web site has information about hundreds of diseases, conditions, and wellness issues. It also has information about clinical research studies that are being conducted on certain diseases and conditions.

National STD and AIDS Hotline

Toll-Free AIDS Hotline: 800-342-2437 (24 hours a day, 7 days a week)
Toll-Free STD Hotline: 800-227-8922
Toll-Free AIDS TTY Service: 800-243-7889
Toll-Free AIDS Spanish Service: 800-344-7432
Website: http://www.ashastd.org/nah

The National STD and AIDS Hotline is a service provided by American Social Health Association and the Centers for Disease Control and Prevention (CDC). The hotline answers questions about the prevention, risk, testing, and treatment of sexually transmitted diseases including HIV/AIDS. It handles approximately a million calls annually.

U.S. Food and Drug Administration (FDA)

5600 Fishers Lane
Rockville, MD 20857-0001
Toll-Free: 888-INFO-FDA (1-888-463-6332)
Website: http://www.fda.gov

FDA is the U.S. Government consumer protection and regulatory agency for food and drugs. Contact this agency for information about the safety of food, medical products, medicines, and cosmetics.

World Health Organization

Avenue Appia 20
1211 Geneva 27
Switzerland
Phone: (011 41 22) 791 21 11
Fax: (011 41 22) 791 31 11
Website: http://www.who.int/en
E-mail: info@who.int

WHO, part of the United Nations, is devoted to improving the health of people around the world. This international organization has health and disease surveillance information in English French and Spanish. A report "Overcoming Antimicrobial Resistance" is available online at www.who.int/infectious-diseases-report/2000/intro.htm.

Chapter 73

Resources for More Information about Vaccines and Vaccine Safety

This chapter includes additional reading and organizational information regarding vaccines and vaccine safety. Sources are listed alphabetically by document title or organization name within each category.

General Vaccine and Vaccine Safety Information

Allied Vaccine Group
Website: http://vaccine.org
E-mail: suggestions@vaccine.org

Epidemiology and Prevention of Vaccine-Preventable Diseases (2004), book
Vaccine Safety (Chapter 15), by the Centers for Disease Control and Prevention
Available online: http://www.cdc.gov/nip/publications/pink/safety.pdf

Immunization Action Coalition
1573 Selby Ave.
St. Paul, MN 55104

This chapter includes excerpts from "Overview of Vaccine Safety," National Immunization Program, Centers for Disease Control and Prevention (CDC) at www.cdc.gov/nip/vacsafe along with additional information and resources. All website and contact information was verified in March 2004. Inclusion does not constitute endorsement.

Phone: 651-647-9009
Fax: 651-647-9131
Website: http://www.immunize.org
E-mail: admin@immunize.org

Immunization Gateway
Website: http://www.immunofacts.com
E-mail: immunofacts@drugfacts.com

Immunization News
links to recently published information on immunizations
Available online: http://www.cdc.gov/nip/news/default.htm

National Immunization Hotline
Toll-Free: 800-232-2522 (English)
Toll-Free: 800-232-0233 (Spanish)
Toll-Free: 800-243-7889 (TTY)

National Immunization Program
Centers for Disease Control and Prevention
1600 Clifton Rd., NE
Mailstop E-05
Atlanta, GA 30333
Toll-Free: 800-232-2522 (English)
Toll-Free: 800-232-0233 (Spanish)
Website: http://www.cdc.gov/nip
E-mail: NIPINFO@cdc.gov

National Network for Immunization Information
301 University Blvd., CH 2.218
Galveston, TX 77555
Phone: 409-772-0199
Fax: 409-747-4995
Website: http://www.immunizationinfo.org
E-mail: nnii@i4ph.org

National Vaccine Program Office
U.S. Department of Health and Human Services
200 Independence Avenue, S.W.
Washington, DC 20201
Toll-Free: 877-696-6775
Phone: 202-619-0257
Website: http://www.hhs.gov/nvpo

Understanding Vaccines (1998), booklet
National Institute on Allergy and Infectious Diseases
Available online: http://www.niaid.nih.gov/publications/vaccine/undvacc.htm

Vaccine Check
Website: http://www.vaccinecheck.com

Vaccine Education Center at The Children's Hospital of Philadelphia
34th Street and Civic Center Blvd.
Philadelphia, PA 19104-4399
Phone: 215-590-9990
Website: http://www.vaccine.chop.edu

Vaccine Page
Website: http://www.vaccines.com

Vaccine Safety: Current and Future Challenges, article
by Robert T. Chen MD, MA, and Beth Hibbs RN, MPH in *Pediatric Annals* July 1998; 27 (7): 445-455
Available online: http://www.cdc.gov/nip/vacsafe/research/peds.htm

Vaccine Safety Forum, Institute of Medicine (1997), book
National Academies Press
Available online: http://www.nap.edu/readingroom/books/vaccine

World Health Organization
Avenue Appia 20
1211 Geneva 27
Switzerland
Phone: (011 41 22) 791 21 11
Fax: (011 41 22) 791 31 11
Website: http://www.who.int
E-mail: info@who.int
Webpage on Vaccine Safety: http://www.who.int/vaccines-diseases

Vaccine Adverse Events

Adverse Effects of Pertussis and Rubella Vaccines (1991), book
by the Institute of Medicine, published by National Academies Press
Available online: http://www.nap.edu/catalog/1815.html

Adverse Events Associated with Childhood Vaccines: Evidence Bearing on Causality (1994), book
by the Institute of Medicine, published by National Academies Press
Available online: http://www.nap.edu/catalog/2138.html

Vaccine Licensure

U.S. Food and Drug Administration (FDA)
5600 Fishers Lane
Rockville, MD 20857-0001
Toll-Free: 888-INFO-FDA (1-888-463-6332)
Website: http://www.fda.gov
Webpage FDA Licensure of Vaccines: http://www.fda.gov/fdac/features/095_vacc.html

Monitoring Vaccine Safety

The Complicated Task of Monitoring Vaccine Safety, article
by Susan S. Ellenberg, PhD and Robert T. Chen, MD, MA in *Journal of the U.S. Public Health Service, Public Health Reports*, January/February, 1997; Vol 112, No. 1; pp. 10-20.
Available online: http://www.cdc.gov/nip/vacsafe/research/phr.htm

The Vaccine Adverse Events Reporting System (VAERS)

Vaccine Adverse Events Reporting System (VAERS)
P.O. Box 1100
Rockville, MD 20849-1100
Toll-Free: 800-822-7967
Fax: 877-721-0366
Website: http://www.vaers.org
E-mail: info@vaers.org
VAERS Form available online: http://www.vaers.org/pdf/vaers_form.pdf

FDA's Web Site on VAERS, webpage
Available online: http://www.fda.gov/cber/vaers/vaers.htm

VAERS Table of Reportable Events
Available online: http://www.vaers.org/reportable.htm

The Vaccine Safety Datalink (VSD) Project

Vaccine Safety Datalink Project: Current and Completed Studies
Available online: http://www.cdc.gov/nip/vacsafe/vsd/research.htm

Vaccine Safety Datalink: Publications and Presentations, References
Available online: http://www.cdc.gov/nip/vacsafe/vsd/references.htm

Vaccine Safety Datalink Project: Vaccine Safety Data-Sharing Process
Available online: http://www.cdc.gov/nip/vacsafe/vsd/default.htm

National Vaccine Injury Compensation Program (NVICP)

National Vaccine Injury Compensation Program
Parklawn Building
5600 Fishers Lane, Room 16C-17
Rockville, Maryland 20857
Phone: 800-338-2382
Website: http://www.hrsa.gov/osp/vicp

Rules of the Court (requirements for filing an NVICP petition)
Clerk, U.S. Court of Federal Claims
717 Madison Place, N.W.
Washington, D.C. 20005
Phone: 202-219-9657
Website: http://www.uscfc.uscourts.gov/osmPage.htm

Risk Communication

Current Vaccine Information Statements (VISs)
Available online: http://www.cdc.gov/nip/publications/vis/default.htm

Instructions for Vaccine Information Statements (VISs)
Available online: http://www.cdc.gov/nip/publications/vis/vis-Instructions.pdf

Risk Communication and Vaccination (1997), book
Institute of Medicine, National Academies Press
Available online: http://www.nap.edu/readingroom/books/rcv

Index

Index

Page numbers followed by 'n' indicate a footnote. Page numbers in *italics* indicate a table or illustration.

B

C

G

H

I

J

K

L

M

O

P

Q

R

S

T

U

V

W

X

Y

Z

Health Reference Series

COMPLETE CATALOG

Adolescent Health Sourcebook

Basic Consumer Health Information about Common Medical, Mental, and Emotional Concerns in Adolescents, Including Facts about Acne, Body Piercing, Mononucleosis, Nutrition, Eating Disorders, Stress, Depression, Behavior Problems, Peer Pressure, Violence, Gangs, Drug Use, Puberty, Sexuality, Pregnancy, Learning Disabilities, and More

Along with a Glossary of Terms and Other Resources for Further Help and Information

Edited by Chad T. Kimball. 658 pages. 2002. 0-7808-0248-9. $78.

"It is written in clear, nontechnical language aimed at general readers. . . . Recommended for public libraries, community colleges, and other agencies serving health care consumers."
—*American Reference Books Annual, 2003*

"Recommended for school and public libraries. Parents and professionals dealing with teens will appreciate the easy-to-follow format and the clearly written text. This could become a 'must have' for every high school teacher." —*E-Streams, Jan '03*

"A good starting point for information related to common medical, mental, and emotional concerns of adolescents." —*School Library Journal, Nov '02*

"This book provides accurate information in an easy to access format. It addresses topics that parents and caregivers might not be aware of and provides practical, useable information." —*Doody's Health Sciences Book Review Journal, Sep-Oct '02*

"Recommended reference source."
—*Booklist, American Library Association, Sep '02*

AIDS Sourcebook, 3rd Edition

Basic Consumer Health Information about Acquired Immune Deficiency Syndrome (AIDS) and Human Immunodeficiency Virus (HIV) Infection, Including Facts about Transmission, Prevention, Diagnosis, Treatment, Opportunistic Infections, and Other Complications, with a Section for Women and Children, Including Details about Associated Gynecological Concerns, Pregnancy, and Pediatric Care

Along with Updated Statistical Information, Reports on Current Research Initiatives, a Glossary, and Directories of Internet, Hotline, and Other Resources

Edited by Dawn D. Matthews. 664 pages. 2003. 0-7808-0631-X. $78.

ALSO AVAILABLE: *AIDS Sourcebook, 1st Edition.* Edited by Karen Bellenir and Peter D. Dresser. 831 pages. 1995. 0-7808-0031-1. $78.

AIDS Sourcebook, 2nd Edition. Edited by Karen Bellenir. 751 pages. 1999. 0-7808-0225-X. $78.

"The 3rd edition of the *AIDS Sourcebook,* part of Omnigraphics' *Health Reference Series,* is a welcome update. . . . This resource is highly recommended for academic and public libraries."
—*American Reference Books Annual, 2004*

"Excellent sourcebook. This continues to be a highly recommended book. There is no other book that provides as much information as this book provides."
—*AIDS Book Review Journal, Dec-Jan 2000*

"Recommended reference source."
—*Booklist, American Library Association, Dec '99*

"A solid text for college-level health libraries."
—*The Bookwatch, Aug '99*

Cited in *Reference Sources for Small and Medium-Sized Libraries, American Library Association, 1999*

Alcoholism Sourcebook

Basic Consumer Health Information about the Physical and Mental Consequences of Alcohol Abuse, Including Liver Disease, Pancreatitis, Wernicke-Korsakoff Syndrome (Alcoholic Dementia), Fetal Alcohol Syndrome, Heart Disease, Kidney Disorders, Gastrointestinal Problems, and Immune System Compromise and Featuring Facts about Addiction, Detoxification, Alcohol Withdrawal, Recovery, and the Maintenance of Sobriety

Along with a Glossary and Directories of Resources for Further Help and Information

Edited by Karen Bellenir. 613 pages. 2000. 0-7808-0325-6. $78.

"This title is one of the few reference works on alcoholism for general readers. For some readers this will be a welcome complement to the many self-help books on the market. Recommended for collections serving general readers and consumer health collections."
—*E-Streams, Mar '01*

"This book is an excellent choice for public and academic libraries."
—*American Reference Books Annual, 2001*

"Recommended reference source."
—*Booklist, American Library Association, Dec '00*

"Presents a wealth of information on alcohol use and abuse and its effects on the body and mind, treatment, and prevention." —*SciTech Book News, Dec '00*

"Important new health guide which packs in the latest consumer information about the problems of alcoholism." —*Reviewer's Bookwatch, Nov '00*

SEE ALSO *Drug Abuse Sourcebook, Substance Abuse Sourcebook*

Allergies Sourcebook, 2nd Edition

Basic Consumer Health Information about Allergic Disorders, Triggers, Reactions, and Related Symptoms, Including Anaphylaxis, Rhinitis, Sinusitis, Asthma, Dermatitis, Conjunctivitis, and Multiple Chemical Sensitivity

Along with Tips on Diagnosis, Prevention, and Treatment, Statistical Data, a Glossary, and a Directory of Sources for Further Help and Information

Edited by Annemarie S. Muth. 598 pages. 2002. 0-7808-0376-0. $78.

ALSO AVAILABLE: *Allergies Sourcebook, 1st Edition.* Edited by Allan R. Cook. 611 pages. 1997. 0-7808-0036-2. $78.

"This book brings a great deal of useful material together. . . . This is an excellent addition to public and consumer health library collections."
—*American Reference Books Annual, 2003*

"This second edition would be useful to laypersons with little or advanced knowledge of the subject matter. This book would also serve as a resource for nursing and other health care professions students. It would be useful in public, academic, and hospital libraries with consumer health collections." —*E-Streams, Jul '02*

■

Alternative Medicine Sourcebook, 2nd Edition

Basic Consumer Health Information about Alternative and Complementary Medical Practices, Including Acupuncture, Chiropractic, Herbal Medicine, Homeopathy, Naturopathic Medicine, Mind-Body Interventions, Ayurveda, and Other Non-Western Medical Traditions

Along with Facts about such Specific Therapies as Massage Therapy, Aromatherapy, Qigong, Hypnosis, Prayer, Dance, and Art Therapies, a Glossary, and Resources for Further Information

Edited by Dawn D. Matthews. 618 pages. 2002. 0-7808-0605-0. $78.

ALSO AVAILABLE: *Alternative Medicine Sourcebook, 1st Edition.* Edited by Allan R. Cook. 737 pages. 1999. 0-7808-0200-4. $78.

"Recommended for public, high school, and academic libraries that have consumer health collections. Hospital libraries that also serve the public will find this to be a useful resource." —*E-Streams, Feb '03*

"Recommended reference source."
—*Booklist, American Library Association, Jan '03*

"An important alternate health reference."
—*MBR Bookwatch, Oct '02*

"A great addition to the reference collection of every type of library." —*American Reference Books Annual, 2000*

Alzheimer's Disease Sourcebook, 3rd Edition

Basic Consumer Health Information about Alzheimer's Disease, Other Dementias, and Related Disorders, Including Multi-Infarct Dementia, AIDS Dementia Complex, Dementia with Lewy Bodies, Huntington's Disease, Wernicke-Korsakoff Syndrome (Alcohol-Reated Dementia), Delirium, and Confusional States

Along with Information for People Newly Diagnosed with Alzheimer's Disease and Caregivers, Reports Detailing Current Research Efforts in Prevention, Diagnosis, and Treatment, Facts about Long-Term Care Issues, and Listings of Sources for Additional Information

Edited by Karen Bellenir. 645 pages. 2003. 0-7808-0666-2. $78.

ALSO AVAILABLE: *Alzheimer's, Stroke & 29 Other Neurological Disorders Sourcebook, 1st Edition.* Edited by Frank E. Bair. 579 pages. 1993. 1-55888-748-2. $78.

ALSO AVAILABLE: *Alzheimer's Disease Sourcebook, 2nd Edition.* Edited by Karen Bellenir. 524 pages. 1999. 0-7808-0223-3. $78.

"This very informative and valuable tool will be a great addition to any library serving consumers, students and health care workers."
—*American Reference Books Annual, 2004*

"This is a valuable resource for people affected by dementias such as Alzheimer's. It is easy to navigate and includes important information and resources."
—*Doody's Review Service, Feb. 2004*

"Recommended reference source."
—*Booklist, American Library Association, Oct '99*

SEE ALSO *Brain Disorders Sourcebook*

■

Arthritis Sourcebook, 2nd Edition

Basic Consumer Health Information about Osteoarthritis, Rheumatoid Arthritis, Other Rheumatic Disorders, Infectious Forms of Arthritis, and Diseases with Symptoms Linked to Arthritis, Featuring Facts about Diagnosis, Pain Management, and Surgical Therapies

Along with Coping Strategies, Research Updates, a Glossary, and Resources for Additional Help and Information

Edited by Amy L. Sutton. 593 pages. 2004. 0-7808-0667-0. $78.

ALSO AVAILABLE: *Arthritis Sourcebook, 1st Edition.* Edited by Allan R. Cook. 550 pages. 1998. 0-7808-0201-2. $78.

". . . accessible to the layperson."
—*Reference and Research Book News, Feb '99*

Asthma Sourcebook

Basic Consumer Health Information about Asthma, Including Symptoms, Traditional and Nontraditional Remedies, Treatment Advances, Quality-of-Life Aids, Medical Research Updates, and the Role of Allergies, Exercise, Age, the Environment, and Genetics in the Development of Asthma

Along with Statistical Data, a Glossary, and Directories of Support Groups, and Other Resources for Further Information

Edited by Annemarie S. Muth. 628 pages. 2000. 0-7808-0381-7. $78.

"A worthwhile reference acquisition for public libraries and academic medical libraries whose readers desire a quick introduction to the wide range of asthma information." —*Choice, Association of College & Research Libraries, Jun '01*

"Recommended reference source."
—*Booklist, American Library Association, Feb '01*

"Highly recommended." —*The Bookwatch, Jan '01*

"There is much good information for patients and their families who deal with asthma daily."
—*American Medical Writers Association Journal, Winter '01*

"This informative text is recommended for consumer health collections in public, secondary school, and community college libraries and the libraries of universities with a large undergraduate population."
—*American Reference Books Annual, 2001*

■

Attention Deficit Disorder Sourcebook

Basic Consumer Health Information about Attention Deficit/Hyperactivity Disorder in Children and Adults, Including Facts about Causes, Symptoms, Diagnostic Criteria, and Treatment Options Such as Medications, Behavior Therapy, Coaching, and Homeopathy

Along with Reports on Current Research Initiatives, Legal Issues, and Government Regulations, and Featuring a Glossary of Related Terms, Internet Resources, and a List of Additional Reading Material

Edited by Dawn D. Matthews. 470 pages. 2002. 0-7808-0624-7. $78.

"Recommended reference source."
—*Booklist, American Library Association, Jan '03*

"This book is recommended for all school libraries and the reference or consumer health sections of public libraries." —*American Reference Books Annual, 2003*

■

Back & Neck Sourcebook, 2nd Edition

Basic Consumer Health Information about Spinal Pain, Spinal Cord Injuries, and Related Disorders, Such as Degenerative Disk Disease, Osteoarthritis, Scoliosis, Sciatica, Spina Bifida, and Spinal Stenosis, and Featuring Facts about Maintaining Spinal Health, Self-Care, Pain Management, Rehabilitative Care, Chiropractic Care, Spinal Surgeries, and Complementary Therapies

Along with Suggestions for Preventing Back and Neck Pain, a Glossary of Related Terms, and a Directory of Resources

Edited by Amy L. Sutton. 600 pages. 2004. 0-7808-0738-3 $78.

ALSO AVAILABLE: *Back & Neck Disorders Sourcebook, 1st Edition.* Edited by Karen Bellenir. 548 pages. 1997. 0-7808-0202-0. $78.

"The strength of this work is its basic, easy-to-read format. Recommended."
—*Reference and User Services Quarterly, American Library Association, Winter '97*

■

Blood & Circulatory Disorders Sourcebook

Basic Information about Blood and Its Components, Anemias, Leukemias, Bleeding Disorders, and Circulatory Disorders, Including Aplastic Anemia, Thalassemia, Sickle-Cell Disease, Hemochromatosis, Hemophilia, Von Willebrand Disease, and Vascular Diseases

Along with a Special Section on Blood Transfusions and Blood Supply Safety, a Glossary, and Source Listings for Further Help and Information

Edited by Karen Bellenir and Linda M. Shin. 554 pages. 1998. 0-7808-0203-9. $78.

"Recommended reference source."
—*Booklist, American Library Association, Feb '99*

"An important reference sourcebook written in simple language for everyday, non-technical users."
—*Reviewer's Bookwatch, Jan '99*

■

Brain Disorders Sourcebook

Basic Consumer Health Information about Strokes, Epilepsy, Amyotrophic Lateral Sclerosis (ALS/Lou Gehrig's Disease), Parkinson's Disease, Brain Tumors, Cerebral Palsy, Headache, Tourette Syndrome, and More

Along with Statistical Data, Treatment and Rehabilitation Options, Coping Strategies, Reports on Current Research Initiatives, a Glossary, and Resource Listings for Additional Help and Information

Edited by Karen Bellenir. 481 pages. 1999. 0-7808-0229-2. $78.

"Belongs on the shelves of any library with a consumer health collection." —*E-Streams, Mar '00*

"Recommended reference source."
—*Booklist, American Library Association, Oct '99*

SEE ALSO *Alzheimer's Disease Sourcebook*

Breast Cancer Sourcebook, 2nd Edition

Basic Consumer Health Information about Breast Cancer, Including Facts about Risk Factors, Prevention, Screening and Diagnostic Methods, Treatment Options, Complementary and Alternative Therapies, Post-Treatment Concerns, Clinical Trials, Special Risk Populations, and New Developments in Breast Cancer Research

Along with Breast Cancer Statistics, a Glossary of Related Terms, and a Directory of Resources for Additional Help and Information

Edited by Sandra J. Judd. 600 pages. 2004. 0-7808-0668-9. $78.

ALSO AVAILABLE: *Breast Cancer Sourcebook, 1st Edition.* Edited by Edward J. Prucha and Karen Bellenir. 580 pages. 2001. 0-7808-0244-6. $78.

"It would be a useful reference book in a library or on loan to women in a support group."
—*Cancer Forum, Mar '03*

"Recommended reference source."
—*Booklist, American Library Association, Jan '02*

"This reference source is highly recommended. It is quite informative, comprehensive and detailed in nature, and yet it offers practical advice in easy-to-read language. It could be thought of as the 'bible' of breast cancer for the consumer." —*E-Streams, Jan '02*

"The broad range of topics covered in lay language make the *Breast Cancer Sourcebook* an excellent addition to public and consumer health library collections."
—*American Reference Books Annual 2002*

"From the pros and cons of different screening methods and results to treatment options, *Breast Cancer Sourcebook* provides the latest information on the subject."
—*Library Bookwatch, Dec '01*

"This thoroughgoing, very readable reference covers all aspects of breast health and cancer. . . . Readers will find much to consider here. Recommended for all public and patient health collections."
—*Library Journal, Sep '01*

SEE ALSO *Cancer Sourcebook for Women, Women's Health Concerns Sourcebook*

■

Breastfeeding Sourcebook

Basic Consumer Health Information about the Benefits of Breastmilk, Preparing to Breastfeed, Breastfeeding as a Baby Grows, Nutrition, and More, Including Information on Special Situations and Concerns Such as Mastitis, Illness, Medications, Allergies, Multiple Births, Prematurity, Special Needs, and Adoption

Along with a Glossary and Resources for Additional Help and Information

Edited by Jenni Lynn Colson. 388 pages. 2002. 0-7808-0332-9. $78.

SEE ALSO *Pregnancy & Birth Sourcebook*

"Particularly useful is the information about professional lactation services and chapters on breastfeeding when returning to work. . . . *Breastfeeding Sourcebook* will be useful for public libraries, consumer health libraries, and technical schools offering nurse assistant training, especially in areas where Internet access is problematic."
—*American Reference Books Annual, 2003*

■

Burns Sourcebook

Basic Consumer Health Information about Various Types of Burns and Scalds, Including Flame, Heat, Cold, Electrical, Chemical, and Sun Burns

Along with Information on Short-Term and Long-Term Treatments, Tissue Reconstruction, Plastic Surgery, Prevention Suggestions, and First Aid

Edited by Allan R. Cook. 604 pages. 1999. 0-7808-0204-7. $78.

"This is an exceptional addition to the series and is highly recommended for all consumer health collections, hospital libraries, and academic medical centers."
—*E-Streams, Mar '00*

"This key reference guide is an invaluable addition to all health care and public libraries in confronting this ongoing health issue."
—*American Reference Books Annual, 2000*

"Recommended reference source."
—*Booklist, American Library Association, Dec '99*

SEE ALSO *Skin Disorders Sourcebook*

■

Cancer Sourcebook, 4th Edition

Basic Consumer Health Information about Major Forms and Stages of Cancer, Featuring Facts about Head and Neck Cancers, Lung Cancers, Gastrointestinal Cancers, Genitourinary Cancers, Lymphomas, Blood Cell Cancers, Endocrine Cancers, Skin Cancers, Bone Cancers, Sarcomas, and Others, and Including Information about Cancer Treatments and Therapies, Identifying and Reducing Cancer Risks, and Strategies for Coping with Cancer and the Side Effects of Treatment

Along with a Cancer Glossary, Statistical and Demographic Data, and a Directory of Sources for Additional Help and Information

Edited by Karen Bellenir. 1,119 pages. 2003. 0-7808-0633-6. $78.

ALSO AVAILABLE: *Cancer Sourcebook, 1st Edition.* Edited by Frank E. Bair. 932 pages. 1990. 1-55888-888-8. $78.

New Cancer Sourcebook, 2nd Edition. Edited by Allan R. Cook. 1,313 pages. 1996. 0-7808-0041-9. $78.

Cancer Sourcebook, 3rd Edition. Edited by Edward J. Prucha. 1,069 pages. 2000. 0-7808-0227-6. $78.

"With cancer being the second leading cause of death for Americans, a prodigious work such as this one, which locates centrally so much cancer-related information, is clearly an asset to this nation's citizens and others." —*Journal of the National Medical Association, 2004*

"This title is recommended for health sciences and public libraries with consumer health collections."
—*E-Streams, Feb '01*

"... can be effectively used by cancer patients and their families who are looking for answers in a language they can understand. Public and hospital libraries should have it on their shelves."
—*American Reference Books Annual, 2001*

"Recommended reference source."
—*Booklist, American Library Association, Dec '00*

Cited in *Reference Sources for Small and Medium-Sized Libraries, American Library Association, 1999*

"The amount of factual and useful information is extensive. The writing is very clear, geared to general readers. Recommended for all levels." —*Choice, Association of College & Research Libraries, Jan '97*

***SEE ALSO** Breast Cancer Sourcebook, Cancer Sourcebook for Women, Pediatric Cancer Sourcebook, Prostate Cancer Sourcebook*

■

Cancer Sourcebook for Women, 2nd Edition

Basic Consumer Health Information about Gynecologic Cancers and Related Concerns, Including Cervical Cancer, Endometrial Cancer, Gestational Trophoblastic Tumor, Ovarian Cancer, Uterine Cancer, Vaginal Cancer, Vulvar Cancer, Breast Cancer, and Common Non-Cancerous Uterine Conditions, with Facts about Cancer Risk Factors, Screening and Prevention, Treatment Options, and Reports on Current Research Initiatives

Along with a Glossary of Cancer Terms and a Directory of Resources for Additional Help and Information

Edited by Karen Bellenir. 604 pages. 2002. 0-7808-0226-8. $78.

***ALSO AVAILABLE:** Cancer Sourcebook for Women, 1st Edition.* Edited by Allan R. Cook and Peter D. Dresser. 524 pages. 1996. 0-7808-0076-1. $78.

"An excellent addition to collections in public, consumer health, and women's health libraries."
—*American Reference Books Annual, 2003*

"Overall, the information is excellent, and complex topics are clearly explained. As a reference book for the consumer it is a valuable resource to assist them to make informed decisions about cancer and its treatments." —*Cancer Forum, Nov '02*

"Highly recommended for academic and medical reference collections." —*Library Bookwatch, Sep '02*

"This is a highly recommended book for any public or consumer library, being reader friendly and containing accurate and helpful information."
—*E-Streams, Aug '02*

"Recommended reference source."
—*Booklist, American Library Association, Jul '02*

***SEE ALSO** Breast Cancer Sourcebook, Women's Health Concerns Sourcebook*

Cardiovascular Diseases & Disorders Sourcebook, 1st Edition

***SEE** Heart Diseases & Disorders Sourcebook, 2nd Edition*

■

Caregiving Sourcebook

Basic Consumer Health Information for Caregivers, Including a Profile of Caregivers, Caregiving Responsibilities and Concerns, Tips for Specific Conditions, Care Environments, and the Effects of Caregiving

Along with Facts about Legal Issues, Financial Information, and Future Planning, a Glossary, and a Listing of Additional Resources

Edited by Joyce Brennfleck Shannon. 600 pages. 2001. 0-7808-0331-0. $78.

"Essential for most collections."
—*Library Journal, Apr 1, 2002*

"An ideal addition to the reference collection of any public library. Health sciences information professionals may also want to acquire the *Caregiving Sourcebook* for their hospital or academic library for use as a ready reference tool by health care workers interested in aging and caregiving." —*E-Streams, Jan '02*

"Recommended reference source."
—*Booklist, American Library Association, Oct '01*

■

Child Abuse Sourcebook

Basic Consumer Health Information about the Physical, Sexual, and Emotional Abuse of Children, with Additional Facts about Neglect, Munchausen Syndrome by Proxy (MSBP), Shaken Baby Syndrome, and Controversial Issues Related to Child Abuse, Such as Withholding Medical Care, Corporal Punishment, and Child Maltreatment in Youth Sports, and Featuring Facts about Child Protective Services, Foster Care, Adoption, Parenting Challenges, and Other Abuse Prevention Efforts

Along with a Glossary of Related Terms and Resources for Additional Help and Information

Edited by Dawn D. Matthews. 620 pages. 2004. 0-7808-0705-7. $78.

■

Childhood Diseases & Disorders Sourcebook

Basic Consumer Health Information about Medical Problems Often Encountered in Pre-Adolescent Children, Including Respiratory Tract Ailments, Ear Infections, Sore Throats, Disorders of the Skin and Scalp, Digestive and Genitourinary Diseases, Infectious Diseases, Inflammatory Disorders, Chronic Physical and Developmental Disorders, Allergies, and More

Along with Information about Diagnostic Tests, Common Childhood Surgeries, and Frequently Used Medications, with a Glossary of Important Terms and Resource Directory

Edited by Chad T. Kimball. 662 pages. 2003. 0-7808-0458-9. $78.

"This is an excellent book for new parents and should be included in all health care and public libraries."
—*American Reference Books Annual, 2004*

■

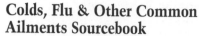

Colds, Flu & Other Common Ailments Sourcebook

Basic Consumer Health Information about Common Ailments and Injuries, Including Colds, Coughs, the Flu, Sinus Problems, Headaches, Fever, Nausea and Vomiting, Menstrual Cramps, Diarrhea, Constipation, Hemorrhoids, Back Pain, Dandruff, Dry and Itchy Skin, Cuts, Scrapes, Sprains, Bruises, and More

Along with Information about Prevention, Self-Care, Choosing a Doctor, Over-the-Counter Medications, Folk Remedies, and Alternative Therapies, and Including a Glossary of Important Terms and a Directory of Resources for Further Help and Information

Edited by Chad T. Kimball. 638 pages. 2001. 0-7808-0435-X. $78.

"A good starting point for research on common illnesses. It will be a useful addition to public and consumer health library collections."
—*American Reference Books Annual 2002*

"Will prove valuable to any library seeking to maintain a current, comprehensive reference collection of health resources. . . . Excellent reference."
—*The Bookwatch, Aug '01*

"Recommended reference source."
—*Booklist, American Library Association, July '01*

■

Communication Disorders Sourcebook

Basic Information about Deafness and Hearing Loss, Speech and Language Disorders, Voice Disorders, Balance and Vestibular Disorders, and Disorders of Smell, Taste, and Touch

Edited by Linda M. Ross. 533 pages. 1996. 0-7808-0077-X. $78.

"This is skillfully edited and is a welcome resource for the layperson. It should be found in every public and medical library."
—*Booklist Health Sciences Supplement, American Library Association, Oct '97*

■

Congenital Disorders Sourcebook

Basic Information about Disorders Acquired during Gestation, Including Spina Bifida, Hydrocephalus, Cerebral Palsy, Heart Defects, Craniofacial Abnormalities, Fetal Alcohol Syndrome, and More

Along with Current Treatment Options and Statistical Data

Edited by Karen Bellenir. 607 pages. 1997. 0-7808-0205-5. $78.

"Recommended reference source."
—*Booklist, American Library Association, Oct '97*

SEE ALSO *Pregnancy & Birth Sourcebook*

■

Consumer Issues in Health Care Sourcebook

Basic Information about Health Care Fundamentals and Related Consumer Issues, Including Exams and Screening Tests, Physician Specialties, Choosing a Doctor, Using Prescription and Over-the-Counter Medications Safely, Avoiding Health Scams, Managing Common Health Risks in the Home, Care Options for Chronically or Terminally Ill Patients, and a List of Resources for Obtaining Help and Further Information

Edited by Karen Bellenir. 618 pages. 1998. 0-7808-0221-7. $78.

"Both public and academic libraries will want to have a copy in their collection for readers who are interested in self-education on health issues."
—*American Reference Books Annual, 2000*

"The editor has researched the literature from government agencies and others, saving readers the time and effort of having to do the research themselves. Recommended for public libraries."
—*Reference and User Services Quarterly, American Library Association, Spring '99*

"Recommended reference source."
—*Booklist, American Library Association, Dec '98*

■

Contagious Diseases Sourcebook

Basic Consumer Health Information about Infectious Diseases Spread by Person-to-Person Contact through Direct Touch, Airborne Transmission, Sexual Contact, or Contact with Blood or Other Body Fluids, Including Hepatitis, Herpes, Influenza, Lice, Measles, Mumps, Pinworm, Ringworm, Severe Acute Respiratory Syndrome (SARS), Streptococcal Infections, Tuberculosis, and Others

Along with Facts about Disease Transmission, Antimicrobial Resistance, and Vaccines, with a Glossary and Directories of Resources for More Information

Edited by Karen Bellenir. 643 pages. 2004. 0-7808-0736-7. $78.

■

Contagious & Non-Contagious Infectious Diseases Sourcebook

Basic Information about Contagious Diseases like Measles, Polio, Hepatitis B, and Infectious Mononucleosis, and Non-Contagious Infectious Diseases like Tetanus and Toxic Shock Syndrome, and Diseases Occurring as Secondary Infections Such as Shingles and Reye Syndrome

Along with Vaccination, Prevention, and Treatment Information, and a Section Describing Emerging Infectious Disease Threats

Edited by Karen Bellenir and Peter D. Dresser. 566 pages. 1996. 0-7808-0075-3. $78.

Death & Dying Sourcebook

Basic Consumer Health Information for the Layperson about End-of-Life Care and Related Ethical and Legal Issues, Including Chief Causes of Death, Autopsies, Pain Management for the Terminally Ill, Life Support Systems, Insurance, Euthanasia, Assisted Suicide, Hospice Programs, Living Wills, Funeral Planning, Counseling, Mourning, Organ Donation, and Physician Training

Along with Statistical Data, a Glossary, and Listings of Sources for Further Help and Information

Edited by Annemarie S. Muth. 641 pages. 1999. 0-7808-0230-6. $78.

"Public libraries, medical libraries, and academic libraries will all find this sourcebook a useful addition to their collections."
—*American Reference Books Annual, 2001*

"An extremely useful resource for those concerned with death and dying in the United States."
—*Respiratory Care, Nov '00*

"Recommended reference source."
—*Booklist, American Library Association, Aug '00*

"This book is a definite must for all those involved in end-of-life care." —*Doody's Review Service, 2000*

■

Dental Care & Oral Health Sourcebook, 2nd Edition

Basic Consumer Health Information about Dental Care, Including Oral Hygiene, Dental Visits, Pain Management, Cavities, Crowns, Bridges, Dental Implants, and Fillings, and Other Oral Health Concerns, Such as Gum Disease, Bad Breath, Dry Mouth, Genetic and Developmental Abnormalities, Oral Cancers, Orthodontics, and Temporomandibular Disorders

Along with Updates on Current Research in Oral Health, a Glossary, a Directory of Dental and Oral Health Organizations, and Resources for People with Dental and Oral Health Disorders

Edited by Amy L. Sutton. 609 pages. 2003. 0-7808-0634-4. $78.

ALSO AVAILABLE: *Oral Health Sourcebook, 1st Edition.* Edited by Allan R. Cook. 558 pages. 1997. 0-7808-0082-6. $78.

"This book could serve as a turning point in the battle to educate consumers in issues concerning oral health."
—*American Reference Books Annual, 2004*

"Unique source which will fill a gap in dental sources for patients and the lay public. A valuable reference tool even in a library with thousands of books on dentistry. Comprehensive, clear, inexpensive, and easy to read and use. It fills an enormous gap in the health care literature." —*Reference and User Services Quarterly, American Library Association, Summer '98*

"Recommended reference source."
—*Booklist, American Library Association, Dec '97*

Depression Sourcebook

Basic Consumer Health Information about Unipolar Depression, Bipolar Disorder, Postpartum Depression, Seasonal Affective Disorder, and Other Types of Depression in Children, Adolescents, Women, Men, the Elderly, and Other Selected Populations

Along with Facts about Causes, Risk Factors, Diagnostic Criteria, Treatment Options, Coping Strategies, Suicide Prevention, a Glossary, and a Directory of Sources for Additional Help and Information

Edited by Karen Belleni. 602 pages. 2002. 0-7808-0611-5. $78.

"*Depression Sourcebook* is of a very high standard. Its purpose, which is to serve as a reference source to the lay reader, is very well served."
—*Journal of the National Medical Association, 2004*

"Invaluable reference for public and school library collections alike." —*Library Bookwatch, Apr '03*

"Recommended for purchase."
—*American Reference Books Annual, 2003*

■

Diabetes Sourcebook, 3rd Edition

Basic Consumer Health Information about Type 1 Diabetes (Insulin-Dependent or Juvenile-Onset Diabetes), Type 2 Diabetes (Noninsulin-Dependent or Adult-Onset Diabetes), Gestational Diabetes, Impaired Glucose Tolerance (IGT), and Related Complications, Such as Amputation, Eye Disease, Gum Disease, Nerve Damage, and End-Stage Renal Disease, Including Facts about Insulin, Oral Diabetes Medications, Blood Sugar Testing, and the Role of Exercise and Nutrition in the Control of Diabetes

Along with a Glossary and Resources for Further Help and Information

Edited by Dawn D. Matthews. 622 pages. 2003. 0-7808-0629-8. $78.

ALSO AVAILABLE: *Diabetes Sourcebook, 1st Edition.* Edited by Karen Bellenir and Peter D. Dresser. 827 pages. 1994. 1-55888-751-2. $78.

Diabetes Sourcebook, 2nd Edition. Edited by Karen Bellenir. 688 pages. 1998. 0-7808-0224-1. $78.

"This edition is even more helpful than earlier versions. . . . It is a truly valuable tool for anyone seeking readable and authoritative information on diabetes."
—*American Reference Books Annual, 2004*

"An invaluable reference." —*Library Journal, May '00*

Selected as one of the 250 "Best Health Sciences Books of 1999." —*Doody's Rating Service, Mar-Apr 2000*

"Provides useful information for the general public."
—*Healthlines, University of Michigan Health Management Research Center, Sep/Oct '99*

". . . provides reliable mainstream medical information . . . belongs on the shelves of any library with a consumer health collection." —*E-Streams, Sep '99*

"Recommended reference source."
—*Booklist, American Library Association, Feb '99*

Diet & Nutrition Sourcebook, 2nd Edition

Basic Consumer Health Information about Dietary Guidelines, Recommended Daily Intake Values, Vitamins, Minerals, Fiber, Fat, Weight Control, Dietary Supplements, and Food Additives

Along with Special Sections on Nutrition Needs throughout Life and Nutrition for People with Such Specific Medical Concerns as Allergies, High Blood Cholesterol, Hypertension, Diabetes, Celiac Disease, Seizure Disorders, Phenylketonuria (PKU), Cancer, and Eating Disorders, and Including Reports on Current Nutrition Research and Source Listings for Additional Help and Information

Edited by Karen Bellenir. 650 pages. 1999. 0-7808-0228-4. $78.

ALSO AVAILABLE: *Diet & Nutrition Sourcebook, 1st Edition.* Edited by Dan R. Harris. 662 pages. 1996. 0-7808-0084-2. $78.

"This book is an excellent source of basic diet and nutrition information." —*Booklist Health Sciences Supplement, American Library Association, Dec '00*

"This reference document should be in any public library, but it would be a very good guide for beginning students in the health sciences. If the other books in this publisher's series are as good as this, they should all be in the health sciences collections."
—*American Reference Books Annual, 2000*

"This book is an excellent general nutrition reference for consumers who desire to take an active role in their health care for prevention. Consumers of all ages who select this book can feel confident they are receiving current and accurate information." —*Journal of Nutrition for the Elderly, Vol. 19, No. 4, '00*

"Recommended reference source."
—*Booklist, American Library Association, Dec '99*

SEE ALSO *Digestive Diseases & Disorders Sourcebook, Eating Disorders Sourcebook, Gastrointestinal Diseases & Disorders Sourcebook, Vegetarian Sourcebook*

■

Digestive Diseases & Disorders Sourcebook

Basic Consumer Health Information about Diseases and Disorders that Impact the Upper and Lower Digestive System, Including Celiac Disease, Constipation, Crohn's Disease, Cyclic Vomiting Syndrome, Diarrhea, Diverticulosis and Diverticulitis, Gallstones, Heartburn, Hemorrhoids, Hernias, Indigestion (Dyspepsia), Irritable Bowel Syndrome, Lactose Intolerance, Ulcers, and More

Along with Information about Medications and Other Treatments, Tips for Maintaining a Healthy Digestive Tract, a Glossary, and Directory of Digestive Diseases Organizations

Edited by Karen Bellenir. 335 pages. 2000. 0-7808-0327-2. $78.

"This title would be an excellent addition to all public or patient-research libraries."
—*American Reference Books Annual, 2001*

"This title is recommended for public, hospital, and health sciences libraries with consumer health collections." —*E-Streams, Jul-Aug '00*

"Recommended reference source."
—*Booklist, American Library Association, May '00*

SEE ALSO *Diet & Nutrition Sourcebook, Eating Disorders Sourcebook, Gastrointestinal Diseases & Disorders Sourcebook*

■

Disabilities Sourcebook

Basic Consumer Health Information about Physical and Psychiatric Disabilities, Including Descriptions of Major Causes of Disability, Assistive and Adaptive Aids, Workplace Issues, and Accessibility Concerns

Along with Information about the Americans with Disabilities Act, a Glossary, and Resources for Additional Help and Information

Edited by Dawn D. Matthews. 616 pages. 2000. 0-7808-0389-2. $78.

"It is a must for libraries with a consumer health section." —*American Reference Books Annual 2002*

"A much needed addition to the Omnigraphics *Health Reference Series*. A current reference work to provide people with disabilities, their families, caregivers or those who work with them, a broad range of information in one volume, has not been available until now. . . . It is recommended for all public and academic library reference collections." —*E-Streams, May '01*

"An excellent source book in easy-to-read format covering many current topics; highly recommended for all libraries." —*Choice, Association of College and Research Libraries, Jan '01*

"Recommended reference source."
—*Booklist, American Library Association, Jul '00*

■

Domestic Violence Sourcebook, 2nd Edition

Basic Consumer Health Information about the Causes and Consequences of Abusive Relationships, Including Physical Violence, Sexual Assault, Battery, Stalking, and Emotional Abuse, and Facts about the Effects of Violence on Women, Men, Young Adults, and the Elderly, with Reports about Domestic Violence in Selected Populations, and Featuring Facts about Medical Care, Victim Assistance and Protection, Prevention Strategies, Mental Health Services, and Legal Issues

Along with a Glossary of Related Terms and Resources for Additional Help and Information

Edited by Dawn D. Matthews. 628 pages. 2004. 0-7808-0669-7. $78.

ALSO AVAILABLE: *Domestic Violence & Child Abuse Sourcebook, 1st Edition.* Edited by Helene Henderson. 1,064 pages. 2001. 0-7808-0235-7. $78.

"Interested lay persons should find the book extremely beneficial. . . . A copy of *Domestic Violence and Child Abuse Sourcebook* should be in every public library in the United States."

—*Social Science & Medicine, No. 56, 2003*

"This is important information. The Web has many resources but this sourcebook fills an important societal need. I am not aware of any other resources of this type." —*Doody's Review Service, Sep '01*

"Recommended for all libraries, scholars, and practitioners." —*Choice, Association of College & Research Libraries, Jul '01*

"Recommended reference source."

—*Booklist, American Library Association, Apr '01*

"Important pick for college-level health reference libraries." —*The Bookwatch, Mar '01*

"Because this problem is so widespread and because this book includes a lot of issues within one volume, this work is recommended for all public libraries."

—*American Reference Books Annual, 2001*

■

Drug Abuse Sourcebook, 2nd Edition

Basic Consumer Health Information about Illicit Substances of Abuse and the Misuse of Prescription and Over-the-Counter Medications, Including Depressants, Hallucinogens, Inhalants, Marijuana, Stimulants, and Anabolic Steroids

Along with Facts about Related Health Risks, Treatment Programs, Prevention Programs, a Glossary of Abuse and Addiction Terms, a Glossary of Drug-Related Street Terms, and a Directory Resources for More Information

Edited by Catherine Ginther. 600 pages. 2004. 0-7808-0740-5. $78.

ALSO AVAILABLE: Drug Abuse Sourcebook, 1st Edition. Edited by Karen Bellenir. 629 pages. 2000. 0-7808-0242-X. $78.

"Containing a wealth of information . . . . This resource belongs in libraries that serve a lower-division undergraduate or community college clientele as well as the general public." —*Choice, Association of College and Research Libraries, Jun '01*

"Recommended reference source."

—*Booklist, American Library Association, Feb '01*

"Highly recommended." —*The Bookwatch, Jan '01*

"Even though there is a plethora of books on drug abuse, this volume is recommended for school, public, and college libraries."

—*American Reference Books Annual, 2001*

SEE ALSO *Alcoholism Sourcebook, Substance Abuse Sourcebook*

Ear, Nose & Throat Disorders Sourcebook

Basic Information about Disorders of the Ears, Nose, Sinus Cavities, Pharynx, and Larynx, Including Ear Infections, Tinnitus, Vestibular Disorders, Allergic and Non-Allergic Rhinitis, Sore Throats, Tonsillitis, and Cancers That Affect the Ears, Nose, Sinuses, and Throat

Along with Reports on Current Research Initiatives, a Glossary of Related Medical Terms, and a Directory of Sources for Further Help and Information

Edited by Karen Bellenir and Linda M. Shin. 576 pages. 1998. 0-7808-0206-3. $78.

"Overall, this sourcebook is helpful for the consumer seeking information on ENT issues. It is recommended for public libraries."

—*American Reference Books Annual, 1999*

"Recommended reference source."

—*Booklist, American Library Association, Dec '98*

■

Eating Disorders Sourcebook

Basic Consumer Health Information about Eating Disorders, Including Information about Anorexia Nervosa, Bulimia Nervosa, Binge Eating, Body Dysmorphic Disorder, Pica, Laxative Abuse, and Night Eating Syndrome

Along with Information about Causes, Adverse Effects, and Treatment and Prevention Issues, and Featuring a Section on Concerns Specific to Children and Adolescents, a Glossary, and Resources for Further Help and Information

Edited by Dawn D. Matthews. 322 pages. 2001. 0-7808-0335-3. $78.

"Recommended for health science libraries that are open to the public, as well as hospital libraries. This book is a good resource for the consumer who is concerned about eating disorders." —*E-Streams, Mar '02*

"This volume is another convenient collection of excerpted articles. Recommended for school and public library patrons; lower-division undergraduates; and two-year technical program students." —*Choice, Association of College & Research Libraries, Jan '02*

"Recommended reference source." —*Booklist, American Library Association, Oct '01*

SEE ALSO *Diet & Nutrition Sourcebook, Digestive Diseases & Disorders Sourcebook, Gastrointestinal Diseases & Disorders Sourcebook*

■

Emergency Medical Services Sourcebook

Basic Consumer Health Information about Preventing, Preparing for, and Managing Emergency Situations, When and Who to Call for Help, What to Expect in the Emergency Room, the Emergency Medical Team, Patient Issues, and Current Topics in Emergency Medicine

Along with Statistical Data, a Glossary, and Sources of Additional Help and Information

Edited by Jenni Lynn Colson. 494 pages. 2002. 0-7808-0420-1. $78.

"Handy and convenient for home, public, school, and college libraries. Recommended."

— *Choice, Association of College and Research Libraries, Apr '03*

"This reference can provide the consumer with answers to most questions about emergency care in the United States, or it will direct them to a resource where the answer can be found."

— *American Reference Books Annual, 2003*

"Recommended reference source."

— *Booklist, American Library Association, Feb '03*

■

Endocrine & Metabolic Disorders Sourcebook

Basic Information for the Layperson about Pancreatic and Insulin-Related Disorders Such as Pancreatitis, Diabetes, and Hypoglycemia; Adrenal Gland Disorders Such as Cushing's Syndrome, Addison's Disease, and Congenital Adrenal Hyperplasia; Pituitary Gland Disorders Such as Growth Hormone Deficiency, Acromegaly, and Pituitary Tumors; Thyroid Disorders Such as Hypothyroidism, Graves' Disease, Hashimoto's Disease, and Goiter; Hyperparathyroidism; and Other Diseases and Syndromes of Hormone Imbalance or Metabolic Dysfunction

Along with Reports on Current Research Initiatives

Edited by Linda M. Shin. 574 pages. 1998. 0-7808-0207-1. $78.

"Omnigraphics has produced another needed resource for health information consumers."

—*American Reference Books Annual, 2000*

"Recommended reference source."

— *Booklist, American Library Association, Dec '98*

■

Environmental Health Sourcebook, 2nd Edition

Basic Consumer Health Information about the Environment and Its Effect on Human Health, Including the Effects of Air Pollution, Water Pollution, Hazardous Chemicals, Food Hazards, Radiation Hazards, Biological Agents, Household Hazards, Such as Radon, Asbestos, Carbon Monoxide, and Mold, and Information about Associated Diseases and Disorders, Including Cancer, Allergies, Respiratory Problems, and Skin Disorders

Along with Information about Environmental Concerns for Specific Populations, a Glossary of Related Terms, and Resources for Further Help and Information

Edited by Dawn D. Matthews. 673 pages. 2003. 0-7808-0632-8. $78.

ALSO AVAILABLE: *Environmentally Induced Disorders Sourcebook, 1st Edition.* Edited by Allan R. Cook. 620 pages. 1997. 0-7808-0083-4. $78.

"This recently updated edition continues the level of quality and the reputation of the numerous other volumes in Omnigraphics' *Health Reference Series.*"

—*American Reference Books Annual, 2004*

"Recommended reference source."

—*Booklist, American Library Association, Sep '98*

"This book will be a useful addition to anyone's library." —*Choice Health Sciences Supplement, Association of College and Research Libraries, May '98*

". . . a good survey of numerous environmentally induced physical disorders . . . a useful addition to anyone's library."

—*Doody's Health Sciences Book Reviews, Jan '98*

". . . provide[s] introductory information from the best authorities around. Since this volume covers topics that potentially affect everyone, it will surely be one of the most frequently consulted volumes in the *Health Reference Series.*" —*Rettig on Reference, Nov '97*

■

Environmentally Induced Disorders Sourcebook, 1st Edition

SEE *Environmental Health Sourcebook, 2nd Edition*

■

Ethnic Diseases Sourcebook

Basic Consumer Health Information for Ethnic and Racial Minority Groups in the United States, Including General Health Indicators and Behaviors, Ethnic Diseases, Genetic Testing, the Impact of Chronic Diseases, Women's Health, Mental Health Issues, and Preventive Health Care Services

Along with a Glossary and a Listing of Additional Resources

Edited by Joyce Brennfleck Shannon. 664 pages. 2001. 0-7808-0336-1. $78.

"Recommended for health sciences libraries where public health programs are a priority."

—*E-Streams, Jan '02*

"Not many books have been written on this topic to date, and the *Ethnic Diseases Sourcebook* is a strong addition to the list. It will be an important introductory resource for health consumers, students, health care personnel, and social scientists. It is recommended for public, academic, and large hospital libraries."

— *American Reference Books Annual 2002*

"Recommended reference source."

— *Booklist, American Library Association, Oct '01*

"Will prove valuable to any library seeking to maintain a current, comprehensive reference collection of health resources. . . . An excellent source of health information about genetic disorders which affect particular ethnic and racial minorities in the U.S."

— *The Bookwatch, Aug '01*

Eye Care Sourcebook, 2nd Edition

Basic Consumer Health Information about Eye Care and Eye Disorders, Including Facts about the Diagnosis, Prevention, and Treatment of Common Refractive Problems Such as Myopia, Hyperopia, Astigmatism, and Presbyopia, and Eye Diseases, Including Glaucoma, Cataract, Age-Related Macular Degeneration, and Diabetic Retinopathy

Along with a Section on Vision Correction and Refractive Surgeries, Including LASIK and LASEK, a Glossary, and Directories of Resources for Additional Help and Information

Edited by Amy L. Sutton. 543 pages. 2003. 0-7808-0635-2. $78.

ALSO AVAILABLE: *Ophthalmic Disorders Sourcebook, 1st Edition.* Edited by Linda M. Ross. 631 pages. 1996. 0-7808-0081-8. $78.

". . . a solid reference tool for eye care and a valuable addition to a collection."
—*American Reference Books Annual, 2004*

■

Family Planning Sourcebook

Basic Consumer Health Information about Planning for Pregnancy and Contraception, Including Traditional Methods, Barrier Methods, Hormonal Methods, Permanent Methods, Future Methods, Emergency Contraception, and Birth Control Choices for Women at Each Stage of Life

Along with Statistics, a Glossary, and Sources of Additional Information

Edited by Amy Marcaccio Keyzer. 520 pages. 2001. 0-7808-0379-5. $78.

"Recommended for public, health, and undergraduate libraries as part of the circulating collection."
—*E-Streams, Mar '02*

"Information is presented in an unbiased, readable manner, and the sourcebook will certainly be a necessary addition to those public and high school libraries where Internet access is restricted or otherwise problematic." —*American Reference Books Annual 2002*

"Recommended reference source."
—*Booklist, American Library Association, Oct '01*

"Will prove valuable to any library seeking to maintain a current, comprehensive reference collection of health resources. . . . Excellent reference."
—*The Bookwatch, Aug '01*

SEE ALSO *Pregnancy & Birth Sourcebook*

■

Fitness & Exercise Sourcebook, 2nd Edition

Basic Consumer Health Information about the Fundamentals of Fitness and Exercise, Including How to Begin and Maintain a Fitness Program, Fitness as a Lifestyle, the Link between Fitness and Diet, Advice for Specific Groups of People, Exercise as It Relates to Specific Medical Conditions, and Recent Research in Fitness and Exercise

Along with a Glossary of Important Terms and Resources for Additional Help and Information

Edited by Kristen M. Gledhill. 646 pages. 2001. 0-7808-0334-5. $78.

ALSO AVAILABLE: *Fitness & Exercise Sourcebook, 1st Edition.* Edited by Dan R. Harris. 663 pages. 1996. 0-7808-0186-5. $78.

"This work is recommended for all general reference collections."
—*American Reference Books Annual 2002*

"Highly recommended for public, consumer, and school grades fourth through college."
—*E-Streams, Nov '01*

"Recommended reference source." —*Booklist, American Library Association, Oct '01*

"The information appears quite comprehensive and is considered reliable. . . . This second edition is a welcomed addition to the series."
—*Doody's Review Service, Sep '01*

"This reference is a valuable choice for those who desire a broad source of information on exercise, fitness, and chronic-disease prevention through a healthy lifestyle." —*American Medical Writers Association Journal, Fall '01*

"Will prove valuable to any library seeking to maintain a current, comprehensive reference collection of health resources. . . . Excellent reference."
—*The Bookwatch, Aug '01*

■

Food & Animal Borne Diseases Sourcebook

Basic Information about Diseases That Can Be Spread to Humans through the Ingestion of Contaminated Food or Water or by Contact with Infected Animals and Insects, Such as Botulism, E. Coli, Hepatitis A, Trichinosis, Lyme Disease, and Rabies

Along with Information Regarding Prevention and Treatment Methods, and Including a Special Section for International Travelers Describing Diseases Such as Cholera, Malaria, Travelers' Diarrhea, and Yellow Fever, and Offering Recommendations for Avoiding Illness

Edited by Karen Bellenir and Peter D. Dresser. 535 pages. 1995. 0-7808-0033-8. $78.

"Targeting general readers and providing them with a single, comprehensive source of information on selected topics, this book continues, with the excellent caliber of its predecessors, to catalog topical information on health matters of general interest. Readable and thorough, this valuable resource is highly recommended for all libraries."
—*Academic Library Book Review, Summer '96*

"A comprehensive collection of authoritative information." —*Emergency Medical Services, Oct '95*

Food Safety Sourcebook

Basic Consumer Health Information about the Safe Handling of Meat, Poultry, Seafood, Eggs, Fruit Juices, and Other Food Items, and Facts about Pesticides, Drinking Water, Food Safety Overseas, and the Onset, Duration, and Symptoms of Foodborne Illnesses, Including Types of Pathogenic Bacteria, Parasitic Protozoa, Worms, Viruses, and Natural Toxins

Along with the Role of the Consumer, the Food Handler, and the Government in Food Safety; a Glossary, and Resources for Additional Help and Information

Edited by Dawn D. Matthews. 339 pages. 1999. 0-7808-0326-4. $78.

"This book is recommended for public libraries and universities with home economic and food science programs." —*E-Streams, Nov '00*

"Recommended reference source."
—*Booklist, American Library Association, May '00*

"This book takes the complex issues of food safety and foodborne pathogens and presents them in an easily understood manner. [It does] an excellent job of covering a large and often confusing topic."
—*American Reference Books Annual, 2000*

■

Forensic Medicine Sourcebook

Basic Consumer Information for the Layperson about Forensic Medicine, Including Crime Scene Investigation, Evidence Collection and Analysis, Expert Testimony, Computer-Aided Criminal Identification, Digital Imaging in the Courtroom, DNA Profiling, Accident Reconstruction, Autopsies, Ballistics, Drugs and Explosives Detection, Latent Fingerprints, Product Tampering, and Questioned Document Examination

Along with Statistical Data, a Glossary of Forensics Terminology, and Listings of Sources for Further Help and Information

Edited by Annemarie S. Muth. 574 pages. 1999. 0-7808-0232-2. $78.

"Given the expected widespread interest in its content and its easy to read style, this book is recommended for most public and all college and university libraries."
—*E-Streams, Feb '01*

"Recommended for public libraries."
—*Reference & User Services Quarterly, American Library Association, Spring 2000*

"Recommended reference source."
—*Booklist, American Library Association, Feb '00*

"A wealth of information, useful statistics, references are up-to-date and extremely complete. This wonderful collection of data will help students who are interested in a career in any type of forensic field. It is a great resource for attorneys who need information about types of expert witnesses needed in a particular case. It also offers useful information for fiction and nonfiction writers whose work involves a crime. A fascinating compilation. All levels." —*Choice, Association of College and Research Libraries, Jan 2000*

"There are several items that make this book attractive to consumers who are seeking certain forensic data. . . . This is a useful current source for those seeking general forensic medical answers."
—*American Reference Books Annual, 2000*

■

Gastrointestinal Diseases & Disorders Sourcebook

Basic Information about Gastroesophageal Reflux Disease (Heartburn), Ulcers, Diverticulosis, Irritable Bowel Syndrome, Crohn's Disease, Ulcerative Colitis, Diarrhea, Constipation, Lactose Intolerance, Hemorrhoids, Hepatitis, Cirrhosis, and Other Digestive Problems, Featuring Statistics, Descriptions of Symptoms, and Current Treatment Methods of Interest for Persons Living with Upper and Lower Gastrointestinal Maladies

Edited by Linda M. Ross. 413 pages. 1996. 0-7808-0078-8. $78.

". . . very readable form. The successful editorial work that brought this material together into a useful and understandable reference makes accessible to all readers information that can help them more effectively understand and obtain help for digestive tract problems."
—*Choice, Association of College & Research Libraries, Feb '97*

SEE ALSO *Diet & Nutrition Sourcebook, Digestive Diseases & Disorders, Eating Disorders Sourcebook*

■

Genetic Disorders Sourcebook, 3rd Edition

Basic Consumer Health Information about Hereditary Diseases and Disorders, Including Facts about the Human Genome, Genetic Inheritance Patterns, Disorders Associated with Specific Genes, such as Sickle Cell Disease, Hemophilia, and Cystic Fibrosis, Chromosome Disorders, such as Down Syndrome, Fragile X Syndrome, and Turner Syndrome, and Complex Diseases and Disorders Resulting from the Interaction of Environmental and Genetic Factors, such as Allergies, Cancer, and Obesity

Along with Facts about Genetic Testing, Suggestions for Parents of Children with Special Needs, Reports on Current Research Initiatives, a Glossary of Genetic Terminology, and Resources for Additional Help and Information

Edited by Karen Bellenir. 777 pages. 2004. 0-7808-0742-1. $78.

ALSO AVAILABLE: *Genetic Disorders Sourcebook, 1st Edition.* Edited by Karen Bellenir. 642 pages. 1996. 0-7808-0034-6. $78.

Genetic Disorders Sourcebook, 2nd Edition. Edited by Kathy Massimini. 768 pages. 2001. 0-7808-0241-1. $78.

"Recommended for public libraries and medical and hospital libraries with consumer health collections."
—*E-Streams, May '01*

"Recommended reference source."

—*Booklist, American Library Association, Apr '01*

"Important pick for college-level health reference libraries." —*The Bookwatch, Mar '01*

"Provides essential medical information to both the general public and those diagnosed with a serious or fatal genetic disease or disorder." —*Choice, Association of College and Research Libraries, Jan '97*

■

Head Trauma Sourcebook

Basic Information for the Layperson about Open-Head and Closed-Head Injuries, Treatment Advances, Recovery, and Rehabilitation

Along with Reports on Current Research Initiatives

Edited by Karen Bellenir. 414 pages. 1997. 0-7808-0208-X. $78.

■

Headache Sourcebook

Basic Consumer Health Information about Migraine, Tension, Cluster, Rebound and Other Types of Headaches, with Facts about the Cause and Prevention of Headaches, the Effects of Stress and the Environment, Headaches during Pregnancy and Menopause, and Childhood Headaches

Along with a Glossary and Other Resources for Additional Help and Information

Edited by Dawn D. Matthews. 362 pages. 2002. 0-7808-0337-X. $78.

"Highly recommended for academic and medical reference collections." —*Library Bookwatch, Sep '02*

■

Health Insurance Sourcebook

Basic Information about Managed Care Organizations, Traditional Fee-for-Service Insurance, Insurance Portability and Pre-Existing Conditions Clauses, Medicare, Medicaid, Social Security, and Military Health Care

Along with Information about Insurance Fraud

Edited by Wendy Wilcox. 530 pages. 1997. 0-7808-0222-5. $78.

"Particularly useful because it brings much of this information together in one volume. This book will be a handy reference source in the health sciences library, hospital library, college and university library, and medium to large public library."

—*Medical Reference Services Quarterly, Fall '98*

Awarded "Books of the Year Award"

—*American Journal of Nursing, 1997*

"The layout of the book is particularly helpful as it provides easy access to reference material. A most useful addition to the vast amount of information about health insurance. The use of data from U.S. government agencies is most commendable. Useful in a library or learning center for healthcare professional students."

—*Doody's Health Sciences Book Reviews, Nov '97*

Health Reference Series Cumulative Index 1999

A Comprehensive Index to the Individual Volumes of the Health Reference Series, Including a Subject Index, Name Index, Organization Index, and Publication Index

Along with a Master List of Acronyms and Abbreviations

Edited by Edward J. Prucha, Anne Holmes, and Robert Rudnick. 990 pages. 2000. 0-7808-0382-5. $78.

"This volume will be most helpful in libraries that have a relatively complete collection of the Health Reference Series." —*American Reference Books Annual, 2001*

"Essential for collections that hold any of the numerous *Health Reference Series* titles."

—*Choice, Association of College and Research Libraries, Nov '00*

■

Healthy Aging Sourcebook

Basic Consumer Health Information about Maintaining Health through the Aging Process, Including Advice on Nutrition, Exercise, and Sleep, Help in Making Decisions about Midlife Issues and Retirement, and Guidance Concerning Practical and Informed Choices in Health Consumerism

Along with Data Concerning the Theories of Aging, Different Experiences in Aging by Minority Groups, and Facts about Aging Now and Aging in the Future; and Featuring a Glossary, a Guide to Consumer Help, Additional Suggested Reading, and Practical Resource Directory

Edited by Jenifer Swanson. 536 pages. 1999. 0-7808-0390-6. $78.

"Recommended reference source."

—*Booklist, American Library Association, Feb '00*

SEE ALSO *Physical & Mental Issues in Aging Sourcebook*

■

Healthy Children Sourcebook

Basic Consumer Health Information about the Physical and Mental Development of Children between the Ages of 3 and 12, Including Routine Health Care, Preventative Health Services, Safety and First Aid, Healthy Sleep, Dental Care, Nutrition, and Fitness, and Featuring Parenting Tips on Such Topics as Bedwetting, Choosing Day Care, Monitoring TV and Other Media, and Establishing a Foundation for Substance Abuse Prevention

Along with a Glossary of Commonly Used Pediatric Terms and Resources for Additional Help and Information.

Edited by Chad T. Kimball. 647 pages. 2003. 0-7808-0247-0. $78.

"It is hard to imagine that any other single resource exists that would provide such a comprehensive guide

of timely information on health promotion and disease prevention for children aged 3 to 12."

—*American Reference Books Annual, 2004*

"The strengths of this book are many. It is clearly written, presented and structured."

—*Journal of the National Medical Association, 2004*

■

Healthy Heart Sourcebook for Women

Basic Consumer Health Information about Cardiac Issues Specific to Women, Including Facts about Major Risk Factors and Prevention, Treatment and Control Strategies, and Important Dietary Issues

Along with a Special Section Regarding the Pros and Cons of Hormone Replacement Therapy and Its Impact on Heart Health, and Additional Help, Including Recipes, a Glossary, and a Directory of Resources

Edited by Dawn D. Matthews. 336 pages. 2000. 0-7808-0329-9. $78.

"A good reference source and recommended for all public, academic, medical, and hospital libraries."

—*Medical Reference Services Quarterly, Summer '01*

"Because of the lack of information specific to women on this topic, this book is recommended for public libraries and consumer libraries."

—*American Reference Books Annual, 2001*

"Contains very important information about coronary artery disease that all women should know. The information is current and presented in an easy-to-read format. The book will make a good addition to any library."

—*American Medical Writers Association Journal, Summer '00*

"Important, basic reference."

—*Reviewer's Bookwatch, Jul '00*

SEE ALSO *Heart Diseases & Disorders Sourcebook, Women's Health Concerns Sourcebook*

■

Heart Diseases & Disorders Sourcebook, 2nd Edition

Basic Consumer Health Information about Heart Attacks, Angina, Rhythm Disorders, Heart Failure, Valve Disease, Congenital Heart Disorders, and More, Including Descriptions of Surgical Procedures and Other Interventions, Medications, Cardiac Rehabilitation, Risk Identification, and Prevention Tips

Along with Statistical Data, Reports on Current Research Initiatives, a Glossary of Cardiovascular Terms, and Resource Directory

Edited by Karen Bellenir. 612 pages. 2000. 0-7808-0238-1. $78.

ALSO AVAILABLE: *Cardiovascular Diseases & Disorders Sourcebook, 1st Edition.* Edited by Karen Bellenir and Peter D. Dresser. 683 pages. 1995. 0-7808-0032-X. $78.

"This work stands out as an imminently accessible resource for the general public. It is recommended for the reference and circulating shelves of school, public, and academic libraries."

—*American Reference Books Annual, 2001*

"Recommended reference source."

—*Booklist, American Library Association, Dec '00*

"Provides comprehensive coverage of matters related to the heart. This title is recommended for health sciences and public libraries with consumer health collections."

—*E-Streams, Oct '00*

SEE ALSO *Healthy Heart Sourcebook for Women*

■

Household Safety Sourcebook

Basic Consumer Health Information about Household Safety, Including Information about Poisons, Chemicals, Fire, and Water Hazards in the Home

Along with Advice about the Safe Use of Home Maintenance Equipment, Choosing Toys and Nursery Furniture, Holiday and Recreation Safety, a Glossary, and Resources for Further Help and Information

Edited by Dawn D. Matthews. 606 pages. 2002. 0-7808-0338-8. $78.

"This work will be useful in public libraries with large consumer health and wellness departments."

—*American Reference Books Annual, 2003*

"As a sourcebook on household safety this book meets its mark. It is encyclopedic in scope and covers a wide range of safety issues that are commonly seen in the home."

—*E-Streams, Jul '02*

■

Hypertension Sourcebook

Basic Consumer Health Information about the Causes, Diagnosis, and Treatment of High Blood Pressure, with Facts about Consequences, Complications, and Co-Occurring Disorders, Such as Coronary Heart Disease, Diabetes, Stroke, Kidney Disease, and Hypertensive Retinopathy, and Issues in Blood Pressure Control, Including Dietary Choices, Stress Management, and Medications

Along with Reports on Current Research Initiatives and Clinical Trials, a Glossary, and Resources for Additional Help and Information

Edited by Dawn D. Matthews and Karen Bellenir. 600 pages. 2004. 0-7808-0674-3. $78.

■

Immune System Disorders Sourcebook

Basic Information about Lupus, Multiple Sclerosis, Guillain-Barré Syndrome, Chronic Granulomatous Disease, and More

Along with Statistical and Demographic Data and Reports on Current Research Initiatives

Edited by Allan R. Cook. 608 pages. 1997. 0-7808-0209-8. $78.

Infant & Toddler Health Sourcebook

Basic Consumer Health Information about the Physical and Mental Development of Newborns, Infants, and Toddlers, Including Neonatal Concerns, Nutrition Recommendations, Immunization Schedules, Common Pediatric Disorders, Assessments and Milestones, Safety Tips, and Advice for Parents and Other Caregivers

Along with a Glossary of Terms and Resource Listings for Additional Help

Edited by Jenifer Swanson. 585 pages. 2000. 0-7808-0246-2. $78.

"As a reference for the general public, this would be useful in any library." —*E-Streams, May '01*

"Recommended reference source."
—*Booklist, American Library Association, Feb '01*

"This is a good source for general use."
—*American Reference Books Annual, 2001*

■

Infectious Diseases Sourcebook

Basic Consumer Health Information about Non-Contagious Bacterial, Viral, Prion, Fungal, and Parasitic Diseases Spread by Food and Water, Insects and Animals, or Environmental Contact, Including Botulism, E. Coli, Encephalitis, Legionnaires' Disease, Lyme Disease, Malaria, Plague, Rabies, Salmonella, Tetanus, and Others, and Facts about Newly Emerging Diseases, Such as Hantavirus, Mad Cow Disease, Monkeypox, and West Nile Virus

Along with Information about Preventing Disease Transmission, the Threat of Bioterrorism, and Current Research Initiatives, with a Glossary and Directory of Resources for More Information

Edited by Karen Bellenir. 634 pages. 2004. 0-7808-0675-1. $78.

■

Injury & Trauma Sourcebook

Basic Consumer Health Information about the Impact of Injury, the Diagnosis and Treatment of Common and Traumatic Injuries, Emergency Care, and Specific Injuries Related to Home, Community, Workplace, Transportation, and Recreation

Along with Guidelines for Injury Prevention, a Glossary, and a Directory of Additional Resources

Edited by Joyce Brennfleck Shannon. 696 pages. 2002. 0-7808-0421-X. $78.

"This publication is the most comprehensive work of its kind about injury and trauma."
—*American Reference Books Annual, 2003*

"This sourcebook provides concise, easily readable, basic health information about injuries. . . . This book is well organized and an easy to use reference resource suitable for hospital, health sciences and public libraries with consumer health collections."
—*E-Streams, Nov '02*

"Practitioners should be aware of guides such as this in order to facilitate their use by patients and their families." —*Doody's Health Sciences Book Review Journal, Sep-Oct '02*

"Recommended reference source."
—*Booklist, American Library Association, Sep '02*

"Highly recommended for academic and medical reference collections." —*Library Bookwatch, Sep '02*

■

Kidney & Urinary Tract Diseases & Disorders Sourcebook

Basic Information about Kidney Stones, Urinary Incontinence, Bladder Disease, End Stage Renal Disease, Dialysis, and More

Along with Statistical and Demographic Data and Reports on Current Research Initiatives

Edited by Linda M. Ross. 602 pages. 1997. 0-7808-0079-6. $78.

■

Learning Disabilities Sourcebook, 2nd Edition

Basic Consumer Health Information about Learning Disabilities, Including Dyslexia, Developmental Speech and Language Disabilities, Non-Verbal Learning Disorders, Developmental Arithmetic Disorder, Developmental Writing Disorder, and Other Conditions That Impede Learning Such as Attention Deficit/ Hyperactivity Disorder, Brain Injury, Hearing Impairment, Klinefelter Syndrome, Dyspraxia, and Tourette Syndrome

Along with Facts about Educational Issues and Assistive Technology, Coping Strategies, a Glossary of Related Terms, and Resources for Further Help and Information

Edited by Dawn D. Matthews. 621 pages. 2003. 0-7808-0626-3. $78.

ALSO AVAILABLE: *Learning Disabilities Sourcebook, 1st Edition.* Edited by Linda M. Shin. 579 pages. 1998. 0-7808-0210-1. $78.

"The second edition of *Learning Disabilities Sourcebook* far surpasses the earlier edition in that it is more focused on information that will be useful as a consumer health resource."
—*American Reference Books Annual, 2004*

"Teachers as well as consumers will find this an essential guide to understanding various syndromes and their latest treatments. [An] invaluable reference for public and school library collections alike."
—*Library Bookwatch, Apr '03*

Named "Outstanding Reference Book of 1999."
—*New York Public Library, Feb 2000*

"An excellent candidate for inclusion in a public library reference section. It's a great source of information. Teachers will also find the book useful. Definitely worth reading."
—*Journal of Adolescent & Adult Literacy, Feb 2000*

"Readable . . . provides a solid base of information regarding successful techniques used with individuals who have learning disabilities, as well as practical suggestions for educators and family members. Clear language, concise descriptions, and pertinent information for contacting multiple resources add to the strength of this book as a useful tool." —*Choice, Association of College and Research Libraries, Feb '99*

"Recommended reference source."
—*Booklist, American Library Association, Sep '98*

"A useful resource for libraries and for those who don't have the time to identify and locate the individual publications." —*Disability Resources Monthly, Sep '98*

■

Leukemia Sourcebook

Basic Consumer Health Information about Adult and Childhood Leukemias, Including Acute Lymphocytic Leukemia (ALL), Chronic Lymphocytic Leukemia (CLL), Acute Myelogenous Leukemia (AML), Chronic Myelogenous Leukemia (CML), and Hairy Cell Leukemia, and Treatments Such as Chemotherapy, Radiation Therapy, Peripheral Blood Stem Cell and Marrow Transplantation, and Immunotherapy

Along with Tips for Life During and After Treatment, a Glossary, and Directories of Additional Resources

Edited by Joyce Brennfleck Shannon. 587 pages. 2003. 0-7808-0627-1. $78.

"Unlike other medical books for the layperson, . . . the language does not talk down to the reader. . . . This volume is highly recommended for all libraries."
—*American Reference Books Annual, 2004*

■

Liver Disorders Sourcebook

Basic Consumer Health Information about the Liver and How It Works; Liver Diseases, Including Cancer, Cirrhosis, Hepatitis, and Toxic and Drug Related Diseases; Tips for Maintaining a Healthy Liver; Laboratory Tests, Radiology Tests, and Facts about Liver Transplantation

Along with a Section on Support Groups, a Glossary, and Resource Listings

Edited by Joyce Brennfleck Shannon. 591 pages. 2000. 0-7808-0383-3. $78.

"A valuable resource."
—*American Reference Books Annual, 2001*

"This title is recommended for health sciences and public libraries with consumer health collections."
—*E-Streams, Oct '00*

"Recommended reference source."
—*Booklist, American Library Association, Jun '00*

■

Lung Disorders Sourcebook

Basic Consumer Health Information about Emphysema, Pneumonia, Tuberculosis, Asthma, Cystic Fibrosis, and Other Lung Disorders, Including Facts about Diagnostic Procedures, Treatment Strategies, Disease Prevention Efforts, and Such Risk Factors as Smoking, Air Pollution, and Exposure to Asbestos, Radon, and Other Agents

Along with a Glossary and Resources for Additional Help and Information

Edited by Dawn D. Matthews. 678 pages. 2002. 0-7808-0339-6. $78.

"This title is a great addition for public and school libraries because it provides concise health information on the lungs."
—*American Reference Books Annual, 2003*

"Highly recommended for academic and medical reference collections." —*Library Bookwatch, Sep '02*

■

Medical Tests Sourcebook, 2nd Edition

Basic Consumer Health Information about Medical Tests, Including Age-Specific Health Tests, Important Health Screenings and Exams, Home-Use Tests, Blood and Specimen Tests, Electrical Tests, Scope Tests, Genetic Testing, and Imaging Tests, Such as X-Rays, Ultrasound, Computed Tomography, Magnetic Resonance Imaging, Angiography, and Nuclear Medicine

Along with a Glossary and Directory of Additional Resources

Edited by Joyce Brennfleck Shannon. 654 pages. 2004. 0-7808-0670-0. $78.

ALSO AVAILABLE: *Medical Tests, 1st Edition.* Edited by Joyce Brennfleck Shannon. 691 pages. 1999. 0-7808-0243-8. $78.

"Recommended for hospital and health sciences libraries with consumer health collections."
—*E-Streams, Mar '00*

"This is an overall excellent reference with a wealth of general knowledge that may aid those who are reluctant to get vital tests performed."
—*Today's Librarian, Jan 2000*

"A valuable reference guide."
—*American Reference Books Annual, 2000*

■

Men's Health Concerns Sourcebook, 2nd Edition

Basic Consumer Health Information about the Medical and Mental Concerns of Men, Including Theories about the Shorter Male Lifespan, the Leading Causes of Death and Disability, Physical Concerns of Special Significance to Men, Reproductive and Sexual Concerns, Sexually Transmitted Diseases, Men's Mental and Emotional Health, and Lifestyle Choices That Affect Wellness, Such as Nutrition, Fitness, and Substance Use

Along with a Glossary of Related Terms and a Directory of Organizational Resources in Men's Health

Edited by Robert Aquinas McNally. 644 pages. 2004. 0-7808-0671-9. $78.

ALSO AVAILABLE: *Men's Health Concerns Sourcebook, 1st Edition.* Edited by Allan R. Cook. 738 pages. 1998. 0-7808-0212-8. $78.

"This comprehensive resource and the series are highly recommended."

—American Reference Books Annual, 2000

"Recommended reference source."

—Booklist, American Library Association, Dec '98

■

Mental Health Disorders Sourcebook, 2nd Edition

Basic Consumer Health Information about Anxiety Disorders, Depression and Other Mood Disorders, Eating Disorders, Personality Disorders, Schizophrenia, and More, Including Disease Descriptions, Treatment Options, and Reports on Current Research Initiatives

Along with Statistical Data, Tips for Maintaining Mental Health, a Glossary, and Directory of Sources for Additional Help and Information

Edited by Karen Bellenir. 605 pages. 2000. 0-7808-0240-3. $78.

ALSO AVAILABLE: *Mental Health Disorders Sourcebook, 1st Edition.* Edited by Karen Bellenir. 548 pages. 1995. 0-7808-0040-0. $78.

"Well organized and well written."

—American Reference Books Annual, 2001

"Recommended reference source."

—Booklist, American Library Association, Jun '00

■

Mental Retardation Sourcebook

Basic Consumer Health Information about Mental Retardation and Its Causes, Including Down Syndrome, Fetal Alcohol Syndrome, Fragile X Syndrome, Genetic Conditions, Injury, and Environmental Sources

Along with Preventive Strategies, Parenting Issues, Educational Implications, Health Care Needs, Employment and Economic Matters, Legal Issues, a Glossary, and a Resource Listing for Additional Help and Information

Edited by Joyce Brennfleck Shannon. 642 pages. 2000. 0-7808-0377-9. $78.

"Public libraries will find the book useful for reference and as a beginning research point for students, parents, and caregivers."

—American Reference Books Annual, 2001

"The strength of this work is that it compiles many basic fact sheets and addresses for further information in one volume. It is intended and suitable for the general public. This sourcebook is relevant to any collection providing health information to the general public."

—E-Streams, Nov '00

"From preventing retardation to parenting and family challenges, this covers health, social and legal issues and will prove an invaluable overview."

—Reviewer's Bookwatch, Jul '00

Movement Disorders Sourcebook

Basic Consumer Health Information about Neurological Movement Disorders, Including Essential Tremor, Parkinson's Disease, Dystonia, Cerebral Palsy, Huntington's Disease, Myasthenia Gravis, Multiple Sclerosis, and Other Early-Onset and Adult-Onset Movement Disorders, Their Symptoms and Causes, Diagnostic Tests, and Treatments

Along with Mobility and Assistive Technology Information, a Glossary, and a Directory of Additional Resources

Edited by Joyce Brennfleck Shannon. 655 pages. 2003. 0-7808-0628-X. $78.

". . . a good resource for consumers and recommended for public, community college and undergraduate libraries."

—American Reference Books Annual, 2004

■

Muscular Dystrophy Sourcebook

Basic Consumer Health Information about Congenital, Childhood-Onset, and Adult-Onset Forms of Muscular Dystrophy, Such as Duchenne, Becker, Emery-Dreifuss, Distal, Limb-Girdle, Facioscapulohumeral (FSHD), Myotonic, and Ophthalmoplegic Muscular Dystrophies, Including Facts about Diagnostic Tests, Medical and Physical Therapies, Management of Co-Occurring Conditions, and Parenting Guidelines

Along with Practical Tips for Home Care, a Glossary, and Directories of Additional Resources

Edited by Joyce Brennfleck Shannon. 577 pages. 2004. 0-7808-0676-X. $78.

■

Obesity Sourcebook

Basic Consumer Health Information about Diseases and Other Problems Associated with Obesity, and Including Facts about Risk Factors, Prevention Issues, and Management Approaches

Along with Statistical and Demographic Data, Information about Special Populations, Research Updates, a Glossary, and Source Listings for Further Help and Information

Edited by Wilma Caldwell and Chad T. Kimball. 376 pages. 2001. 0-7808-0333-7. $78.

"The book synthesizes the reliable medical literature on obesity into one easy-to-read and useful resource for the general public."

—American Reference Books Annual 2002

"This is a very useful resource book for the lay public."

—Doody's Review Service, Nov '01

"Well suited for the health reference collection of a public library or an academic health science library that serves the general population." *—E-Streams, Sep '01*

"Recommended reference source."

—Booklist, American Library Association, Apr '01

" Recommended pick both for specialty health library collections and any general consumer health reference collection." *— The Bookwatch, Apr '01*

Ophthalmic Disorders Sourcebook, 1st Edition

SEE *Eye Care Sourcebook, 2nd Edition*

■

Oral Health Sourcebook

SEE *Dental Care & Oral Health Sourcebook, 2nd Ed.*

■

Osteoporosis Sourcebook

Basic Consumer Health Information about Primary and Secondary Osteoporosis and Juvenile Osteoporosis and Related Conditions, Including Fibrous Dysplasia, Gaucher Disease, Hyperthyroidism, Hypophosphatasia, Myeloma, Osteopetrosis, Osteogenesis Imperfecta, and Paget's Disease

Along with Information about Risk Factors, Treatments, Traditional and Non-Traditional Pain Management, a Glossary of Related Terms, and a Directory of Resources

Edited by Allan R. Cook. 584 pages. 2001. 0-7808-0239-X. $78.

"This would be a book to be kept in a staff or patient library. The targeted audience is the layperson, but the therapist who needs a quick bit of information on a particular topic will also find the book useful."
—*Physical Therapy, Jan '02*

"This resource is recommended as a great reference source for public, health, and academic libraries, and is another triumph for the editors of Omnigraphics."
—*American Reference Books Annual 2002*

"Recommended for all public libraries and general health collections, especially those supporting patient education or consumer health programs."
—*E-Streams, Nov '01*

"Will prove valuable to any library seeking to maintain a current, comprehensive reference collection of health resources. . . . From prevention to treatment and associated conditions, this provides an excellent survey."
—*The Bookwatch, Aug '01*

"Recommended reference source."
—*Booklist, American Library Association, July '01*

SEE ALSO *Women's Health Concerns Sourcebook*

■

Pain Sourcebook, 2nd Edition

Basic Consumer Health Information about Specific Forms of Acute and Chronic Pain, Including Muscle and Skeletal Pain, Nerve Pain, Cancer Pain, and Disorders Characterized by Pain, Such as Fibromyalgia, Shingles, Angina, Arthritis, and Headaches

Along with Information about Pain Medications and Management Techniques, Complementary and Alternative Pain Relief Options, Tips for People Living with Chronic Pain, a Glossary, and a Directory of Sources for Further Information

Edited by Karen Bellenir. 670 pages. 2002. 0-7808-0612-3. $78.

ALSO AVAILABLE: *Pain Sourcebook, 1st Edition.* Edited by Allan R. Cook. 667 pages. 1997. 0-7808-0213-6. $78.

"A source of valuable information. . . . This book offers help to nonmedical people who need information about pain and pain management. It is also an excellent reference for those who participate in patient education."
—*Doody's Review Service, Sep '02*

"The text is readable, easily understood, and well indexed. This excellent volume belongs in all patient education libraries, consumer health sections of public libraries, and many personal collections."
—*American Reference Books Annual, 1999*

"A beneficial reference." —*Booklist Health Sciences Supplement, American Library Association, Oct '98*

"The information is basic in terms of scholarship and is appropriate for general readers. Written in journalistic style . . . intended for non-professionals. Quite thorough in its coverage of different pain conditions and summarizes the latest clinical information regarding pain treatment." —*Choice, Association of College and Research Libraries, Jun '98*

"Recommended reference source."
—*Booklist, American Library Association, Mar '98*

■

Pediatric Cancer Sourcebook

Basic Consumer Health Information about Leukemias, Brain Tumors, Sarcomas, Lymphomas, and Other Cancers in Infants, Children, and Adolescents, Including Descriptions of Cancers, Treatments, and Coping Strategies

Along with Suggestions for Parents, Caregivers, and Concerned Relatives, a Glossary of Cancer Terms, and Resource Listings

Edited by Edward J. Prucha. 587 pages. 1999. 0-7808-0245-4. $78.

"An excellent source of information. Recommended for public, hospital, and health science libraries with consumer health collections." —*E-Streams, Jun '00*

"Recommended reference source."
—*Booklist, American Library Association, Feb '00*

"A valuable addition to all libraries specializing in health services and many public libraries."
—*American Reference Books Annual, 2000*

■

Physical & Mental Issues in Aging Sourcebook

Basic Consumer Health Information on Physical and Mental Disorders Associated with the Aging Process, Including Concerns about Cardiovascular Disease, Pulmonary Disease, Oral Health, Digestive Disorders, Musculoskeletal and Skin Disorders, Metabolic Changes, Sexual and Reproductive Issues, and Changes in Vision, Hearing, and Other Senses

Along with Data about Longevity and Causes of Death, Information on Acute and Chronic Pain, Descriptions of Mental Concerns, a Glossary of Terms, and Resource Listings for Additional Help

Edited by Jenifer Swanson. 660 pages. 1999. 0-7808-0233-0. $78.

"This is a treasure of health information for the layperson." — *Choice Health Sciences Supplement, Association of College & Research Libraries, May 2000*

"Recommended for public libraries."
—*American Reference Books Annual, 2000*

"Recommended reference source."
—*Booklist, American Library Association, Oct '99*

SEE ALSO *Healthy Aging Sourcebook*

■

Podiatry Sourcebook

Basic Consumer Health Information about Foot Conditions, Diseases, and Injuries, Including Bunions, Corns, Calluses, Athlete's Foot, Plantar Warts, Hammertoes and Clawtoes, Clubfoot, Heel Pain, Gout, and More

Along with Facts about Foot Care, Disease Prevention, Foot Safety, Choosing a Foot Care Specialist, a Glossary of Terms, and Resource Listings for Additional Information

Edited by M. Lisa Weatherford. 380 pages. 2001. 0-7808-0215-2. $78.

"Recommended reference source."
—*Booklist, American Library Association, Feb '02*

"There is a lot of information presented here on a topic that is usually only covered sparingly in most larger comprehensive medical encyclopedias."
—*American Reference Books Annual 2002*

■

Pregnancy & Birth Sourcebook, 2nd Edition

Basic Consumer Health Information about Conception and Pregnancy, Including Facts about Fertility, Infertility, Pregnancy Symptoms and Complications, Fetal Growth and Development, Labor, Delivery, and the Postpartum Period, as Well as Information about Maintaining Health and Wellness during Pregnancy and Caring for a Newborn

Along with Information about Public Health Assistance for Low-Income Pregnant Women, a Glossary, and Directories of Agencies and Organizations Providing Help and Support

Edited by Amy L. Sutton. 626 pages. 2004. 0-7808-0672-7. $78.

ALSO AVAILABLE: *Pregnancy & Birth Sourcebook, 1st Edition.* Edited by Heather E. Aldred. 737 pages. 1997. 0-7808-0216-0. $78.

"A well-organized handbook. Recommended."
—*Choice, Association of College and Research Libraries, Apr '98*

"Recommended reference source."
—*Booklist, American Library Association, Mar '98*

"Recommended for public libraries."
—*American Reference Books Annual, 1998*

SEE ALSO *Congenital Disorders Sourcebook, Family Planning Sourcebook*

■

Prostate Cancer Sourcebook

Basic Consumer Health Information about Prostate Cancer, Including Information about the Associated Risk Factors, Detection, Diagnosis, and Treatment of Prostate Cancer

Along with Information on Non-Malignant Prostate Conditions, and Featuring a Section Listing Support and Treatment Centers and a Glossary of Related Terms

Edited by Dawn D. Matthews. 358 pages. 2001. 0-7808-0324-8. $78.

"Recommended reference source."
—*Booklist, American Library Association, Jan '02*

"A valuable resource for health care consumers seeking information on the subject. . . .All text is written in a clear, easy-to-understand language that avoids technical jargon. Any library that collects consumer health resources would strengthen their collection with the addition of the *Prostate Cancer Sourcebook*."
—*American Reference Books Annual 2002*

■

Public Health Sourcebook

Basic Information about Government Health Agencies, Including National Health Statistics and Trends, Healthy People 2000 Program Goals and Objectives, the Centers for Disease Control and Prevention, the Food and Drug Administration, and the National Institutes of Health

Along with Full Contact Information for Each Agency

Edited by Wendy Wilcox. 698 pages. 1998. 0-7808-0220-9. $78.

"Recommended reference source."
—*Booklist, American Library Association, Sep '98*

"This consumer guide provides welcome assistance in navigating the maze of federal health agencies and their data on public health concerns."
—*SciTech Book News, Sep '98*

■

Reconstructive & Cosmetic Surgery Sourcebook

Basic Consumer Health Information on Cosmetic and Reconstructive Plastic Surgery, Including Statistical Information about Different Surgical Procedures, Things to Consider Prior to Surgery, Plastic Surgery Techniques and Tools, Emotional and Psychological Considerations, and Procedure-Specific Information

Along with a Glossary of Terms and a Listing of Resources for Additional Help and Information

Edited by M. Lisa Weatherford. 374 pages. 2001. 0-7808-0214-4. $78.

"An excellent reference that addresses cosmetic and medically necessary reconstructive surgeries. . . . The

style of the prose is calm and reassuring, discussing the many positive outcomes now available due to advances in surgical techniques."

—*American Reference Books Annual 2002*

"Recommended for health science libraries that are open to the public, as well as hospital libraries that are open to the patients. This book is a good resource for the consumer interested in plastic surgery."

—*E-Streams, Dec '01*

"Recommended reference source."

—*Booklist, American Library Association, July '01*

■

Rehabilitation Sourcebook

Basic Consumer Health Information about Rehabilitation for People Recovering from Heart Surgery, Spinal Cord Injury, Stroke, Orthopedic Impairments, Amputation, Pulmonary Impairments, Traumatic Injury, and More, Including Physical Therapy, Occupational Therapy, Speech/ Language Therapy, Massage Therapy, Dance Therapy, Art Therapy, and Recreational Therapy

Along with Information on Assistive and Adaptive Devices, a Glossary, and Resources for Additional Help and Information

Edited by Dawn D. Matthews. 531 pages. 1999. 0-7808-0236-5. $78.

"This is an excellent resource for public library reference and health collections."

—*American Reference Books Annual, 2001*

"Recommended reference source."

—*Booklist, American Library Association, May '00*

■

Respiratory Diseases & Disorders Sourcebook

Basic Information about Respiratory Diseases and Disorders, Including Asthma, Cystic Fibrosis, Pneumonia, the Common Cold, Influenza, and Others, Featuring Facts about the Respiratory System, Statistical and Demographic Data, Treatments, Self-Help Management Suggestions, and Current Research Initiatives

Edited by Allan R. Cook and Peter D. Dresser. 771 pages. 1995. 0-7808-0037-0. $78.

"Designed for the layperson and for patients and their families coping with respiratory illness. . . . an extensive array of information on diagnosis, treatment, management, and prevention of respiratory illnesses for the general reader." —*Choice, Association of College and Research Libraries, Jun '96*

"A highly recommended text for all collections. It is a comforting reminder of the power of knowledge that good books carry between their covers."

—*Academic Library Book Review, Spring '96*

"A comprehensive collection of authoritative information presented in a nontechnical, humanitarian style for patients, families, and caregivers." —*Association of Operating Room Nurses, Sep/Oct '95*

SEE ALSO *Lung Disorders Sourcebook*

Sexually Transmitted Diseases Sourcebook, 2nd Edition

Basic Consumer Health Information about Sexually Transmitted Diseases, Including Information on the Diagnosis and Treatment of Chlamydia, Gonorrhea, Hepatitis, Herpes, HIV, Mononucleosis, Syphilis, and Others

Along with Information on Prevention, Such as Condom Use, Vaccines, and STD Education; And Featuring a Section on Issues Related to Youth and Adolescents, a Glossary, and Resources for Additional Help and Information

Edited by Dawn D. Matthews. 538 pages. 2001. 0-7808-0249-7. $78.

ALSO AVAILABLE: *Sexually Transmitted Diseases Sourcebook, 1st Edition.* Edited by Linda M. Ross. 550 pages. 1997. 0-7808-0217-9. $78.

"Recommended for consumer health collections in public libraries, and secondary school and community college libraries."

—*American Reference Books Annual 2002*

"Every school and public library should have a copy of this comprehensive and user-friendly reference book."

—*Choice, Association of College & Research Libraries, Sep '01*

"This is a highly recommended book. This is an especially important book for all school and public libraries." —*AIDS Book Review Journal, Jul-Aug '01*

"Recommended reference source."

—*Booklist, American Library Association, Apr '01*

"Recommended pick both for specialty health library collections and any general consumer health reference collection." —*The Bookwatch, Apr '01*

■

Skin Disorders Sourcebook

Basic Information about Common Skin and Scalp Conditions Caused by Aging, Allergies, Immune Reactions, Sun Exposure, Infectious Organisms, Parasites, Cosmetics, and Skin Traumas, Including Abrasions, Cuts, and Pressure Sores

Along with Information on Prevention and Treatment

Edited by Allan R. Cook. 647 pages. 1997. 0-7808-0080-X. $78.

". . . comprehensive, easily read reference book."

—*Doody's Health Sciences Book Reviews, Oct '97*

SEE ALSO *Burns Sourcebook*

■

Sleep Disorders Sourcebook

Basic Consumer Health Information about Sleep and Its Disorders, Including Insomnia, Sleepwalking, Sleep Apnea, Restless Leg Syndrome, and Narcolepsy

Along with Data about Shiftwork and Its Effects, Information on the Societal Costs of Sleep Deprivation, Descriptions of Treatment Options, a Glossary of Terms, and Resource Listings for Additional Help

Edited by Jenifer Swanson. 439 pages. 1998. 0-7808-0234-9. $78.

"This text will complement any home or medical library. It is user-friendly and ideal for the adult reader."
—American Reference Books Annual, 2000

"A useful resource that provides accurate, relevant, and accessible information on sleep to the general public. Health care providers who deal with sleep disorders patients may also find it helpful in being prepared to answer some of the questions patients ask."
—Respiratory Care, Jul '99

"Recommended reference source."
—Booklist, American Library Association, Feb '99

■

Smoking Concerns Sourcebook

Basic Consumer Health Information about Nicotine Addiction and Smoking Cessation, Featuring Facts about the Health Effects of Tobacco Use, Including Lung and Other Cancers, Heart Disease, Stroke, and Respiratory Disorders, Such as Emphysema and Chronic Bronchitis

Along with Information about Smoking Prevention Programs, Suggestions for Achieving and Maintaining a Smoke-Free Lifestyle, Statistics about Tobacco Use, Reports on Current Research Initiatives, a Glossary of Related Terms, and Directories of Resources for Additional Help and Information

Edited by Karen Bellenir. 625 pages. 2004. 0-7808-0323-X. $78.

■

Sports Injuries Sourcebook, 2nd Edition

Basic Consumer Health Information about the Diagnosis, Treatment, and Rehabilitation of Common Sports-Related Injuries in Children and Adults

Along with Suggestions for Conditioning and Training, Information and Prevention Tips for Injuries Frequently Associated with Specific Sports and Special Populations, a Glossary, and a Directory of Additional Resources

Edited by Joyce Brennfleck Shannon. 614 pages. 2002. 0-7808-0604-2. $78.

ALSO AVAILABLE: *Sports Injuries Sourcebook, 1st Edition.* Edited by Heather E. Aldred. 624 pages. 1999. 0-7808-0218-7. $78.

"This is an excellent reference for consumers and it is recommended for public, community college, and undergraduate libraries."
—American Reference Books Annual, 2003

"Recommended reference source."
—Booklist, American Library Association, Feb '03

Stress-Related Disorders Sourcebook

Basic Consumer Health Information about Stress and Stress-Related Disorders, Including Stress Origins and Signals, Environmental Stress at Work and Home, Mental and Emotional Stress Associated with Depression, Post-Traumatic Stress Disorder, Panic Disorder, Suicide, and the Physical Effects of Stress on the Cardiovascular, Immune, and Nervous Systems

Along with Stress Management Techniques, a Glossary, and a Listing of Additional Resources

Edited by Joyce Brennfleck Shannon. 610 pages. 2002. 0-7808-0560-7. $78.

"Well written for a general readership, the *Stress-Related Disorders Sourcebook* is a useful addition to the health reference literature."
—American Reference Books Annual, 2003

"I am impressed by the amount of information. It offers a thorough overview of the causes and consequences of stress for the layperson. . . . A well-done and thorough reference guide for professionals and nonprofessionals alike."
—Doody's Review Service, Dec '02

■

Stroke Sourcebook

Basic Consumer Health Information about Stroke, Including Ischemic, Hemorrhagic, Transient Ischemic Attack (TIA), and Pediatric Stroke, Stroke Triggers and Risks, Diagnostic Tests, Treatments, and Rehabilitation Information

Along with Stroke Prevention Guidelines, Legal and Financial Information, a Glossary, and a Directory of Additional Resources

Edited by Joyce Brennfleck Shannon. 606 pages. 2003. 0-7808-0630-1. $78.

"This volume is highly recommended and should be in every medical, hospital, and public library."
—American Reference Books Annual, 2004

■

Substance Abuse Sourcebook

Basic Health-Related Information about the Abuse of Legal and Illegal Substances Such as Alcohol, Tobacco, Prescription Drugs, Marijuana, Cocaine, and Heroin; and Including Facts about Substance Abuse Prevention Strategies, Intervention Methods, Treatment and Recovery Programs, and a Section Addressing the Special Problems Related to Substance Abuse during Pregnancy

Edited by Karen Bellenir. 573 pages. 1996. 0-7808-0038-9. $78.

"A valuable addition to any health reference section. Highly recommended."
—The Book Report, Mar/Apr '97

". . . a comprehensive collection of substance abuse information that's both highly readable and compact. Families and caregivers of substance abusers will find

the information enlightening and helpful, while teachers, social workers and journalists should benefit from the concise format. Recommended."

—*Drug Abuse Update, Winter '96/'97*

SEE ALSO *Alcoholism Sourcebook, Drug Abuse Sourcebook*

Surgery Sourcebook

Basic Consumer Health Information about Inpatient and Outpatient Surgeries, Including Cardiac, Vascular, Orthopedic, Ocular, Reconstructive, Cosmetic, Gynecologic, and Ear, Nose, and Throat Procedures and More

Along with Information about Operating Room Policies and Instruments, Laser Surgery Techniques, Hospital Errors, Statistical Data, a Glossary, and Listings of Sources for Further Help and Information

Edited by Annemarie S. Muth and Karen Bellenir. 596 pages. 2002. 0-7808-0380-9. $78.

"Large public libraries and medical libraries would benefit from this material in their reference collections."

—*American Reference Books Annual, 2004*

"Invaluable reference for public and school library collections alike." —*Library Bookwatch, Apr '03*

Transplantation Sourcebook

Basic Consumer Health Information about Organ and Tissue Transplantation, Including Physical and Financial Preparations, Procedures and Issues Relating to Specific Solid Organ and Tissue Transplants, Rehabilitation, Pediatric Transplant Information, the Future of Transplantation, and Organ and Tissue Donation

Along with a Glossary and Listings of Additional Resources

Edited by Joyce Brennfleck Shannon. 628 pages. 2002. 0-7808-0322-1. $78.

"Along with these advances [in transplantation technology] have come a number of daunting questions for potential transplant patients, their families, and their health care providers. This reference text is the best single tool to address many of these questions. . . . It will be a much-needed addition to the reference collections in health care, academic, and large public libraries."

—*American Reference Books Annual, 2003*

"Recommended for libraries with an interest in offering consumer health information." —*E-Streams, Jul '02*

"This is a unique and valuable resource for patients facing transplantation and their families."

—*Doody's Review Service, Jun '02*

Traveler's Health Sourcebook

Basic Consumer Health Information for Travelers, Including Physical and Medical Preparations, Transportation Health and Safety, Essential Information about Food and Water, Sun Exposure, Insect and Snake Bites, Camping and Wilderness Medicine, and Travel with Physical or Medical Disabilities

Along with International Travel Tips, Vaccination Recommendations, Geographical Health Issues, Disease Risks, a Glossary, and a Listing of Additional Resources

Edited by Joyce Brennfleck Shannon. 613 pages. 2000. 0-7808-0384-1. $78.

"Recommended reference source."

—*Booklist, American Library Association, Feb '01*

"This book is recommended for any public library, any travel collection, and especially any collection for the physically disabled."

—*American Reference Books Annual, 2001*

Vegetarian Sourcebook

Basic Consumer Health Information about Vegetarian Diets, Lifestyle, and Philosophy, Including Definitions of Vegetarianism and Veganism, Tips about Adopting Vegetarianism, Creating a Vegetarian Pantry, and Meeting Nutritional Needs of Vegetarians, with Facts Regarding Vegetarianism's Effect on Pregnant and Lactating Women, Children, Athletes, and Senior Citizens

Along with a Glossary of Commonly Used Vegetarian Terms and Resources for Additional Help and Information

Edited by Chad T. Kimball. 360 pages. 2002. 0-7808-0439-2. $78.

"Organizes into one concise volume the answers to the most common questions concerning vegetarian diets and lifestyles. This title is recommended for public and secondary school libraries." —*E-Streams, Apr '03*

"Invaluable reference for public and school library collections alike." —*Library Bookwatch, Apr '03*

"The articles in this volume are easy to read and come from authoritative sources. The book does not necessarily support the vegetarian diet but instead provides the pros and cons of this important decision. The *Vegetarian Sourcebook* is recommended for public libraries and consumer health libraries."

—*American Reference Books Annual, 2003*

Women's Health Concerns Sourcebook, 2nd Edition

Basic Consumer Health Information about the Medical and Mental Concerns of Women, Including Maintaining Health and Wellness, Gynecological Concerns, Breast Health, Sexuality and Reproductive Issues, Menopause, Cancer in Women, the Leading Causes of Death and Disability among Women, Physical Concerns of Special Significance to Women, and Women's Mental and Emotional Health

Along with a Glossary of Related Terms and Directories of Resources for Additional Help and Information

Edited by Amy L. Sutton. 748 pages. 2004. 0-7808-0673-5. $78.

ALSO AVAILABLE: *Women's Health Concerns Sourcebook, 1st Edition.* Edited by Heather E. Aldred. 567 pages. 1997. 0-7808-0219-5. $78.

"Handy compilation. There is an impressive range of diseases, devices, disorders, procedures, and other physical and emotional issues covered . . . well organized, illustrated, and indexed." —*Choice, Association of College and Research Libraries, Jan '98*

SEE ALSO *Breast Cancer Sourcebook, Cancer Sourcebook for Women, Healthy Heart Sourcebook for Women, Osteoporosis Sourcebook*

■

Workplace Health & Safety Sourcebook

Basic Consumer Health Information about Workplace Health and Safety, Including the Effect of Workplace Hazards on the Lungs, Skin, Heart, Ears, Eyes, Brain, Reproductive Organs, Musculoskeletal System, and Other Organs and Body Parts

Along with Information about Occupational Cancer, Personal Protective Equipment, Toxic and Hazardous Chemicals, Child Labor, Stress, and Workplace Violence

Edited by Chad T. Kimball. 626 pages. 2000. 0-7808-0231-4. $78.

"As a reference for the general public, this would be useful in any library." —*E-Streams, Jun '01*

"Provides helpful information for primary care physicians and other caregivers interested in occupational medicine. . . . General readers; professionals." —*Choice, Association of College & Research Libraries, May '01*

"Recommended reference source." —*Booklist, American Library Association, Feb '01*

"Highly recommended." —*The Bookwatch, Jan '01*

■

Worldwide Health Sourcebook

Basic Information about Global Health Issues, Including Malnutrition, Reproductive Health, Disease Dispersion and Prevention, Emerging Diseases, Risky Health Behaviors, and the Leading Causes of Death

Along with Global Health Concerns for Children, Women, and the Elderly, Mental Health Issues, Research and Technology Advancements, and Economic, Environmental, and Political Health Implications, a Glossary, and a Resource Listing for Additional Help and Information

Edited by Joyce Brennfleck Shannon. 614 pages. 2001. 0-7808-0330-2. $78.

"Named an Outstanding Academic Title." —*Choice, Association of College & Research Libraries, Jan '02*

"Yet another handy but also unique compilation in the extensive Health Reference Series, this is a useful work because many of the international publications reprinted or excerpted are not readily available. Highly recommended." —*Choice, Association of College & Research Libraries, Nov '01*

"Recommended reference source." —*Booklist, American Library Association, Oct '01*

Teen Health Series

Helping Young Adults Understand, Manage, and Avoid Serious Illness

Cancer Information for Teens

Health Tips about Cancer Awareness, Prevention, Diagnosis, and Treatment

Including Facts about Frequently Occurring Cancers, Cancer Risk Factors, and Coping Strategies for Teens Fighting Cancer or Dealing with Cancer in Friends or Family Members

Edited by Wilma R. Caldwell. 428 pages. 2004. 0-7808-0678-6. $58.

■

Diet Information for Teens

Health Tips about Diet and Nutrition

Including Facts about Nutrients, Dietary Guidelines, Breakfasts, School Lunches, Snacks, Party Food, Weight Control, Eating Disorders, and More

Edited by Karen Bellenir. 399 pages. 2001. 0-7808-0441-4. $58.

"Full of helpful insights and facts throughout the book. . . . An excellent resource to be placed in public libraries or even in personal collections."
—*American Reference Books Annual 2002*

"Recommended for middle and high school libraries and media centers as well as academic libraries that educate future teachers of teenagers. It is also a suitable addition to health science libraries that serve patrons who are interested in teen health promotion and education." —*E-Streams, Oct '01*

"This comprehensive book would be beneficial to collections that need information about nutrition, dietary guidelines, meal planning, and weight control. . . . This reference is so easy to use that its purchase is recommended." —*The Book Report, Sep-Oct '01*

"This book is written in an easy to understand format describing issues that many teens face every day, and then provides thoughtful explanations so that teens can make informed decisions. This is an interesting book that provides important facts and information for today's teens." —*Doody's Health Sciences Book Review Journal, Jul-Aug '01*

"A comprehensive compendium of diet and nutrition. The information is presented in a straightforward, plain-spoken manner. This title will be useful to those working on reports on a variety of topics, as well as to general readers concerned about their dietary health."
—*School Library Journal, Jun '01*

Drug Information for Teens

Health Tips about the Physical and Mental Effects of Substance Abuse

Including Facts about Alcohol, Anabolic Steroids, Club Drugs, Cocaine, Depressants, Hallucinogens, Herbal Products, Inhalants, Marijuana, Narcotics, Stimulants, Tobacco, and More

Edited by Karen Bellenir. 452 pages. 2002. 0-7808-0444-9. $58.

"A clearly written resource for general readers and researchers alike." —*School Library Journal*

"The chapters are quick to make a connection to their teenage reading audience. The prose is straightforward and the book lends itself to spot reading. It should be useful both for practical information and for research, and it is suitable for public and school libraries."
—*American Reference Books Annual, 2003*

"Recommended reference source."
—*Booklist, American Library Association, Feb '03*

"This is an excellent resource for teens and their parents. Education about drugs and substances is key to discouraging teen drug abuse and this book provides this much needed information in a way that is interesting and factual." —*Doody's Review Service, Dec '02*

■

Fitness Information for Teens

Health Tips about Exercise, Physical Well-Being, and Health Maintenance

Including Facts about Aerobic and Anaerobic Conditioning, Stretching, Body Shape and Body Image, Sports Training, Nutrition, and Activities for Non-Athletes

Edited by Karen Bellenir. 425 pages. 2004. 0-7808-0679-4. $58.

■

Mental Health Information for Teens

Health Tips about Mental Health and Mental Illness

Including Facts about Anxiety, Depression, Suicide, Eating Disorders, Obsessive-Compulsive Disorders, Panic Attacks, Phobias, Schizophrenia, and More

Edited by Karen Bellenir. 406 pages. 2001. 0-7808-0442-2. $58.

"In both language and approach, this user-friendly entry in the *Teen Health Series* is on target for teens needing information on mental health concerns." —*Booklist, American Library Association, Jan '02*

"Readers will find the material accessible and informative, with the shaded notes, facts, and embedded glossary insets adding appropriately to the already interesting and succinct presentation."

—*School Library Journal, Jan '02*

"This title is highly recommended for any library that serves adolescents and parents/caregivers of adolescents." —*E-Streams, Jan '02*

"Recommended for high school libraries and young adult collections in public libraries. Both health professionals and teenagers will find this book useful."

—*American Reference Books Annual 2002*

"This is a nice book written to enlighten the society, primarily teenagers, about common teen mental health issues. It is highly recommended to teachers and parents as well as adolescents."

—*Doody's Review Service, Dec '01*

■

Sexual Health Information for Teens

Health Tips about Sexual Development, Human Reproduction, and Sexually Transmitted Diseases

Including Facts about Puberty, Reproductive Health, Chlamydia, Human Papillomavirus, Pelvic Inflammatory Disease, Herpes, AIDS, Contraception, Pregnancy, and More

Edited by Deborah A. Stanley. 391 pages. 2003. 0-7808-0445-7. $58.

"This work should be included in all high school libraries and many larger public libraries. . . . highly recommended."

—*American Reference Books Annual 2004*

"Sexual Health approaches its subject with appropriate seriousness and offers easily accessible advice and information."

—*School Library Journal, Feb. 2004*

Skin Health Information For Teens

Health Tips about Dermatological Concerns and Skin Cancer Risks

Including Facts about Acne, Warts, Hives, and Other Conditions and Lifestyle Choices, Such as Tanning, Tattooing, and Piercing, That Affect the Skin, Nails, Scalp, and Hair

Edited by Robert Aquinas McNally. 430 pages. 2003. 0-7808-0446-5. $58.

"This volume, as with others in the series, will be a useful addition to school and public library collections."

—*American Reference Books Annual 2004*

"This volume serves as a one-stop source and should be a necessity for any health collection."

—*Library Media Connection*

■

Sports Injuries Information For Teens

Health Tips about Sports Injuries and Injury Protection

Including Facts about Specific Injuries, Emergency Treatment, Rehabilitation, Sports Safety, Competition Stress, Fitness, Sports Nutrition, Steroid Risks, and More

Edited by Joyce Brennfleck Shannon. 425 pages. 2003. 0-7808-0447-3. $58.

"This work will be useful in the young adult collections of public libraries as well as high school libraries."

—*American Reference Books Annual 2004*

Health Reference Series

Adolescent Health Sourcebook
AIDS Sourcebook, 3rd Edition
Alcoholism Sourcebook
Allergies Sourcebook, 2nd Edition
Alternative Medicine Sourcebook, 2nd Edition
Alzheimer's Disease Sourcebook, 3rd Edition
Arthritis Sourcebook
Asthma Sourcebook
Attention Deficit Disorder Sourcebook
Back & Neck Disorders Sourcebook
Blood & Circulatory Disorders Sourcebook
Brain Disorders Sourcebook
Breast Cancer Sourcebook
Breastfeeding Sourcebook
Burns Sourcebook
Cancer Sourcebook, 4th Edition
Cancer Sourcebook for Women, 2nd Edition
Caregiving Sourcebook
Child Abuse Sourcebook
Childhood Diseases & Disorders Sourcebook
Colds, Flu & Other Common Ailments Sourcebook
Communication Disorders Sourcebook
Congenital Disorders Sourcebook
Consumer Issues in Health Care Sourcebook
Contagious & Non-Contagious Infectious Diseases Sourcebook
Death & Dying Sourcebook
Dental Care & Oral Health Sourcebook, 2nd Edition
Depression Sourcebook
Diabetes Sourcebook, 3rd Edition
Diet & Nutrition Sourcebook, 2nd Edition
Digestive Diseases & Disorder Sourcebook
Disabilities Sourcebook
Domestic Violence Sourcebook, 2nd Edition
Drug Abuse Sourcebook
Ear, Nose & Throat Disorders Sourcebook
Eating Disorders Sourcebook
Emergency Medical Services Sourcebook
Endocrine & Metabolic Disorders Sourcebook
Environmentally Health Sourcebook, 2nd Edition
Ethnic Diseases Sourcebook
Eye Care Sourcebook, 2nd Edition
Family Planning Sourcebook
Fitness & Exercise Sourcebook, 2nd Edition
Food & Animal Borne Diseases Sourcebook
Food Safety Sourcebook
Forensic Medicine Sourcebook
Gastrointestinal Diseases & Disorders Sourcebook
Genetic Disorders Sourcebook, 2nd Edition
Head Trauma Sourcebook
Headache Sourcebook
Health Insurance Sourcebook
Health Reference Series Cumulative Index 1999
Healthy Aging Sourcebook
Healthy Children Sourcebook

saved the lives of *thy w.* *2 Sam* 19:5
gold is mine, and *thy w.* *1 Ki* 20:3
deliver me *thy w.* and children. 5
Lord will smite thy people and *thy w.* *2 Chr* 21:14
bring *thy w.* and children. *Jer* 38:23
thy w. and concubines. *Dan* 5:23

your **wives**

take waggons for *your w.* *Gen* 45:19
come not at *your w.* *Ex* 19:15*
your w. shall be widows. 22:24
golden earrings of *your w.* 32:2
your w. and your little ones and your cattle. *Deut* 3:19; *Josh* 1:14
your w.: shouldest enter into covenant with the Lord. *Deut* 29:11
fight for *your w.* and. *Neh* 4:14
wickedness of *your w.* *Jer* 44:9
Lord, saying; Ye and *your w.* 25
you to put away *your w.* *Mat* 19:8
husbands, love *your w.* *Eph* 5:25
Col 3:19

wizard

a *w.* shall surely be put. *Lev* 20:27
be found among you a *w.* *Deut* 18:11

wizards

nor seek after *w.* to be. *Lev* 19:31
the soul that turneth after *w.* 20:6
Saul had put *w.* out of the land. *1 Sam* 28:3, 9
Manasseh dealt with *w.* *2 Ki* 21:6
2 Chr 33:6
Josiah put the *w.* and. *2 Ki* 23:24
Seek unto *w.* that peep. *Isa* 8:19
shall seek to idols and *w.* 19:3

woe

w. to thee, Moab ! *Num* 21:29
Jer 48:46
w. unto us, for there hath. *1 Sam* 4:7
8; *Jer* 4:13; 6:4; *Lam* 5:16
who hath *w.*? who hath ? *Pr* 23:29
w. to him that is alone. *Eccl* 4:10
w. to thee, O land, when. 10:16
w. to their soul, for they. *Isa* 3:9
w. unto the wicked! it shall be. 11
w. to the multitude of. 17:12
w. to the land shadowing. 18:1
w. to the crown of pride, to. 28:1
w. to Ariel. 29:1
w. to the rebellious children. 30:1
w. to thee that spoilest. 33:1
w. to him that striveth with. 45:9
w. to him that saith to fatherless. 10
w. unto thee, O Jerusalem. *Jer* 13:27
w. to him that buildeth by. 22:13
w. to the pastors that destroy. 23:1
w. to Nebo. 48:1
written, mourning and *w.* *Ezek* 2:10
w. to foolish prophets, that. 13:3
w. to women that sew pillows. 18
w. w. to thee. 16:23
w. to bloody city. 24:6, 9; *Nah* 3:1
Howl, *W.* worth the day! *Ezek* 30:2
w. be to the shepherds that. 34:2
w. to you that desire the. *Amos* 5:18
w. to him that increaseth. *Hab* 2:6
w. to him that coveteth an evil. 9
w. to him that buildeth a town. 12
w. to him that giveth his. 15
w. to him that saith to the wood. 19
w. to the inhabitants of. *Zeph* 2:5
w. to her that is filthy. 3:1
w. to the idol shepherd. *Zech* 11:17
w. unto thee, Chorazin! *w.* unto thee. *Mat* 11:21; *Luke* 10:13
w. unto the world because of offences, *w.* *Mat* 18:7; *Luke* 17:1
w. unto you scribes and. *Mat* 23:13
14, 15 23, 25, 27, 29; *Luke* 11:44
w. unto you, ye blind guides, which say. *Mat* 23:16
but *w.* unto that man by. 26:24
Mark 14:21; *Luke* 22:22
w. unto you that are rich. *Luke* 6:24
w. to you that are full, *w.* to you. 25
w. unto you when all men speak. 26
but *w.* unto you Pharisees. 11:42, 43
he said, *W.* to you also. 46, 47, 52
I heard an angel flying, saying, *W. w. w.* *Rev* 8:13; 12:12
one *w.* **is past.** 9:12
the second *w.* **is past.** 11:14

woe *is me*

w. is me, that I sojourn. *Ps* 120:5
w. is me! for I am undone. *Isa* 6:5
w. is me now, for my soul. *Jer* 4:31
w. is me for my hurt. 10:19
w. is me, my mother. 15:10
w. is me, for the Lord hath. 45:3
w. is me! for I am as when. *Mi* 7:1

woe *unto me*

if I be wicked, *w. unto me.* *Job* 10:15
My leanness, *w. unto me.* *Isa* 24:16
w. unto me if I preach. *1 Cor* 9:16

woe *to them*

w. to them that join house to house. *Isa* 5:8
w. to them that rise up early in. 11
w. to them that draw iniquity. 18
w. to them that call evil good. 20
w. to them that are wise in their. 21
w. to them that are mighty to. 22
w. to them that decree. 10:1
w. to them that seek deep to. 29:15
w. to them that go down into. 31:1
w. to them, for their day. *Jer* 50:27
w. to them, for they have. *Hos* 7:13
w. to them when I depart from. 9:12
w. to them that are at. *Amos* 6:1
w. to them that devise. *Mi* 2:1
w. to them which are with child, and to them that give. *Mat* 24:19
Mark 13:17; *Luke* 21:23
w. unto them! for they have gone in the way of Cain. *Jude* 11

woeful

neither I desired the *w.* day. *Jer* 17:16

woes

behold, there come two *w.* *Rev* 9:12

wolf

In a country where a large part of wealth consisted of flocks of sheep the habits of wolves became thoroughly well known, and were often used as symbols of such habits and actions of mankind as might bear a resemblance to them, as Gen 49:27.

Isaiah describing the tranquillity of the reign of the Messiah, *says,* The *wolf* shall dwell with the lamb, and the leopard shall lie down with the kid, *etc.,* Isa 11:6. *Persecutors are elsewhere compared to wolves,* Mat 10:16, Behold, I send you forth as sheep in the midst of *wolves.*

shall ravin as a *w.* *Gen* 49:27
the *w.* shall dwell with. *Isa* 11:6
the *w.* and the lamb shall. 65:25
a *w.* of the evenings shall. *Jer* 5:6
but he that is an hireling, seeth the *w.* coming: and the *w.* *John* 10:12

wolves

her princes are like *w.* *Ezek* 22:27
fiercer than evening *w.* *Hab* 1:8
her judges evening *w.* *Zeph* 3:3
they are ravening *w.* *Mat* 7:15
as sheep in the midst of *w.* 10:16
as lambs among *w.* *Luke* 10:3
grievous *w.* shall enter in. *Acts* 20:29

woman

Woman *was created to be a companion and helper to man. She was equal to him in that authority and jurisdiction that God gave them over all other animals. But after the fall, God made her subject to the government of man,* Gen 3:16.

Weak and ineffectual men are sometimes spoken of as women, Isa 3:12; 19:16.

and the rib, taken from man, made he a *w.* *Gen* 2:22
she shall be called *W.*, she was. 23
between thee and the *w.* 3:15
the *w.* will not come. 24:5, 39
let the same be the *w.* the Lord. 44
and hurt a *w.* with child. *Ex* 21:22
nor shall a *w.* stand. *Lev* 18:23
with mankind as with a *w.* 20:13*
he shall set the *w.* *Num* 5:18, 30
the *w.* shall be a curse among. 27
brought a Midianitish *w.* in. 25:6
Phinehas thrust the *w.* through. 8
if a *w.* vow a vow unto the Lord. 30:3
now kill every *w.* that hath. 31:17
I took this *w.* and found. *Deut* 22:14
the *w.* took the two men. *Josh* 2:4
bring out thence the *w.* 6:22
Sisera into the hand of a *w.* *Judg* 4:9
a certain *w.* cast a piece of a millstone. 9:53; *2 Sam* 11:21
men say not of me, a *w.* *Judg* 9:54
man that spakest to the *w.*? 13:11
is there never a *w.* among ? 14:3
Samson loved a *w.* in the. 16:4
the *w.* in the dawning of the. 19:26
the *w.* was left of her sons. *Ruth* 1:5
know thou art a virtuous *w.* 3:11
w. like Rachel and Leah. 4:11
Hannah said, I am a *w.* of a sorrowful spirit. *1 Sam* 1:15
I am the *w.* that stood by thee. 26
Lord give thee seed of this *w.* 2:20
seek me a *w.* that hath a. 28:7
me concerning this *w.* *2 Sam* 3:8
from the roof David saw a *w.* 11:2
put now this *w.* out from me. 13:17
the *w.* spread a covering over. 17:19
then *w.* went unto all people. 20:22
I and this *w.* dwell in. *1 Ki* 3:17
herself to be another *w.* 14:5
the son of the *w.* fell sick. 17:17
where was a great *w.* *2 Ki* 4:8
there cried a *w.* saying, Help. 6:26
this is the *w.* 8:5
see this cursed *w.* 9:34
Athaliah that wicked *w.* *2 Chr* 24:7
if my heart have been deceived by a *w.* *Job* 31:9
pain as of a *w.* in travail. *Ps* 48:6
Isa 13:8; 21:3; 26:17; *Jer* 4:31
6:24; 13:21; 22:23; 30:6; 31:8
48:41; 49:22, 24; 50:43
thee from the evil *w.* *Pr* 6:24
met him a *w.* subtle of heart. 7:10
a foolish *w.* is clamorous. 9:13
a virtuous *w.* is a crown. 12:4; 31:10
every wise *w.* buildeth her. 14:1
than with a brawling *w.* in. 21:9, 19
who can find a virtuous *w.*? 31:10
a *w.* that feareth the Lord shall. 30
the *w.* whose heart is snares and nets. *Eccl* 7:26
but a *w.* among all those have I. 28
cry like a travailing *w.* *Isa* 42:14
or to the *w.*, What hast thou? 45:10
can a *w.* forget her sucking ? 49:15
Lord hath called thee as a *w.* 54:6*
of Zion to a delicate *w.* *Jer* 6:2
created a new thing, a *w.* 31:22
Jerusalem is a menstruous *w.* *Lam* 1:17
imperious whorish *w.* *Ezek* 16:30†
unto her, as they go in to a *w.* 23:44
uncleanness of a removed *w.* 36:17
go yet, love a *w.* beloved. *Hos* 3:1
the sorrows of a travailing *w.* shall come upon. 13:13; *Mi* 4:9, 10
this is a *w.* that sitteth in. *Zech* 5:7
whoso looketh on a *w.* to lust after her. *Mat* 5:28
a *w.* which was diseased with an issue. 9:20; *Mark* 5:25; *Luke* 8:43
leaven, which a *w.* took. *Mat* 13:33
O *w.*, great is thy faith, be it. 15:28
and last of all the *w.* died also. 22:27
Mark 12:22; *Luke* 20:32
Why trouble ye the *w.*? *Mat* 26:10
this that this *w.* hath done shall. 13
if a *w.* shall put away. *Mark* 10:12
manner of *w.* this is ? *Luke* 7:39
Simon, Seest thou this *w.*? 44
ought not this *w.*, being a daughter of Abraham ? 13:16
w. what have I to do with thee ? *John* 2:4
askest drink of me who am a *w.*? 4:9
on him for the saying of the *w.* 39
brought to him a *w.* taken in. 8:3, 4
when Jesus saw none but the *w.* 10
he saith to his mother, *W.* 19:26
Dorcas: this *w.* was full. *Acts* 9:36
and a *w.* **named Damaris.** 17:34

the natural use of the *w.* *Rom* 1:27
the *w.* which hath an husband is. 7:2
for a man not to touch a *w.* *1 Cor* 7:1
every *w.* have her own husband. 2
but every *w.* that prayeth. 11:5
if the *w.* be not covered, let her. 6
the *w.* is the glory of the man. 7
man is not of the *w.*; but the *w.* 8
neither man for the *w.*; but the *w.* 9
the *w.* ought to have power on. 10
nevertheless, neither is the man without the *w.*, nor the *w.* 11
as the *w.* is of the man, even so is the man also by the *w.* 12
comely that a *w.* pray uncovered? 13
if a *w.* have long hair, it is a glory. 15
forth his Son, made of a *w.* *Gal* 4:4
then destruction cometh as travail on a *w.* *1 Thes* 5:3
I suffer not a *w.* to teach. *1 Tim* 2:12
the *w.* being deceived, was in the. 14
sufferest that *w.* Jezebel. *Rev* 2:20
there appeared *w.* clothed with. 12:1
the *w.* fled. 6
the earth helped the *w.* 16
dragon was wroth with the *w.* 17
I saw a *w.* sit on a scarlet. 17:3
a *w.* drunken. 6
I will tell the mystery of the *w.* 7
see **born, man, strange**

young **woman**

the seed which Lord shall give thee of this *young w.* *Ruth* 4:12

womankind

with mankind as with *w.* *Lev* 18:22

womb

two nations are in thy *w.* *Gen* 25:23
there were twins in her *w.* 24; 38:27
Lord opened Leah's *w.* 29:31
God opened Rachel's *w.* 30:22
of breasts, and of *w.* 49:25
openeth the *w.* is mine. *Ex* 13:2
are given me, instead of such as open every *w.*, even. *Num* 8:16
bless the fruit of thy *w.* *Deut* 7:13
Nazarite from the *w.* *Judg* 13:5, 7
any more sons in my *w.*? *Ruth* 1:11
had shut up her *w.* *1 Sam* 1:5, 6
why died I not from the *w.*? *Job* 3:11
brought me forth of the *w.* 10:18
the *w.* shall forget him, he. 24:20
that made me in the *w.* make him? fashion us in the *w.*? 31:15
if it had issued out of the *w.* 38:8
out of whose *w.* came the ice? 29
who took me out of the *w.* *Ps* 22:9
I was cast upon thee from the *w.* 10
are estranged from the *w.* 58:3
I been holden up from the *w.* 71:6
from the *w.* of the morning. 110:3
the barren *w.* saith not, It. *Pr* 30:16
what, the son of my *w.*? 31:2
nor how bones grow in *w.* *Eccl* 11:5
Lord formed thee from the *w.* *Isa* 44:2, 24; 49:5
which are carried from the *w.* 46:3
a transgressor from the *w.* 48:8
called me from the *w.* 49:1
compassion on the son of her *w.*? 15
bring forth, and shut the *w.*? 66:9
camest forth out of the *w.* *Jer* 1:5
because he slew me not from the *w.*; or my mother's *w.* to be. 20:17
why came I forth of the *w.*? 18
pass through the fire all that openeth the *w.* *Ezek* 20:26
their glory shall fly away from the birth and *w.* *Hos* 9:11*
give them a miscarrying *w.* 14
brother by the heel in the *w.* 12:3
shalt conceive in thy *w.* *Luke* 1:31
leaped in her *w.* for joy. 41, 44
he was conceived in the *w.* 2:21
every male that openeth the *w.* 23
see **fruit, mother**

wombs

fast closed up all the *w.* *Gen* 20:18
blessed are the *w.* that. *Luke* 23:29

women

the time that *w.* go out to. *Gen* 24:11
all the *w.* went out after. *Ex* 15:20
w. that were wise hearted. 35:25
all the *w.* whose heart stirred. 26
ten *w.* shall bake your bread in one oven. *Lev* 26:26
Moses said, Have ye saved all the *w.* alive? *Num* 31:15
the *w.* and little ones. *Deut* 20:14
the law before the *w.* *Josh* 8:35
blessed above *w.* shall Jael wife of. *Judg* 5:24
they saved alive of the *w.* of. 21:14
they lay with the *w.* *1 Sam* 2:22
as thy sword hath made *w.* 15:33
the *w.* came out of the cities. 18:6
the *w.* answered one another as. 7
kept themselves from *w.* 21:4
of a truth *w.* have been kept. 5
Amalekites had taken the *w.* 30:2
passing the love of *w.* *2 Sam* 1:26
the king left ten *w.* to keep. 15:16
then came two *w.* that. *1 Ki* 3:16
and rip up their *w.* with child. *2 Ki* 8:12, 15, 16
where the *w.* wove hangings. 23:7
even him did outlandish *w.* cause to sin. *Neh* 13:26
made a feast for the *w.* *Esth* 1:9
loved Esther above all the *w.* 2:17
little children and *w.* 3:13; 8:11
no *w.* found so fair as. *Job* 42:15
among thy honourable *w.* *Ps* 45:9
give not thy strength to *w.* *Pr* 31:3
O thou fairest among *w.* *S of S* 1:8 5:9; 6:1
as for my people, *w.* rule. *Isa* 3:12
in that day seven *w.* shall take. 4:1
day Egypt shall be like to *w.* 19:16
the *w.* come, and set them. 27:11
rise up, ye *w.* that are at ease. 32:9
careless *w.* 10
tremble, ye *w.* that are at ease. 11
the *w.* knead their dough. *Jer* 7:18
mourning and cunning *w.* 9:17
word of the Lord, O ye *w.* 20
w. left, shall be brought to. 38:22
Jeremiah said to all the *w.* 44:24
they shall become as *w.* and. 50:37
men of Babylon became as *w.* 51:30
shall the *w.* eat children? *Lam* 2:20
the pitiful *w.* have sodden. 4:10
they ravished *w.* in Zion, and. 5:11
there sat *w.* weeping. *Ezek* 8:14
maids, little children, and *w.* 9:6
woe to *w.* that sew pillows to. 13:18
is in thee from other *w.* 16:34
I will judge thee as *w.* that. 38
there were two *w.*, daughters. 23:2
judge after the manner of *w.* 45
w. may be taught not to do after. 48
he shall give him the daughter of *w.* *Dan* 11:17
nor shall regard the desire of *w.* 37
their *w.* with child shall. *Hos* 13:16
because they have ripped up *w.* with child. *Amos* 1:13
the *w.* of my people have. *Mi* 2:9
in the midst of thee are *w.* *Nah* 3:13
two *w.* and had wings. *Zech* 5:9
old *w.* shall dwell in the streets. 8:4
the houses rifled, the *w.* shall. 14:2
that are born of *w.* there hath not risen a greater. *Mat* 11:11; *Luke* 7:28
they that had eaten were 5000 men, besides *w.* *Mat* 14:21; 15:38
two *w.* grinding at the mill. 24:41 *Luke* 17:35
and many *w.* were then. *Mat* 27:55
blessed art thou among *w.* *Luke* 1:28, 42
certain *w.* also made us. 24:22
and found it even so as the *w.* 24
in prayer with the *w.* *Acts* 1:14
stirred up the devout *w.* 13:50
we spake to the *w.* which. 16:13
of the chief *w.* not a few. 17:4, 12
their *w.* did change the. *Rom* 1:26
let your *w.* keep silence. *1 Cor* 14:34
shame for *w.* to speak in churches. 35
help those *w.* which laboured with me. *Phil* 4:3
w. adorn themselves in. *1 Tim* 2:9
which becometh *w.* professing. 10
let the *w.* learn in silence with. 11
intreat the elder *w.* as mothers. 5:2
that the younger *w.* marry. 14*
captive silly *w.* laden. *2 Tim* 3:6
aged *w.* behave as becometh. *Tit* 2:3
they may teach the younger *w.* 4
w. received their dead. *Heb* 11:35
the holy *w.* adorned. *1 Pet* 3:5
they had hair as hair of *w.* *Rev* 9:8
that are not defiled with *w.* 14:4
see **children, men, singing, strange**

womenservants

gave *w.* to Abraham. *Gen* 20:14
had menservants and *w.* 32:5*

won

out of the spoils *w.* in. *1 Chr* 26:27
a brother offended is harder to be *w.* *Pr* 18:19
w. by the conversation. *1 Pet* 3:1*

wonder

give thee a sign or a *w.* *Deut* 13:1
and the sign or the *w.* come. 2
upon thee for a sign and a *w.* 28:46
him to enquire of the *w.* *2 Chr* 32:31
I am as a *w.* to many. *Ps* 71:7
walked barefoot for a *w.* *Isa* 20:3
marvellous work and a *w.* 29:14
they were filled with *w.* *Acts* 3:10
a great *w.* in heaven. *Rev* 12:1*, 3*

wonder, *verb*

stay yourselves, and *w.*; cry. *Isa* 29:9
the prophets shall *w.* *Jer* 4:9
behold ye, regard and *w.* *Hab* 1:5
behold, ye despisers, *w.* *Acts* 13:41
dwell on the earth shall *w.* *Rev* 17:8

wondered

he *w.* there was no. *Isa* 59:16
I *w.* that there was none. 63:5
for they are men *w.* at. *Zech* 3:8*
all they that heard it *w.* *Luke* 2:18
they all *w.* at the gracious. 4:22
believed not for joy, and *w.* 24:41
Moses *w.* *Acts* 7:31
Simon [Magus] *w.* 8:13*
all the world *w.* after. *Rev* 13:3
I saw her, I *w.* with great. 17:6

wonderful

make thy plagues *w.* *Deut* 28:59
thy love to me was *w.* *2 Sam* 1:26
house . . . shall be *w.* great. *2 Chr* 2:9
things too *w.* for me. *Job* 42:3
thy testimonies are *w.* *Ps* 119:129
knowledge is too *w.* for me. 139:6
there be three things that are too *w.* *Pr* 30:18
his name shall be called *W.* *Isa* 9:6
for thou hast done *w.* things. 25:1
of hosts who is *w.* in counsel. 28:29
a *w.* thing is committed. *Jer* 5:30
when they saw the *w.* *Mat* 21:15
see **works**

wonderfully

when he had wrought *w.* *1 Sam* 6:6
thee for I am *w.* made. *Ps* 139:14
Jerusalem came down *w.* *Lam* 1:9
he shall destroy *w.* and. *Dan* 8:24

wondering

the man *w.* at her, held. *Gen* 24:21*
Peter *w.* at that which was come to pass. *Luke* 24:12
ran together greatly *w.* *Acts* 3:11

wonderously, wondrously

angel did *w.*: Manoah. *Judg* 13:19*
the Lord hath dealt *w.* *Joel* 2:26

wonders

my hand and smite Egypt with all my *w.* *Ex* 3:20; 7:3; 11:9 *Deut* 6:22; 7:19; 26:8; 34:11
see thou do those *w.* *Ex* 4:21
did these *w.* 11:10
fearful in praises, doing *w.*? 15:11
hath God assayed to go and take a nation by *w.*? *Deut* 4:34
to-morrow the Lord will do *w.* among you. *Josh* 3:5
remember his *w.* *1 Chr* 16:12 *Ps* 105:5
thou shewedst *w.* upon. *Neh* 9:10
nor were mindful of thy *w.* 17 *Ps* 78:11, 43
doeth *w.* without number. *Job* 9:10
remember thy *w.* of old. *Ps* 77:11
thou art the God that doest *w.* 14
shew *w.* to the dead? 88:10

shall thy *w.* be known in the? *Ps* 88:12
shall praise thy *w.* O Lord. 89:5
his *w.* among all people. 96:3*
they shewed his *w.* in the. 105:27
our fathers understood not thy *w.* in Egypt. 106:7
see his works and his *w.* 107:24
who sent *w.* into the midst of. 135:9
who alone doeth great *w.* 136:4
I and the children are for *w.* in Israel. *Isa* 8:18
who hath set signs and *w.* *Jer* 32:20
brought forth thy people with *w.* 21
to shew the signs and *w.* *Dan* 4:2
signs! how mighty his *w.*! 3
he worketh *w.* in heaven. 6:27
it be to the end of these *w.*? 12:6
I will shew *w.* in heaven. *Joel* 2:30
Acts 2:19
false prophets, and shall shew great *w.* *Mat* 24:24; *Mark* 13:22
Except ye see signs and *w.* *John* 4:48
approved of God by *w.* *Acts* 2:22
fear on every soul, many signs and *w.* were. 43; 5:12; 14:3; 15:12
that *w.* may be done by the. 4:30
Stephen did great *w.* among. 6:8
after he had shewed *w.* in the land of Egypt. 7:36
obedient through *w.* *Rom* 15:19
an apostle wrought in *w.* *2 Cor* 12:12
is with signs and lying *w.* *2 Thes* 2:9
witness with signs and *w.* *Heb* 2:4
he doeth great *w.*, so that he maketh fire come down. *Rev* 13:13*

wondrous

sing psalms, talk ye of all his *w.*
1 Chr 16:9; *Ps* 26:7; 105:2
119:27; 145:5
consider the *w.* works. *Job* 37:14
dost thou know the *w.* works? 16
I declared thy *w.* works. *Ps* 71:17
the God of Israel, who only doeth *w.* things. 72:18; 86:10
that thy name is near, thy *w.* 75:1
they believed not for his *w.* 78:32
who had done *w.* works in. 106:22
that I may behold *w.* things. 119:18
according to his *w.* works. *Jer* 21:2

wont

if the ox were *w.* to push. *Ex* 21:29
was I ever *w.* to do so to thee?
Num 22:30
where David and his men were *w.* to haunt. *1 Sam* 30:31
were *w.* to speak in. *2 Sam* 20:18
seven times more than *w.* *Dan* 3:19
the governor was *w.* to. *Mat* 27:15
as he was *w.*, he taught. *Mark* 10:1
he went as he was *w.* to. *Luke* 22:39*
where prayer was *w.* to. *Acts* 16:13

wood

Abraham took *w.* and put. *Gen* 22:6
Behold the fire and the *w.* 7
whether there be *w.* *Num* 13:20
things that are made of *w.* 31:20
make thee an ark of *w.* *Deut* 10:1
goeth into a *w.* to hew *w.* 19:5*
from the hewer of thy *w.* 29:11
Josh 9:21, 23, 27; *Jer* 46:22
the mountain is a *w.* *Josh* 17:18*
and they clave the *w.* *1 Sam* 6:14
they of the land came to a *w.* 14:25
went to David into the *w.* 23:16
the *w.* devoured more. *2 Sam* 18:8*
lay the bullock on *w.* *1 Ki* 18:23
she bears out of the *w.* *2 Ki* 2:24
I have prepared *w.* for things of *w.*
1 Chr 29:2
the boar out of the *w.* *Ps* 80:13
it in the fields of the *w.* 132:6
as when one cleaveth *w.* 141:7
where no *w.* is, there the. *Pr* 26:20
as *w.* to fire, so is a contentious. 21
he that cleaveth *w.* shall. *Eccl* 10:9
itself as if it were no *w.* *Isa* 10:15
thereof is fire and much *w.* 30:33
they that set up the *w.* of. 45:20
will bring silver, for *w.* brass. 60:17
I will make my words fire, this people *w.* *Jer* 5:14
the children gather *w.*, the. 7:18
the yokes of *w.* but shalt. 28:13
shall *w.* be taken thereof to do any work? *Ezek* 15:3
heap on *w.* 24:10
no *w.* out of the field. 39:10
dwell solitary in the *w.* *Mi* 7:14*
that saith to the *w.* Awake. *Hab* 2:19
go up, bring *w.* and build. *Hag* 1:8
hearth of fire among the *w.* *Zech* 12:6
on this foundation, *w.*, hay. *1 Cor* 3:12
but also vessels of *w.* *2 Tim* 2:20
see **offering, stone**

woods

sleep safely in the *w.* *Ezek* 34:25

woof

be in the warp or *w.* *Lev* 13:48
be spread in the warp or the *w.* 51
whether warp or *w.* 52
be not spread, wash the *w.* 53, 58
rend it out of the warp or *w.* 56
of leprosy in the warp or *w.* 59

wool

I will put a fleece of *w.* *Judg* 6:37
100,000 rams with *w.* *2 Ki* 3:4
giveth snow like *w.* *Ps* 147:16
she seeketh *w.* and flax. *Pr* 31:13
like crimson, shall be as *w.* *Isa* 1:18
like *w.*: but my righteousness. 51:8
was thy merchant in *w.* *Ezek* 27:18
ye clothe you with the *w.* 34:3
and no *w.* shall come upon. 44:17
the hair of his head like *w.* *Dan* 7:9
Rev 1:14
lovers that give me my *w.* *Hos* 2:5
I will recover my *w.* and my flax. 9

woollen

whether *w.* or linen. *Lev* 13:47, 59
the warp or woof of *w.* 48, 52
mingled of linen and *w.* come upon thee. 19:19*; *Deut* 22:11

word

(Word, *the Greek* logos, *is sometimes used of Jesus Christ,* John 1. The word of God *is a name often given to the scriptures, and the law of God*)

go and bring me *w.* again. *Gen* 37:14
Mat 2:8
O my lord, let me speak a *w.*
Gen 44:18; *2 Sam* 14:12
according to *w.* of Moses. *Ex* 8:13
Israel did according to the *w.* 12:35
Levi did according to the *w.* 32:28
Lev 10:7
they brought back *w.* *Num* 13:26
lodge here, I will bring you *w.* 22:8
Deut 1:22
yet the *w.* I shall say to. *Num* 22:20
the *w.* I shall speak. 35
the *w.* God putteth. 38
the Lord put a *w.* in Balaam's. 23:5
they brought us *w.* again. *Deut* 1:25
ye shall not add unto the *w.* I. 4:2
but by every *w.* that proceedeth out.
8:3*; *Mat* 4:4
presume to speak a *w.* *Deut* 18:20
how shall we know the *w.*? 21
Jer 28:9
by their *w.* shall every controversy be tried. *Deut* 21:5
the *w.* is nigh thee. 30:14; *Rom* 10:8
remember the *w.* Moses. *Josh* 1:13
not a *w.* which Joshua read not. 8:35
I brought him *w.* 14:7
brought them *w.* 22:32
the *w.* of Samuel came. *1 Sam* 4:1
not answer Abner a *w.* *2 Sam* 3:11
in all places spake I a *w.* 7:7
1 Chr 17:6
the *w.* thou hast spoken concerning thy servant. *2 Sam* 7:25
till there come *w.* from you. 15:28
speak ye not a *w.* of bringing. 19:10
the king's *w.* prevailed. 24:4
1 Chr 21:4
brought the king *w.* again. *1 Ki* 2:30
2 Ki 22:9, 20; *2 Chr* 34:16, 28
w. that I have heard is good.
1 Ki 2:42*
hath not failed one *w.* of all. 8:56
the people answered not a *w.* 18:21
Isa 36:21
he smote according to the *w.* of Elisha. *2 Ki* 6:18
hear the *w.* of the great king. 18:28
mindful of the *w.* which he commanded. *1 Chr* 16:15; *Ps* 105:8
advise what *w.* I shall. *1 Chr* 21:12*
remember, the *w.* that thou. *Neh* 1:8
he did according to the *w.* *Esth* 1:21
as the *w.* went out of the king's. 7:8
none spake a *w.* to Job. *Job* 2:13
by the *w.* of thy lips, I have. *Ps* 17:4
the Lord gave the *w.* 68:11
remember the *w.* unto thy. 119:49
mine eyes fail for the *w.* of thy. 123
not a *w.* in my tongue. 139:4
a good *w.* maketh the. *Pr* 12:25
whoso despiseth the *w.* shall. 13:13
simple believe the *w.* but. 14:15
w. spoken in due season, how! 15:23
a *w.* fitly spoken is like apples. 25:11
where the *w.* of a king is. *Eccl* 8:4
despised *w.* of the Holy. *Isa* 5:24
speak *w.* and it shall not stand. 8:10
the Lord sent a *w.* to Jacob, it. 9:8
man an offender for a *w.* 29:21
thine ears shall hear a *w.* 30:21
counsellor could answer a *w.* 41:28
that confirmeth the *w.* of. 44:26
w. is gone out of my mouth. 45:23
should know how to speak a *w.* 50:4
become wind, and the *w.* *Jer* 5:13
let your ear receive *w.* 9:20; 10:1
nor shall the *w.* perish from. 18:18
for every man's *w.* shall be. 23:36
them, diminish not a *w.* 26:2
for I have pronounced the *w.* 34:5
king said, Is there any *w.*? 37:17
for the *w.* thou hast spoken. 44:16
therefore hear the *w.* at my mouth.
Ezek 3:17; 33:7
the *w.* that I shall speak. 12:25
the *w.* that I have spoken shall. 28
would confirm the *w.* 13:6
hear what is *w.* that cometh. 33:30
changed the king's *w.* *Dan* 3:28
the demand is by the *w.* of. 4:17
while the *w.* was in the king's. 31
for *w.* came to the king. *Jonah* 3:6
to the *w.* I covenanted. *Hag* 2:5
speak the *w.* only, he shall. *Mat* 8:8
whoso speaketh a *w.* against the Son of man. 12:32; *Luke* 12:10
every idle *w.* men. *Mat* 12:36
when any one heareth the *w.* of the kingdom. 13:19, 20, 22, 23
Mark 4:16, 18, 20; *Luke* 8:15
or persecution ariseth because of the *w.*, he. *Mat* 13:21; *Mark* 4:17
he answered her not a *w.*
Mat 15:23
that every *w.* may be established.
18:16; *2 Cor* 13:1
able to answer him a *w.* *Mat* 22:46
he answered him to never a *w.* 27:14
to bring his disciples *w.* 28:8
sower soweth the *w.* *Mark* 4:14
Peter called to mind the *w.* 14:72
the Lord confirming the *w.* 16:20
saying, What a *w.* is this! *Luke* 4:36
say in a *w.* and my servant shall. 7:7
Jesus, a prophet mighty in *w.* 24:19
the *W.* and the *W.* was with God, and the *W.* was God. *John* 1:1
the *W.* was made flesh, and. 14
they believed the *w.* that Jesus said.
2:22; 4:50
w. I have spoken shall judge. 12:48
w. which ye hear is not mine. 14:24
ye are clean through the *w.* I. 15:3
remember the *w.* that I said. 20
that *w.* might be fulfilled, written. 25
believe on me through their *w.* 17:20
the *w.* which God sent to. *Acts* 10:36
if ye have any *w.* of exhortation, say on. 13:15
to you is the *w.* of this salvation. 26
by my mouth, should hear *w.* 15:7
they received the *w.* with all. 17:11
I commend you to the *w.* of. 20:32
Paul had spoken one *w.* 28:25
that is, the *w.* of faith. *Rom* 10:8
make Gentiles obedient by *w.* 15:18
kingdom of God is not in *w.*
1 Cor 4:20

w. of wisdom, to another the *w.* of knowledge. *1 Cor* 12:8
w. toward you was not. *2 Cor* 1:18
God committed to us the *w.* of. 5:19
such as we are in *w.* by letters. 10:11
law is fulfilled in one *w.* *Gal* 5:14
let him that is taught in the *w.* 6:6
washing of water by the *w.* *Eph* 5:26
are bold to speak the *w.* *Phil* 1:14
holding forth the *w.* of life to. 2:16
heard in the *w.* of the truth. *Col* 1:5
let the *w.* of Christ dwell in. 3:16
whatsoever ye do in *w.* or deed. 17
our gospel came not to you in *w.* only. *1 Thes* 1:5
having received the *w.* in much. 6
w. . . , ye receive it not as *w.* of men, but as it is in truth, *w.* of God. 2:13
not by Spirit, nor by *w.* *2 Thes* 2:2
have been taught, whether by *w.* 15
and stablish you in every good *w.* 17
if any man obey not our *w.* by. 3:14
be thou an example of believers in *w.* *1 Tim* 4:12
they who labour in the *w.* 5:17
their *w.* will eat as doth. *2 Tim* 2:17
preach *w.*; be instant in season. 4:2
holding fast the faithful *w.* *Tit* 1:9
upholding all things by the *w.* of his power. *Heb* 1:3
if the *w.* spoken by angels was. 2:2
but the *w.* preached did not. 4:2
is unskilful in the *w.* of. 5:13
but the *w.* of the oath, which. 7:28
intreated *w.* should not be. 12:19
brethren, suffer the *w.* of. 13:22
meekness the ingrafted *w.* *Jas* 1:21
be ye doers of the *w.* and not. 22
if any be a hearer of the *w.* and. 23
if any man offend not in *w.*, the. 3:2
the sincere milk of the *w.* *1 Pet* 2:2
who stumble at the *w.* being. 8
not the *w.*, may without the *w.* 3:1
we have a more sure *w.* of prophecy. *2 Pet* 1:19
the heavens by the same *w.* are. 3:7
handled, of the *w.* of life. *1 John* 1:1
let us not love in *w.* but in. 3:18
the Father, the *W.* and. 5:7
because thou hast kept *w.* *Rev* 3:10
they overcame by the *w.* of. 12:11

word *of God*

that I may shew thee the *w. of God.* *1 Sam* 9:27
the *w. of God* came to Shemaiah, *1 Ki* 12:22
the *w. of God* came to Nathan. *1 Chr* 17:3
every *w. of God* is pure. *Pr* 30:5
the *w. of* our *God* shall. *Isa* 40:8
making the *w. of God.* *Mark* 7:13
w. of God came unto John. *Luke* 3:2
alone, but by every *w. of God.* 4:4
on him to hear the *w. of God.* 5:1
the seed is the *w. of God.* 8:11
these that hear the *w. of God.* 21
they that hear the *w. of God.* 11:28
gods to whom *w. of God.* *John* 10:35
they spake the *w. of God.* *Acts* 4:31
should leave the *w. of God.* 6:2
the *w. of God* increased. 7; 12:24
Samaria had received the *w. of God.* 8:14
Gentiles had received the *w. of God.* 11:1
desired to hear the *w. of God.* 13:7
city came to hear the *w. of God.* 44
w. of God should have been first. 46
mightily grew the *w. of God.* 19:20
not as though the *w. of God* hath taken none effect. *Rom* 9:6
hearing by the *w. of God.* 10:17
came the *w. of God* out from you? *1 Cor* 14:36
corrupt the *w. of God.* *2 Cor* 2:17
not handling the *w. of God.* 4:2
and the sword of the Spirit, which is the *w. of God.* *Eph* 6:17
which is given me to fulfil the *w. of God.* *Col* 1:25
received the *w. of God.* *1 Thes* 2:13
it is sanctified by the *w. of God* and prayer. *1 Tim* 4:5
but the *w. of God* is not bound. *2 Tim* 2:9
the *w. of God* be not blasphemed. *Tit* 2:5
the *w. of God* is quick. *Heb* 4:12
tasted the good *w. of God.* 6:5
framed by the *w. of God.* 11:3
spoken to you the *w. of God.* 13:7
being born again by the *w. of God.* *1 Pet* 1:23
by the *w. of God* the heavens were of old. *2 Pet* 3:5
are strong, and the *w. of God* abideth in you. *1 John* 2:14
record of the *w. of God.* *Rev* 1:2
isle of Patmos, for the *w. of God.* 9
that were slain for *w. of God.* 6:9
name is called the *w. of God.* 19:13
beheaded for the *w. of God.* 20:4

see **heard**

his **word**

at *his w.* shall they go out, and at *his w.* they shall come. *Num* 27:21
he shall not break *his w.* 30:2
the Lord stablish *his w.* *1 Sam* 1:23
his w. was in my tongue. *2 Sam* 23:2
may continue *his w.* *1 Ki* 2:4
the Lord hath performed *his w.* that he spake. 8:20; *2 Chr* 6:10
to enquire of *his w.* *2 Ki* 1:16
might perform *his w.* *2 Chr* 10:15
in God I will praise *his w.*, in God I have put my trust. *Ps* 56:4, 10
unto the voice of *his w.* 103:20
the time that *his w.* came. 105:19
rebelled not against *his w.* 28
they believed not *his w.* but. 106:24
he sent *his w.* and healed. 107:20
I wait for the Lord and in *his w.* do I hope. 130:5
his w. runneth very swiftly. 147:15
sendeth out *his w.* and melteth. 18
he sheweth *his w.* unto Jacob. 19
wind fulfilling *his w.* 148:8
that tremble at *his w.* *Isa* 66:5
but *his w.* was in my heart as a fire. *Jer* 20:9
he hath fulfilled *his w.* *Lam* 2:17
that executeth *his w.* *Joel* 2:11
out the spirits with *his w.* *Mat* 8:16
for *his w.* was with power. *Luke* 4:32
many believed because of *his* own *w.* *John* 4:41
ye have not *his w.* abiding. 5:38
gladly received *his w.* *Acts* 2:41
but hath in due times manifested *his w.* *Tit* 1:3
whoso keepeth *his w.* *1 John* 2:5

see **Lord**

my **word**

whether *my w.* shall come to pass. *Num* 11:23
ye rebelled against *my w.* 20:24
will I perform *my w.* *1 Ki* 6:12
rain, but according to *my w.* 17:1
so shall *my w.* be that goeth forth out of my mouth. *Isa* 55:11
him that trembleth at *my w.* 66:2
hasten *my w.* to perform. *Jer* 1:12
my w., let him speak *my w.* 23:28
is not *my w.* like as a fire? 29
the prophets that steal *my w.* 30
I will perform *my* good *w.* 29:10
but *my w.* shall not pass. *Mat* 24:35
he that heareth *my w.* *John* 5:24
continue in *my w.*, then are ye. 8:31
kill me because *my w.* hath. 37
ye cannot hear *my w.* 43
thou hast kept *my w.*, and hast not denied my name. *Rev* 3:8

this **word**

is not *this* the *w.* that? *Ex* 14:12
since the Lord spake *this w.* to Moses. *Josh* 14:10
they sent *this w.* to the king. *2 Sam* 19:14*
hast not spoken *this w.* *1 Ki* 2:23
this is the *w.* that the Lord hath spoken of him. *2 Ki* 19:21
Isa 16:13; 24:3; 37:22
shall alter *this w.* *Ezra* 6:11
should do according to *this w.* 10:5
not according to *this w.* *Isa* 8:20
because ye despise *this w.* *Isa* 30:12
ye speak *this w.* *Jer* 5:14; 23:38
proclaim there *this w.* and say. 7:2
speak unto them *this w.* 13:12
thou say *this w.* to them. 14:17
down, and speak there *this w.* 22:1
in the reign of Jehoiakim *this w.* came. 26:1; 27:1; 34:8; 36:1
hear now *this w.* 28:7; *Amos* 3:1
4:1; 5:1
spoken *this w.* to me. *Dan* 10:11
this is the *w.* of the Lord. *Zech* 4:6
him audience to *this w.* *Acts* 22:22
for *this* is *w.* of promise. *Rom* 9:9
this w., Yet once more. *Heb* 12:27
this is the *w.* which is. *1 Pet* 1:25

thy **word**

be according to *thy w.* *Gen* 30:34
according to *thy w.* shall my. 41:40
Be it according to *thy w.* *Ex* 8:10
I have pardoned, according to *thy w.* *Num* 14:20
have observed *thy w.* *Deut* 33:9
done according to *thy w.* *1 Ki* 3:12
let *thy w.* I pray thee, be. 8:26
done all these things at *thy w.* 18:36
let *thy w.* I pray thee, be like the word of one of. 22:13; *2 Chr* 18:12
heed according to *thy w.* *Ps* 119:9
thy w. have I hid in mine heart. 11
statutes, I will not forget *thy w.* 16
live, and keep *thy w.* 17, 101
quicken me according to *thy w.* 25, 107, 154
strengthen thou me according to *thy w.* 28, 116
stablish *thy w.* 38
salvation according to *thy w.* 41
I trust in *thy w.* 42
comfort in affliction, for *thy w.* 50
be merciful to me according to *thy w.* 58, 65, 76
but now have I kept *thy w.* 67
I have hoped in *thy w.* 74, 147
I hope in *thy w.* 81, 114
mine eyes fail for *thy w.* 82
ever, O Lord, *thy w.* is settled. 89
thy w. is a lamp. 105
order my steps in *thy w.*, let not. 133
thy w. is pure. 140
that I might meditate in *thy w.* 148
because they kept not *thy w.* 158
thy w. is true. 160
standeth in awe of *thy w.* 161
I rejoice at *thy w.* 162
give me understanding according to *thy w.* 169
deliver me according to *thy w.* 170
my tongue shall speak of *thy w.* 172
thou hast magnified *thy w.* 138:2
thy w. was to me the joy. *Jer* 15:16
drop *thy w.* toward the south. *Ezek* 20:46
drop *thy w.* toward the holy. 21:2
drop not *thy w.* against. *Amos* 7:16
made naked, even *thy w.* *Hab* 3:9
according to *thy w.* *Luke* 1:38
in peace, according to *thy w.* 2:29
nevertheless at *thy w.* I will let. 5:5
and they have kept *thy w.* *John* 17:6
I have given them *thy w.* 14
thy w. is truth. 17
with all boldness they may speak *thy w.* *Acts* 4:29

see **truth**

words

shalt put *w.* in his mouth. *Ex* 4:15
let them not regard vain *w.* 5:9
returned the *w.* of the people. 19:8
the gift perverteth the *w.* of the righteous. 23:8; *Deut* 16:19
the *w.* which were in the first tables. *Ex* 34:1
Moses wrote the *w.* of the covenant. 28; *Deut* 10:2
I sent to Sihon with *w.* *Deut* 2:26
go aside from any of the *w.* 28:14
keep the *w.* of his covenant. 29:9
2 Ki 23:3, 24; *2 Chr* 34:31
hear, O earth, the *w.* of. *Deut* 32:1
Ps 54:2; 78:1; *Pr* 7:24
Saul was afraid of the *w.* of Samuel. *1 Sam* 28:20

the w. of men of Judah were fiercer. 2 Sam 19:43
w. of prophets declare good to the king. 1 Ki 22:13; 2 Chr 18:12
Elisha telleth the w. 2 Ki 6:12
but they are but vain w. 18:20
Isa 36:5
sing praises with the w. 2 Chr 29:30
the people rested on the w. 32:8
he sent letters with w. of peace and truth. Esth 9:30
ye imagine to reprove w.? Job 6:26
shall w. of thy mouth be like ? 8:2
not the ear try w.? 12:11; 34:3
thou lettest such w. go out. 15:13
shall vain w. have an end ? 16:3
I could heap up w. against you. 4
ere ye make an end of w.? 18:2
ye break me in pieces with w.? 19:2
I would know the w. he would. 23:5
I have esteemed the w. of his. 12
he multiplieth w. without. 35:16
darkeneth counsel by w.? 38:2
let the w. of my mouth. Ps 19:14
why so far from the w. of ? 22:1
the w. of his mouth are iniquity. 36:3
thou lovest all devouring w. 52:4
w. of his mouth were smoother than butter. 55:21
for w. of their lips, let them. 59:12
to understand the w. of. Pr 1:6
decline not from the w. 4:5; 5:7
thou art snared with the w. of. 6:2
in multitude of w. there wanteth not sin. 10:19
w. of the wicked are to lie in wait for blood. 12:6
w. of the pure are pleasant w. 15:26
the w. of a man's mouth are as. 18:4
w. of a talebearer are as wounds. 8; 26:22
he pursueth them with w. 19:7
he causeth thee to err from w. 27
he overthroweth the w. of the. 22:12
bow down thine ear, hear the w. 17
certainty of the w. of truth; that thou mightest answer the w. of. 21
thou shalt lose thy sweet w. 23:8
will not be corrected by w. 29:19
a fool's voice is known by multitude of w. Eccl 5:3; 10:14
the w. of a wise man's mouth. 10:12
find out acceptable w.: that which was written, even w. of truth. 12:10
the w. of the wise are as goads. 11
become as the w. of a book sealed. Isa 29:11
it may be God will hear the w. 37:4
uttering from the heart w. of. 59:13
w. of this covenant. Jer 11:2, 6
because of the Lord, and the w. 23:9
w. of Jonadab son of Rechab. 35:14
remnant shall know whose w. 44:28
whose w. thou canst not. Ezek 3:6
shall speak great w. against most High. Dan 7:25
shut up the w. 12:4
the w. are closed up. 9
I have slain them by the w. of my mouth. Hos 6:5
take with you w. and turn to. 14:2
good and comfortable w. Zech 1:13
should ye not hear the w.? 7:7
saying the same w. Mat 26:44
Mark 14:39
wondered at gracious w. Luke 4:22
the w. that I speak unto you, they are spirit. John 6:63
to whom we go ? thou hast the w. 68
I have given to them the w. 17:8
with many other w. did. Acts 2:40
Moses was mighty in w. and. 7:22
was warned to hear w. of thee. 10:22
Peter, who shall tell thee w. 11:14
to this agree the w. of the prophets. 15:15
have troubled you with w. 24
but if it be a question of w. 18:15
to remember the w. of the. 20:35
most of all for the w. he spake. 38
but I speak forth w. of truth. 26:25
by good w. deceive hearts of the simple. Rom 16:18*
not with wisdom of w. 1 Cor 1:17
2:4, 13
except ye utter w. easy to. 14:9*
I had rather speak five w. with. 19
deceive you with vain w. Eph 5:6
nourished up in w. of faith and doctrine. 1 Tim 4:6
that they strive not about w. to no profit. 2 Tim 2:14
greatly withstood our w. 4:15
be mindful of the w. spoken by prophets. 2 Pet 3:2
hear the w. of this prophecy. Rev 1:3; 22:18
take away from the w. of this. 22:19

all the words

all the w. of Joseph. Gen 45:27
Moses told Aaron all the w. of the Lord. Ex 4:28
Moses told the people all the w. 24:3; Num 11:24
Moses wrote all the w. of the Lord. Ex 24:4
on the tables were written all the w. Deut 9:10
keep all the w. 17:19
write on stones all the w. 27:3, 8
that confirmeth not all the w. 26
not observe to do all the w. 28:58
may do all the w. of this law. 29:29
and observe to do all the w. 31:12
Moses spake all the w. of. 32:44
set your hearts to all the w. 46
he read all the w. of the law, the blessings and. Josh 8:34
Samuel told all the w. of the Lord. 1 Sam 8:10
Lord will hear all the w. of Rabshakeh. 2 Ki 19:4; Isa 37:17
Josiah read all the w. of the covenant. 2 Ki 23:2; 2 Chr 34:30
all the w. of my mouth. Pr 8:8
unto all the w. spoken. Eccl 7:21
bring on them all the w. Jer 11:8
speak all the w. that I command thee. 26:2
to all the w. of Jeremiah. 20
write all the w. I have spoken. 30:2; 36:2
Baruch wrote all the w. of the Lord. 36:4, 32
had ended all the w. of Lord. 43:1
speak to the people all the w. of this life. Acts 5:20

words *of God*

hath said, which heard the w. of God. Num 24:4, 16
Heman the king's seer in the w. of God. 1 Chr 25:5
every one that trembleth at the w. of God. Ezra 9:4
they rebelled against the w. of God. Ps 107:11
he whom God sent, speaketh w. of God. John 3:34
of God, heareth the w. of God. 8:47
until the w. of God be fulfilled. Rev 17:17

see **heard**

his words

they hated him yet the more for his w. Gen 37:8
thou heardest his w. out of the fire. Deut 4:36
Jephthah uttered all his w. before the Lord. Judg 11:11
he let none of his w. fall to the ground. 1 Sam 3:19
but they despised his w. 2 Chr 36:16
and lay up his w. in thine. Job 22:22
he hath not directed his w. 32:14
his w. were without wisdom. 34:35
for he multiplieth his w. against. 37
his w. softer than oil. Ps 55:21
then believed they his w. 106:12
knowledge spareth his w. Pr 17:27
seest thou a man that is hasty in his w.? 29:20
add thou not unto his w., lest. 30:6
will not call back his w. Isa 31:2
heed to any of his w. Jer 18:18
he hath confirmed his w. Dan 9:12
the land is not able to bear all his w. Amos 7:10
the disciples were astonished at his w. Mark 10:24
to catch him in his w. 12:13
Luke 20:20
not take hold of his w. Luke 20:26*
they remembered his w. 24:8

see **lord**

my words

he said, Hear now my w. Num 12:6
Job 34:2
make them hear my w. Deut 4:10
therefore lay up my w. in. 11:18
and I will put my w. in his. 18:18
whosoever will not hearken to my w. 19; Jer 29:19; 35:13
and they uttered my w. Neh 6:19
therefore my w. are swallowed up. Job 6:3
Oh that my w. were now written! 19:23
after my w. they spake not. 29:22
hearken to all my w. 33:1; 34:16
Acts 2:14
my w. shall be of the uprightness of my heart. Job 33:3; 36:4
give ear to my w. O Lord. Ps 5:1
seeing thou castest my w. 50:17
every day they wrest my w. 56:5
they shall hear my w.: for they.141:6
known my w. unto you. Pr 1:23
if thou wilt receive my w. 2:1
let thine heart retain my w. 4:4
attend to my w. 4:20
keep my w. 7:1
I have put my w. in thy mouth, and say unto Zion. Isa 51:16; Jer 1:9
my w. which I have put. Isa 59:21
I will make my w. in thy mouth fire. Jer 5:14
have not hearkened to my w. 6:19
refused to hear my w. 11:10; 13:10
will cause thee to hear my w. 18:2
they might not hear my w. 19:15
my people to hear my w. 23:22
ye have not heard my w. 25:8
bring upon that land all my w. 13
I will bring my w. on this city. 39:16
you may know my w. shall. 44:29
thou shalt speak my w. unto them Ezek 2:7; 3:4, 10
there shall none of my w. 12:28
do not my w. do good to ? Mi 2:7
my w. did they not take hold of your fathers ? Zech 1:6
whosoever shall be ashamed of me and my w. Mark 8:38; Luke 9:26
but my w. shall not pass away. Mark 13:31; Luke 21:33
thou believest not my w. Luke 1:20
shall ye believe my w.? John 5:47
if any man hear my w. and. 12:47
he that receiveth not my w. 48
will keep my w. 14:23
my w. abide in you. 15:7

their words

their w. pleased Hamor. Gen 34:18
I believed not their w. 2 Chr 9:6
through all the earth, their w. to end of the world. Ps 19:4; Rom 10:18
be not afraid of their w. Ezek 2:6
their w. seemed to them as idle tales. Luke 24:11

these words

according to these w. Gen 39:17
to the tenor of these w. 43:7
these are the w. thou shalt speak. Ex 19:6, 7
God spake all these w. 20:1
Deut 5:22
Lord said, Write thou these w. Ex 34:27; Jer 36:17
these are the w. which the Lord. Ex 35:1; Deut 6:6; 29:1
as he had made an end of speaking all these w. Num 16:31
Deut 32:45; 1 Sam 24:16
observe, hear all these w. Deut 12:28; Zech 8:9
David laid up these w. 1 Sam 21:12
his servants with these w. 24:7

to all *these w.*, and this vision, so did. *2 Sam* 7:17; *1 Chr* 17:15
thy master and to thee to speak *these w.*? *2 Ki* 18:27; *Isa* 36:12
the man of God proclaimed *these w.* *2 Ki* 23:16
go proclaim *these w.* *Jer* 3:12
speak all *these w.* unto. 7:27; 26:15
all *these w.* 16:10
ye will not hear *these w.* 22:5
prophesy thou all *these w.* 25:30
Let no man know of *these w.* 38:24
when he had written *these w.* 45:1
51:60
thou shalt read all *these w.* 51:61
these are the *w.* I spake. *Luke* 24:44
these w. spake his parents, because they feared Jews. *John* 9:22
these are not *w.* of him that. 10:21*
hear *these w.*; Jesus of. *Acts* 2:22
while Peter yet spake *these w.* 10:44
besought *these w.* might be preached to them. 13:42
when he had said *these w.* 28:29
comfort one another with *these w.* *1 Thes* 4:18
for *these w.* are true. *Rev* 21:5

thy **words**

shall receive of *thy w.* *Deut* 33:3
will not hearken to *thy w.* *Josh* 1:18
do not according to *thy w.* *Judg* 11:10
Manoah said, Now let *thy w.* 13:12
transgressed *thy w.* *1 Sam* 15:24
hearkened to *thy w.* 28:21
thy w.' sake hast thou done all these great things. *2 Sam* 7:21
that God, and *thy w.* be true. 28
in and confirm *thy w.* *1 Ki* 1:14
hast performed *thy w.* *Neh* 9:8
thy w. upheld him that was falling. *Job* 4:4
said I would keep *thy w.* *Ps* 119:57
how sweet are *thy w.* to my! 103
entrance of *thy w.* giveth light. 130
enemies have forgotten *thy w.* 139
shalt lose *thy* sweet *w.* *Pr* 23:8
despise the wisdom of *thy w.* 9
therefore let *thy w.* be few. *Eccl* 5:2
thy w. were found, and I did eat them. *Jer* 15:16
hear *thy w.* but do them not. *Ezek* 33:31, 32
the first day *thy w.* were heard, and I am come for *thy w.* *Dan* 10:12
for by *thy w.* thou shalt be justified, and by *thy w.* thou. *Mat* 12:37

your **words**

that *your w.* be proved. *Gen* 42:16
bring Benjamin, so shall *your w.* 20
let it be according unto *your w.* 44:10; *Josh* 2:21
the voice of *your w.* *Deut* 1:34; 5:28
I waited for *your w.*; I gave ear. *Job* 32:11
that heareth *your w.* *Isa* 41:26
to God according to *your w.* *Jer* 42:4
multiplied *your w.* against me. *Ezek* 35:13
ye have wearied the Lord with *your w.* *Mal* 2:17
your w. have been stout. 3:13
you nor hear *your w.* *Mat* 10:14

work

Is taken, [1] *For such business as is proper to every man's calling, which may be done in six days.* Ex 20:9, Six days shalt thou labour and do all thy *work.* [2] *For any thought, word, or outward action, whether good or evil,* Eccl 12:14, God shall bring every *work* into judgement. [3] Work *is put for miracle,* John 7:21.

The *works* of God, denote, [1] *His* work *of creation.* [2] *His* works *of providence in preserving and governing the world.* [3] *His* work *of redemption, and particularly the faith of true believers is called* the work of God.

By good works *are to be understood all manner of duties inward and outward, thoughts as well as words and actions, toward God or man, which are commanded in the law of God, and proceed from a pure heart and faith unfeigned.*

let there more *w.* be laid on the men. *Ex* 5:9
no manner of *w.* shall be done. 12:16; 20:10; *Lev* 16:29; 23:3, 28, 31; *Num* 29:7
shew them *w.* that they. *Ex* 18:20
whoso doeth any *w.* therein shall be cut off. 31:14, 15; *Lev* 23:30
six days shall *w.* be. *Ex* 35:2; 20:9
sufficient for all the *w.* and. 36:7
convocation, ye shall do no servile *w.* *Lev* 23:7, 8, 21, 25, 35, 36; *Num* 28:18, 25, 26; 29:1, 12, 35
the *w.* of men's hands. *Deut* 4:28; 27:15; *2 Ki* 19:18; *2 Chr* 32:19; *Ps* 115:4; 135:15
in it thou shalt not do any *w.* *Deut* 5:14; 16:8; *Jer* 17:22, 24
that the Lord may bless thee in all *w.* *Deut* 14:29; 24:19; 28:12; 30:9
do no *w.* with the firstling of. 15:19
anger through the *w.* of your hands. 31:29; *1 Ki* 16:7; *Jer* 32:30
bless the Lord and accept *w.* 33:11
officers which were over the *w.* *1 Ki* 5:16; 9:23; *1 Chr* 29:6; *2 Chr* 2:18
another court of the like *w.* *1 Ki* 7:8
into the hands of them that did the *w.* *2 Ki* 12:11; 22:5*, 9
employed in that *w.* day. *1 Chr* 9:33
to minister as every day's *w.* 16:37
Solomon young, and the *w.* is great. 29:1; *Neh* 4:19
every *w.* that he began. *2 Chr* 31:21
the men did the *w.* faithfully. 34:12
then ceased the *w.* of. *Ezra* 4:24
this *w.* goeth fast on, prospereth. 5:8
let the *w.* of this house of God. 6:7
hands in the *w.* of house of God. 22
neither is it a *w.* of one day. 10:13
put not their necks to *w.* *Neh* 3:5
slay them, and cause the *w.* 4:11
why should the *w.* cease whilst? 6:3
they perceived this *w.* was. 16
fathers gave to the *w.* 7:70
thou hast blessed the *w.* *Job* 1:10
thou shouldest despise the *w.* 10:3
thou wilt have a desire to *w.* 14:15
go they forth to their *w.* 24:5
for the *w.* of a man shall he render unto him. 34:11; *1 Pet* 1:17
are all the *w.* of his hands. *Job* 34:19
he sheweth them their *w.* and. 36:9
when I consider the *w.* of thy fingers. *Ps* 8:3, 6
the wicked is snared in the *w.* 9:16
firmament sheweth his handy *w.* 19:1
after the *w.* of their hands. 28:4
we heard what *w.* thou didst. 44:1
establish thou the *w.* of our. 90:17
proved me and saw my *w.* 95:9
I hate the *w.* of them that. 101:3
the heavens are the *w.* of thy. 102:25
on the *w.* of thy hands. 143:5
worketh a deceitful *w.* *Pr* 11:18
time there for every *w.* *Eccl* 3:17
why should God destroy the *w.*? 5:6
I applied my heart to every *w.* 8:9
according to *w.* of the wicked, according to the *w.* of the. 14
there is no *w.* in the grave. 9:10
God will bring every *w.* into. 12:14
w. of the hands of a cunning workman. *S of S* 7:1
they worship the *w.* of their own hands. *Isa* 2:8; 37:19; *Jer* 1:16; 10:3, 9, 15; 51:18
he shall not look to the *w.* *Isa* 17:8
neither shall there be any *w.* 19:15
blessed be Assyria the *w.* of. 25
do his *w.*, his strange *w.* 28:21
shall the *w.* say of him that? 29:16*
he seeth his children, and the *w.* 23
the *w.* of righteousness shall. 32:17
concerning the *w.* of my hands command me. 45:11
my *w.* is with my God. 49:4*
they shall inherit the *w* of my. 60:21
will direct their *w.* in truth. 61:8*
all are the *w.* of thy hands. *Isa* 64:8
mine elect shall long enjoy *w.* 65:22
great in counsel and mighty in *w.* *Jer* 32:19
recompense her according to her *w.* 50:29; *Lam* 3:64
be taken to do any *w.*? *Ezek* 15:3
is it meet for any *w.*? 4
it was meet for no *w.* 5
w. of an imperious whorish. 16:30
w. of the craftsman. *Hos* 13:2
we will say no more to the *w.* 14:3
shalt no more worship *w.* *Mi* 5:13
for I will work a *w.* in. *Hab* 1:5
and so is every *w.* of. *Hag* 2:14
there do no mighty *w.* *Mark* 6:5
I have done one *w.* and. *John* 7:21
finished the *w.* thou gavest me. 17:4
if this *w.* be of men it will. *Acts* 5:38
for the *w.* whereunto I have. 13:2
wonder, for I work a *w.* in your days, a *w.* which ye will not believe. 41
the *w.* which they fulfilled. 14:26
not with them to the *w.* 15:38
which shew *w.* of the law. *Rom* 2:15
a short *w.* will the Lord make. 9:28
otherwise *w.* is no more *w.* 11:6*
every man's *w.* shall be. *1 Cor* 3:13
if any man's *w.* abide. 14
if *w.* be burnt. 15
are not ye my *w.* in the Lord? 9:1
he gave some for the *w.* *Eph* 4:12
for the *w.* of Christ he. *Phil* 2:30
that God may fulfil the *w.* of faith. *2 Thes* 1:11
every good word and *w.* 2:17
do the *w.* of an evangelist. *2 Tim* 4:5
patience have her perfect *w.* *Jas* 1:4
but a doer of the *w.* shall be. 25
see **evil, needle**

work, *verb*

go and *w.* *Ex* 5:18
six days thou shalt *w.* 34:21
whoso doeth *w.* therein shall. 35:2
they did *w.* wilily and went. *Josh* 9:4
the Lord will *w.* for us. *1 Sam* 14:6
sold thyself to *w.* evil. *1 Ki* 21:20, 25
people had a mind to *w.* *Neh* 4:6
left hand, where he doth *w.* *Job* 23:9
in heart ye *w.* wickedness. *Ps* 58:2
time for thee, Lord, to *w.* 119:126
w. a deceitful work. *Pr* 11:18
they that *w.* in flax, shall. *Isa* 19:9
I will *w.* and who shall let it? 43:13
ye *w.* abomination and. *Ezek* 33:26
he shall *w.* deceitfully. *Dan* 11:23
woe to them that *w.* evil. *Mi* 2:1
I will *w.* a work in your days, which. *Hab* 1:5; *Acts* 13:41
w. for I am with you. *Hag* 2:4
they that *w.* wickedness. *Mal* 3:15
son, go *w.* to-day in. *Mat* 21:28
six days in which men ought to *w.* *Luke* 13:14
my Father worketh hitherto, and I *w.* *John* 5:17
that we might *w.* the works? 6:28
What dost thou *w.*? 30
w. the works of him that sent me ... cometh when no man can *w.* 9:4
sin by the law did *w.* in. *Rom* 7:5
we know that all things *w.* 8:28
to *w.* all uncleanness. *Eph* 4:19
w. out your own salvation. *Phil* 2:12
study to *w.* with your own hands. *1 Thes* 4:11
of iniquity doth *w.* *2 Thes* 2:7
if any would not *w.*, neither. 3:10
that with quietness they *w.* 12
see **iniquity**

work *of God,* **works** *of God*

tables were the *w. of God.* *Ex* 32:16
wondrous *w. of God.* *Job* 37:14
declare the *w. of God.* *Ps* 64:9
come and see the *w. of God.* 66:5
not forget the *w. of God.* 78:7
consider the *w. of God.* *Eccl* 7:13
beheld all the *w. of God.* 8:17
knowest not the *w. of God.* 11:5
work the *w. of God.* *John* 6:28
this is the *w. of God* that ye. 29
the *w. of God* should be made manifest in him. 9:3

speak the *w. of God.* Acts 2:11
destroy not *w. of God.* Rom 14:20
see **good, great**

his **work**

God ended *his w.* Gen 2:2
rested from *his w.* 3
every man from *his w.* Ex 36:4
he is the rock, *his w.* Deut 32:4
an old man came from *his w.* at even. Judg 19:16
asses and put to *his w.* 1 Sam 8:16
and wrought all *his w.* 1 Ki 7:14
with the king for *his w.* 1 Chr 4:23
of Israel he made no servants for *his w.* 2 Chr 8:9
Baasha let *his w.* cease, he. 16:5
every man to *his w.* Neh 4:15
for the reward of *his w.* Job 7:2*
that thou magnify *his w.* 36:24
that all men may know *his w.* 37:7
renderest to every man according to *his w.* Ps 62:12; Pr 24:29
man goeth forth to *his w.* Ps 104:23
his w. is honourable and. 111:3
all the weights of the bag are *his w.* Pr 16:11
whether *his w.* be pure or. 20:11
but as for the pure *his w.* is. 21:8
let him hasten *his w.* that. Isa 5:19
performed *his* whole *w.* 10:12
may do *his w., his* strange *w.* 28:21
behold, *his w.* is before him. 40:10* 62:11*
an instrument for *his w.* 54:16
giveth him not for *his w.* Jer 22:13*
the maker of *his w.* Hab 2:18
to every man *his w.* Mark 13:34
my meat is to finish *his w.* John 4:34
every man prove *his* own *w.* Gal 6:4
give every man as *his w.* Rev 22:12
see **Lord**

our **work**

this shall comfort us concerning *our w.* Gen 5:29

thy **work**

six days do all *thy w.* Ex 20:9 23:12; Deut 5:13
Lord recompense *thy w.* Ruth 2:12
meditate also of all *thy w.* Ps 77:12
let *thy w.* appear unto thy. 90:16
made me glad through *thy w.* 92:4
prepare *thy w.* without. Pr 24:27
or *thy w.,* He hath no hands? Isa 45:9
for *thy w.* shall be rewarded, saith the Lord. Jer 31:16
revive *thy w.* in the midst. Hab 3:2

your **work**

not aught of *your w.* Ex 5:11
for *your w.* shall be rewarded. 2 Chr 15:7
ye are of nothing, *your w.* is of nought. Isa 41:24
remembering *your w.* of faith, and labour of love. 1 Thes 1:3
God is not unrighteous to forget *your w.* Heb 6:10

worker

was a *w.* in brass. 1 Ki 7:14

workers

w. with familiar spirits. 2 Ki 23:24
we then as *w.* together. 2 Cor 6:1
false apostles, deceitful *w.* 11:13
beware of evil *w.* Phil 3:2
see **iniquity**

worketh

lo, all these things *w.* God. Job 33:29
he that walketh uprightly, and *w.* righteousness. Ps 15:2
he that *w.* deceit shall not. 101:7
w. a deceitful work. Pr 11:18*
a flattering mouth *w.* ruin. 26:28
w. willingly with her hands. 31:13
what profit hath he that *w.*? Eccl 3:9
the smith with his tongs *w.* in the coals, and he *w.* it. Isa 44:12
thou meetest him that *w.* 64:5
he *w.* signs and wonders. Dan 6:27
my Father *w.* hitherto. John 5:17
he that *w.* righteousness. Acts 10:35
glory and peace to every one that *w.* good. Rom 2:10
to him that *w.* is the reward. Rom 4:4
to him that *w.* not, but believeth. 5
because the law *w.* wrath, for. 15
knowing that tribulation *w.* 5:3
love *w.* no ill to his neighbour. 13:10
God that *w.* all in all. 1 Cor 12:6
all these *w.* that one and the. 11
for he *w.* the work of the. 16:10
so then death *w.* in us. 2 Cor 4:12
w. for us a more exceeding. 17
w. repentance to salvation, but the sorrow of the world *w.* death. 7:10
w. miracles among you. Gal 3:5
but faith, which *w.* by love. 5:6
who *w.* all things after. Eph 1:11
the spirit that now *w.* in the. 2:2
the power that *w.* in us. 3:20
for it is God that *w.* in you. Phil 2:13
his working, which *w.* in. Col 1:29
effectually *w.* in you. 1 Thes 2:13
of your faith *w.* patience. Jas 1:3
the wrath of man *w.* not. 20
nor whatsoever *w.* abomination. Rev 21:27

workfellow

Timothy my *w.* saluteth. Rom 16:21*

working

like a sharp razor, *w.* Ps 52:2
w. salvation in the midst of. 74:12
who is excellent in *w.* Isa 28:29*
be shut the six *w.* days. Ezek 46:1
the Lord *w.* with them. Mark 16:20
men with men *w.* that. Rom 1:27
sin *w.* death in me by that. 7:13
and labour, *w.* with our. 1 Cor 4:12
not we power to forbear *w.*? 9:6
to another the *w.* of miracles. 12:10
according to the *w.* of. Eph 1:19
given me by the effectual *w.* 3:7
according to the effectual *w.* 4:16
w. with his hands the. 28
according to the *w.* whereby he is able. Phil 3:21
his *w.* which worketh in. Col 1:29
is after the *w.* of Satan. 2 Thes 2:9
w. not at all, but are. 3:11
w. in you that which is. Heb 13:21
spirits of devils *w.* miracles. Rev 16:14

workman

wisdom to work all manner of work of the cunning *w.* Ex 35:35; 38:23
the work of a cunning *w.* S of S 7:1
the *w.* melteth a graven. Isa 40:19
he seeketh to him a cunning *w.* 20
work of the *w.* with the axe. Jer 10:3
the *w.* made it therefore. Hos 8:6
w. is worthy of his meat. Mat 10:10*
a *w.* that needeth not be. 2 Tim 2:15

workmanship

and in all manner of *w.* Ex 31:3, 5 35:31
to all the *w.* thereof. 2 Ki 16:10
the *w.* of tabrets was. Ezek 28:13
for we are his *w.* created in Christ Jesus. Eph 2:10

workmen

they gave that to the *w.* to repair. 2 Ki 12:14, 15; 2 Chr 34:10, 17
there are *w.* with thee. 1 Chr 22:15
number of *w.* 25:1
w. wrought. 2 Chr 24:13
to set forward the *w.* in. Ezra 3:9
the *w.*, they are of men. Isa 44:11
called with the *w.* of like occupation. Acts 19:25

works

fulfil your *w.* and your. Ex 5:13
the Lord hath sent me to do all these *w.* Num 16:28
the Lord blessed thee in all the *w.* Deut 2:7; 16:15
which knew not the *w.* Judg 2:10
according to all the *w.* they have done. 1 Sam 8:8
w. the man of God did. 1 Ki 13:11
me to anger with all the *w.* of their hands. 2 Ki 22:17; 2 Chr 34:25
from their wicked *w.* Neh 9:35
have done abominable *w.* Ps 14:1
concerning the *w.* of men, by the word of thy lips. 17:4
I will triumph in the *w.* of. 92:4
the *w.* of the Lord are great. Ps 111:2
the *w.* of his hands are verity. 7
forsake not the *w.* of. 138:8
to practise wicked *w.* with. 141:4
let her own *w.* praise her. Pr 31:31
I have seen the *w.* Eccl 1:14; 2:11
wrought all our *w.* in us. Isa 26:12
have done all these *w.* Jer 7:13
to anger with the *w.* of your hands to. 25:6, 7; 44:8
according to their deeds and the *w.* 25:14; Rev 2:23
w. may be abolished. Ezek 6:6
honour him whose *w.* Dan 4:37
the *w.* of the house of. Mi 6:16
John heard in prison the *w.* Mat 11:2
shew him greater *w.* John 5:20
the *w.* which the Father hath given me, the same *w.* that I do. 36
thy disciples may see the *w.* 7:3
because I testify that the *w.* 7
if children, ye would do the *w.* 8:39
I must work the *w.* of him. 9:4
w. that I do in my Father's. 10:25
of these *w.* do ye stone me? 32
if I do not the *w.* 37
believe the *w.* 38
he doeth the *w.* 14:10
believe me for the very *w.*' 11
the *w.* that I do, shall he do; . . . *w.* 12
not done among them the *w.* 15:24
they rejoiced in the *w.* Acts 7:41
Gentiles should do *w.* meet. 26:20
by what law? of *w.*? Rom 3:27
if Abraham were justified by *w.* 4:2
imputeth righteousness without *w.* 6
not of *w.* but of him that. 9:11
but as it were by the *w.* of. 32
is it no more of *w.*: . . . but if it be of *w.*, is it no more of grace. 11:6
let us therefore cast off the *w.* 13:12
is not justified by the *w.* of the law, for by the *w.* of the law. Gal 2:16
Spirit by the *w.* of the law? 3:2
doeth he it by the *w.* of the law? 5
as many as are of *w.* of the law. 10
the *w.* of the flesh are manifest. 5:19
not of *w.* lest any man. Eph 2:9
unfruitful *w.* of darkness. 5:11
in your mind by wicked *w.* Col 1:21
to esteem them in love for their *w.*'s sake. 1 Thes 5:13
saved us, not according to our *w.* 2 Tim 1:9; Tit 3:5
but in *w.* they deny God. Tit 1:16
the heavens are the *w.* Heb 1:10
thou didst set him over the *w.* 2:7
your fathers . . . saw my *w.* forty. 3:9
although the *w.* were finished. 4:3
of repentance from dead *w.* 6:1
purge conscience from dead *w.* 9:14
if he have not *w.* can? Jas 2:14
faith without *w.* is dead. 17, 20, 26
w.: shew me thy faith without *w.* 18
Abraham justified by *w.*? 2:21
by *w.* was faith made perfect. 22
ye see then that by *w.* a man. 24
was not the harlot justified by *w.*? 25
the earth and the *w.* 2 Pet 3:10
that he might destroy *w.* 1 John 3:8
keepeth my *w.* to the end. Rev 2:26
yet repented not of the *w.* of. 9:20
double according to her *w.* 18:6
see **evil, good, work** *of God*

his **works**

his w. have been to thee very good. 1 Sam 19:4
Hezekiah prospered in all *his w.* 2 Chr 32:30
and all *his w.* are done. Ps 33:4
forgat *his w.* and his wonders. 78:11; 106:13
bless the Lord, all *his w.* 103:22
Lord shall rejoice in *his w.* 104:31
let them declare *his w.* with. 107:22
people the power of *his w.* 111:6
mercies are over all *his w.* 145:9
the Lord is holy in all *his w.* 17
possessed me before *his w.* Pr 8:22
to every man according to *his w.*? 24:12; Mat 16:27; 2 Tim 4:14
rejoice in *his* own *w.* Eccl 3:22
righteous in all *his w.* Dan 9:14

to God are all *his w.* *Acts* 15:18
seventh day from all *his w.* *Heb* 4:4
ceased from *his* own *w.*? 10
faith wrought with *his w.*? *Jas* 2:22
of a good conversation *his w.* 3:13
see **Lord, marvellous, mighty**

their **works**

let the people from *their w.*? *Ex* 5:4
shalt not do after *their w.* 23:24
according to these *their w.* *Neh* 6:14
he knoweth *their w.* *Job* 34:25
considereth all *their w.* *Ps* 33:15
and they learned *their w.* 106:35
defiled with *their* own *w.* 39
and *their w.* are in the hand of God. *Eccl* 9:1
their w. are in the dark. *Isa* 29:15
they are vanity, *their w.* 41:29
nor shall they cover themselves with *their w.*: *their w.* are works. 59:6
their w. and their thoughts. 66:18
forget any of *their w.* *Amos* 8:7
God saw *their w.* that. *Jonah* 3:10
not ye after *their w.* *Mat* 23:3
all *their w.* they do to be seen. 5
be according to *their w.* *2 Cor* 11:15
and *their w.* do follow. *Rev* 14:13
the dead judged according to *their w.* 20:12, 13

thy **works**

according to *thy w.*? *Deut* 3:24
bless thee in all *thy w.* 15:10
Lord hath broken *thy w.* *2 Chr* 20:37
tell of all *thy* wondrous *w.* *Ps* 26:7
145:4
How terrible art thou in *thy w.*! 66:3
that I may declare all *thy w.* 73:28
nor any works like unto *thy w.* 86:8
O Lord, how great are *thy w.*! 92:5
satisfied with fruit of *thy w.* 104:13
how manifold are *thy w.*! 24
I meditate on all *thy w.* 143:5
all *thy w.* shall praise thee. 145:10
commit *thy w.* unto the. *Pr* 16:3
now God accepteth *thy w.* *Eccl* 9:7
I will declare *thy w.* *Isa* 57:12
hast trusted in *thy w.* *Jer* 48:7
faith without *thy w.* *Jas* 2:18
I know *thy w.* *Rev* 2:2, 9, 13, 19
3:1, 8, 15
I have not found *thy w.* perfect. 3:2

wonderful **works**

Lord, are thy *wonderful w.* *Ps* 40:5
his *wonderful w.* that he. 78:4
Lord for his *wonderful w.* to the children of men! 107:8, 15, 21, 31
made his *wonderful w.* to be. 111:4
in thy name have done many *wonderful w.* *Mat* 7:22
do hear them speak in our tongues the *wonderful w.* of. *Acts* 2:11
see **wondrous**

world

To the Eastern people of earliest times the world *was very small, including little except Mesopotamia, Canaan, Arabia, and parts of Egypt. During Old Testament times it remained much the same, extending a little to the East, as the nations there grew to power; and other parts of Asia and Africa became somewhat known to the adventurous. Few knew more than rumours of Italy and even Greece. In the time of Christ* the world *really meant the Roman Empire, with parts of Asia and Africa which were more or less under its sway. All outside of this was vague. In Bible language* world *is frequently used for the inhabitants of the world, and, in the New Testament, of mortal existence in distinction from spiritual life.*

The Revised Versions often substitute the word earth.

he hath set the *w.* *1 Sam* 2:8
the foundations of the *w.* were discovered. *2 Sam* 22:16; *Ps* 18:15
the *w.* also shall not. *1 Chr* 16:30
chased out of the *w.* *Job* 18:18
disposed the whole *w.*? *Job* 34:13
do on the face of the *w.* 37:12
he shall judge the *w.* in righteousness. *Ps* 9:8; 96:13; 98:9
soul from the men of the *w.* 17:14
their words to end of the *w.* 19:4
Rom 10:18
all the ends of the *w.* *Ps* 22:27
the earth and the *w.* is the Lord's. 24:1; 98:7; *Nah* 1:5
let the inhabitants of the *w.* *Ps* 33:8
all ye inhabitants of the *w.* 49:1
for the *w.* is mine. 50:12
the lightnings lightened the *w.* 77:18
97:4
thou hast founded the *w.* 89:11
formed the earth and the *w.* 90:2
the *w.* also is established, it. 93:1
w. also shall be established. 96:10
not made the dust of the *w.* *Pr* 8:26
also he hath set the *w.* *Eccl* 3:11†
I will punish the *w.* for. *Isa* 13:11
is this he that made the *w.*? 14:17
the face of the *w.* with cities. 21
w. languisheth and fadeth. 24:4
the face of the *w.* with fruit. 27:6
let the *w.* hear, and all that. 34:1
ye shall not be confounded, *w.* 45:17
the devil sheweth him all the kingdoms of *w.* *Mat* 4:8; *Luke* 4:5
ye are the light of the *w.* *Mat* 5:14
the field is the *w.*; good seed. 13:38
it be in the end of this *w.* 40, 49
gain the whole *w.* and lose his own? 16:26; *Mark* 8:36; *Luke* 9:25
woe to the *w.* because of. *Mat* 18:7
gospel of kingdom shall be preached in all the *w.* 24:14; *Mark* 14:9
which have been since the *w.* began. *Luke* 1:70†; *Acts* 3:21†
a decree that all the *w.* *Luke* 2:1
worthy to obtain that *w.* 20:35
in the *w.*, the *w.* was made by him, and *w.* *John* 1:10; *Acts* 17:24
taketh away the sin of *w.* *John* 1:29
God so loved the *w.* that he. 3:16
that the *w.* through him might. 17
Christ, the Saviour of the *w.* 4:42; *1 John* 4:14
that giveth life unto the *w.* *John* 6:33
I give for the life of the *w.* 51
things, shew thyself to the *w.* 7:4
the *w.* cannot hate you, but me. 7
I am the light of the *w.* 8:12; 9:5
the *w.* is gone after him. 12:19
not to judge, but to save the *w.* 47
the Spirit, whom the *w.* 14:17
a little while and the *w.* seeth. 19
thou wilt manifest thyself unto us and not unto the *w.*? 22
I give, not as the *w.* giveth. 27
that the *w.* may know I love. 14:31
if *w.* hate you. 15:18; *1 John* 3:13
if ye were of the *w.*, the *w.* *John* 15:19
but the *w.* shall rejoice. 16:20
the *w.* and go to the Father. 28
I have overcome the *w.* 33
with thee before the *w.* was. 17:5
men thou gavest me out of the *w.* 6
I pray not for the *w.* but for them. 9
w. hated them, because they are not of the *w.* 14
not take them out of the *w.* 15
the *w.*, even as I am not of *w.* 16
that the *w.* may believe thou. 21, 23
O Father, the *w.* hath not known. 25
I spake openly to the *w.* 18:20
suppose *w.* could not contain. 21:25
turned the *w.* upside down. *Acts* 17:6
Diana, whom Asia and the *w.* worshippeth. 19:27
a mover of sedition among all the Jews throughout the *w.* 24:5
your faith is spoken of through the whole *w.* *Rom* 1:8
how shall God judge the *w.*? 3:6
that all the *w.* may become guilty. 19
should be heir of the *w.* 4:13
of them be the riches of the *w.* 11:12
of them be the reconciling of *w.* 15
the *w.* by wisdom knew. *1 Cor* 1:21
God ordained before the *w.* 2:7
received not the spirit of the *w.* 12
or the *w.*, or life, or death. 3:22
are made a spectacle to *w.* *1 Cor* 4:9
we are made as the filth of *w.* 13
must ye needs go out of the *w.* 5:10
saints shall judge the *w.*? 6:2
things that are in the *w.* 7:33, 34
I will eat no flesh while the *w.* 8:13*
not be condemned with the *w.* 11:32
God reconciling the *w.* *2 Cor* 5:19
Jesus, by whom the *w.* is crucified to me, and I to the *w.* *Gal* 6:14
in Christ before the *w.* began. *2 Tim* 1:9*; *Tit* 1:2*
subjection the *w.* to come. *Heb* 2:5
have tasted the powers of the *w.* 6:5*
the *w.* was not worthy. 11:38
unspotted from the *w.* *Jas* 1:27
the tongue is a fire, a *w.* of. 3:6
the friendship of the *w.* is enmity with God? A friend of the *w.* is. 4:4
spared not the old *w.*, bringing in the flood upon the *w.* *2 Pet* 2:5
whereby the *w.* that then was. 3:6
propitiation for sins of *w.* *1 John* 2:2
love not the *w.* 15
but is of the *w.* 16
the *w.* passeth away, and the. 17
the *w.* knoweth us not, because. 3:1
w.: therefore speak they of the *w.* 4:5
of God, overcometh the *w.* 5:4, 5
we are of God, and whole *w.* lieth. 19
shall come upon all the *w.* *Rev* 3:10
deceiveth the whole *w.* 12:9
and all the *w.* wondered after. 13:3
see **foundation**

in, or *into the* **world**

who prosper *in the w.* *Ps* 73:12*
preached *in the* whole *w.* *Mat* 26:13
hundred-fold, and *in the w.* to come eternal. *Mark* 10:30; *Luke* 18:30
lighteth every man that cometh *into the w.* *John* 1:9
he was *in the w.* and the world. 10
God sent not his Son *into the w.* to condemn the world. 3:17
light is come *into the w.* and men. 19
prophet that should come *into the w.* 6:14; 11:27
in the w., I am the light of world. 9:5
I am come a light *into the w.* 12:46
in w. ye shall have tribulation. 16:33
I am no more *in the w.*, but these are *in the w.* 17:11
while I was with them *in the w.* 12
cause came I *into the w.* 18:37
as by one man sin entered *into the w.* *Rom* 5:12
until the law, sin was *in the w.* 13
an idol is nothing *in the w.* *1 Cor* 8:4
having no hope, without God *in the w.* *Eph* 2:12
gospel is come to you as it is *in* all *the w.* *Col* 1:6
Christ Jesus came *into the w.* to save sinners. *1 Tim* 1:15
and believed on *in the w.* 3:16
he cometh *into the w.* *Heb* 10:5
afflictions that are *in the w.* *1 Pet* 5:9
things that are *in the w.* *1 John* 2:15
false prophets are gone out *into the w.* 4:1
even now already is it *in the w.* 3
greater than he that is *in the w.* 4
Son *into the w.* that we might live. 9
many deceivers are entered *into the w.* *2 John* 7

this **world**

forgiven him in *this w.* *Mat* 12:32
the care of *this w.* choke the word. 13:22; *Mark* 4:19
for the children of *this w.* are wiser than. *Luke* 16:8
The children of *this w.* marry. 20:34
ye are of *this w.*; I am not of *this w.* *John* 8:23
I am come into *this w.* 9:39
he that hateth life in *this w.* 12:25
is the judgement of *this w.*; now shall the prince of *this w.* be cast. 31
he should depart out of *this w* 13:1
for prince of *this w.* cometh. 14:30
because the prince of *this w.* 16:11
My kingdom is not of *this w.*: if my kingdom were of *this w.* 18:36

be not conformed to this w.: but be ye. Rom 12:2
of this w.? hath not God made foolish the wisdom of this w.? 1 Cor 1:20
not the wisdom of this w. 2:6
seemeth to be wise in this w. 3:18
wisdom of this w. is foolishness. 19
the fornicators of this w. 5:10
they that use this w. as not. 7:31
the god of this w. hath blinded the minds. 2 Cor 4:4
he might deliver us from this present evil w. Gal 1:4
not only in this w., but in. Eph 1:21
to the course of this w. 2:2
the rulers of the darkness of this w. 6:12
nothing into this w. 1 Tim 6:7
that are rich in this w. 17
loved this present w. 2 Tim 4:10
godly in this present w. Tit 2:12
chosen the poor of this w. Jas 2:5
but whoso hath this w.'s. 1 John 3:17
is, so are we in this w. 4:17

worldly

denying ungodliness and w. Tit 2:12
the first covenant had a w. Heb 9:1

worlds

by whom also he made the w. Heb 1:2
the w. were framed by the. 11:3

worm

was there any w. therein. Ex 16:24
I have said to the w., Thou. Job 17:14
the w. shall feed sweetly on. 24:20
much less man that is a w. 25:6
but I am a w. and no man. Ps 22:6
the w. is spread under. Isa 14:11
fear not, thou w. Jacob, and. 41:14
w. shall eat them like wool. 51:8
for their w. shall not die, nor their fire. 66:24; Mark 9:44, 46, 48
God prepared a w., it smote the gourd. Jonah 4:7

worms

their manna bred w. Ex 16:20
grapes, for the w. shall. Deut 28:39
my flesh is clothed with w. Job 7:5
though w. destroy this body. 19:26
they shall lie down, and w. 21:26
worm under thee, and the w. cover. Isa 14:11
out of their holes like w. Mi 7:17
Herod was eaten of w. Acts 12:23

wormwood

a root that beareth w. Deut 29:18
her end is bitter as w., sharp as a sword. Pr 5:4
I will feed them with w. Jer 9:15
23:15
made me drunken with w. Lam 3:15
remembering my misery, the w. 19
who turn judgement to w. Amos 5:7
star is called w. and the third part of the waters became w. Rev 8:11

worse

we will deal w. with thee. Gen 19:9
be w. than all that befell. 2 Sam 19:7
Omri did w. than all. 1 Ki 16:25*
Judah was put to the w. before. 2 Ki 14:12; 2 Chr 25:22
the Syrians were put to the w. 1 Chr 19:16, 19
people be put to the w. 2 Chr 6:24*
Manasseh made Jerusalem do w. 33:9*
they did w. than their fathers. Jer 7:26; 16:12
see your faces w. liking? Dan 1:10
the rent is made w. Mat 9:16
Mark 2:21
the last state of that man is w. than first. Mat 12:45; Luke 11:26
last error shall be w. Mat 27:64
bettered, but grew w. Mark 5:26
then that which is w. John 2:10
sin no more, lest a w. thing. 5:14
eat not, are we the w. 1 Cor 8:8
for the better, but for the w. 11:17
denied the faith, and is w. 1 Tim 5:8
shall wax w. and w. 2 Tim 3:13
the latter end is w. 2 Pet 2:20

worship

lad will go yonder and w. Gen 22:5
to Lord, and w. ye afar off. Ex 24:1
for thou shalt w. no other god. 34:14
be driven to w. them. Deut 4:19
if thou w. other gods. 8:19; 11:16
30:17
before Lord, and w. before the Lord. 26:10; Ps 22:27, 29; 86:9
man went up early to w. 1 Sam 1:3
turn again, that I may w. 15:25, 30
the people went to w. 1 Ki 12:30
to w. in house of Rimmon. 2 Ki 5:18
ye fear, and him shall ye w. 17:36*
hath said to Judah, Ye shall w. 18:22
2 Chr 32:12; Isa 36:7
w. the Lord in the beauty of holiness. 1 Chr 16:29; Ps 29:2; 66:4; 96:9
Mat 4:10; Luke 4:8
I will w. toward thy holy temple. Ps 5:7; 138:2
he is thy Lord, and w. thou. 45:11
neither shalt thou w. any. 81:9
O come let us w. and bow. 95:6
w. him, all ye gods. 97:7
w. at his footstool, for. 99:5; 132:7
exalt the Lord, and w. at his. 99:9
they w. the work of their hands. Isa 2:8, 20; 46:6
w. the Lord in the holy mount. 27:13
princes also shall w. because. 49:7
all flesh shall come to w. 66:23
that enter in at these gates to w. Jer 7:2; 26:2
they that w. other gods, be. 13:10
go not after other gods to w. 25:6
we w. her without our men? 44:19
he shall w. at threshold. Ezek 46:2
the people of the land shall w. 3
he that entereth to w. by the. 9
w. the golden image. Dan 3:5, 10, 15
not w. the image. 12, 18, 28
do not ye w. the golden image? 3:14
if ye w. 15
no more w. the work of. Mi 5:13
them that w. the host. Zeph 1:5
men shall w. him, every one. 2:11
to w. the King the Lord of hosts. Zech 14:16, 17
star, and come to w. him. Mat 2:2
that I may come and w. him also. 8
if thou wilt fall down and w. me. 4:9; Luke 4:7
in vain do they w. me. Mat 15:9
Mark 7:7
Jerusalem is the place where men ought to w. John 4:20
ye w. ye know not what: we know what we w.: for salvation. 4:22
they shall w. the Father in. 23, 24
certain Greeks came up to w. 12:20
God gave up to w. Acts 7:42*, 43
came to Jerusalem to w. 8:27
whom ye ignorantly w. 17:23
persuaded men to w. God. 18:13
to Jerusalem to w. God. 24:11
they call heresy, so w. I the. 14*
down, he will w. God. 1 Cor 14:25
which w. God in spirit. Phil 3:3
the angels of God w. him. Heb 1:6
make them come and w. Rev 3:9
and w. him that liveth for ever. 4:10
that they should not w. devils. 9:20
of God, and them w. therein. 11:1
all on the earth shall w. 13:8, 12
they that would not w. the image. 15
w. him that made heaven, earth. 14:7
if any man w. the beast and. 9
who w. the beast, have no rest. 11
all nations shall come and w. 15:4
I fell at his feet to w. 19:10; 22:8
w. God. 22:9

worshipped

Abraham bowed and w. the Lord. Gen 24:26, 48
Abraham's servant w. the Lord. 52
Israel bowed and w. Ex 4:31
12:27; 33:10
a calf, and w. it. 32:8; Ps 106:19
Moses w. Ex 34:8
other gods, and w. Deut 17:3; 29:26
1 Ki 9:9; 2 Ki 21:21; 2 Chr 7:22
Jer 1:16; 8:2; 16:11; 22:9
Gideon w. Judg 7:15
Hannah w. before Lord. 1 Sam 1:19
Samuel w. 28
Saul w. the Lord. 15:31
then David arose and w. 2 Sam 12:20; 15:32
and w. Ashtaroth. 1 Ki 11:33
Baal and w. him. 16:31; 22:53
w. all the host of heaven and served. 2 Ki 17:16; 21:3; 2 Chr 33:3
congregation bowed down and w. the Lord. 1 Chr 29:20; 2 Chr 7:3
29:28, 29, 30
all people w. the Lord. Neh 8:6; 9:3
Job w. Job 1:20
w. the sun. Ezek 8:16
king w. Daniel. Dan 2:46
w. the golden image. 3:7
fell down and w. Christ. Mat 2:11
a leper came and w. him. 8:2
a certain ruler w. him. 9:18
were in the ship w. him. 14:33
woman came and w. him. 15:25
fell down and w. his lord. 18:26
by the feet and w. him. 28:9
his disciples w. him. 17; Luke 24:52
out of the tombs and w. Mark 5:6
and bowing knees, w. him. 15:19
our fathers w. in this. John 4:20
blind man believed, and w. him. 9:38
fell down and w. Peter. Acts 10:25
Lydia w. God. 16:14
neither is w. with men's. 17:25*
Justus w. God. 18:7
w. the creature more. Rom 1:25
above all that is w. 2 Thes 2:4
Jacob w. Heb 11:21
the twenty-four elders w. Rev 5:14
11:16; 19:4
the angels w. God. 7:11
they w. the dragon, they w. 13:4
a sore fell on them which w. 16:2
them that w. his image. 19:20
souls that had not w. the beast. 20:4

worshipper

if any man be a w. of God. John 9:31
the city of Ephesus is a w. of Diana. Acts 19:35*

worshippers

destroy the w. of Baal. 2 Ki 10:19
all the w. of Baal came. 21
that there be none but the w. 23
then the true w. shall. John 4:23
the w. once purged. Heb 10:2

worshippeth

host of heaven w. thee. Neh 9:6
yea, he maketh a god, and w. it. Isa 44:15, 17
falleth not down and w. Dan 3:6, 11
Asia and the world w. Acts 19:27

worshipping

as he was w. in the house of Nisroch. 2 Ki 19:37; Isa 37:38
fell before the Lord, w. 2 Chr 20:18
mother of Zebedee's children came w. Mat 20:20
beguile you in w. of angels. Col 2:18

worst

I will bring the w. of the. Ezek 7:24

worth

as much money as it is w. Gen 23:9
the land is w. four hundred. 15
priest shall reckon the w. Lev 27:23
hath been w. a double. Deut 15:18
but thou art w. ten thousand of us. 2 Sam 18:3
give the w. of thy vineyard. 1 Ki 21:2
thy speech nothing w. Job 24:25
heart of wicked is little w. Pr 10:20
howl ye, Woe w. the day! Ezek 30:2

worthies

he shall recount his w. Nah 2:5

worthily

do thou w. in Ephratah. Ruth 4:11

worthy

I am not w. of the least. Gen 32:10
if the wicked man be w. Deut 25:2
he gave a w. portion. 1 Sam 1:5*
Lord liveth, ye are w. to die. 26:16
who is w. to be praised. 2 Sam 22:4
Ps 18:3

shew himself a *w.* man. *1 Ki* 1:52
this man is *w.* to die. *Jer* 26:11
he is not *w.* 16
whose shoes I am not *w.* *Mat* 3:11
Lord, I am not *w.* that thou shouldest come under. 8:8; *Luke* 7:6
for the workman is *w.* of his meat. *Mat* 10:10
enquire who in it is *w.* and. 11
be *w.* . . . but if it be not *w.* 13
me, he is not *w.* of me. 37, 38
which were bidden were not *w.* 22:8
I am not *w.* to unloose. *Mark* 1:7
Luke 3:16; *John* 1:27; *Acts* 13:25
bring forth fruits *w.* of. *Luke* 3:8
that he was *w.* for whom. 7:4
nor thought I myself *w.* to come. 7
for the labourer is *w.* of his. 10:7
commit things *w.* of stripes. 12:48
I am no more *w.* to be. 15:19, 21
shall be accounted *w.* to. 20:35
be accounted *w.* to escape. 21:36*
very *w.* deeds are done. *Acts* 24:2
are not *w.* to be compared with the glory. *Rom* 8:18
that ye walk *w.* of the. *Eph* 4:1
that ye might walk *w.* of. *Col* 1:10
would walk *w.* of God. *1 Thes* 2:12
w. of all acceptation. *1 Tim* 1:15; 4:9
the labourer is *w.* of his reward. 5:18
sorer punishment, suppose ye, shall he be thought *w.*? *Heb* 10:29
of whom the world was not *w.* 11:38
blaspheme that *w.* name? *Jas* 2:7*
in white, for they are *w.* *Rev* 3:4
thou art *w.* to receive glory. 4:11
5:12
Who is *w.* to open the book? 5:2
found *w.* to open the book. 4
thou art *w.* to take the book and. 9
to drink, for they are *w.* 16:6
see **count, counted, death**

wot, -teth

(*The American Revision everywhere, and the English Revision usually, put here the modern word* know, *which has the same meaning*)
I *w.* not who hath done. *Gen* 21:26
my master *w.* not what is with. 39:8
w. ye not that such a man? 44:15
as for this Moses, we *w.* *Ex* 32:1
23; *Acts* 7:40
I *w.* he whom thou blessest is blessed. *Num* 22:6
the men went I *w.* not. *Josh* 2:5
I *w.* that through ignorance ye did it. *Acts* 3:17
w. ye not what the scripture saith? *Rom* 11:2
I shall choose I *w.* not. *Phil* 1:22

would

I *w.* it might be according. *Gen* 30:34
I *w.* there were a sword. *Num* 22:29
whosoever *w.*, he consecrated him *1 Ki* 13:33
do with them as they *w.* *Neh* 9:24
Jews did what they *w.* to. *Esth* 9:5
not hearken, and Israel *w.* *Ps* 81:11
but ye *w.* none of my. *Pr* 1:25
they *w.* none of my counsel. 30
whom he *w.* he slew, and whom he *w.* he kept alive, and whom he *w.* he set up, and *w.* *Dan* 5:19
whatsoever ye *w.* that men should. *Mat* 7:12; *Luke* 6:31
to release a prisoner whom they *w.* *Mat* 27:15
calleth to him whom he *w.*, and they came unto him. *Mark* 3:13
we *w.* thou shouldest do for us. 10:35
what *w.* ye that I should do? 36
fishes as much as they *w.* *John* 6:11
reason *w.* that I should. *Acts* 18:14
what I *w.* that I do not. *Rom* 7:15
for the good that I *w.* I do not. 19
I *w.* that all men were. *1 Cor* 7:7
I *w.* that ye all spake with. 14:5
not find you such as I *w.* *2 Cor* 12:20
w. that we should remember. *Gal* 2:10
I *w.* they were cut off which. 5:12
do the things that ye *w.* 17
I *w.* ye knew what great. *Col* 2:1
forbiddeth them that *w.* *3 John* 10
I know thy works, I *w.* *Rev* 3:15

would *God*

w. God we had died in Egypt, when. *Ex* 16:3; *Num* 14:2
w. God that all the Lord's people were prophets! *Num* 11:29
w. God we had died when our. 20:3
w. God it were even, *w. God* it were morning! *Deut* 28:67
w. to *God* we had dwelt on the other side Jordan! *Josh* 7:7
w. God this people were. *Judg* 9:29
w. God I had died for. *2 Sam* 18:33
w. God my lord were. *2 Ki* 5:3
w. God that all were such as I am. *Acts* 26:29
I *w.* to *God* ye did reign. *1 Cor* 4:8
w. to *God* ye could bear with me. *2 Cor* 11:1

would *not*

if I knew, then *w. not* I tell it thee? *1 Sam* 20:9
his armourbearer *w. not.* 31:4
1 Chr 10:4
he *w. not,* nor did he eat with them. *2 Sam* 12:17
but Amnon *w. not* hearken. 13:16
howbeit David *w. not* go, but. 25
but Joab *w. not* come to. 14:29
but Jehoshaphat *w. not.* *1 Ki* 22:49
which Lord *w. not* pardon. *2 Ki* 24:4
yet *w.* they *not* give ear. *Neh* 9:30
yet *w.* I *not* believe he. *Job* 9:16
and ye *w. not.* *Isa* 30:15
Mat 23:37; *Luke* 13:34
besought him to have patience, he *w. not.* *Mat* 18:30
were bidden: they *w. not* come. 22:3
we *w. not* have been partakers with them. 23:30
w. not have suffered his house. 24:43
tasted, he *w. not* drink. 27:34
he *w. not* that any man. *Mark* 9:30
angry, and *w. not* go in. *Luke* 15:28
he *w. not* for a while, but. 18:4
he *w. not* lift so much as his. 13
who *w. not* that I should reign. 19:27
he *w. not* walk in Jewry. *John* 7:1
that he *w. not* delay to. *Acts* 9:38
when he *w. not* be persuaded. 21:14
I do that which I *w. not.* *Rom* 7:16
I *w. not,* brethren, that ye should be. 11:25; *1 Cor* 10:1
I *w. not* ye should have fellowship. *1 Cor* 10:20
you, such as ye *w. not.* *2 Cor* 12:20
because we *w. not* be chargeable to you. *1 Thes* 2:9
then *w.* he *not* afterward. *Heb* 4:8

wouldest

Caleb said, What *w.* thou? *Josh* 15:18; *1 Ki* 1:16
walkedst whither thou *w.* *John* 21:18

wouldest *not*

whither thou *w. not.* *John* 21:18
offering thou *w. not.* *Heb* 10:5, 8

wound, *substantive*

give *w.* for *w.*, stripe for. *Ex* 21:25
blood ran out of the *w.* *1 Ki* 22:35
my *w.* is incurable without transgression. *Job* 34:6
a *w.* and dishonour. *Pr* 6:33
the blueness of a *w.* cleanseth. 20:30
the stroke of their *w.* *Isa* 30:26
woe is me, for my *w.* is. *Jer* 10:19
and why is my *w.* incurable? 15:18
w. is grievous. 30:12; *Nah* 3:19
thee with *w.* of an enemy. *Jer* 30:14
Judah saw his *w.* . . . yet could he not cure your *w.* *Hos* 5:13
they that eat have laid a *w.* *Ob* 7*
her *w.* is incurable, it is. *Mi* 1:9
and his deadly *w.* was healed. *Rev* 13:3*, 12*, 14*

wound

alive; I *w.* and I heal. *Deut* 32:39
God shall *w.* the head. *Ps* 68:21*
he shall *w.* the heads over. 110:6*
when ye *w.* their weak. *1 Cor* 8:12

wound, *verb*

they *w.* body of Jesus. *John* 19:40*
young men *w.* up Ananias. *Acts* 5:6*

wounded

is *w.* in the stones. *Deut* 23:1
w. of the Philistines. *1 Sam* 17:52
Saul was *w.* of the archers. 31:3*
1 Chr 10:3*
I have *w.* mine enemies. *2 Sam* 22:39*; *Ps* 18:38*
in smiting he *w.* him. *1 Ki* 20:37
carry me out, for I am *w.* 22:34
2 Chr 18:33
the Syrians *w.* Joram. *2 Ki* 8:28
for I am sore *w.* *2 Chr* 35:23
soul of the *w.* crieth out. *Job* 24:12
suddenly shall they be *w.* *Ps* 64:7
of those whom thou hast *w.* 69:26
my heart is *w.* within me. 109:22
cast down many *w.* *Pr* 7:26
a *w.* spirit who can bear? 18:14*
found me, they *w.* me. *S of S* 5:7
art thou not it that *w.*? *Isa* 51:9*
but he was *w.* for our. 53:5
I *w.* thee with the wound. *Jer* 30:14
but *w.* men among them. 37:10
through all the land the *w.* 51:52
when they swooned as *w.* *Lam* 2:12
when the *w.* cry, shall? *Ezek* 26:15
the *w.* shall be judged in the. 28:23
groanings of a deadly *w.* 30:24
when they fall on the sword, shall not be *w.* *Joel* 2:8*
I was *w.* in the house. *Zech* 13:6
cast stones and they *w.* him in the head. *Mark* 12:4; *Luke* 20:12
thieves, which *w.* him. *Luke* 10:30
they fled out of that house naked and *w.* *Acts* 19:16
heads, as it were *w.* *Rev* 13:3*

woundedst

thou *w.* the head out of. *Hab* 3:13

woundeth

he *w.*, and his hands make. *Job* 5:18

wounding

slain a man to my *w.* *Gen* 4:23

wounds, *substantive*

went back to be healed of the *w.* *2 Ki* 8:29; 9:15; *2 Chr* 22:6
he multiplied my *w.* *Job* 9:17
my *w.* stink, are corrupt. *Ps* 38:5
and bindeth up their *w.* 147:3
words of a talebearer are as *w.* *Pr* 18:8*; 26:22*
who hath woe? who hath *w.*? 23:29
faithful are *w.* of friend, but. 27:6
in it, but *w.*, bruises, and. *Isa* 1:6
continually is grief and *w.* *Jer* 6:7
I will heal thee of thy *w.* saith. 30:17
what are these *w.* in thy hands? *Zech* 13:6
bound up his *w.* *Luke* 10:34

wove

the women *w.* hangings. *2 Ki* 23:7

woven

ephod have binding of *w.* work. *Ex* 28:32; 39:22
made coats of fine linen *w.* 39:27
the coat was without seam, *w.* *John* 19:23

wrap

he can *w.* himself in it. *Isa* 28:20
a reward; so they *w.* it up. *Mi* 7:3*

wrapped

Tamar *w.* herself and sat. *Gen* 38:14
Goliath's sword is *w.* *1 Sam* 21:9
Elijah *w.* his face in. *1 Ki* 19:13
mantle and *w.* it together. *2 Ki* 2:8
roots are *w.* about the heap. *Job* 8:17
sinews of his stones are *w.* 40:17*
the sword is *w.* up for. *Ezek* 21:15*
the weeds were *w.* about. *Jonah* 2:5
Joseph *w.* the body in a clean linen cloth. *Mat* 27:59; *Mark* 15:46*
Luke 23:53
Mary *w.* him in swaddling clothes. *Luke* 2:7
babe *w.* in swaddling clothes. 12
napkin *w.* together in a. *John* 20:7*

wrath

(Generally the Revised Versions use the more modern terms anger, vexation, indignation, fury)

cursed be their *w.* for it. *Gen* 49:7
lest *w.* come upon all. *Lev* 10:6
that no *w.* be on the congregation. *Num* 1:53; 18:5
for there is *w.* gone out from. 16:46
remember, how thou provokedst the Lord thy God to *w.* *Deut* 9:7, 22
the Lord rooted them out in anger and *w.* 29:28
were it not I feared the *w.* 32:27
let them live, lest *w.* *Josh* 9:20
and *w.* fell on all the. 22:20
if the king's *w.* arise. *2 Sam* 11:20
turned not from great *w.* *2 Ki* 23:26
because there fell *w.* *1 Chr* 27:24
therefore is *w.* upon thee. *2 Chr* 19:2
they trespass not, and so *w.* 10
w. came upon Judah for. 24:18
and there is fierce *w.* 28:13
that his fierce *w.* may turn. 29:10
therefore there was *w.* upon. 32:25
provoked God to *w.* *Ezra* 5:12
should there be *w.* against ? 7:23
yet ye bring more *w.* *Neh* 13:18
shall arise too much *w.* *Esth* 1:18
when the *w.* of the king was. 2:1
not, then Haman full of *w.* 3:5
was the king's *w.* pacified. 7:10
for *w.* killeth the foolish man. *Job* 5:2
w. bringeth the punishments. 19:29
he shall drink of the *w.* of. 21:20
hypocrites in heart heap up *w.* 36:13
because there is *w.*, beware. 18
forsake *w.* *Ps* 37:8
in *w.* they hate me. 55:3
surely the *w.* of man shall praise thee, the remainder of *w.* 76:10
stretch thy hand against *w.* of. 138:7
of the wicked is *w.* *Pr* 11:23
a fool's *w.* presently known. 12:16
that is slow to *w.* is of great. 14:29
a soft answer turneth away *w.* 15:1
w. of a king is as messengers. 16:14
king's *w.* is as the roaring. 19:12
a man of great *w.* shall suffer. 19
bosom pacifieth strong *w.* 21:14
who dealeth in proud *w.* 24
but a fool's *w.* is heavier. 27:3
w. is cruel, and anger is. 4
but wise men turn away *w.* 29:8
forcing of *w.* bringeth forth. 30:33
much *w.* with his sickness. *Eccl* 5:17
day of Lord cometh with *w.* *Isa* 13:9
he who smote the people in *w.* 14:6
in a little *w.* I hid my face. 54:8
fight against you in *w.* *Jer* 21:5
driven them in great *w.* 32:37
in that ye provoke me to *w.* 44:8
w. is on all the multitude. *Ezek* 7:12
and he reserveth *w.* for. *Nah* 1:2
O Lord, in *w.* remember. *Hab* 3:2
not deliver in day of *w.* *Zeph* 1:18
therefore came a great *w.* *Zech* 7:12
fathers provoked me to *w.* 8:14
to flee from *w.* to come. *Mat* 3:7; *Luke* 3:7
they were filled with *w.* *Luke* 4:28; *Acts* 19:28
be *w.* on this people. *Luke* 21:23
but treasurest up *w.* against the day of *w.* *Rom* 2:5
that obey unrighteousness, *w.* 8
because the law worketh *w.* 4:15
we shall be saved from *w.* 5:9
endured the vessels of *w.* fitted. 9:22
but rather give place unto *w.* 12:19
minister of God to execute *w.* 13:4
be subject, not only for *w.* 5
works of flesh are *w.*, strife. *Gal* 5:20
by nature the children of *w.* *Eph* 2:3
not sun go down upon your *w.* 4:26
let all *w.*, anger, and clamour. 31
provoke not your children to *w.* 6:4
put off all these; *w.*, malice. *Col* 3:8
who delivered us from the *w.* to come. *1 Thes* 1:10
for *w.* is come on them to. 2:16
hath not appointed us to *w.* 5:9
holy hands, without *w.* *1 Tim* 2:8
Moses not fearing the *w.* of the king. *Heb* 11:27
slow to speak, slow to *w.* *Jas* 1:19
w. of man worketh not. 20
and hide us from the *w.* *Rev* 6:16
come down, having great *w.* 12:12
she made all nations drink wine of *w.* 14:8; 18:3

day of **wrath**

his goods flow away in the *day of* his *w.* *Job* 20:28
the wicked brought forth to the *day of w.* 21:30
Lord strike through kings in *day of* his *w.* *Ps* 110:5
profit not in the *day of w.* *Pr* 11:4
that day is a *day of w.* *Zeph* 1:15
w. against the *day of w.* *Rom* 2:5
the great *day of* his *w.* is. *Rev* 6:17

wrath *of God*

the fierce *w. of God* is. *2 Chr* 28:11
till the *w. of God* be turned from us. *Ezra* 10:14
the *w. of God* came. *Ps* 78:31
but the *w. of God* abideth. *John* 3:36
the *w. of God* is revealed. *Rom* 1:18
things, *w. of God* cometh on the children. *Eph* 5:6; *Col* 3:6
shall drink of the wine of the *w. of God.* *Rev* 14:10
into winepress of the *w. of God.* 19
is filled up the *w. of God.* 15:1
golden vials full of the *w. of God.* 7
vials of the *w. of God* on earth. 16:1
winepress of the *w. of God.* 19:15

his **wrath**

Lord overthrew in *his w.* *Deut* 29:23
nor executedst *his w.* *1 Sam* 28:18
turned not from *his w.* *2 Ki* 23:26
his fierce *w.* may turn away. *2 Chr* 29:10; 30:8
his w. is against them. *Ezra* 8:22
from the banquet in *his w.* *Esth* 7:7
he teareth me in *his w.* *Job* 16:9
the fury of *his w.* on him. 20:23
he speak to them in *his w.* *Ps* 2:5
swallow them up in *his w.* 21:9
take them away in *his w.* 58:9
did not stir up all *his w.* 78:38
the fierceness of *his w.* 49
stood to turn away *his w.* 106:23
his w. against him that. *Pr* 14:35
turn away *his w.* from him. 24:18
Moab's pride and *his w.* *Isa* 16:6
the Lord hath forsaken the generation of *his w.* *Jer* 7:29
at *his w.* the earth shall. 10:10
I know *his w.*, saith the Lord. 48:30
hath thrown down in *his w.* *Lam* 2:2
affliction by the rod of *his w.* 3:1
because he kept *his w.* *Amos* 1:11
God willing to shew *his w.* *Rom* 9:22
of fierceness of *his w.* *Rev* 16:19

see **kindled,** *wrath of the* **Lord**

my **wrath**

my w. shall wax hot. *Ex* 22:24
let me alone, that *my w.* 32:10
hath turned *my w.* away. *Num* 25:11
my w. shall not be poured out on Jerusalem. *2 Chr* 12:7
to whom I sware in *my w.* *Ps* 95:11
against the people of *my w.* *Isa* 10:6
for in *my w.* I smote thee. 60:10
for *my w.* is on all the multitude. *Ezek* 7:14
thus will I accomplish *my w.* 13:15
thee in fire of *my w.* 21:31; 22:21
them with the fire of *my w.* 22:31
of *my w.* have I spoken. 38:19
I will pour out *my w.* on. *Hos* 5:10
I took him away in *my w.* 13:11
so sware in *my w.* they. *Heb* 3:11
as I have sworn in *my w.*, if they. 4:3

thy **wrath**

thou sentest *thy w.* which. *Ex* 15:7
doth *thy w.* wax hot against ? 32:11
turn from *thy* fierce *w.* and. 12
keep me secret until *thy w.* be past. *Job* 14:13
cast abroad the rage of *thy w.* 40:11
rebuke me not in *thy w.* *Ps* 38:1
pour out *thy w.* on the heathen. 79:6
taken away all *thy w.* *Ps* 85:3
thy w. lieth hard on me. 88:7
thy fierce *w.* goeth over me. 16
how long shall *thy w.* burn ? 89:46
and by *thy w.* are we troubled. 90:7
days are passed away in *thy w.* 9
according to thy fear, so is *thy w.* 11
thine indignation and *thy w.* 102:10
I stood to turn away *thy w.* *Jer* 18:20
was *thy w.* against the sea. *Hab* 3:8
thy w. is come, and time. *Rev* 11:18

wrathful

let thy *w.* anger take. *Ps* 69:24
a *w.* man stirreth up. *Pr* 15:18

wraths

be envyings, *w.*, strifes. *2 Cor* 12:20

wreath

two rows of pomegranates on each *w.* *2 Chr* 4:13*

wreathed

my transgressions are *w.* *Lam* 1:14*

wreathen

two chains at the ends, of *w.* work. *Ex* 28:14, 22, 24, 25; 39:15, 17, 18
pillar of *w.* work he carried away. *2 Ki* 25:17*

wreaths

w. of chain work for. *1 Ki* 7:17
two *w.* to cover the. *2 Chr* 4:12*
pomegranates on the two *w.* 13*

wrest

many, to *w.* judgement. *Ex* 23:2
thou shalt not *w.* the judgement of thy poor. 6
thou shalt not *w.* judgement; neither take a gift. *Deut* 16:19
day they *w.* my words. *Ps* 56:5
they that are unstable *w.* *2 Pet* 3:16

wrestle

we *w.* not against flesh. *Eph* 6:12

wrestled

wrestlings have I *w.* with. *Gen* 30:8
there *w.* a man with him. 32:24
thigh was out of joint as he *w.* 25

wrestlings

with great *w.* have I wrestled with my sister. *Gen* 30:8

wretched

O *w.* man that I am ! *Rom* 7:24
knowest not thou art *w.* *Rev* 3:17

wretchedness

let me not see my *w.* *Num* 11:15

wring

the priest shall *w.* off his head. *Lev* 1:15; 5:8
all the wicked shall *w.* *Ps* 75:8†

wringed

Gideon *w.* the dew out. *Judg* 6:38

wringing

the *w.* of the nose bringeth forth blood. *Pr* 30:33

wrinkle

a glorious church not having spot or *w.* *Eph* 5:27

wrinkles

hast filled me with *w.* *Job* 16:8*

write

I will *w.* on these tables. *Ex* 34:1; *Deut* 10:2
W. thou these words. *Ex* 34:27
w. thou every man's. *Num* 17:2
thou shalt *w.* Aaron's name on. 3
w. them on posts. *Deut* 6:9; 11:20
then let him *w.* her a bill of divorcement, and. 24:1, 3; *Mark* 10:4
w. on the stones the. *Deut* 27:3, 8
now therefore *w.* ye this. 31:19
Uzziah did Isaiah *w.* *2 Chr* 26:22
we might *w.* the names. *Ezra* 5:10
sure covenant and *w.* it. *Neh* 9:38
w. ye also for the Jews. *Esth* 8:8
w. them on the table. *Pr* 3:3; 7:3
w. in the great roll with. *Isa* 8:1
that *w.* grievousness which. 10:1
few, that a child may *w.* them. 19
now go, *w.* it before them. 30:8
saith the Lord, *W.* ye. *Jer* 22:30
w. the words I have spoken. 30:2; 36:2, 17, 28

I will w. it in their hearts. Jer 31:33
Heb 8:10
son of man, w. the name. Ezek 24:2
w. upon the sticks for. 37:16
w. it in their sight, that they. 43:11
w. the vision and make it. Hab 2:2
it seemed good to me to w. to thee in order. Luke 1:3
take thy bill and w. fifty. 16:6
w. fourscore. 7
and the prophets did w. John 1:45
w. not, King of the Jews, but. 19:21
that we w. to them that. Acts 15:20
thing to w. unto my lord, that I might have somewhat to w. 25:26
I w. not these things to. 1 Cor 4:14
things I w. are the. 14:37
for we w. none other things to you. 2 Cor 1:13
to this end also did I w., that. 2:9
it is superfluous for me to w. to. 9:1
I w. to them which heretofore. 13:2
therefore I w. these things, being. 10
now the things I w. unto. Gal 1:20
to w. the same things. Phil 3:1
not that I w. to you. 1 Thes 4:9; 5:1
so I w. 2 Thes 3:17
these things I w. 1 Tim 3:14
minds will I w. them. Heb 10:16
I now w. unto you. 2 Pet 3:1
1 John 2:1
these things w. we to. 1 John 1:4
brethren, I w. no new. 2:7
again, a new commandment I w. 8
I w. to you, little children. 12, 13
I w. to you, fathers, I w. to you. 13
having many things to w. 2 John 12
ink and pen w. to you. 3 John 13
diligence to w. of common salvation, it was needful for me to w. Jude 3
what thou seest, w. Rev 1:11, 19
unto the angel of the church of . . . w. 2:1, 8, 12, 18; 3:1, 7, 14
I will w. on him the name of my God . . . I will w. upon him my new. 3:12
to w.: a voice saying, w. not. 10:4
W., Blessed are the dead which. 14:13
W., Blessed are they which. 19:9
w.: for these words are true. 21:5
see **book**

writer

handle the pen of the w. Judg 5:14*
the pen of a ready w. Ps 45:1
a man with a w.'s inkhorn by his side. Ezek 9:2, 3

writest

for thou w. bitter things. Job 13:26
sticks whereon thou w. Ezek 37:20

writeth

count, when he w. up. Ps 87:6

writing

and the w. was the w. of. Ex 32:16
plate of the holy crown a w. 39:30
according to the first w. Deut 10:4
made an end of w. the law. 31:24
the Lord made me understand in w. 1 Chr 28:19
Huram answered in w. 2 Chr 2:11
came a w. from Jehoram. 21:12
prepare according to the w. of. 35:4
Cyrus put the proclamation in w. 36:22; Ezra 1:1
the w. of the letter was in. Ezra 4:7
unto all provinces according to the w. Esth 1:22; 3:12; 8:9; 9:27
copy of the w. was published. 3:14
to Hatach a copy of the w. 4:8
the w. in the king's name may. 8:8
the w. of Hezekiah, when. Isa 38:9
not written in the w. of. Ezek 13:9
whosoever shall read this w. Dan 5:7
could not read the w. 8
should read this w. 15
if thou canst read the w. thou. 16
yet I will read the w. to the king. 17
this is the w. that was. 24, 25
sign the w. 6:8
king Darius signed the w. 9
when Daniel knew that the w. 10
give her a w. of divorcement. Mat 5:31; 19:7
the w. was, Jesus of. John 19:19

hand-writing

blotting out the hand-w. Col 2:14

writings

if ye believe not his w. John 5:47

writing table

asked for a w. table. Luke 1:63

written

w. with the finger of God. Ex 31:18
Deut 9:10
elders did as it was w. 1 Ki 21:11
these w. by name smote. 1 Chr 4:41
the passover as it was w. 2 Chr 30:5
a letter wherein was w. Ezra 5:7
therein was a record thus w. 6:2
weight of the vessels was w. 8:34
sent an open letter, wherein was w. Neh 6:6
they found w. in the law. 8:14
and therein was found w. 13:1
it be w. among the laws. Esth 1:19
let it be w. that they may be. 3:9
of king Ahasuerus was it w. 12
found w. that Mordecai told of. 6:2
let it be w. to reverse Haman's. 8:5
let them not be w. with. Ps 69:28
be w. for the generation to. 102:18
on them the judgement w. 149:9
have not I w. to thee excellent things? Pr 22:20
that which was w. was. Eccl 12:10
shall be w. in the earth. Jer 17:13
hast w., saying, The king? 36:29
the roll was w. within. Ezek 2:10
nor w. in the writing of house. 13:9
writing that was w. Dan 5:24, 25
set up his accusation w. Mat 27:37
is it not w., My house? Mark 11:17
of his accusation was w. 15:26
Luke 23:38; John 19:20
place where it was w. Luke 4:17
rejoice that your names are w. 10:20
all things w. shall be accomplished. 18:31; 21:22
disciples remembered that it was w. John 2:17
Is it not w. in your law, I said? 10:34
but these are w. that ye might. 20:31
w. every one, the world could not contain the books . . . be w. 21:25
fulfilled all that was w. Acts 13:29
the Gentiles, we have w. 21:25
the work of the law w. Rom 2:15
now it was not w. for his sake. 4:23
they are w. for our admonition. 1 Cor 10:11
ye are our epistle w. in our. 2 Cor 3:2
w. not with ink, but with the. 3
if the ministration of death w. in. 7
I Paul have w. with. Philem 19
firstborn w. in heaven. Heb 12:23*
things which are w. therein. Rev 1:3
and in the stone a new name w. 2:17
not w. in the book of life. 13:8
having his Father's name w. 14:1
upon her head was a name w. 17:5
name w. on his thigh. 19:12, 16
names of the twelve tribes w. 21:12

is written

observe to do all that is w. Josh 1:8
that which is w. concerning us. 2 Ki 22:13
for writing which is w. in. Esth 8:8
every one that is w. among. Isa 4:3
sin of Judah is w. with. Jer 17:1
oath that is w. in the law. Dan 9:11
what is w. in the law? Luke 10:26
What is this then that is w.? 20:17
this that is w. must be. 22:37
be fulfilled that is w. John 15:25
to think of men above that which is w. 1 Cor 4:6
for our sakes, no doubt, this is w. 9:10
the saying that is w., Death. 15:54

it is written

as it is w. in the law of. Josh 8:31
1 Ki 2:3; 2 Chr 23:18; 25:4; 31:3
35:12; Ezra 3:2, 4; 6:18
Neh 8:15; 10:34, 36; Dan 9:13
it is w. of me. Ps 40:7; Heb 10:7
it is w. before me. Isa 65:6
thus it is w. by the prophet. Mat 2:5; Luke 24:46
this is he of whom it is w. Mat 11:10; Luke 7:27
as it is w. of him. Mat 26:24
Mark 9:13; 14:21
it is w. Mat 26:31; Mark 14:27
Luke 4:8; Acts 23:5
and how it is w. of the. Mark 9:12
as it is w. in the law. Luke 2:23
according as it is w. Rom 11:8
1 Cor 1:31; 2 Cor 4:13
for it is w. Rom 12:19; 14:11
Gal 3:10
not himself, but as it is w. Rom 15:3
so it is w., The first man. 1 Cor 15:45
because it is w., Be ye holy; for I am holy. 1 Pet 1:16

I have, or have I written

commandment, I have w. Ex 24:12
I have w. to him great. Hos 8:12
Pilate said, What I have w. I have w. John 19:22
I have w. to you fathers. 1 John 2:14
these things have I w. 26; 5:13

were written

of them that were w. Num 11:26
words were now w. Job 19:23
fulfilled which were w. Luke 24:44
things were w. of him. John 12:16
were w. aforetime were w. for our learning. Rom 15:4
see **book, chronicle**

wrong

Sarai said, My w. be. Gen 16:5
to him that did the w. Ex 2:13
against him what is w. Deut 19:16
thou doest me w. to war. Judg 11:27
seeing there is no w. in. 1 Chr 12:17
no man to do them w.: yea, he reproved kings for. 16:21; Ps 105:14
not done w. to the king. Esth 1:16
behold, I cry out of w. Job 19:7
do no w., do no violence. Jer 22:3
buildeth his chambers by w. 13*
seen my w.: judge thou. Lam 3:59
therefore w. judgement. Hab 1:4*
Friend, I do thee no w. Mat 20:13
one of them suffer w. Acts 7:24
why do ye w. one to another? 26
neighbour w. thrust him away. 27
if it were a matter of w. 18:14
the Jews have I done no w. 25:10
do ye not rather take w.? 1 Cor 6:7
nay, ye do w. and defraud your. 8
that had done the w. nor for his cause that suffered w. 2 Cor 7:12
I was not burdensome to you? forgive me this w. 12:13
w. shall receive for the w. Col 3:25

wronged

receive us, we have w. 2 Cor 7:2
if he hath w. thee, or. Philem 18

wrongeth

he that sinneth against me w. his own soul. Pr 8:36

wrongfully

the devices ye w. Job 21:27
let not mine enemies w. Ps 35:19
they that hate me w. are. 38:19
being mine enemies w. 69:4
me w., help thou me. 119:86
they have oppressed the stranger w. Ezek 22:29
endure grief, suffering w. 1 Pet 2:19

wrote

Moses w. all the words of the Lord and rose. Ex 24:4; Deut 31:9
Lord w. upon the tables words of. Ex 34:28; Deut 4:13; 5:22; 10:4
and Moses w. their. Num 33:2
Moses w. this song the. Deut 31:22
Joshua w. upon the. Josh 8:32
Samuel w. the manner of the kingdom. 1 Sam 10:25
David w. a letter to Joab. 2 Sam 11:14, 15
Jezebel w. letters in. 1 Ki 21:8, 9
Jehu w. 2 Ki 10:1, 6
Shemaiah w. 1 Chr 24:6
Hezekiah w. letters to. 2 Chr 30:1
Sennacherib w. to rail on the. 32:17
they w. an accusation. Ezra 4:6
Rehum w. 8, 9

Y

they brought a rate *y.* *by* *y.* *1 Ki* 10:25; *2 Chr* 9:24
as he had done *y.* *by* *y.* *2 Ki* 17:4
wood offering *y.* *by* *y.* *Neh* 10:34
firstfruits of all trees *y.* *by* *y.* 35
which they offered *y.* *by* *y.* *Heb* 10:1

year *to* year

ordinance from *y.* *to* *y.* *Ex* 13:10
coat to him from *y.* *to* *y.* *1 Sam* 2:19
Samuel went from *y.* *to* *y.* in. 7:16
your God from *y.* *to* *y.* *2 Chr* 24:5
add ye *y.* *to* *y.*; let them. *Isa* 29:1
from *y.* *to* *y.* to worship. *Zech* 14:16

yearly

as a *y.* hired servant. *Lev* 25:53
daughters of Israel went *y.* to lament. *Judg* 11:40
of the Lord in Shiloh *y.* 21:19
Elkanah went up *y.* to. *1 Sam* 1:3
to offer the *y.* sacrifice. 21; 2:19
there is a *y.* sacrifice there. 20:6
keep 14th day of month Adar, and fifteenth of same *y.* *Esth* 9:21

yearn

for his bowels did *y.* *Gen* 43:30

yearned

for her bowels *y.* upon. *1 Ki* 3:26

years

for seasons, days, and *y.* *Gen* 1:14
these are the days of the *y.* 25:7
an old man and full of *y.* 8
an hundred thirty seven *y.* 17
few and evil have the *y.* of. 47:9
according to the number of *y.* *Lev* 25:15, 16, 50, 52
the money according to the *y.* 27:18
consider the *y.* of many. *Deut* 32:7
Joshua was old and stricken in *y.* *Josh* 13:1
been with me these *y.* *1 Sam* 29:3
David was old and stricken in *y.* *1 Ki* 1:1
not be dew nor rain these *y.* 17:1
Asa had no war in those *y.* *2 Chr* 14:6
after certain *y.* he went down. 18:2
are thy *y.* as man's days? *Job* 10:5
the number of *y.* is hidden to. 15:20
when a few *y.* are come, I. 16:22
and multitude of *y.* should. 32:7
they shall spend their *y.* in. 36:11
nor can number of his *y.* be. 26
and my *y.* are spent. *Ps* 31:10
wilt prolong his *y.* as many. 61:6
I considered the *y.* of ancient. 77:5
I will remember the *y.* of the. 10
their *y.* did he consume in. 78:33
for a thousand *y.* in thy sight are but. 90:4; *2 Pet* 3:8
we spend our *y.* as a tale. *Ps* 90:9
our *y.* are threescore *y.* and ten. 10
according to the *y.* wherein we. 15
thy *y.* are throughout all. 102:24
thou art the same, thy *y.* shall. 27
the *y.* of thy life shall be many. *Pr* 4:10; 9:11
lest thou give thy *y.* unto. 5:9
the *y.* of the wicked shall be. 10:27
evil days come not, nor *y.* *Eccl* 12:1
the *y.* of an hireling. *Isa* 21:16
of the residue of my *y.* 38:10
I shall go softly all my *y.* 15
I have laid on thee the *y.* *Ezek* 4:5
art come even unto thy *y.* 22:4
in latter *y.* thou shalt come. 38:8
by books the number of the *y.* *Dan* 9:2
in the end of *y.* they shall join. 11:6
continue more *y.* than the king. 8
shall come after certain *y.* 13
even to the *y.* of many. *Joel* 2:2
I will restore the *y.* the locusts. 25
in the midst of the *y.* *Hab* 3:2
the offering be pleasant as in the former *y.* *Mal* 3:4
well stricken in *y.* *Luke* 1:7, 18
days and months, and *y.* *Gal* 4:10
thy *y.* shall not fail. *Heb* 1:12
by faith Moses, when he was come to *y.*, refused. 11:24
bound Satan a thousand *y.* *Rev* 20:2
till the thousand *y.* should be. 3
reigned with Christ a thousand *y.* 4
when the thousand *y.* are expired. 7

see numeral words in their places, as **hundred, two, three.** *Also* **many, old, sin**

yell

like lions, they shall *y.* *Jer* 51:38*

yelled

roared and *y.* on him. *Jer* 2:15

yellow

behold, if there be in it a *y.* thin hair. *Lev* 13:30
if there be in it no *y.* hair. 32
priests shall not seek for *y.* hair. 36
covered with *y.* gold. *Ps* 68:13

yesterday

fulfilled your task *y.*? *Ex* 5:14
why came not the son of Jesse to meat *y.*? *1 Sam* 20:27
thou camest but *y.* *2 Sam* 15:20
I have seen *y.* the blood. *2 Ki* 9:26
we are but of *y.* and know. *Job* 8:9
a thousand years in thy sight are but as *y.* *Ps* 90:4
y. at the seventh hour. *John* 4:52
didst the Egyptian *y.*? *Acts* 7:28
Jesus Christ, the same *y.* *Heb* 13:8

yesternight

behold, I lay *y.* with my. *Gen* 19:34
your fathers spake to me *y.* 31:29
affliction, and rebuked thee *y.* 42

yet

y. did not the butler. *Gen* 40:23
as *y.* exaltest thyself. *Ex* 9:17
knowest thou not *y.* that Egypt? 10:7
if ye will not *y.* hearken. *Lev* 26:18
y. for all that, when they be. 44
y. in this thing ye did. *Deut* 1:32
y. they are thy people and. 9:29
ye are not as *y.* come to the. 12:9
y. the Lord hath not given you. 29:4
as *y.* I am as strong. *Josh* 14:11
Lord said, The people are *y.* too many. *Judg* 7:4
y. ye have forsaken me and. 10:13
y. honour me now before the elders. *1 Sam* 15:30
y. he hath made with me an everlasting covenant. *2 Sam* 23:5
y. hast not been as my. *1 Ki* 14:8
y. I have left me 7000. 19:18
there is *y.* one by whom we. 22:8
as *y.* the people did sacrifice. 43
2 Ki 14:4
y. the Lord would not destroy Judah. *2 Ki* 8:19
them from his presence as *y.* 13:23
as *y.* the people had not prepared. *2 Chr* 20:33
people did *y.* corruptly. 27:2
not cleansed, *y.* did they eat. 30:18
temple was not *y.* laid. *Ezra* 3:6
y. our God hath not forsaken us. 9:9; *Neh* 9:19
y. required not I bread. *Neh* 5:18
y. ye bring more wrath upon. 13:18
y. all this availeth me. *Esth* 5:13
while he was *y.* *Job* 1:16, 17, 18
then should I *y.* have comfort. 6:10
though he slay me, *y.* will I. 13:15
y. he shall perish for ever. 20:7
when the Almighty was *y.* 29:5
y. he knoweth it not in great. 35:15
y. have I set my king on my. *Ps* 2:6
y. have I not seen the righteous forsaken. 37:25
I shall *y.* praise him. 42:5, 11
43:5; 71:14
this is come, *y.* have we. 44:17
y. have I not declined. 119:51, 157
y. do I not forget thy statutes. 83
109, 141
y. will not his foolishness. *Pr* 27:22
y. is not washed from their. 30:12
better is he which hath not *y.* been. *Eccl* 4:3
kiss thee, *y.* I should. *S of S* 8:1
y. a remnant of them. *Isa* 10:22
for the Lord will *y.* choose. 14:1
y. gleaning grapes shall be. 17:6
while it is *y.* in his hand, he. 28:4
this is the rest, *y.* they would. 12
y. he also is wise, and will. 31:2
Israel be not gathered, *y.* shall. 49:5
they may forget, *y.* will I not. *Isa* 49:15
he was oppressed, *y.* he. 53:7
I will *y.* plead with you. *Jer* 2:9
y. return to me. 3:1
y. they prosper. 5:28
y. my mind could not be. 15:1
prophets, *y.* they ran: *y.* they. 23:21
y. they were not afraid, nor. 36:24
though they cry, *y.* will. *Ezek* 8:18
y. will I be to them as a little. 11:16
said, I am a god, *y.* thou art a. 28:2
I will *y.* for this be enquired. 36:37
y. made we not our prayer before God. *Dan* 9:13
because it is *y.* for a time. 11:35
y. he shall come to his end. 45
grey hairs are upon him, *y.* *Hos* 7:9
y. I am the Lord thy God from. 13:4
given you want of bread, *y.* have ye not returned to me. *Amos* 4:6
8, 9, 10, 11; *Hag* 2:17
he shall say, Is there *y.*? *Amos* 6:10
y. I will look toward thy. *Jonah* 2:4
y. forty days and Nineveh. 3:4
was my saying, when I was *y.* 4:2
are there *y.* the treasures? *Mi* 6:10
y. was she carried away. *Nah* 3:10
y. I will rejoice in the Lord, I will joy. *Hab* 3:18
y. is she thy companion. *Mal* 2:14
do not ye *y.* understand, that? *Mat* 15:17; 16:9; *Mark* 8:17
I kept, what lack I *y.*? *Mat* 19:20
but the end is not *y.* 24:6
Mark 13:7
time of figs was not *y.* *Mark* 11:13
words I spake while *y.* *Luke* 24:44
unto her, Mine hour is not *y.* come. *John* 2:4; 7:6, 30; 8:20
for the Holy Ghost was not *y.* 7:39
though he were dead *y.* shall. 11:25
for as *y.* they knew not the. 20:9
as *y.* the Holy Ghost was fallen upon none of them. *Acts* 8:16
he had *y.* being uncircumcised. *Rom* 4:11, 12
we were *y.* without strength. 5:6
while we were *y.* sinners. 8
why doth he *y.* hope for? 8:24
Why doth he *y.* find fault? 9:19
ye are *y.* carnal. *1 Cor* 3:3
y. so as by fire. 15
to the married I command, *y.* not I, but the Lord. 7:10
y. for all that will they not. 14:21
y. not I, but the grace of God. 15:10
your faith is vain, ye are *y.* 17
that he will *y.* deliver. *2 Cor* 1:10
to spare you I came not as *y.* 23
y. true, as unknown, *y.* known. 6:8
y. not I, but Christ. *Gal* 2:20
in vain? if it be *y.* in vain. 3:4
I, brethren, if I *y.* preach. 5:11
when I was *y.* with you. *2 Thes* 2:5
y. is he not crowned. *2 Tim* 2:5
we see not *y.* all things. *Heb* 2:8
like as we are, *y.* without sin. 4:15
for he was *y.* in the loins of. 7:10
and by it he being dead *y.* 11:4
warned of things not seen as *y.* 7
keep the whole law, *y.* *Jas* 2:10
y. if thou kill. 11
y. ye have not. 4:2
it doth not *y.* appear. *1 John* 3:2
and is not, and *y.* is. *Rev* 17:8
and the other is not *y.* come. 10
received no kingdom as *y.* 12
see **alive**

yield

the ground, it shall not henceforth *y.* her strength. *Gen* 4:12
fat, shall *y.* royal dainties. 49:20
that it may *y.* to you the increase. *Lev* 19:25
y. her increase, trees *y.* fruit. 26:4
for your land shall not *y.* her. 20
but *y.* yourselves to the Lord. *2 Chr* 30:8
the land shall *y.* her increase. *Ps* 67:6; 85:12
plant vineyards, which may *y.* 107:37
speech she caused him to *y.* *Pr* 7:21

vineyard shall y. one bath, and the seed of an homer shall y. *Isa* 5:10
the bud shall y. no meal: if so be it y. the stranger shall. *Hos* 8:7
the fig tree and vine y. *Joel* 2:22
fields shall y. no meat. *Hab* 3:17
but do not thou y. unto. *Acts* 23:21
nor y. ye your members as instruments of . . . sin, y. *Rom* 6:13*
that to whom ye y. yourselves servants. 16*
y. your members servants to. 19*
no fountain y. salt water. *Jas* 3:12

yielded
his sons, y. up the ghost. *Gen* 49:33
rod of Aaron y. almonds. *Num* 17:8
y. their bodies that they. *Dan* 3:28
Jesus cried again, and y. *Mat* 27:50
then Sapphira y. up the. *Acts* 5:10
ye have y. your members. *Rom* 6:19

yieldeth
it y. much increase. *Neh* 9:37
wilderness y. food for. *Job* 24:5
y. the peaceable fruit of. *Heb* 12:11

yielding
bring forth herb y. seed, tree y. fruit. *Gen* 1:11, 12
given you every tree y. seed. 29
for y. pacifieth great. *Eccl* 10:4
see **fruit**

yoke
This term is used both literally and figuratively in the Bible. Figuratively it is used [1] *Of the yoke of bondage, or slavery,* Lev 26:13; *Deut* 28:48. [2] *Of the yoke of afflictions and crosses,* Lam 3:27. [3] *Of the yoke of punishment for sin,* Lam 1:14. [4] *Of the yoke of Christ's service,* Mat 11:29, 30.
that thou shalt break his y. *Gen* 27:40; *Jer* 30:8
I have broken the bands of your y. *Lev* 26:13; *Ezek* 34:27
a red heifer without blemish, on which never came y. *Num* 19:2
Deut 21:3; *1 Sam* 6:7
he shall put a y. of iron upon thy neck. *Deut* 28:48; *Jer* 28:14
Saul took a y. of oxen. *1 Sam* 11:7
an half acre, which a y. of. 14:14
y. grievous, make his heavy y. *1 Ki* 12:4, 10, 11, 14; *2 Chr* 10:4
with twelve y. of oxen. *1 Ki* 19:19
he took a y. of oxen, and slew. 21
Job had five hundred y. *Job* 1:3
he had a thousand y. of oxen. 42:12
thou hast broken the y. of his burden. *Isa* 9:4; 10:27; 14:25
hast very heavily laid thy y. 47:6
and that ye break every y. 58:6
I have broken thy y. *Jer* 2:20
altogether broken the y. 5:5
not put their neck under the y. 27:8
bring their neck under the y. 11, 12
broken the y. of the king. 28:2; 4, 11
Hananiah had broken the y. 12*
unaccustomed to the y. 31:18
husbandman and his y. 51:23
the y. of my transgressions. *Lam* 1:14
good for a man to bear the y. 3:27
they that take off the y. *Hos* 11:4
now will I break his y. *Nah* 1:13
take my y. upon you. *Mat* 11:29
my y. is easy. 30
bought five y. of oxen. *Luke* 14:19
to put a y. on the disciples' neck. *Acts* 15:10
be not entangled with the y. *Gal* 5:1
as are under the y. *1 Tim* 6:1

yoked
be not unequally y. with. *2 Cor* 6:14

yokefellow
I intreat thee also, true y. *Phil* 4:3

yokes
make thee bonds and y. *Jer* 27:2*
y. of wood; but make y. of iron. 28:13
break the y. of Egypt. *Ezek* 30:18

yonder
I and the lad will go y. *Gen* 22:5
scatter thou the fire y. *Num* 16:37
while I meet the Lord y. 23:15
y. is that Shunammite. *2 Ki* 4:25
Remove hence to y. place. *Mat* 17:20
here, while I go and pray y. 26:36

you
a space between y. and ark. *Josh* 3:4
and shake my head at y. *Job* 16:4
your iniquities have separated between y. and your God. *Isa* 59:2
and I will put a new spirit within y. *Ezek* 11:19; 36:26, 27
are about y., bear shame. 36:7, 36
I am pressed under y. *Amos* 2:13
y. only have I known of all. 3:2
he that heareth y. heareth me; and he that despiseth y. *Luke* 10:16
and y. yourselves thrust out. 13:28
the name of God is blasphemed through y. *Rom* 2:24
lest they come and find y. unprepared. *2 Cor* 9:4
gospel in the regions beyond y. 10:16
for I seek not yours but y. 12:14
y. hath he quickened. *Eph* 2:1
y. that were sometime alienated and enemies. *Col* 1:21
y., being dead in your sins, hath he quickened. 2:13
see **tell**

after **you**
with you, and seed *after* y. *Gen* 9:9
inheritance for your children *after* y. *Lev* 25:46; *1 Chr* 28:8
draw out a sword *after* y. *Lev* 26:33
as they pursued *after* y. *Deut* 11:4
that shall rise up *after* y. 29:22
behold, I come *after* y. *1 Sam* 25:19
shall follow close *after* y. *Jer* 42:16
which long *after* y. *2 Cor* 9:14
Phil 1:8
longed *after* y. *Phil* 2:26

against **you**
I have sinned *against* y. *Ex* 10:16
I will set my face *against* y. *Lev* 26:17; *Jer* 44:11
they murmur *against* y. *Num* 17:5
came out *against* y. *Deut* 1:44
earth to witness *against* y. this day, that ye shall soon. 4:26; 30:19
I testify *against* y. that ye. 8:19
the Lord was wroth *against* y. 9:19
11:17; *Josh* 23:16
Jericho fought *against* y. *Josh* 24:11
the Lord is witness *against* y. *1 Sam* 12:5; *Mi* 1:2
Ammonites came *against* y. *1 Sam* 12:12
hand of Lord shall be *against* y. 15
counselled *against* y. *2 Sam* 17:21
to cry alarm *against* y. *2 Chr* 13:12
heap up words *against* y. *Job* 16:4
I devise a device *against* y. *Jer* 18:11
will fight *against* y. in anger. 21:5
of evil pronounced *against* y. 26:13
Chaldeans that fight *against* y. 37:10
the king of Babylon shall not come *against* y. 19
cannot do any thing *against* y. 38:5
words shall stand *against* y. 44:29
conceived a purpose *against* y. 49:30
I am *against* y. *Ezek* 13:8
enemy said *against* y. 36:2
Lord hath spoken *against* y. *Amos* 3:1; 5:1; *Zeph* 2:5
I will raise up *against* y. a nation. *Amos* 6:14
take up a parable *against* y. *Mi* 2:4
manner of evil *against* y. *Mat* 5:11
go into the village over *against* y. 21:2; *Mark* 11:2; *Luke* 19:30
the very dust of your city we do wipe off *against* y. *Luke* 10:11
be a witness *against* y. *Jas* 5:3
whereas they speak *against* y. as evil doers. *1 Pet* 2:12

among or *amongst* **you**
strange gods that are *among* y. *Gen* 35:2; *Josh* 24:23; *1 Sam* 7:3
tabernacle *amongst* y. *Lev* 26:11
I will walk *among* y. and will. 12
I will send wild beasts *among* y. 22
I will send pestilence *among* y. 25
despised the Lord who is *among* y. *Num* 11:20; 14:42; *Deut* 6:15
7:21; *Josh* 3:10
who is there *among* y.? *2 Chr* 36:23
Ezra 1:3
who *among* y. will give? *Isa* 42:23
who is *among* y. that feareth? 50:10
purge out from *among* y. *Ezek* 20:38
who is left *among* y. that? *Hag* 2:3
who is there *among* y.? *Mal* 1:10
it shall not be so *among* y. *Mat* 20:26; *Mark* 10:43
among y. let him be your servant. *Mat* 20:27; 23:11; *Luke* 22:26
he that is least *among* y. *Luke* 9:48
but I am *among* y. as he. 22:27
standeth one *among* y. *John* 1:26
he that is without sin *among* y. 8:7
brethren, look ye out *among* y. seven men. *Acts* 6:3
and whosoever *among* y. 13:26
let them who *among* y. are. 25:5
some fruit *among* y. *Rom* 1:13
every man that is *among* y. 12:3
no divisions *among* y. *1 Cor* 1:10
contentions *among* y. 11; 11:18
to know any thing *among* y. 2:2
is *among* y. envying, strife. 3:3
if any man *among* y. seemeth. 18
there is fornication *among* y. 5:1
taken away from *among* y. 2
how say some *among* y. that? 15:12
Christ who was preached *among* y. *2 Cor* 1:19
in presence am base *among* y. 10:1
will humble me *among* y. 12:21
not be once named *among* y. *Eph* 5:3
what manner of men were *among* y. *1 Thes* 1:5
if any man *among* y. *Jas* 1:26
is any *among* y. afflicted? 5:13
is any sick *among* y.? 14
feed the flock of God which is *among* y. *1 Pet* 5:2
false teachers *among* y. *2 Pet* 2:1
who was slain *among* y. *Rev* 2:13
see **sojourneth**

before **you**
the land shall be *before* y. *Gen* 34:10
God did send me *before* y. 45:5, 7
for evil is *before* y. *Ex* 10:10
these the nations are defiled which I cast out *before* y. *Lev* 18:24
20:23; *Num* 33:52, 55; *Deut* 11:23
Josh 3:10; 9:24; 23:5, 9; 24:8
12; *Judg* 6:9
men of the land done which were *before* y. *Lev* 18:27, 28, 30
shall fall *before* y. 26:7, 8
are there *before* y. *Num* 14:43
shall be subdued *before* y. 32:29
set the land *before* y. *Deut* 1:8
Lord who goeth *before* y. shall. 30
set *before* y. this day. 4:8; 11:32
I set *before* y. a blessing and a curse. 11:26; 30:19
dried up Jordan *before* y. *Josh* 4:23
I sent the hornet *before* y. 24:12
behold, he is *before* y. *1 Sam* 9:12
the king walketh *before* y. 12:2
my statutes which I have set *before* y. *2 Chr* 7:19; *Jer* 26:4; 44:10
Lord will go *before* y. *Isa* 52:12
behold, I set *before* y. the. *Jer* 21:8
so persecuted they the prophets which were *before* y. *Mat* 5:12
kingdom of God *before* y. 21:31
risen again, I will go *before* y. 26:32
28:7; *Mark* 14:28; 16:7
eat such things as are set *before* y. *Luke* 10:8; *1 Cor* 10:27
doth this man stand here *before* y. whole. *Acts* 4:10

by **you**
I will not be enquired of *by* y. *Ezek* 20:3, 31
I trust to be brought on my way *by* y. *Rom* 15:24
if the world shall be judged *by* y. *1 Cor* 6:2

was refreshed by y. all. 2 Cor 7:13
shall be enlarged by y. 10:15

concerning you

what Lord will command concerning y. Num 9:8
which the Lord spake concerning y. Josh 23:14
hath said concerning y. Jer 42:19
this is the will of God concerning y. 1 Thes 5:18

for you

as for y. Gen 44:17; 50:20 Num 14:32; Deut 1:40; Josh 23:9 Job 17:10
one ordinance shall be for y. Num 15:15, 16
all that he did for y. Deut 1:30 4:34; 1 Sam 12:24
as for y. O house of Israel. Ezek 20:39; 34:17
behold I am for y. and I will. 36:9
but one decree for y. Dan 2:9
to what end is it for y.? Amos 5:18
is it not for y. to know judgement? Mi 3:1
is it time for y., to dwell? Hag 1:4
commandment is for y. Mal 2:1
more tolerable for Tyre and Sidon, than for y. Mat 11:22; Luke 10:14
kingdom prepared for y. Mat 25:34
that I should do for y. Mark 10:36
this is my body which is given for y. Luke 22:19
blood shed for y. 20; 1 Cor 11:24
prepare a place for y. John 14:2, 3
I will pray the Father for y. 16:26
is not for y. to know the times or the seasons. Acts 1:7
therefore have I called for y. 28:20
God through Christ for y. Rom 1:8
was Paul crucified for y.? 1 Cor 1:13
care for y. appear. 2 Cor 7:12; 8:16
by their prayer for y. 9:14; Phil 1:4 Col 1:3, 9; 4:12; 2 Thes 1:11
and be spent for y. 2 Cor 12:15
I cease not to give thanks for y. Eph 1:16; 1 Thes 1:2; 3:9 2 Thes 1:3; 2:13
at my tribulations for y. Eph 3:13 Col 1:24
is not grievous, but for y. Phil 3:1
which is laid up for y. Col 1:5
which is given to me for y. 25
great conflict I have for y. 2:1
that he hath a great zeal for y. 4:13
is unprofitable for y. Heb 13:17
reserved in heaven for y. 1 Pet 1:4
on him, for he careth for y. 5:7

from you

sent me away from y. Gen 26:27
we are very far from y. Josh 9:22
not removed from y. 1 Sam 6:3
come word from y. 2 Sam 15:28
wrath turn away from y. 2 Chr 30:8
turn away his face from y. 9
will hide mine eyes from y. Isa 1:15
have hid his face from y. 59:2
good things from y. Jer 5:25
which are gone from y. 34:21
keep nothing back from y. 42:4
cast away from y. your. Ezek 18:31
remove far from y. the. Joel 2:20
I have withholden the rain from y. Amos 4:7
kingdom of God shall be taken from y. Mat 21:43
no man taketh from y. John 16:22
who is taken up from y. Acts 1:11
but seeing ye put it from y. 13:46
word of God out from y. 1 Cor 14:36
of commendation from y. 2 Cor 3:1
let evil speaking be put away from y. Eph 4:31
for from y. sounded out. 1 Thes 1:8
but we being taken from y. 2:17
and he will flee from y. Jas 4:7

in you

be any truth in y. Gen 42:16
let him also rejoice in y. Judg 9:19
sanctified in y. Ezek 20:41; 36:23
will put breath in y. 37:6, 14
I have no pleasure in y. saith the Lord. Mal 1:10
but the Spirit which speaketh in y. Mat 10:20
works which were done in y. 11:21
not his word abiding in y. John 5:38
not the love of God in y. 42
the flesh, ye have no life in y. 6:53
he shall be in y. 14:17
and I in y. 20; 15:4
if my words abide in y. 15:7 1 John 2:14, 24
the Spirit dwelleth in y. Rom 8:9 1 John 2:27
and if Christ be in y. Rom 8:10
as much as lieth in y., live. 12:18
Christ is confirmed in y. 1 Cor 1:6
Holy Ghost which is in y. 6:19
God is in y. of a truth. 14:25
having confidence in y. all. 2 Cor 2:3 7:16; 8:22; Gal 5:10
but life in y. 2 Cor 4:12
he was comforted in y. 7:7
he would finish in y. the same. 8:6
exceeding grace of God in y. 9:14
is not weak, but mighty in y. 13:3
that Jesus Christ is in y.? 5
I travail, till Christ be formed in y. Gal 4:19
one God . . . who is above all, and through all, and in y. all. Eph 4:6
let this mind be in y. which. Phil 2:5
it is God which worketh in y. 13
which bringeth forth fruit, as it doth also in y. Col 1:6
which is Christ in y., the hope. 27
Christ dwell in y. richly. 3:16
worketh in y. 1 Thes 2:13
so that we glory in y. 2 Thes 1:4
Christ may be glorified in y. 12
every good thing in y. Philem 6
working in y. that which is well-pleasing. Heb 13:21
the hope that is in y. 1 Pet 3:15
if these things be in y. 2 Pet 1:8
which thing is true in him and in y. 1 John 2:8
greater is he that is in y. than. 4:4

of you

why should I be deprived of y. both? Gen 27:45
may be done of y. Ex 12:16
unto me every one of y. Deut 1:22
faint because of y. Josh 2:9
to these nations because of y. 23:3
that all of y. have conspired against me. 1 Sam 22:8
O people, every one of y. 1 Ki 22:28
what Ezra requires of y. Ezra 7:21
though there were of y. cast out unto uttermost part of heaven. Neh 1:9
ye shall be slain all of y. Ps 62:3
that escape of y. shall. Ezek 6:9
he shall receive of y. Mi 1:11
which of y. by taking thought can add one cubit? Mat 6:27; Luke 12:25
doth not each one of y.? Luke 13:15
of y. convinceth me of? John 8:46
I speak not of y. all, I know. 13:18
which God did by him in the midst of y. Acts 2:22
in turning every one of y. 3:26
which was set at nought of y. 4:11
faith both of y. and me. Rom 1:12
declared to me of y. 1 Cor 1:11
such were some of y. but ye. 6:11
the feet, I have no need of y. 12:21
every one of y. hath a psalm. 14:26
let every one of y. lay by him. 16:2
and our hope of y. is. 2 Cor 1:7
boasted any thing to him of y. 7:14
suffer, if a man take of y. 11:20
did I make a gain of y.? 12:17
Did Titus make a gain of y.? 18
this only would I learn of y. Gal 3:2
for as many of y. as have been. 27
voice, for I stand in doubt of y. 4:20
brother, who is one of y. Col 4:9, 12
neither of y. sought we. 1 Thes 2:6
every one of y. should know. 4:4
no evil thing to say of y. Tit 2:8
the hire which is of y. kept. Jas 5:4
they speak evil of y. 1 Pet 3:16; 4:4

on, or upon you

plague shall not be upon y. Ex 12:13
bestow upon y. a blessing. Ex 32:29
oil of the Lord is upon y. Lev 10:7
they said, Ye take too much upon y. Num 16:3, 7
not set his love upon y. Deut 7:7
things are come upon y. Josh 23:15
they will be upon y. Neh 4:12
of the Lord be upon y. Ps 129:8
upon y. the spirit of sleep. Isa 29:10
he may have mercy upon y. 30:18 Jer 42:12
I will visit upon y. the. Jer 23:2
this thing is come upon y. 40:3
I will blow upon y. in. Ezek 22:21
days shall come upon y. Amos 4:2
before the fierce anger of the Lord come upon y. Zeph 2:2
upon y. may come the. Mat 23:35
of God is come upon y. Luke 11:20
and so that day come upon y. 21:34
I send the promise of my Father upon y. 24:49
darkness come upon y. John 12:35
Holy Ghost is come upon y. Acts 1:8
not cast a snare upon y. 1 Cor 7:35
upon y. labour in vain. Gal 4:11
howl for your miseries that shall come upon y. Jas 5:1
of God resteth upon y. 1 Pet 4:14
I will put upon y. none. Rev 2:24

over you

I will even appoint over y. Lev 26:16
hate you shall reign over y. 17
rejoiced over y. to do you good, he will rejoice over y. Deut 28:63
rule over y. nor my son rule over y.: Lord shall rule over y. Judg 8:23
seventy reign over y. or one? 9:2
ye anoint me king over y. 15
that shall reign over y. 1 Sam 8:11
I have made a king over y. 12:1
the Lord hath set a king over y. 13
David to be king over y. 2 Sam 3:17
chief priest is over y. 2 Chr 19:11
watchmen over y. saying. Jer 6:17
fury poured out will I rule over y. Ezek 20:33
heaven over y. is stayed. Hag 1:10
me a divider over y.? Luke 12:14
not have dominion over y. Rom 6:14
of this power over y. 1 Cor 9:12
over y. with godly zeal. 2 Cor 11:2
we were comforted over y. in affliction. 1 Thes 3:7
know them which are over y. 5:12
remember them which have the rule over y. Heb 13:7
obey them that have the rule over y. 17
salute them that have the rule over y. 24

to or unto you

every herb to y. it shall. Gen 1:29
and take our daughters unto y. 34:9
and will be to y. a God. Ex 6:7
children shall say unto y. 12:26
not make unto y. gods of gold. 20:23
it shall be unto y. most holy. 30:36
I will also do this unto y. Lev 26:16
they shall be to y. for an. Num 10:8
be to y. a memorial. 10
unto y. for a fringe. 15:39
I shall do unto y. as I thought. 33:56
to them, and they to y. Josh 23:12
as they have been to y. 1 Sam 4:9
unto y. O men, I call. Pr 8:4
this iniquity shall be to y. Isa 30:13
to y. it is commanded. Dan 3:4
unto y. that fear my name. Mal 4:2
that men should do to y. Mat 7:12 Luke 6:31
to your faith be it unto y. Mat 9:29
because it is given unto y. to know. 13:11; Mark 4:11; Luke 8:10
unto y. that hear shall. Mark 4:24
unto y. is born this day a Saviour. Luke 2:11
to them which do good to y. 6:33
I appoint unto y. a kingdom. 22:29
for the promise is unto y. Acts 2:39
unto y. first, God having raised. 3:26
therefore came I unto y. 10:29
to y. is the word of this. 13:26

doubtless I am *to y.* *1 Cor* 9:2
word of God *unto y.* only? 14:36
to reach even *unto y.* *2 Cor* 10:13
we are come as far as *to y.* 14
but *to y.* of salvation. *Phil* 1:28
unto y. it is given not only to. 29
our gospel came not *unto y.* in word. *1 Thes* 1:5
to y. who are troubled. *2 Thes* 1:7
unto y. that believe. *1 Pet* 2:7
but *unto y.* I say, and. *Rev* 2:24
see **say, told**

toward **you**

good work *toward y.* *Jer* 29:10
thoughts I think *toward y.* 11
judgement is *toward y.* *Hos* 5:1
our word *toward y.* was. *2 Cor* 1:18
is more abundant *toward y.* 7:15
all grace abound *toward y.* 9:8
being absent am bold *toward y.* 10:1
by the power of God *toward y.* 13:4
abound in love one toward another, as we do *toward y.* *1 Thes* 3:12

with **you**

then we will dwell *with y.* *Gen* 34:16
but God shall be *with y.* 48:21
my bones hence *with y.* *Ex* 13:19
that I have talked *with y.* 20:22
Aaron and Hur are *with y.* 24:14
with y. shall be a man. *Num* 1:4
where I will meet *with y.* 17:4
it may be well *with y.* *Deut* 5:33
no part *with y.* 12:12
God goeth *with y.* 20:4
nor *with y.* only do I make. 29:14
neither will I be *with y.* *Josh* 7:12
said, The Lord be *with y.* *Ruth* 2:4
and mother be *with y.* *1 Sam* 22:3
me, and I will go *with y.* 23:23
what have I to do *with y.*? *2 Sam* 16:10; 19:22
go forth *with y.* myself. 18:2
master's sons are *with y.* *2 Ki* 10:2
see there be *with y.* none of. 23
and it shall be well *with y.* 25:24
Jer 40:9
Lord your God *with y.*? *1 Chr* 22:18
there are *with y.* golden calves. *2 Chr* 13:8
the Lord is *with y.* while ye. 15:2
for the Lord, who is *with y.* in. 19:6
the Lord will be *with y.* 20:17
with y., even *with y.*, sins? 28:10
let us build *with y.*: for we. *Ezra* 4:2
lest I deal *with y.* after. *Job* 42:8
do *with y.* as this potter? *Jer* 18:6
I am *with y.* 42:11; *Hag* 1:13; 2:4
will I plead *with y.* *Ezek* 20:35, 36
when I have wrought *with y.* 44
the Lord shall be *with y.* *Amos* 5:14
with y., for God is *with y.* *Zech* 8:23
how long shall I be *with y.*? *Mat* 17:17
Mark 9:19; *Luke* 9:41
the poor always *with y.*, but me ye. *Mat* 26:11; *John* 12:8
I drink it new *with y.* in. *Mat* 26:29
I am *with y.* alway, unto the. 28:20
you, while I was *with y.* *Luke* 24:44
yet a little while am I *with y.*, then I go to. *John* 7:33; 12:35; 13:33
Have I been so long *with y.*? 14:9
that he may abide *with y.* 16
he dwelleth *with y.* 17
being present *with y.* 25
peace I leave *with y.* 27
because I was *with y.* 16:4
I should bear *with y.* *Acts* 18:14
I have been *with y.* at all. 20:18
comforted together *with y.* *Rom* 1:12
I may *with y.* be refreshed. 15:32
now the God of peace be *with y.* all. 33; *2 Cor* 13:11; *Phil* 4:9
the grace of our Lord Jesus Christ be *with y.* *Rom* 16:20, 24
1 Cor 16:23; *Phil* 4:23; *Col* 4:18
1 Thes 5:28; *2 Thes* 3:18
2 Tim 1:2; 4:22; *Tit* 3:15
Heb 13:25; *2 John* 3; *Rev* 22:21
was *with y.* in weakness. *1 Cor* 2:3
that we also might reign *with y.* 4:8
see that he may be *with y.* 16:10
my love be *with y.* all in Christ. 24
establisheth us *with y.* *2 Cor* 1:21
and present us *with y.* *2 Cor* 4:14
hearts to die and live *with y.* 7:3
when I was present *with y.* 11:9
Gal 4:18, 20
I joy and rejoice *with y.* *Phil* 2:17
am I *with y.* in the spirit. *Col* 2:5
glorified, as it is *with y.* *2 Thes* 3:1
the Lord be *with y.* all. 16
God dealeth *with y.* as. *Heb* 12:7
peace be *with y.* all. *1 Pet* 5:14
spots and blemishes, while they feast *with y.* *2 Pet* 2:13

young

have not cast their *y.* *Gen* 31:38
the flocks and herds with *y.* 33:13
nothing cast their *y.* *Ex* 23:26
not kill it and her *y.* *Lev* 22:28
take the dam with the *y.* *Deut* 22:6
let the dam go and take the *y.* 7
shew favour to the *y.* 28:50
eagle fluttereth over her *y.* 32:11
had a *y.* son Micha. *2 Sam* 9:12
my son is *y.* *1 Chr* 22:5; 29:1
when Rehoboam was *y.* *2 Chr* 13:7
Josiah, while he was yet *y.* 34:3
ewes great with *y.* *Ps* 78:71
where she may lay her *y.* 84:3
those that are with *y.* *Isa* 40:11
for the *y.* of the flock. *Jer* 31:12
cropped off the top of his *y.* twigs. *Ezek* 17:4, 22
whose *y.* daughter had. *Mark* 7:25*
when *y.* thou girdedst. *John* 21:18
see **child, children, man, men, old**

young *ass*, or *asses*

the shoulders of *y. asses.* *Isa* 30:6
the *y. asses* shall eat clean. 24
he found a *y. ass*, sat. *John* 12:14
see **bullock**

young *bullocks*

shall offer two *y. bullocks.* *Num* 28:11, 19, 27
need, both *y. bullocks.* *Ezra* 6:9

young *calf*

take thee a *y. calf* for. *Lev* 9:2*

young *cow*

man shall nourish a *y. cow.* *Isa* 7:21

young *dromedaries*

he sent letters by riders on *y. dromedaries.* *Esth* 8:10*

young *eagles*

y. eagles shall eat it. *Pr* 30:17

young *hart*

my beloved is like a *y. hart.* *S of S* 2:9, 17; 8:14
see **lion, lions**

young *one*

her eye shall be evil toward her *y. one.* *Deut* 28:57
neither shall seek the *y. one*, nor heal. *Zech* 11:16*

young *ones*

whether they be *y. ones.* *Deut* 22:6
when his *y. ones* cry to. *Job* 38:41
bring forth their *y. ones.* 39:3
their *y. ones* are in good liking. 4
is hardened against her *y. ones.* 16
the eagles' *y. ones* also suck. 30
their *y. ones* shall lie. *Isa* 11:7
give suck to their *y. ones.* *Lam* 4:3

young *pigeon*

dove, and a *y. pigeon.* *Gen* 15:9
bring a *y. pigeon* for a. *Lev* 12:6

young *pigeons*

offering of *y. pigeons.* *Lev* 1:14
a lamb, he shall bring two *y. pigeons.* 5:7; 12:8; 14:22, 30; 15:14, 29
Num 6:10; *Luke* 2:24
if he be not able to bring two *y. pigeons.* *Lev* 5:11

young *ravens*

food to *y. ravens* which cry. *Ps* 147:9

young *roes*

thy breasts are like two *y. roes.* *S of S* 4:5; 7:3

young *unicorn*

Sirion like a *y. unicorn.* *Ps* 29:6

young *virgin*

for my lord a *y. virgin.* *1 Ki* 1:2

young *virgins*

found 400 *y. virgins.* *Judg* 21:12
let fair *y. virgins* be sought. *Esth* 2:2
together all the *y. virgins.* 3

young *woman*

thee of this *y. woman.* *Ruth* 4:12

young *women*

they may teach *y. women.* *Tit* 2:4

younger

Noah knew what his *y.* son. *Gen* 9:24*
firstborn said to the *y.* 19:31, 34
and the *y.* she also bare a son. 38
the elder shall serve the *y.* 25:23
Rom 9:12
on Jacob her *y.* son. *Gen* 27:15
called Jacob her *y.* son. 42
the name of the *y.* daughter. 29:16
seven years for the *y.* 18
to give the *y.* before firstborn. 26
is this your *y.* brother? 43:29*
his right hand on the *y.* 48:14
his *y.* brother shall be greater. 19
Caleb's *y.* brother. *Judg* 1:13; 3:9
is not her *y.* sister fairer? 15:2
Saul's *y.* daughter. *1 Sam* 14:49
cast lots over against their *y.* brethren. *1 Chr* 24:31
that are *y.* than I, have me in derision. *Job* 30:1
y. sister is Sodom. *Ezek* 16:46
sisters, thine elder and *y.* 61
y. said, Father, give me. *Luke* 15:12
the *y.* son gathered all, and took. 13
let him be as the *y.* 22:26
intreat the *y.* men as. *1 Tim* 5:1
the *y.* women as sisters, with all. 2
the *y.* widows refuse, for when. 11
that the *y.* women marry. 14
likewise, ye *y.* submit. *1 Pet* 5:5

youngest

the *y.* is this day with our father. *Gen* 42:13, 32
except your *y.* brother come. 15, 20
34; 44:23, 26
they sat, the *y.* according. 43:33
in the sack's mouth of the *y.* 44:2
eldest, and left off at the *y.* 12
in his *y.* son shall he set up gates of it. *Josh* 6:26; *1 Ki* 16:34
yet Jotham the *y.* son. *Judg* 9:5
remaineth yet the *y.* *1 Sam* 16:11
David was the *y.*: the eldest. 17:14
save Jehoahaz the *y.* *2 Chr* 21:17
his *y.* son king in his stead. 22:1

yours

the land of Egypt is *y.* *Gen* 45:20
feet tread shall be *y.* *Deut* 11:24
answered, Our life for *y.* *Josh* 2:14
the battle is not *y.* but. *2 Chr* 20:15
in land that is not *y.* *Jer* 5:19
y. is the kingdom of God. *Luke* 6:20
they will keep *y.* also. *John* 15:20
for all things are *y.* *1 Cor* 3:21, 22
lest this liberty of *y.* become. 8:9
refreshed my spirit and *y.* 16:18
for I seek not *y.* but you. *2 Cor* 12:14

yourselves

wash, and rest *y.* under. *Gen* 18:4
be not angry with *y.* that ye. 45:5
gather *y.* together. 49:1, 2; *Jer* 6:1
Ezek 39:17; *Joel* 3:11; *Zeph* 2:1
Rev 19:17
take heed unto *y.* *Ex* 19:12
Deut 2:4; 4:15, 23; 11:16
Josh 23:11; *Jer* 17:21
as for the perfume, ye shall not make to *y.* *Ex* 30:37
consecrate *y.* to-day to the. 32:29
ye shall not make *y.* abominable, neither shall ye make *y.* *Lev* 11:43
sanctify *y.* 11:44; 20:7; *Num* 11:18
Josh 3:5; 7:13; *1 Sam* 16:5
1 Chr 15:12; *2 Chr* 29:5; 35:6
ye defile *y.* *Lev* 11:44; 18:24, 30
nor make to *y.* molten gods. 19:4
lift you up *y.*? *Num* 16:3
separate *y.* from this. 21
Moses saying, Arm some of *y.* 31:3
women-children keep for *y.* 18
purify both *y.* and your. 19

lest ye corrupt y. Deut 4:16, 25
mightier nations than y. 11:23
not cut y. for the dead. 14:1
present y. in the tabernacle. 31:14
ye will utterly corrupt y. 29
hide y. there three days. Josh 2:16
keep y. from the accursed thing, lest ye make y. accursed. 6:18
take for a prey unto y. 8:2
nor serve them, nor bow y. unto. 23:7
and bowed y. to them. 16
ye are witnesses against y. that ye have chosen. 24:22
not fall upon me y. Judg 15:12
quit y. like men, O ye. 1 Sam 4:9
present y. before the Lord. 10:19
Saul said, Disperse y. 14:34
you one bullock for y. 1 Ki 18:25
set y. in array, and they set. 20:12
2 Chr 20:17; Jer 50:14
have consecrated y. 2 Chr 29:31
but yield y. unto the Lord. 30:8
to give over y. to die by. 32:11
prepare y. by the houses of. 35:4
separate y. from the. Ezra 10:11
their daughters for y. Neh 13:25
that ye make y. strange. Job 19:3
if ye will indeed magnify y. 5
all ye y. have seen it. 27:12
and offer up for y. a burnt. 42:8
associate y., O ye people: gird y. Isa 8:9; Joel 1:13
stay y. Isa 29:9
shew y. men. 46:8
are in darkness, shew y. 49:9
for iniquities have ye sold y. 50:1
that compass y. about with. 11
ye have sold y. for nought. 52:3
against whom do ye sport y. 57:4
by inflaming y. with idols under. 5
in their glory shall ye boast y. 61:6
circumcise y. to the Lord. Jer 4:4
humble y. 13:18; Jas 4:10; 1 Pet 5:6
wallow y. in ashes, ye. Jer 25:34
innocent blood upon y. 26:15
saith the Lord, deceive not y. 37:9
that ye might cut y. off and. 44:8
repent and turn y. Ezek 14:6
18:30, 32
defile not y. with the idols. 20:7, 18
ye pollute y. with all your idols. 31
then shall ye lothe y. 43; 36:31
keepers of my charge for y. 44:8
to y. in righteousness. Hos 10:12
your God ye made to y. Amos 5:26
eat for y. and drink for y. Zech 7:6
think not to say within y. Mat 3:9
Luke 3:8
lay not up for y. Mat 6:19
lay up for y. 20
Why reason ye among y.? 16:8
neither go in y. 23:13; Luke 11:52
child of hell than y. Mat 23:15
ye be witnesses unto y. 31
go ye rather, and buy for y. 25:9
come ye y. apart into. Mark 6:31
that ye disputed among y.? 9:33
have salt in y. and peace one. 50
but take heed to y.: they shall deliver you up. 13:9; Luke 17:3; 21:34
Acts 5:35; 20:28
ye y. touch not the. Luke 11:46
provide y. bags which wax. 12:33
ye y. like unto men that wait for. 36
why even of y. judge ye not? 57
kingdom, ye y. thrust out. 13:28
make to y. friends of the. 16:9
ye are they which justify y. 15
he said, Go shew y. unto the. 17:14
know of y. that summer is. 21:30
and divide it among y. 22:17
but weep for y. and for. 23:28
ye y. bear me witness. John 3:28
said, Murmur not among y. 6:43
do ye enquire among y. of? 16:19
signs God did, as you y. Acts 2:22
save y. from this untoward. 40
seeing ye judge y. unworthy. 13:46
from which if ye keep y. ye. 15:29
trouble not y. for his life. 20:10
you y. know, that these hands. 34
reckon ye also y. to be. Rom 6:11
but yield y. unto God, as those. 13
whom ye yield y. servants to. 16
dearly beloved, avenge not y., but rather give place. Rom 12:19
put from y. that wicked. 1 Cor 5:13
ye not rather suffer y. to be? 6:7
ye may give y. to fasting and. 7:5
judge in y.: is it comely that? 11:13
I beseech, that ye submit y. 16:16
yea, what clearing of y., in all things ye have approved y. 2 Cor 7:11
seeing ye y. are wise. 11:19
examine y. whether ye be in. 13:5
faith, and that not of y. Eph 2:8
speaking to y. in psalms. 5:19
submitting y. one to another. 21
wives, submit y. unto your. Col 3:18
y., brethren, know our entrance in unto you. 1 Thes 2:1
y. know that we are appointed. 3:3
ye y. are taught of God, to. 4:9
y. know that the day of the Lord. 5:2
wherefore comfort y. together. 11
and be at peace among y. 13, 15
that ye withdraw y. 2 Thes 3:6
y. knowing how ye ought to follow us. 7
knowing in y. ye have. Heb 10:34
remember, as being y. also. 13:3
and submit y.: for they watch for. 17
ye not then partial in y.? Jas 2:4
submit y. to God. 4:7
not fashioning y. to. 1 Pet 1:14
submit y. to every ordinance. 2:13
arm y. likewise with the same. 4:1
fervent charity among y. 8
ye younger, submit y. unto. 5:5
keep y. from idols. 1 John 5:21
look to y. that we lose not. 2 John 8
building up y. on your most. Jude 20
keep y. in the love of God, looking. 21

youth

is evil from his y. Gen 8:21
youngest according to his y. 43:33
about cattle, from our y. 46:34
father's house, as in her y. Lev 22:13
being in her father's house in her y. Num 30:3, 16
the y. drew not a sword, because yet a y. Judg 8:20
thou art but a y., and he a man of war from his y. 1 Sam 17:33
for he was but a y. 42
whose son is this y.? 55
befell thee from thy y. 2 Sam 19:7
fear the Lord from my y. 1 Ki 18:12
the iniquities of my y. Job 13:26
are full of the sin of his y. 20:11
as I was in the days of my y. 29:4*
on my right hand rise the y. 30:12*
from my y. he was brought up. 31:18
return to the days of his y. 33:25
hypocrites die in y. and. 36:14
not the sins of my y. Ps 25:7
thou art my trust from my y. 71:5
hast taught me from my y. 17
and ready to die from my y. 88:15
the days of his y. hast thou. 89:45
so that thy y. is renewed. 103:5
thou hast the dew of thy y. 110:3
so are the children of thy y. 127:4
afflicted me from my y. 129:1
as plants grown up in y. 144:12
the guide of her y. Pr 2:17
with the wife of thy y. 5:18
O young man in thy y. Eccl 11:9
for childhood and y. are vanity. 10*
Creator in the days of thy y. 12:1
hast laboured from thy y. Isa 47:12
thy merchants from thy y. 15
forget the shame of thy y. 54:4
hath called thee as a wife of y. 6
the kindness of thy y. Jer 2:2
thou art the guide of my y. 3:4
of our fathers from our y. 24
we and our fathers from our y. 25
been thy manner from thy y. 22:21
bear the reproach of my y. 31:19
evil before me from their y. 32:30
been at ease from his y. 48:11
bear the yoke in his y. Lam 3:27
been polluted from my y. Ezek 4:14
remembered days of thy y. 16:22, 43
my covenant in days of thy y. 60
whoredoms in their y. 23:3
her y. they lay with her and. 8
the days of her y. Ezek 23:19, 21
as in the days of her y. Hos 2:15
for the husband of her y. Joel 1:8
to keep cattle from my y. Zech 13:5
and the wife of thy y. Mal 2:14
let none deal treacherously against the wife of his y. 15
all these have I kept from my y. up; what lack I yet? Mat 19:20
Mark 10:20; Luke 18:21
life from my y. know all. Acts 26:4
let no man despise thy y. 1 Tim 4:12

youthful

flee also y. lusts, but. 2 Tim 2:22

youths

I discerned among the y. Pr 7:7
even the y. shall faint. Isa 40:30

you-ward

which to y.-ward is not. 2 Cor 13:3
grace given me to y.-ward. Eph 3:2

Z

Zacchaeus

Z. make haste and. Luke 19:5

Zachariah, Zechariah

Z. son of Jeroboam reigned. 2 Ki 14:29; 15:8, 11
Abi daughter of Z. 18:2; 2 Chr 29:1
chief of the Reubenites; Jeiel, Z. 1 Chr 5:7
Z. porter of the door. 9:21; 15:18
20, 24; 26:2
Geder, Ahio, Z. and Mickloth. 9:37
next to Asaph, Z. 16:5
Z. son of Isshiah. 24:25
Z. the fourth son of Hosah. 26:11
Z. the son of Shelemiah, a wise. 14
was Iddo the son of Z. 27:21
Jehoshaphat sent to Z. 2 Chr 17:7
on Jahaziel son of Z. 20:14
Jehiel and Z. the sons of. 21:2
Spirit of God came upon Z. 24:20
sought God in the days of Z. 26:5
of the sons of Asaph, Z. 29:13
Z. of the Kohathites was. 34:12
Hilkiah, Z. rulers of the house. 35:8
Z. the son of Iddo prophesied to. Ezra 5:1; 6:14; Neh 12:16
sons of Pharosh, Z. Ezra 8:3
Z. the son of Bebai. 11
Elam, Z. 10:26
on Ezra's left hand stood Z. Neh 8:4
Z. the son of Amariah. 11:4
Z. the son of Shiloni. 5
Z., the son of Pashur. 12
Z. the son of Jonathan. 12:35
Z. with trumpets. 41
Z. the son of Jeberechiah. Isa 8:2
Z. the son of Barachiah. Zech 1:1
7:1; Mat 23:35; Luke 11:51
see also Zacharias, p. 783

Zadok

Z. and Abimelech. 2 Sam 8:17
Z. and Abiathar carried the. 15:29
hast thou not with thee Z. and? 35
Z. and Abiathar were priests. 20:25
1 Ki 4:4
but Z. was not with Adonijah. 1 Ki 1:8, 26
Z. and Nathan have anointed. 45
and Z. the priest. 2:35; 1 Chr 29:22
Azariah the son of Z. 1 Ki 4:2
Jerusha the daughter of Z. was. 2 Ki 15:33; 2 Chr 27:1
Ahitub begat Z. 1 Chr 6:8; 12:53
9:11; 18:16
Z. a young man, mighty man. 12:28
both Z. of the sons of Eleazar. 24:3
of the Aaronites, Z. was. 27:17
priest of the house of Z. 2 Chr 31:10
Shallum, the son of Z. Ezra 7:2
Z. repaired. Neh 3:4, 29
Z. sealed. 10:21
of the priests, the son of Z. 11:11
made Z. the scribe treasurer. 13:13

these are the sons of *Z*. *Ezek* 40:46 43:19; 44:15
priests sanctified of sons of *Z*. 48:11

Zalmunna

after Zebah and *Z*. *Judg* 8:5
Zebah and *Z*. in thy hand. 6, 15
arose and slew Zebah and *Z*. 21
princes as Zebah and *Z*. *Ps* 83:11

Zarah, *see also* **Zerah**

Judah's son was called *Z*. *Gen* 38:30; 46:12
Tamar bare Pharez and *Z*. *1 Chr* 2:4; *Mat* 1:3
the sons of *Z*., Zimri, and. *1 Chr* 2:6

Zarephath

get thee to *Z*. *1 Ki* 17:9
he went to *Z*. 10
Israel shall possess to *Z*. *Ob* 20

zeal

to slay them in his *z*. *2 Sam* 21:2
come and see my *z*. for. *2 Ki* 10:16
the *z*. of the Lord shall do this. 19:31 *Isa* 37:32
the *z*. of thy house hath eaten me up and. *Ps* 69:9; *John* 2:17
my *z*. hath consumed. *Ps* 119:139
the *z*. of the Lord will. *Isa* 9:7
and he was clad with *z*. as. 59:17
where is thy *z*. and thy? 63:15
have spoken it in my *z*. *Ezek* 5:13
that they have *z*. of God. *Rom* 10:2
yea, what *z*.! *2 Cor* 7:11
your *z*. provoked many. 9:2
concerning *z*., persecuting. *Phil* 3:6
hath a great *z*. for you. *Col* 4:13*

zealous

was *z*. for my sake. *Num* 25:11*
he was *z*. for his God and made. 13*
are all *z*. of the law. *Acts* 21:20
Paul was *z*. towards God. 22:3 *Gal* 1:14
are *z*. of spiritual gifts. *1 Cor* 14:2
purify a peculiar people, *z*. *Tit* 2:14
I rebuke and chasten: be *z*. *Rev* 3:19

zealously

they *z*. affect you, but. *Gal* 4:17
it is good to be *z*. affected in a. 18

Zebah, *see* **Zalmunna**

Zebedee

ship with *Z*. their father. *Mat* 4:21
apostles, James and John the sons of *Z*. 10:2; 26:37; *Mark* 1:19; 3:17 10:35; *Luke* 5:10; *John* 21:2
mother of *Z*.'s children. *Mat* 20:20 27:56
they left their father *Z*. *Mark* 1:20

Zeboim

king of *Z*. *Gen* 14:2
overthrow of *Z*. *Deut* 29:23
the valley of *Z*. to the. *1 Sam* 13:18
Benjamin dwelt at *Z*. *Neh* 11:34
how shall I set thee at *Z*.? *Hos* 11:8

Zebul

the son of Jerubbaal, and *Z*. his officer. *Judg* 9:28
Z. thrust out Gaal and his. 41

Zebulun

Leah called his name *Z*. *Gen* 30:20
Reuben, Simeon, Judah, *Z*. 35:23
the sons of *Z*. 46:14; *Num* 1:30 26:26
Z. shall dwell at the. *Gen* 49:13
of *Z*.: Eliab the son of Helon. *Num* 1:9; 2:7; 7:24; 10:16
mount Ebal to curse; Reuben, Gad, Asher, *Z*. *Deut* 27:13
of *Z*. he said, Rejoice, *Z*. in. 33:18
third lot came up for *Z*. *Josh* 19:10
nor did *Z*. drive out the. *Judg* 1:30
Barak called *Z*. and Naphtali. 4:10
out of *Z*. they that handle. 5:14
Z. and Naphtali were a people that jeoparded their lives. 18
he sent messengers to *Z*. 6:35
buried in the country of *Z*. 12:12
of *Z*. Ishmaiah was the. *1 Chr* 27:19
divers of *Z*. humbled. *2 Chr* 30:11
the princes of *Z*. and. *Ps* 68:27
afflicted the land of *Z*. *Isa* 9:1
Z. a portion. *Ezek* 48:26
one gate of *Z*. 33
in the borders of *Z*. *Mat* 4:13
the land of *Z*. and Nephthalim. 15

tribe of **Zebulun**

the *tribe of Z*. 57,400. *Num* 1:31
then the *tribe of Z*.: Eliab. 2:7; 10:16
tribe of Z., Gaddiel to spy. 13:10
prince of the *tribe of Z*. to. 34:25
out of the *tribe of Z*. twelve cities. *Josh* 21:7, 34; *1 Chr* 6:63, 77
of the *tribe of Z*. were sealed 12,000. *Rev* 7:8

Zedekiah

Z. made horns of iron. *1 Ki* 22:11 *2 Chr* 18:10
Z. smote Micaiah on the cheek. *1 Ki* 22:24; *2 Chr* 18:23
changed his name to *Z*. *2 Ki* 24:17
sons of *Z*. and put out the eyes of *Z*. 25:7; *Jer* 39:6, 7; 52:10, 11
son of Josiah, *Z*. *1 Chr* 3:15
sons of Jehoiakim: *Z*. 16
Z. his brother king. *2 Chr* 36:10
I will deliver *Z*. and his. *Jer* 21:7
Lord make thee like *Z*. and. 29:22
Z. shall not escape from the. 32:4
he shall lead *Z*. to Babylon. 5
the army overtook *Z*. 39:5; 52:8

Zeeb, *see* **Oreb**

Zelophehad

Z. had no sons, but daughters. *Num* 26:33; *Josh* 17:3
the daughters of *Z*. speak. *Num* 27:7
daughters of *Z*. were married. 36:11

Zelotes, *see* **Simon**

Zelzah

Rachel's sepulchre at *Z*. *1 Sam* 10:2

Zenas

bring *Z*. the lawyer and. *Tit* 3:13

Zephaniah

the captain took *Z*. second priest. *2 Ki* 25:18; *Jer* 52:24
Z. of the sons of the. *1 Chr* 6:36
Zedekiah sent *Z*. to. *Jer* 21:1
letters in thy name to *Z*. 29:25
Z. read this letter in the ears. 29
Z. the son of Maaseiah. 37:3
the word came to *Z*. *Zeph* 1:1
house of Josiah son of *Z*. *Zech* 6:10
be to Hen the son of *Z*. 14

Zerah, *see also* **Zarah**

the son of Reuel, *Z*. *Gen* 36:13, 17 *1 Chr* 1:37
Jobab the son of *Z*. reigned. *Gen* 36:33; *1 Chr* 1:44
of *Z*. the family. *Num* 26:13, 20
of Zabdi, the son of *Z*. *Josh* 7:1
did not Achan the son of *Z*.? 22:20
sons of Simeon were *Z*. *1 Chr* 4:24
Z. son of Iddo. 6:21
Ethni the son of *Z*. 41
of the sons of *Z*. Jeuel dwelt in. 9:6
Z. the Ethiopian came. *2 Chr* 14:9
of the children of *Z*. *Neh* 11:24

Zeresh

Haman called for *Z*. his. *Esth* 5:10

Zerubbabel

of Pedaiah, *Z*., sons of *Z*. *1 Chr* 3:19
which came up with *Z*. *Ezra* 2:2 *Neh* 12:1
Z. the son of. *Ezra* 3:2, 8; 5:2
Israel in the days of *Z*. *Neh* 12:47
Lord by Haggai to *Z*. *Hag* 1:1
then *Z*. obeyed the voice of. 12
stirred up the spirit of *Z*. 14
yet now be strong, O *Z*. 2:4
speak to *Z*. of Judah. 21
word of the Lord unto *Z*. *Zech* 4:6
before *Z*. thou shalt become. 7
the hands of *Z*. have laid. 9

Zeruiah

three sons of *Z*. there. *2 Sam* 2:18
the sons of *Z*. be too hard. 3:39
Joab son of *Z*. 8:16; *1 Chr* 18:15
What have I do with you, ye sons of *Z*.? *2 Sam* 16:10; 19:22
whose sisters were *Z*. *1 Chr* 2:16

Ziba

art thou *Z*.? *2 Sam* 9:2
Z. had fifteen sons. 10
the king said to *Z*., Thine are. 16:4
I said, Thou and *Z*. divide. 19:29

Zibeon

Anah the daughter of *Z*. the Hivite. *Gen* 36:2, 14
these are the children of *Z*. 24 *1 Chr* 1:40
duke *Z*. *Gen* 36:29

Zidon

border shall be to *Z*. *Gen* 49:13
chased them to great *Z*. *Josh* 11:8
Kanah, even unto great *Z*. 19:28
and served the gods of *Z*. *Judg* 10:6
because it was far from *Z*. 18:28
which belongeth to *Z*. *1 Ki* 17:9
drink unto them of *Z*. *Ezra* 3:7
whom the merchants of *Z*. *Isa* 23:2
be thou ashamed, O *Z*.: the sea. 4
O thou virgin, daughter of *Z*. 12
all the kings of *Z*. *Jer* 25:22
yokes to the king of *Z*. 27:3
to cut off from Tyre and *Z*. 47:4
the inhabitants of *Z*. *Ezek* 27:8
set thy face against *Z*. and. 28:21
I am against thee, O *Z*. 22
what have ye to do with me, O Tyre, and *Z*.? *Joel* 3:4
Z. though it be very wise. *Zech* 9:2

Zidonians

Z. and Amalekites did. *Judg* 10:12
after the manner of the *Z*. 18:7
but king Solomon loved women of *Z*. *1 Ki* 11:1
Ashtoreth, goddess of the *Z*. 33
Z. that are gone down. *Ezek* 32:30

Zif

the month of *Z*. which is. *1 Ki* 6:1
was laid in the month *Z*. 37

Ziklag

Achish gave *Z*. to. *1 Sam* 27:6
we burnt *Z*. 30:14
abode two days in *Z*. *2 Sam* 1:1
I slew them in *Z*. 4:10
they dwelt at *Z*. *1 Chr* 4:30 *Neh* 11:28
came to David to *Z*. 12:1, 20

Zilpah

Laban gave to Leah, *Z*. *Gen* 29:24
Leah gave *Z*. her maid. 30:9
Z. Leah's maid bare Jacob. 10, 12
the sons of *Z*., Gad. 35:26; 46:18
was with the sons of *Z*. 37:2

Zimri

that was slain was *Z*. *Num* 25:14
Z. conspired against. *1 Ki* 16:9, 16
Z. reigned seven days in Tirzah. 15
had *Z*. peace, who slew? *2 Ki* 9:31
the sons of Zorah, *Z*. *1 Chr* 2:6
Z. the son of Jehoadah. 8:36
Jarah begat *Z*. 9:42
I made all the kings of *Z*. *Jer* 25:25

Zin

from wilderness of *Z*. *Num* 13:21
to the desert of *Z*. 20:1; 33:36
ye rebelled in the desert of *Z*. 27:14; *Deut* 32:51

Zion, Sion

David took strong hold of *Z*. the. *2 Sam* 5:7; *1 Chr* 11:5
the city of David, which is *Z*. *1 Ki* 8:1; *2 Chr* 5:2
king on my holy hill of *Z*. *Ps* 2:6
walk about *Z*. and go round. 48:12
thy good pleasure unto *Z*. 51:18
for God will save *Z*. and. 69:35
the Lord loveth the gates of *Z*. 87:2
he said of *Z*., This and that man. 5
Z. heard and was glad. 97:8
arise and have mercy on *Z*. 102:13
Lord shall build up *Z*. 16
turned the captivity of *Z*. 126:1
turned back that hate *Z*. 129:5
the Lord hath chosen *Z*. 132:13
dew on the mountains of *Z*. 133:3
when we remembered *Z*. 137:1
Sing us one of the songs of *Z*. 3
reign, even thy God, O *Z*. 146:10
praise the Lord, O Jerusalem, praise thy God, O *Z*. 147:12
let the children of *Z*. be. 149:2
Z. shall be redeemed. *Isa* 1:27
shout, thou inhabitant of *Z*. 12:6
that the Lord hath founded *Z*. 14:32
the Lord hath filled *Z*. with. 33:5

look on *Z*. *Isa* 33:20
for controversy of *Z*. 34:8
come to *Z*. with songs. 35:10
O *Z*. that bringest good tidings. 40:9
the first shall say to *Z*. 41:27
but *Z*. said, The Lord hath. 49:14
for the Lord shall comfort *Z*. 51:3
come with singing unto *Z*. 11
and say unto *Z*., Thou art my. 16
put on thy strength, O *Z*. 52:1
saith unto *Z*., Thy God reigneth! 7
Lord shall bring again *Z*. 8
Redeemer shall come to *Z*. 59:20
call thee the *Z*. of the holy. 60:14
for *Z*.'s sake will I not hold. 62:1
Z. is a wilderness, Jerusalem. 64:10
as soon as *Z*. travailed, she. 66:8
I will bring you to *Z*. *Jer* 3:14
set up the standard toward *Z*. 4:6
Judah? thy soul lothed *Z*. 14:19
Z. shall be plowed like a field. 26:18; *Mi* 3:12
this is *Z*. whom no man. *Jer* 30:17
arise ye, and let us go up to *Z*. 31:6
and sing in the height of *Z*. 12
they shall ask the way to *Z*. 50:5
shall the inhabitant of *Z*. say. 51:35
the ways of *Z*. do mourn. *Lam* 1:4
Z. spreadeth forth her hands, and. 17
the precious sons of *Z*. 4:2
because the mountain of *Z*. 5:18
be glad, ye children of *Z*. *Joel* 2:23
Lord will roar from *Z*. *Amos* 1:2
they build up *Z*. with. *Mi* 3:10
for the law shall go forth of *Z*. 4:2
say, Let our eye look upon *Z*. 11
I am jealous for *Z*. *Zech* 1:14
The Lord shall yet comfort *Z*. 17
deliver thyself, O *Z*. 2:7
jealous for *Z*. 8:2
Lord, I am returned to *Z*. 3
raised up thy sons, O *Z*. 9:13
see **daughter, daughters**

in **Zion**

praises to the Lord, who dwelleth *in Z*. *Ps* 9:11; 76:2; *Joel* 3:21
praise waiteth for thee, O God, *in Z*. *Ps* 65:1
every one *in Z*. appeareth. 84:7
Lord is great *in Z*.; he is high. 99:2
name of the Lord *in Z*. 102:21
that is left *in Z*. shall be. *Isa* 4:3
my people that dwellest *in Z*. 10:24
I lay *in Z*. for a foundation a stone, a tried stone. 28:16; *1 Pet* 2:6
people shall dwell *in Z*. *Isa* 30:19
the Lord, whose fire is *in Z*. 31:9
the sinners *in Z*. are afraid. 33:14
I will place salvation *in Z*. 46:13
unto them that mourn *in Z*. 61:3
is not Lord *in Z*.? is not? *Jer* 8:19
declare *in Z*. the vengeance. 50:28
let us declare *in Z*. the work. 51:10
that they have done *in Z*. 24
sabbaths be forgotten *in Z*. *Lam* 2:6
hath kindled a fire *in Z*. 4:11
they ravished the women *in Z*. 5:11
blow ye the trumpet *in Z*. and sound. *Joel* 2:1, 15
your God dwelling *in Z*. 3:17
that are at ease *in Z*. *Amos* 6:1
behold, I lay *in Z*. a. *Rom* 9:33

mount **Zion**

a remnant, they that escape out of *mount Z*. *2 Ki* 19:31; *Isa* 37:32
joy of whole earth *mount Z*. *Ps* 48:2
let *mount Z*. rejoice. 11
this *mount Z*. wherein thou. 74:2
the *mount Z*. which he loved. 78:68
as *mount Z*. which cannot be. 125:1
of *mount Z*. a cloud. *Isa* 4:5
dwelleth in *mount Z*. 8:18; 18:7
his work upon *mount Z*. 10:12
shall reign in *mount Z*. 24:23
fight against *mount Z*. 29:8
fight for *mount Z*. 31:4
in *mount Z*. shall be deliverance. *Joel* 2:32; *Ob* 17
come up on *mount Z*. *Ob* 21
reign over them in *mount Z*. *Mi* 4:7
are come unto *mount Z*. *Heb* 12:22
lo, a Lamb stood on the *mount Z*. *Rev* 14:1

out of **Zion**

Oh that the salvation of Israel were come *out of Z*.! *Ps* 14:7; 53:6
the Lord strengthen thee *out of Z*. 20:2; 110:2
bless thee *out of Z*. 128:5; 134:3
blessed be the Lord *out of Z*. 135:21
for *out of Z*. shall go. *Isa* 2:3
wailing is heard *out of Z*. *Jer* 9:19
shall roar *out of Z*. *Joel* 3:16
shall come *out of Z*. *Rom* 11:26

Zippor, *see* Balak

Zipporah

Jethro gave Moses *Z*. *Ex* 2:21
Z. took a sharp stone. 4:25
Jethro took *Z*. 18:2

Zoan

seven years before *Z*. *Num* 13:22
things did he in *Z*. *Ps* 78:12, 43
princes of *Z*. are fools. *Isa* 19:11, 13
for his princes were at *Z*. 30:4
I will set fire in *Z*. and. *Ezek* 30:14

Zoar

of Bela, which is *Z*. *Gen* 14:2, 8
the city was called *Z*. 19:22
city of palm trees to *Z*. *Deut* 34:3
fugitives shall flee unto *Z*. *Isa* 15:5
their voice from *Z*. *Jer* 48:34

Zobah

against the kings of *Z*. *1 Sam* 14:47
Hadadezer the king of *Z*. *2 Sam* 8:3
1 Ki 11:24; *1 Chr* 18:3, 9
Igal son of Nathan of *Z*. *2 Sam* 23:36
fled from the king of *Z*. *1 Ki* 11:23

Zophar

Z. the Naamathite. *Job* 2:11; 11:1
20:1; 42:9

Zorah

coast of inheritance of Dan, was *Z*. *Josh* 19:41
man of *Z*. named Manoah. *Judg* 13:2
Spirit moved Samson between *Z*. 25
buried Samson between *Z*. 16:31
the Danites sent from *Z*. 18:2
unto their brethren to *Z*. 8
Rehoboam built *Z*. and. *2 Chr* 11:10

Zorobabel

Salathiel begat *Z*. *Mat* 1:12
Z. begat Abiud. 13
Rhesa the son of *Z*. *Luke* 3:27

Zuar, *see* Nathanael

Zur

Cozbi the daughter of *Z*. *Num* 25:15
Z. a prince of Midian slain. 31:8
Josh 13:21
Z. the son of. *1 Chr* 8:30; 9:36

Zurishaddai, *see* Shelumiel

Zuzims

the kings smote the *Z*. *Gen* 14:5

APPENDIX

A List of Proper Names, seldom mentioned in Scripture, and not included in the body of the Concordance

ABDIEL. *1 Chr* 5:15
Abelshittim. *Num* 33:49
Abez. *Josh* 19:20
Abi. *2 Ki* 18:2
Abiasaph. *Ex* 6:24
Abida. *Gen* 25:4; *1 Chr* 1:33
Abiel. (1) *1 Sam* 9:1; 14:51. (2) *1 Chr* 11:32
Abihud. *1 Chr* 8:3
Abilene. *Luke* 3:1
Abimael. *Gen* 10:26-28; *1 Chr* 1:20-22
Abishalom. *1 Ki* 15:2, 10
Abishua. (1) *1 Chr* 6:4, 5, 50; *Ezra* 7:5. (2) *1 Chr* 8:4
Abishur. *1 Chr* 2:28, 29
Abital. *2 Sam* 3:4; *1 Chr* 3:3
Abitub. *1 Chr* 8:11
Accad. *Gen* 10:10
Achaz (Ahaz). *Mat* 1:9
Achbor. (1) *Gen* 36:38, 39; *1 Chr* 1:49. (2) *2 Ki* 22:12, 14. (3) *Jer* 26:22; 36:12
Adadah. *Josh* 15:21, 22
Adah. (1) *Gen* 4:19, 20, 23. (2) *Gen* 36:2, 4, 10, 12, 16
Adaiah. (1) *2 Ki* 22:1. (2) *1 Chr* 6:41. (3) *1 Chr* 8:12-21. (4) *1 Chr* 9:10-12; *Neh* 11:12. (5) *2 Chr* 23:1. (6) *Ezra* 10:29. (7) *Ezra* 10:34-39. (8) *Neh* 11:5
Adalia. *Esth* 9:8
Adamah. *Josh* 19:35, 36
Adami. *Josh* 19:33
Adbeel. *Gen* 25:13; *1 Chr* 1:29
Addan (Addon). *Ezra* 2:59; *Neh* 7:61
Addar. (1) *Josh* 15:3. (2) *1 Chr* 8:3
Ader. *1 Chr* 8:15
Adiel. (1) *1 Chr* 4:36. (2) *1 Chr* 9:12. (3) *1 Chr* 27:25
Adin. (1) *Ezra* 2:15; *Neh* 7:20. (2) *Ezra* 8:6. (3) *Neh* 10:14-16
Adina. *1 Chr* 11:42
Adino. *2 Sam* 23:8
Adithaim. *Josh* 15:33-36
Adlai. *1 Chr* 27:29
Admatha. *Esth* 1:14
Adna. (1) *Ezra* 10:30. (2) *Neh* 12:12-15
Adnah. (1) *1 Chr* 12:20. (2) *2 Chr* 17:14
Adoniram. *1 Ki* 4:6; 5:14
Adonizedek. *Josh* 10:1, 3
Adoraim. *2 Chr* 11:5-9
Adoram. (1) *2 Sam* 20:24. (2) *1 Ki* 12:18
Aeneas. *Acts* 9:33, 34
Aenon. *John* 3:23
Aharah. *1 Chr* 8:1
Aharhel. *1 Chr* 4:8
Ahasai. *Neh* 11:13
Ahasbai. *2 Sam* 23:34
Ahban. *1 Chr* 2:29
Aher. *1 Chr* 7:12
Ahi. (1) *1 Chr* 5:15. (2) *1 Chr* 7:34
Ahiam. *2 Sam* 23:33; *1 Chr* 11:35
Ahian. *1 Chr* 7:19
Ahiezer. (1) *Num* 1:12; 2:25; 7:66, 71; 10:25. (2) *1 Chr* 12:3
Ahihud. (1) *Num* 34:27. (2) *1 Chr* 8:7
Ahilud. *2 Sam* 8:16; 20:24; *1 Ki* 4:3, 12; *1 Chr* 18:15
Ahimoth. *1 Chr* 6:25
Ahinadab. *1 Ki* 4:14
Ahira. *Num* 1:15; 2:29; 7:78, 83; 10:27
Ahiram. *Num* 26:38
Ahishahar. *1 Chr* 7:10
Ahishar. *1 Ki* 4:6
Ahlab. *Judg* 1:31
Ahlai. (1) *1 Chr* 2:31. (2) *1 Chr* 11:41
Ahoah. *1 Chr* 8:4
Ahumai. *1 Chr* 4:2
Ahuzam. *1 Chr* 4:6
Ahuzzath. *Gen* 26:26
Aiah, Ajah. (1) *Gen* 36:24; *1 Chr* 1:40. (2) *2 Sam* 3:7; 21:8, 10, 11
Aija. *Neh* 11:31
Aijalon, Ajalon. (1) *Josh* 19:42; 21:24; *Judg* 1:35. (2) *Judg* 12:12. (3) *1 Sam* 14:31; *1 Chr* 8:13; *2 Chr* 11:10; 28:18. (4) *1 Chr* 6:69
Aijeleth Shahar. *Ps* 22 title
Akan (Jakan). *Gen* 36:27; *1 Chr* 1:42
Akkub. (1) *1 Chr* 3:24. (2) *1 Chr* 9:17; *Neh* 11:19; 12:25. (3) *Ezra* 2:42; *Neh* 7:45. (4) *Ezra* 2:45. (5) *Neh* 8:7
Akrabbim. *Num* 34:4; *Josh* 15:3
Alameth. *1 Chr* 7:8
Alammelech. *Josh* 19:26
Alamoth. *1 Chr* 15:20; *Ps* 46 title
Alemeth. (1) *1 Chr* 6:60. (2) *1 Chr* 8:36; 9:42
Aliah (Alva). *Gen* 36:40; *1 Chr* 1:51
Alian (Alvan). *Gen* 36:23; *1 Chr* 1:40
Allon. (1) *Josh* 19:33. (2) *1 Chr* 4:37
Allon Bachuth. *Gen* 35:8
Almodad. *Gen* 10:26; *1 Chr* 1:20
Almon. *Josh* 21:18
Almon-Diblathaim. *Num* 33:46, 47
Aloth. *1 Ki* 4:16
Altaschith. *Ps* 57 title; 58 title; 59 title; 75 title
Alvan. *See* Alian
Amad. *Josh* 19:26
Amal. *1 Chr* 7:35
Amam. *Josh* 15:26
Amariah. (1) *1 Chr* 6:7, 52; *Ezra* 7:3. (2) *1 Chr* 6:11. (3) *1 Chr* 23:19; 24:23. (4) *2 Chr* 19:11. (5) *2 Chr* 31:15. (6) *Ezra* 10:42 (7) *Neh* 10:3; 12:2, 13. (8) *Neh* 11:4. (9) *Zeph* 1:1
Amasai. (1) *1 Chr* 6:25, 35; *2 Chr* 29:12. (2) *1 Chr* 12:18. (3) *1 Chr* 15:24
Amashai. *Neh* 11:13
Amasiah. *2 Chr* 17:16
Ami. *Ezra* 2:57
Amittai. *2 Ki* 14:25; *Jonah* 1:1
Ammiel. (1) *Num* 13:12. (2) *2 Sam* 9:4, 5; 17:27. (3) *1 Chr* 3:5. (4) *1 Chr* 26:5
Ammihud. (1) *Num* 1:10; 2:18; 7:48, 53; 10:22; *1 Chr* 7:26. (2) *Num* 34:20. (3) *Num* 34:28. (4) *2 Sam* 13:37. (5) *1 Chr* 9:4
Ammihur. *2 Sam* 13:37
Ammishaddai. *Num* 1:12; 2:25; 7:66, 71; 10:25
Ammizabad. *1 Chr* 27:6
Amok. *Neh* 12:7, 20
Amraphel. *Gen* 14:1, 9
Amzi. (1) *1 Chr* 6:46. (2) *Neh* 11:12
Anab. *Josh* 11:21; 15:50
Anaharath. *Josh* 19:19
Anaiah. (1) *Neh* 8:4. (2) *Neh* 10:22
Anamim. *Gen* 10:13; *1 Chr* 1:11
Anan. *Neh* 10:26
Anani. *1 Chr* 3:24
Ananiah. *Neh* 3:23
Anath. *Judg* 3:31; 5:6
Anem. *1 Chr* 6:73
Aniam. *1 Chr* 7:19
Anim. *Josh* 15:50
Antothijah. *1 Chr* 8:24
Anub. *1 Chr* 4:8
Aphekah. *Josh* 15:53
Aphiah. *1 Sam* 9:1
Aphik. *Josh* 13:4; 19:30; *Judg* 1:31
Aphrah. *Mi* 1:10
Aphses. *1 Chr* 24:15
Appaim. *1 Chr* 2:30, 31
Apphia. *Philem* 2
Ara. *1 Chr* 7:38
Arabah. *Josh* 18:18
Arad. (1) *Num* 21:1; 33:40. (2) *1 Chr* 8:15. (3) *Josh* 12:14. *Judg* 1:16
Arah. (1) *1 Chr* 7:39. (2) *Ezra* 2:5; *Neh* 7:10. (3) *Neh* 6:18
Aramnaharaim. *Ps* 60 title
Aramzobah. *Ps* 60 title
Aran. *Gen* 36:28; *1 Chr* 1:42
Archi. *Josh* 16:2
Ard. (1) *Gen* 46:21. (2) *Num* 26:40
Ardon. *1 Chr* 2:18
Areli. *Gen* 46:16; *Num* 26:17
Aridai. *Esth* 9:9
Aridatha. *Esth* 9:8
Arieh. *2 Ki* 15:25
Arisai. *Esth* 9:9
Armoni. *2 Sam* 21:8
Arnan. *1 Chr* 3:21
Arod. *Num* 26:17
Arodi. *Gen* 46:16
Aruboth. *1 Ki* 4:10
Arumah. *Judg* 9:41
Arvad. *Ezek* 27:8, 11
Arza. *1 Ki* 16:9
Asareel. *1 Chr* 4:16
Asarelah. *1 Chr* 25:2
Aser. *Luke* 2:36; *Rev* 7:6

Ashan. Josh 15:42; 19:7; 1 Chr 4:32; 6:59
Ashbea. 1 Chr 4:21
Ashbel. Gen 46:21; Num 26:38; 1 Chr 8:1
Ashdoth Pisgah. Deut 3:17; 4:49; Josh 12:3; 13:20
Ashima. 2 Ki 17:30
Ashkenaz. (1) Gen 10:3; 1 Chr 1:6. (2) Jer 51:27
Ashnah. (1) Josh 15:33. (2) Josh 15:43
Ashpenaz. Dan 1:3
Ashteroth Karnaim. Gen 14:5
Ashvath. 1 Chr 7:33
Asiel. 1 Chr 4:35
Asnah. Ezra 2:50
Aspatha. Esth 9:7
Asriel. (1) Num 26:31; Josh 17:2. (2) 1 Chr 7:14
Asshurim. Gen 25:3
Assir. (1) Ex 6:24; 1 Chr 6:22. (2) 1 Chr 6:23, 37. (3) 1 Chr 3:17
Assos. Acts 20:13, 14
Asuppim. 1 Chr 26:15, 17
Atarah. 1 Chr 2:26
Ataroth. (1) Num 32:3, 34. (2) Josh 16:5. (3) Josh 16:2, 7. (4) 1 Chr 2:54. (5) Num 32:35
Ater. (1) Ezra 2:16; Neh 7:21. (2) Ezra 2:42; Neh 7:45. (3) Neh 10:17
Athaiah. Neh 11:4
Athlai. Ezra 10:28
Attai. (1) 1 Chr 2:35, 36. (2) 1 Chr 12:11. (3) 2 Chr 11:20
Ava. 2 Ki 17:24
Avim. (1) Deut 2:23; Josh 13:3. (2) Josh 18:23
Avith. Gen 36:35; 1 Chr 1:46
Azal. Zech 14:5
Azaliah. 2 Ki 22:3; 2 Chr 34:8
Azaniah. Neh 10:9
Azareel. (1) 1 Chr 12:6. (2) 1 Chr 25:18. (3) 1 Chr 27:22. (4) Ezra 10:41. (5) Neh 11:13; 12:36
Azaz. 1 Chr 5:8
Azaziah. (1) 1 Chr 15:21. (2) 1 Chr 27:20. (3) 2 Chr 31:13
Azbuk. Neh 3:16
Azel. 1 Chr 8:37, 38; 9:43, 44
Azem. Josh 15:29; 19:3; 1 Chr 4:29
Azgad. (1) Ezra 2:12; Neh 7:17. (2) Ezra 8:12. (3) Neh 10:15
Aziel. 1 Chr 15:20
Aziza. Ezra 10:27
Azmaveth. (1) 2 Sam 23:31; 1 Chr 11:33. (2) 1 Chr 8:36; 9:42. (3) 1 Chr 12:3. (4) Ezra 2:24; Neh 12:29. (5) 1 Chr 27:25
Azmon. Num 34:4, 5; Josh 15:4
Aznoth Tabor. Josh 19:34
Azor. Mat 1:13, 14
Azotus. Acts 8:40
Azriel. (1) 1 Chr 5:24. (2) 1 Chr 27:19. (3) Jer 36:26
Azrikam. (1) 1 Chr 3:23. (2) 1 Chr 8:38; 9:44. (3) 1 Chr 9:14; Neh 11:15. (4) 2 Chr 28:7
Azubah. (1) 1 Ki 22:42; 2 Chr 20:31. (2) 1 Chr 2:18, 19
Azur (Azzur). (1) Neh 10:17. (2) Jer 28:1. (3) Ezek 11:1
Azzah. Deut 2:23; 1 Ki 4:24; Jer 25:20
Azzan. Num 34:26

BAALAH. Josh 15:9
Baalath. Josh 19:44; 1 Ki 9:18; 2 Chr 8:6
Baalath-beer. Josh 19:8
Baale. 2 Sam 6:2
Baal-gad. Josh 11:17; 12:7; 13:5
Baal-hanan. (1) Gen 36:38, 39; 1 Chr 1:49, 50. (2) 1 Chr 27:28
Baal-hazor. 2 Sam 13:23
Baal-hermon. Judg 3:3; 1 Chr 5:23
Baara. 1 Chr 8:8
Baaseiah. 1 Chr 6:40
Bakbakkar. 1 Chr 9:15
Bakbuk. Ezra 2:51; Neh 7:53
Bakbukiah. Neh 11:17; 12:9, 25
Bamoth. Num 21:19, 20
Bamoth-baal. Josh 13:17
Bani. (1) 2 Sam 23:36. (2) 1 Chr 6:46. (3) 1 Chr 9:4. (4) Ezra 2:10; 10:29. (5) Ezra 10:34. (6) Ezra 10:38. (7) Neh 3:17; 8:7; 9:4, 5. (8) Neh 9:4; 10:13. (9) Neh 10:14. (10) Neh 11:22
Barachiah. Zech 1:1, 7
Bariah. 1 Chr 3:22
Barkos. Ezra 2:53; Neh 7:55
Bashan-havoth-jair. Deut 3:14
Basmath. 1 Ki 4:15
Bath-rabbim. S of S 7:4
Bathshua. 1 Chr 3:5
Bavai. Neh 3:18
Bazlith. Ezra 2:52; Neh 7:54
Bealiah. 1 Chr 12:5
Bealoth. Josh 15:24
Bebai. (1) Ezra 2:11; Neh 7:16. (2) Ezra 8:11; 10:28. (3) Neh 10:15
Bechorath. 1 Sam 9:1
Bedad. Gen 36:35; 1 Chr 1:46
Bedeiah. Ezra 10:35
Beeliada. 1 Chr 14:7
Beer. (1) Num 21:16. (2) Judg 9:21
Beera. 1 Chr 7:37
Beerah. 1 Chr 5:6
Beer-elim. Isa 15:8
Beeri. (1) Gen 26:34. (2) Hos 1:1
Beer-lahai-roi. Gen 16:14; 24:62; 25:11
Beeroth. (1) Deut 10:6. (2) Josh 9:17; 18:25; 2 Sam 4:2; Ezra 2:25; Neh 7:29
Beeshterah. Josh 21:27
Bela. (1) Gen 14:2, 8. (2) Gen 36:32, 33; 1 Chr 1:43, 44. (3) Gen 46:21; Num 26:38, 40; 1 Chr 7:6, 7; 8:1, 3. (4) 1 Chr 5:8
Ben. 1 Chr 15:18
Beneberak. Josh 19:45
Benejaakan. Num 33:31, 32
Benhail. 2 Chr 17:7
Benhanan. 1 Chr 4:20
Beninu. Neh 10:13
Beno. 1 Chr 24:26, 27
Benzoheth. 1 Chr 4:20
Beon. Num 32:3
Bera. Gen 14:2
Beraiah. 1 Chr 8:21
Berechiah. (1) 1 Chr 3:20. (2) 1 Chr 6:39; 15:17. (3) 1 Chr 9:16. (4) 1 Chr 15:23. (5) 2 Chr 28:12. (6) Neh 3:4, 30; 6:18
Bered. (1) Gen 16:14. (2) 1 Chr 7:20
Beri. 1 Chr 7:36
Beriah. (1) Gen 46:17; Num 26:44, 45; 1 Chr 7:30, 31. (2) 1 Chr 7:23. (3) 1 Chr 8:13, 16. (4) 1 Chr 23:10, 11
Berodach-baladan. See Merodach-baladan
Berothah. Ezek 47:16
Besai. Ezra 2:49; Neh 7:52
Besodeiah. Neh 3:6
Betah. 2 Sam 8:8
Beten. Josh 19:25
Bethanath. Josh 19:38; Judg 1:33
Bethanoth. Josh 15:59
Betharabah. Josh 15:6, 61; 18:22
Betharam. Josh 13:27
Betharbel. Hos 10:14
Bethazmaveth. Neh 7:28
Bethbaalmeon. Josh 13:17
Bethbarah. Judg 7:24
Bethbirei. 1 Chr 4:31
Bethcar. 1 Sam 7:11
Bethdagon. (1) Josh 15:41. (2) Josh 19:27
Bethemek. Josh 19:27
Bethgader. 1 Chr 2:51
Bethharan. Num 32:36
Bethhoglah. Josh 15:6; 18:19, 21
Bethjeshimoth. Num 33:49; Josh 12:3; 13:20; Ezek 25:9
Bethlebaoth. Josh 19:6
Bethmaachah. 2 Sam 20:14, 15, 18; 2 Ki 15:29
Bethmarcaboth. Josh 19:5; 1 Chr 4:31
Bethmeon. Jer 48:23
Bethnimrah. Num 32:36; Josh 13:27
Bethpalet. Josh 15:27; Neh 11:26
Bethpazzez. Josh 19:21
Bethrapha. 1 Chr 4:12
Bethrehob. Judg 18:28; 2 Sam 10:6
Bethshean. Josh 17:11, 16; Judg 1:27; 1 Ki 4:12; 1 Chr 7:29
Bethshittah. Judg 7:22
Bethtappuah. Josh 15:53
Bethul. Josh 19:4
Bethzur. (1) Josh 15:58; 2 Chr 11:7; Neh 3:16. (2) 1 Chr 2:45
Betonim. Josh 13:26
Bezai. (1) Ezra 2:17; Neh 7:23. (2) Neh 10:18
Bezer. (1) Deut 4:43; Josh 20:8; 21:36; 1 Chr 6:78. (2) 1 Chr 7:37
Bigtha. Esth 1:10
Bigvai. (1) Ezra 2:2; Neh 7:7. (2) Ezra 2:14; Neh 7:19. (3) Ezra 8:14. (4) Neh 10:16
Bileam. 1 Chr 6:70
Bilgah. (1) 1 Chr 24:14. (2) Neh 12:5, 18
Bilgai. Neh 10:8
Bilhan. (1) Gen 36:27; 1 Chr 1:42. (2) 1 Chr 7:10
Bilshan. Ezra 2:2; Neh 7:7
Bimhal. 1 Chr 7:33
Binea. 1 Chr 8:37; 9:43
Binnui. (1) Ezra 8:33. (2) Ezra 10:30. (3) Ezra 10:38. (4) Neh 3:24; 10:9. (5) Neh 7:15. (6) Neh 12:8
Birsha. Gen 14:2
Birzavith. 1 Chr 7:31
Bishlam. Ezra 4:7
Bithiah. 1 Chr 4:18
Bithron. 2 Sam 2:29
Bizjothjah. Josh 15:28
Biztha. Esth 1:10
Bocheru. 1 Chr 8:38; 9:44
Bohan. Josh 15:6; 18:17
Bozez. 1 Sam 14:4
Bozkath. Josh 15:39; 2 Ki 22:1
Bunah. 1 Chr 2:25
Bunni. (1) Neh 9:4. (2) Neh 11:15. (3) Neh 10:15

CALAH. Gen 10:11, 12
Calcol. 1 Chr 2:6
Canneh. Ezek 27:23
Caphtorim. Gen 10:14; Deut 2:23; 1 Chr 1:12
Carcas. Esth 1:10
Careah. 2 Ki 25:23
Carshena. Esth 1:14
Casluhim. Gen 10:14; 1 Chr 1:12
Chanaan (see Canaan). Acts 7:11; 13:19
Chedorlaomer. Gen 14:1, 4, 5, 9, 17
Chelal. Ezra 10:30
Chellub. (1) 1 Chr 4:11. (2) 1 Chr 27:26
Chelluh. Ezra 10:35
Chelubai. 1 Chr 2:9
Chenaanah. (1) 1 Ki 22:11, 24; 2 Chr. 18:10, 23. (2) 1 Chr 7:10
Chenani. Neh 9:4
Chephar-haammonia. Josh 18:24
Chephirah. Josh 9:17; 18:26; Ezra 2:25; Neh 7:29
Cheran. Gen 36:26; 1 Chr 1:41
Chesalon. Josh 15:10
Chesed. Gen 22:22
Chesil. Josh 15:30
Chesulloth. Josh 19:18
Chezib. Gen 38:5
Chidon. 1 Chr 13:9
Chinnereth. Num 34:11; Deut 3:17; Josh 11:2; 12:3; 13:27; 19:35; 1 Ki 15:20
Chislon. Num 34:21
Chisloth-tabor. Josh 19:12
Chorashan. 1 Sam 30:30
Chozeba. 1 Chr 4:22
Chub. Ezek 30:5
Chun. 1 Chr 18:8

Cinneroth. *1 Ki* 15:20
Clauda. *Acts* 27:16
Claudia. *2 Tim* 4:21
Claudius. (1) *Acts* 11:28; 18:2. (2) *Acts* 23:26
Clement. *Phil* 4:3
Cnidus. *Acts* 27:7
Colhozeh. (1) *Neh* 3:15. (2) *Neh* 11:5
Conaniah (Cononiah). (1) *2 Chr* 31:12; 31:13. (2) *2 Chr* 35:9
Coos. *Acts* 21:1
Core. *Jude* 11
Cosam. *Luke* 3:28
Coz. *1 Chr* 4:8
Cuthah or Cuth. *2 Ki* 17:24, 30

DABAREH. *Josh* 21:28
Dalaiah. *1 Chr* 3:24
Dalphon. *Esth* 9:7
Danjaan. *2 Sam* 24:6
Dannah. *Josh* 15:49
Dara. *1 Chr* 2:6
Darda. *1 Ki* 4:31
Debir. (1) *Josh* 10:3. (2) *Josh* 10:38, 39; 11:21; 12:13; 15:7, 15, 49; 21:15; *Judg* 1:11; *1 Chr* 6:58. (3) *Josh* 13:26
Dekar. *1 Ki* 4:9
Delaiah. (1) *1 Chr* 24:18. (2) *Ezra* 2:60; *Neh* 7:62. (3) *Neh* 6:10. (4) *Jer* 36:12, 25
Derbe. *Acts* 14:6, 20; 16:1; 20:4
Deuel. *Num* 1:14; 2:14; 7:42, 47; *Deut* 10:20
Diblaim. *Hos* 1:3
Diblath. *Ezek* 6:14
Dibri. *Lev* 24:11
Diklah. *Gen* 10:27; *1 Chr* 1:21
Dilean. *Josh* 15:38
Dimnah. *Josh* 21:35
Dimonah. *Josh* 15:22
Dinhabah. *Gen* 36:32; *1 Chr* 1:43
Dishan. *Gen* 36:21, 28, 30; *1 Chr* 1:38, 42
Dishon. (1) *Gen* 36:21, 26, 30; *1 Chr* 1:38. (2) *Gen* 36:25; *1 Chr* 1:38, 41
Dizahab. *Deut* 1:1
Dodai. *1 Chr* 27:4
Dodanim. *Gen* 10:4; *1 Chr* 1:7
Dodavah. *2 Chr* 20:37
Dodo. (1) *Judg* 10:1. (2) *2 Sam* 23:9; *1 Chr* 11:12. (3) *2 Sam* 23:24; *1 Chr* 11:26
Dophkah. *Num* 33:12, 13

EBIASAPH. *1 Chr* 6:23, 37; 9:19
Ebronah. *Num* 33:34
Eder. (1) *Gen* 35:21. (2) *Josh* 15:21. (3) *1 Chr* 23:23; 24:30
Edrei. (1) *Num* 21:33; *Deut* 1:4; 3:1, 10; *Josh* 12:4; 13:12, 31. (2) *Josh* 19:37
Ehi. *Gen* 46:21
Eker. *1 Chr* 2:27
Eladah. *1 Chr* 7:20
Elasah. (1) *Ezra* 10:22. (2) *Jer* 29:3
Eldaah. *Gen* 25:4; *1 Chr* 1:33
Elead. *1 Chr* 7:21
Eleph. *Josh* 18:28
Eliadah. *1 Ki* 11:23
Eliah. (1) *1 Chr* 8:27. (2) *Ezra* 10:26
Eliahba. *2 Sam* 23:32; *1 Chr* 11:33
Eliasaph. (1) *Num* 1:14; 2:14; 7:42, 47; 10:20. (2) *Num* 3:24
Eliathah. *1 Chr* 25:4, 27
Elidad. *Num* 34:21
Eliel. (1) *1 Chr* 6:34. (2) *1 Chr* 5:24. (3) *1 Chr* 8:20. (4) *1 Chr* 8:22. (5) *1 Chr* 11:46. (6) *1 Chr* 11:47. (7) *1 Chr* 12:11. (8) *1 Chr* 15:9. (9) *1 Chr* 15:11. (10) *2 Chr* 31:13
Elienai. *1 Chr* 8:20
Elika. *2 Sam* 23:25
Elioenai. (1) *1 Chr* 3:23, 24. (2) *1 Chr* 4:36. (3) *1 Chr* 7:8. (4) *Ezra* 10:22. (5) *Ezra* 10:27. (6) *Neh* 12:41. (7) *1 Chr* 26:3 (8) *Ezra* 8:4
Eliphal. *1 Chr* 11:35
Elipheleh. *1 Chr* 15:18, 21
Elishaphat. *2 Chr* 23:1
Elizaphan. (1) *Num* 3:30; *1 Chr* 15:8 (2) *Num* 34:25 (3) *2 Chr* 29:13
Elizur. *Num* 1:5; 2:10; 7:30, 35; 10:18
Ellasar. *Gen* 14:1, 9
Elnaam. *1 Chr* 11:46
Eloi. *Mark* 15:34
Elon-beth-hanan. *1 Ki* 4:9
Eloth. *1 Ki* 9:26; *2 Chr* 8:17; 26:2
Elpaal. *1 Chr* 8:11, 12, 18
Elpalet. *1 Chr* 14:5
Elparan. *Gen* 14:6
Eltekeh. *Josh* 19:44; 21:23
Eltekon. *Josh* 15:59
Eltolad. *Josh* 15:30; 19:4
Eluzai. *1 Chr* 12:5
Elzabad. (1) *1 Chr* 12:12. (2) *1 Chr* 26:7
Elzaphan. (1) *Ex* 6:22; *Lev* 10:4. (2) *Num* 34:25
Enam. *Josh* 15:34
Enan. *Num* 1:15; 2:29; 7:78, 83; 10:27
Engannim. (1) *Josh* 15:34. (2) *Josh* 19:21; 21:29
Enhaddah. *Josh* 19:21
Enhakkore. *Judg* 15:19
Enhazor. *Josh* 19:37
Enmishpat. *Gen* 14:7
Enrimmon. *Neh* 11:29
Enshemesh. *Josh* 15:7; 18:17
Entappuah. *Josh* 17:7
Ephai. *Jer* 40:8
Epher. (1) *Gen* 25:4; *1 Chr* 1:33. (2) *1 Chr* 4:17. (3) *1 Chr* 5:24
Ephlal. *1 Chr* 2:37
Ephod. *Num* 34:23
Eran. *Num* 26:36
Erech. *Gen* 10:10
Eri. *Gen* 46:16; *Num* 26:16
Eshbaal. *1 Chr* 8:33; 9:39
Eshban. *Gen* 36:26; *1 Chr* 1:41
Eshean. *Josh* 15:52
Eshek. *1 Chr* 8:39
Eshtaol. *Josh* 15:33; 19:41; *Judg* 13:25; 16:31; 18:2, 8, 11
Eshtemoa. (1) *Josh* 15:50; 21:14; *1 Sam* 30:28; *1 Chr* 6:57. (2) *1 Chr* 4:17, 19
Eshton. *1 Chr* 4:11, 12
Ethbaal. *1 Ki* 16:31
Ether. *Josh* 15:42; 19:7
Ethnan. *1 Chr* 4:7
Ethni. *1 Chr* 6:41
Evi. *Num* 31:8; *Josh* 13:21
Ezar. *1 Chr* 1:38
Ezbai. *1 Chr* 11:37
Ezbon. (1) *Gen* 46:16. (2) *1 Chr* 7:7
Ezekias. *Mat* 1:9, 10
Ezem. *1 Chr* 4:29
Ezer. (1) *1 Chr* 7:21. (2) *Neh* 12:42. (3) *1 Chr* 4:4. (4) *1 Chr* 12:9. (5) *Neh* 3:19. (6) *Gen* 36:21, 27, 30; *1 Chr* 1:38, 42
Ezion-gaber (Ezion-geber). *Num* 33:35, 36; *Deut* 2:8; *1 Ki* 9:26; 22:48; *2 Chr* 8:17; 20:36
Ezri. *1 Chr* 27:26

GAASH. *Josh* 24:30; *Judg* 2:9; *2 Sam* 23:30; *1 Chr* 11:32
Gaba. *Josh* 18:24; *Ezra* 2:26; *Neh* 7:30
Gabbai. *Neh* 11:8
Gaddi. *Num* 13:11
Gaddiel. *Num* 13:10
Gadi. *2 Ki* 15:14, 17
Gaham. *Gen* 22:24
Gahar. *Ezra* 2:47; *Neh* 7:49
Galal. (1) *1 Chr* 9:15. (2) *1 Chr* 9:16; *Neh* 11:17
Gamul. *1 Chr* 24:17
Gareb. (1) *2 Sam* 23:38; *1 Chr* 11:40. (2) *Jer* 31:39.
Gashmu. *Neh* 6:6
Gatam. *Gen* 36:11, 16; *1 Chr* 1:36
Gath-hepher. *2 Ki* 14:25
Gath-rimmon. (1) *Josh* 19:45. (2) *Josh* 21:25; *1 Chr* 6:69
Gazez. (1) *1 Chr* 2:46. (2) *1 Chr* 2:46
Gazzam. *Ezra* 2:48; *Neh* 7:51
Geber. (1) *1 Ki* 4:13. (2) *1 Ki* 4:19
Geder. *Josh* 12:13
Gederah. *Josh* 15:36
Gederoth. *Josh* 15:41; *2 Chr* 28:18
Gederothaim. *Josh* 15:36
Gedor. (1) *Josh* 15:58. (2) *1 Chr* 12:7. (3) *1 Chr* 8:31; 9:37. (4) *1 Chr* 4:4, 18. (5) *1 Chr* 4:39
Geliloth. *Josh* 18:17
Gemalli. *Num* 13:12
Genubath. *1 Ki* 11:20
Gesham. *1 Chr* 2:47
Geshem. *Neh* 2:19; 6:1, 2
Gether. *Gen* 10:23; *1 Chr* 1:17
Geuel. *Num* 13:15
Gezer. *Josh* 10:33; 12:12; 16:3, 10; 21:21; *Judg* 1:29; *1 Ki* 9:15, 16, 17; *1 Chr* 6:67; 7:28; 20:4
Gibbar. *Ezra* 2:20
Gibethon. *Josh* 19:44; 21:23; *1 Ki* 15:27; 16:15, 17
Gibea. *1 Chr* 2:49
Giddalti. *1 Chr* 25:4, 29
Giddel. (1) *Ezra* 2:47; *Neh* 7:49. (2) *Ezra* 2:56; *Neh* 7:58.
Gidom. *Judg* 20:45
Gilalia. *Neh* 12:36
Giloh. *Josh* 15:51; *2 Sam* 15:12
Gimzo. *2 Chr* 28:18
Ginath. *1 Ki* 16:21, 22
Ginnethon. *Neh* 10:6; 12:4, 16
Gispa. *Neh* 11:21
Gittah-hepher. *Josh* 19:13
Gittaim. (1) *2 Sam* 4:3. (2) *Neh* 11:33
Goath. *Jer* 31:39
Gudgodah. *Deut* 10:7
Guni. (1) *Gen* 46:24; *Num* 26:48; *1 Chr* 7:13. (2) *1 Chr* 5:15
Gurbaal. *2 Chr* 26:7

HAAHASHTARI. *1 Chr* 4:6
Habaiah. *Ezra* 2:61; *Neh* 7:63
Habakkuk. *Hab* 1:1; 3:1
Habaziniah. *Jer* 35:3
Habor. *2 Ki* 17:6; 18:11; *1 Chr* 5:26
Hachaliah. *Neh* 1:1; 10:1
Hachmoni. *1 Chr* 27:32
Hadad. (1) *Gen* 36:35, 36; *1 Chr* 1:46, 47. (2) *1 Ki* 11:14, 17, 19, 21, 25. (3) *1 Chr* 1:30. (4) *1 Chr* 1:50, 51
Hadar. (1) *Gen* 25:15. (2) *Gen* 36:39
Hadashah. *Josh* 15:37
Hadattah. *Josh* 15:25
Hadid. *Ezra* 2:33; *Neh* 7:37; 11:34
Hadlai. *2 Chr* 28:12
Hagab. *Ezra* 2:46
Hagabah. *Ezra* 2:45; *Neh* 7:48
Haggeri. *1 Chr* 11:38
Haggi. *Gen* 46:16; *Num* 26:15
Haggiah. *1 Chr* 6:30
Hai. *Gen* 12:8; 13:3
Hakkatan. *Ezra* 8:12
Hakkoz. *1 Chr* 24:10
Hakupha. *Ezra* 2:51; *Neh* 7:53
Halah. *2 Ki* 17:6; 18:11; *1 Chr* 5:26
Halak. *Josh* 11:17; 12:7
Halhul. *Josh* 15:58
Hali. *Josh* 19:25
Halohesh. (1) *Neh* 3:12. (2) *Neh* 10:24
Hamath-zobah. *2 Chr* 8:3
Hammath. *Josh* 19:35
Hammelech. *Jer* 36:26; 38:6
Hammoleketh. *1 Chr* 7:18
Hammon. (1) *Josh* 19:28. (2) *1 Chr* 6:76
Hammoth-dor. *Josh* 21:32
Hamonah. *Ezek* 39:16
Hamuel. *1 Chr* 4:26
Hamul. *Gen* 46:12; *Num* 26:21; *1 Chr* 2:5
Hamutal. *2 Ki* 23:31; 24:18; *Jer* 52:1

Hanan. (1) *1 Chr* 8:23. (2) *1 Chr* 8:38; 9:44. (3) *1 Chr* 11:43. (4) *Ezra* 2:46; *Neh* 7:49. (5) *Neh* 8:7. (6) *Neh* 10:10; 13:13. (7) *Neh* 10:22. (8) *Neh* 10:26. (9) *Jer* 35:4
Hanes. *Isa* 30:4
Hannathon. *Josh* 19:14
Hanniel. (1) *Num* 34:23. (2) *1 Chr* 7:39
Haphraim. *Josh* 19:19
Haradah. *Num* 33:24, 25
Hareph. *1 Chr* 2:51
Hareth. *1 Sam* 22:5
Harhaiah. *Neh* 3:8
Harhas. *2 Ki* 22:14
Harhur. *Ezra* 2:51; *Neh* 7:53
Harim. (1) *1 Chr* 24:8; *Ezra* 2:39; 10:21; *Neh* 3:11; 7:42. (2) *Ezra* 2:32; *Neh* 7:35. (3) *Ezra* 10:31. (4) *Neh* 10:5. (5) *Neh* 10:27. (6) *Neh* 12:15
Hariph. (1) *Neh* 7:24. (2) *Neh* 10:19
Harnepher. *1 Chr* 7:36
Haroeh. *1 Chr* 2:52
Harsha. *Ezra* 2:52; *Neh* 7:54
Harum. *1 Chr* 4:8
Harumaph. *Neh* 3:10
Haruz. *2 Ki* 21:19
Hasadiah. *1 Chr* 3:20
Hasenuah. *1 Chr* 9:7
Hashabiah. (1) *1 Chr* 6:45. (2) *1 Chr* 9:14. (3) *1 Chr* 25:3. (4) *1 Chr* 26:30. (5) *1 Chr* 27:17. (6) *2 Chr* 35:9. (7) *Ezra* 8:19. (8) *Ezra* 8:24. (9) *Neh* 3:17. (10) *Neh* 10:11. (11) *Neh* 11:15. (12) *Neh* 11:22. (13) *Neh* 12:21. (14) *Neh* 12:24
Hashbadana. *Neh* 8:4
Hashem. *1 Chr* 11:34
Hashmonah. *Num* 33:29, 30
Hashub. (1) *1 Chr* 9:14; *Neh* 11:15. (2) *Neh* 3:11. (3) *Neh* 3:23. (4) *Neh* 10:23
Hashubah. *1 Chr* 3:20
Hashum. (1) *Ezra* 2:19; 10:33; *Neh* 7:22. (2) *Neh* 8:4. (3) *Neh* 10:18
Hasrah. *2 Chr* 34:22
Hassenaah. *Neh* 3:3
Hasupha. *Ezra* 2:43; *Neh* 7:46
Hatach. *Esth* 4:5, 6, 9, 10
Hathath. *1 Chr* 4:13
Hatipha. *Ezra* 2:54; *Neh* 7:56
Hatita. *Ezra* 2:42; *Neh* 7:45
Hattil. *Ezra* 2:57; *Neh* 7:59
Hattush. (1) *1 Chr* 3:22. (2) *Ezra* 8:2; *Neh* 3:10; 10:4. (3) *Neh* 12:2
Hauran. *Ezek* 47:16, 18
Havilah. (1) *Gen* 10:7; *1 Chr* 1:9. (2) *Gen* 10:29; *1 Chr* 1:23. (3) *Gen* 2:11. (4) *Gen* 25:18; *1 Sam* 15:7
Havoth-jair. *Num* 32:41; *Deut* 3:14; *Judg* 10:4
Hazaiah. *Neh* 11:5
Hazar-addar. *Num* 34:4
Hazar-enan. *Num* 34:9, 10; *Ezek* 47:17; 48:1
Hazar-gaddah. *Josh* 15:27
Hazar-hatticon. *Ezek* 47:16
Hazarmaveth. *Gen* 10:26; *1 Chr* 1:20
Hazarshual. *Josh* 15:28; 19:3; *1 Chr* 4:28; *Neh* 11:27
Hazarsusah. *Josh* 19:5
Hazerim. *Deut* 2:23
Hazezon-tamar. *Gen* 14:7; *2 Chr* 20:2
Haziel. *1 Chr* 23:9
Hazo. *Gen* 22:22
Heber. (1) *1 Chr* 4:18. (2) *1 Chr* 5:13. (3) *1 Chr* 8:17. (4) *1 Chr* 8:22. (*See also* p. 296)
Helah. *1 Chr* 4:5, 7
Helbah. *Judg* 1:31
Heleb. *2 Sam* 23:29
Heled. *1 Chr* 11:30
Helek. *Num* 26:30; *Josh* 17:2
Helem. (1) *1 Chr* 7:35. (2) *Zech* 6:14
Heleph. *Josh* 19:33
Helez. (1) *2 Sam* 23:26; *1 Chr* 11:27; 27:10. (2) *1 Chr* 2:39
Helkai. *Neh* 12:15
Helkath. *Josh* 19:25; 21:31
Helon. *Num* 1:9; 2:7; 7:24, 29; 10:16
Hemam (Homam). *Gen* 36:22; *1 Chr* 1:39
Hemath. (1) *Amos* 6:14. (2) *1 Chr* 2:55
Hemdan. *Gen* 36:26
Hena. *2 Ki* 18:34; 19:13; *Isa* 37:13
Henadad. *Ezra* 3:9; *Neh* 3:18, 24; 10:9
Hepher. (1) *Num* 26:32; 27:1; *Josh* 17:2, 3. (2) *1 Chr* 4:6. (3) *1 Chr* 11:36. (4) *Josh* 12:17; *1 Ki* 4:10
Heres. *Judg* 1:35
Heresh. *1 Chr* 9:15
Hesed. *1 Ki* 4:10
Heshmon. *Josh* 15:27
Hethlon. *Ezek* 47:15; 48:
Hezeki. *1 Chr* 8:17
Hezion. *1 Ki* 15:18
Hezir. (1) *1 Chr* 24:15. (2) *Neh* 10:20
Hezrai. *2 Sam* 23:35
Hezro. *1 Chr* 11:37
Hiddai. *2 Sam* 23:30
Hierapolis. *Col.* 4:13
Hilen. *1 Chr* 6:58
Hillel. *Judg* 12:13, 15
Hirah. *Gen* 38:1, 12
Hizkiah. *Zeph* 1:1
Hizkijah. *Neh* 10:17
Hobah. *Gen* 14:15
Hod. *1 Chr* 7:37
Hodaiah. *1 Chr* 3:24
Hodaviah. (1) *1 Chr* 5:24. (2) *1 Chr* 9:7. (3) *Ezra* 2:40
Hodesh. *1 Chr* 8:9
Hodevah. *Neh* 7:43
Hodiah. (1) *1 Chr* 4:19. (2) *Neh* 8:7; 9:5; 10:10, 13. (3) *Neh* 10:18
Hoglah. *Num* 26:33; 27:1; 36:11; *Josh* 17:3
Hoham. *Josh* 10:3
Holon. (1) *Josh* 15:51; 21:15 (2) *Jer* 48:21
Homam. *1 Chr* 1:39
Horam. *Josh* 10:33
Horem. *Josh* 19:38
Hori. (1) *Gen* 36:22, 30; *1 Chr* 1:39. (2) *Num* 13:5
Horim. *Gen* 14:6; 36:20, 21, 29; *Deut* 2:12, 22
Hosah. (1) *Josh* 19:29. (2) *1 Chr* 16:38; 26:10, 11, 16
Hoshaiah. (1) *Neh* 12:32. (2) *Jer* 42:1; 43:2
Hoshama. *1 Chr* 3:18
Hotham. (1) *1 Chr* 7:32. (2) *1 Chr* 11:44
Hothir. *1 Chr* 25:4, 28
Hukkok. *Josh* 19:34
Hukok. *1 Chr* 6:75
Hul. *Gen* 10:23; *1 Chr* 1:17
Huldah. *2 Ki* 22:14; *2 Chr* 34:22
Humtah. *Josh* 15:54
Hupham. *Num* 26:39
Huppah. *1 Chr* 24:13
Huppim. *Gen* 46:21; *1 Chr* 7:12, 15
Huram. (1) *1 Chr* 8:5. (2) *2 Chr* 2:3, 11, 12. (3) *2 Chr* 4:11, 16
Hushah. *1 Chr* 4:4
Husham. *Gen* 36:34, 35; *1 Chr* 1:45, 46
Hushim. (1) *Gen* 46:23. (2) *1 Chr* 7:12. (3) *1 Chr* 8:8, 11
Huz. *Gen* 22:21

IBLEAM. *Josh* 17:11; *Judg* 1:27; *2 Ki* 9:27
Ibneiah. *1 Chr* 9:8
Ibnijah. *1 Chr* 9:8
Ibri. *1 Chr* 24:27
Ibzan. *Judg* 12:8, 10
Idalah. *Josh* 19:15
Idbash. *1 Chr* 4:3
Igal. (1) *Num* 13:7. (2) *2 Sam* 23:36
Igeal. *1 Chr* 3:22
Iim. (1) *Num* 33:45. (2) *Josh* 15:29
Ijeabarim. *Num* 21:11; 33:44
Ijon. *1 Ki* 15:20; *2 Ki* 15:29; *2 Chr* 16:4
Ikkesh. *2 Sam* 23:26; *1 Chr* 11:28; 27:9
Ilai. *1 Chr* 11:29
Imla. *1 Ki* 22:8, 9; *2 Chr* 18:7, 8
Immer. (1) *1 Chr* 9:12; *Ezra* 2:37; 10:20; *Neh* 7:40; 11:13. (2) *1 Chr* 24:14. (3) *Ezra* 2:59; *Neh* 7:61. (4) *Neh* 3:29. (5) *Jer* 20:1
Imna. *1 Chr* 7:35
Imnah. (1) *1 Chr* 7:30. (2) *2 Chr* 31:14
Imrah. *1 Chr* 7:36
Imri. (1) *1 Chr* 9:4. (2) *Neh* 3:2
Ir. *1 Chr* 7:12
Iram. *Gen* 36:43; *1 Chr* 1:54
Iri. *1 Chr* 7:7
Irnahash. *1 Chr* 4:12
Irpeel. *Josh* 18:27
Irshemesh. *Josh* 19:41
Iru. *1 Chr* 4:15
Iscah. *Gen* 11:29
Ishbah. *1 Chr* 4:17
Ishbak. *Gen* 25:2; *1 Chr* 1:32
Ishbibenoh. *2 Sam* 21:16
Ishi. (1) *1 Chr* 2:31. (2) *1 Chr* 4:20. (3) *1 Chr* 4:42. (4) *1 Chr* 5:24. (5) *Hos* 2:16
Ishiah. (1) *1 Chr* 7:3. (2) *1 Chr* 24:21. (3) *1 Chr* 24:25. (4) *Ezra* 10:31
Ishma. *1 Chr* 4:3
Ishmaiah. *1 Chr* 27:19
Ishmerai. *1 Chr* 8:18
Ishod. *1 Chr* 7:18
Ishpan. *1 Chr* 8:22
Ishtob. *2 Sam* 10:6, 8
Ishuah. *Gen* 46:17; *1 Chr* 7:30
Ishui. (1) *Gen* 46:17; *Num* 26:44; *1 Chr* 7:30. (2) *1 Sam* 14:49
Ismachiah. *2 Chr* 31:13
Ismaiah. *1 Chr* 12:4
Ispah. *1 Chr* 8:16
Ithai. *1 Chr* 11:31
Ithmah. *1 Chr* 11:46
Ithnan. *Josh* 15:23
Ithra. *2 Sam* 17:25
Ithran. (1) *Gen* 36:26; *1 Chr* 1:41. (2) *1 Chr* 7:37
Ithream. *2 Sam* 3:5; *1 Chr* 3:3
Ittah-kazin. *Josh* 19:13
Ittai. *2 Sam* 15:19, 21, 22; 18:2, 5, 12
Izhar. *Ex* 6:18. 21; *Num* 3:19; 16:1; *1 Chr* 6:2, 18, 38; 23:12, 18
Izrahiah. *1 Chr* 7:3
Izri. *1 Chr* 25:11

JAAKAN. *Deut* 10:6; *1 Chr* 1:42
Jaakobah. *1 Chr* 4:36
Jaala. *Ezra* 2:56; *Neh* 7:58
Jaanai. *1 Chr* 5:12
Jaareoregim. *2 Sam* 21:19
Jaasau. *Ezra* 10:37
Jaasiel. (1) *1 Chr* 11:47. (2) *1 Chr* 27:21
Jaazer. *Num* 21:32; 32:35; *Josh* 13:25; 21:39; *2 Sam* 24:5; *1 Chr* 6:81; 26:31; *Jer* 48:32
Jaaziah. *1 Chr* 24:26, 27
Jaaziel. *1 Chr* 15:18
Jabneel. (1) *Josh* 15:11. (2) *Josh* 19:33
Jabneh. *2 Chr* 26:6
Jachan. *1 Chr* 5:13
Jada. *1 Chr* 2:28, 32
Jadau. *Ezra* 10:43
Jaddua. (1) *Neh* 10:21. (2) *Neh* 12:11, 22
Jadon. *Neh* 3:7
Jagur. *Josh* 15:21
Jahath. (1) *1 Chr* 4:2. (2) *1 Chr* 6:20, 43. (3) *1 Chr* 23:10, 11. (4) *1 Chr* 24:22. (5) *2 Chr* 32:12
Jahaziah. *Ezra* 10:15
Jahaziel. (1) *1 Chr* 12:4. (2) *1 Chr* 16:6. (3) *1 Chr* 23:19; 24:23. (4) *2 Chr* 20:14. (5) *Ezra* 8:5
Jahdai. *1 Chr* 2:47

Jahdiel. 1 Chr 5:24
Jahdo. 1 Chr 5:14
Jahleel. Gen 46:14; Num 26:26
Jahmai. 1 Chr 7:2
Jahzah. 1 Chr 6:78
Jahzeel. Gen 46:24; Num 26:48; 1 Chr 7:13
Jahzerah. 1 Chr 9:12
Jakim. (1) 1 Chr 8:19. (2) 1 Chr 24:12
Jalon. 1 Chr 4:17
Jamin. (1) Gen 46:10; Ex 6:15; Num 26:12; 1 Chr 4:24. (2) 1 Chr 2:27. (3) Neh 8:7
Jamlech. 1 Chr 4:34
Janoah. 2 Ki 15:29
Janohah. Josh 16:6, 7
Janum. Josh 15:53
Japhia. (1) Josh 10:3. (2) Josh 19:12. (3) 2 Sam 5:15; 1 Chr 3:7; 14:6
Japhlet. 1 Chr 7:32, 33
Japhleti. Josh 16:3
Japho. Josh 19:46
Jarah. 1 Chr 9:42
Jaresiah. 1 Chr 8:27
Jarha. 1 Chr 2:34, 35
Jarib. (1) 1 Chr 4:24. (2) Ezra 8:16. (3) Ezra 10:18
Jarmuth. (1) Josh 10:3, 5, 23; 12:11; 15:35; Neh 11:29. (2) Josh 21:29
Jaroah. 1 Chr 5:14
Jashen. 2 Sam 23:32
Jashobeam. (1) 1 Chr 11:11; 27:2. (2) 1 Chr 12:6
Jashub. (1) Num 26:24; 1 Chr 7:1. (2) Ezra 10:29
Jashubilehem. 1 Chr 4:22
Jathniel. 1 Chr 26:2
Jattir. Josh 15:48; 21:14; 1 Sam 30:27; 1 Chr 6:57
Jaziz. 1 Chr 27:31
Jearim. Josh 15:10
Jeaterai. 1 Chr 6:21
Jeberechiah. Isa 8:2
Jebus. Josh 18:16, 28; Judg 19:10, 11; 1 Chr 11:4, 5
Jecamiah. 1 Chr 3:18
Jecholiah. 2 Ki 15:2; 2 Chr 26:3
Jechonias. Mat 1:11, 12
Jedaiah. (1) 1 Chr 4:37. (2) Neh 3:10
Jedaiah. (1) 1 Chr 9:10; 24:7; Ezra 2:36; Neh 7:39. (2) Neh 11:10; 12:6, 19; Zech 6:10, 14. (3) Neh 12:7, 21
Jediael. (1) 1 Chr 7:6, 10, 11. (2) 1 Chr 11:45. (3) 1 Chr 12:20. (4) 1 Chr 26:2
Jedidah. 2 Ki 22:1
Jeezer. Num 26:30
Jehaleleel. (1) 1 Chr 4:16. (2) 2 Chr 29:12
Jehdeiah. (1) 1 Chr 24:20. (2) 1 Chr 27:30
Jehezekel. 1 Chr 24:16
Jehiah. 1 Chr 15:24
Jehiel. (1) 1 Chr 15:18, 20; 16:5. (2) 1 Chr 23:8; 29:8. (3) 1 Chr 27:32. (4) 2 Chr 21:2. (5) 2 Chr 29:14. (6) 2 Chr 31:13. (7) 2 Chr 35:8. (8) Ezra 8:9. (9) Ezra 10:2. (10) Ezra 10:21. (11) Ezra 10:26
Jehieli. 1 Chr 26:21, 22
Jehizkiah. 2 Chr 28:12
Jehoadah. 1 Chr 8:36
Jehoaddan. 2 Ki 14:2; 2 Chr 25:1
Jehohanan. (1) 1 Chr 26:3. (2) 2 Chr 17:15. (3) 2 Chr 23:1. (4) Ezra 10:28. (5) Neh 12:13. (6) Neh 12:42.
Jehoiarib. (1) 1 Chr 9:10. (2) 1 Chr 24:7
Jehonathan. (1) 1 Chr 27:25. (2) 2 Chr 17:8. (3) Neh 12:18
Jehoshabeath. 2 Chr 22:11
Jehosheba. 2 Ki 11:2
Jehozabad. (1) 2 Ki 12:21; 2 Chr 24:26. (2) 1 Chr 26:4. (3) 2 Chr 17:18
Jehozadak. 1 Chr 6:14, 15
Jehubbah. 1 Chr 7:34
Jehucal. Jer 37:3; 38:1
Jehud. Josh 19:45
Jehudi. Jer 36:14, 21, 23
Jehudijah. 1 Chr 4:18
Jehush. 1 Chr 8:39
Jeiel. (1) 1 Chr 5:7. (2) 1 Chr 9:35. (3) 1 Chr 11:44. (4) 1 Chr 15:18, 21; 16:5. (5) 2 Chr 20:14. (6) 2 Chr 26:11. (7) 2 Chr 29:13. (8) 2 Chr 35:9. (9) Ezra 8:13. (10) Ezra 10:43
Jekabzeel. Neh 11:25
Jekameam. 1 Chr 23:19; 24:23
Jekamiah. 1 Chr 2:41
Jekuthiel. 1 Chr 4:18
Jemima. Job 42:14
Jemuel. Gen 46:10; Ex 6:15
Jerah. Gen 10:26; 1 Chr 1:20
Jered. 1 Chr 4:18
Jeremai. Ezra 10:33
Jeremoth. (1) 1 Chr 8:14. (2) Ezra 10:26. (3) Ezra 10:27. (4) 1 Chr 23:23. (5) 1 Chr 25:22
Jeriah. 1 Chr 23:19; 24:23; 26:31
Jeribai. 1 Chr 11:46
Jeriel. 1 Chr 7:2
Jerioth. 1 Chr 2:18
Jeroham. (1) 1 Sam 1:1; 1 Chr 6:27, 34. (2) 1 Chr 8:27. (3) 1 Chr 9:8. (4) 1 Chr 9:12; Neh 11:12. (5) 1 Chr 12:7. (6) 1 Chr 27:22. (7) 2 Chr 23:1
Jeruel. 2 Chr 20:16
Jerusha. 2 Ki 15:33; 2 Chr 27:1
Jesaiah. (1) 1 Chr 3:21. (2) 1 Chr 25:3, 15. (3) 1 Chr 26:25. (4) Ezra 8:7. (5) Ezra 8:19. (6) Neh 11:7
Jeshanah. 2 Chr 13:19
Jesharelah. 1 Chr 25:14
Jeshebeah. 1 Chr 24:13
Jesher. 1 Chr 2:18
Jeshimon. (1) Num 21:20; 23:28. (2) 1 Sam 23:24; 26:1
Jeshishai. 1 Chr 5:14
Jeshohaiah. 1 Chr 4:36
Jesiah. (1) 1 Chr 12:6. (2) 1 Chr 23:20
Jesimiel. 1 Chr 4:36
Jesui. Num 26:44
Jether. (1) Judg 8:20. (2) 1 Ki 2:5, 32; 1 Chr 2:17. (3) 1 Chr 2:32. (4) 1 Chr 4:17. (5) 1 Chr 7:38
Jetheth. Gen 36:40; 1 Chr 1:51
Jethlah. Josh 19:42
Jetur. (1) Gen 25:15; 1 Chr 1:31. (2) 1 Chr 5:19
Jeuel. 1 Chr 9:6
Jeush. (1) Gen 36:5, 14, 18; 1 Chr 1:35. (2) 1 Chr 7:10. (3) 1 Chr 23:10, 11. (4) 2 Chr 11:19
Jeuz. 1 Chr 8:10
Jezaniah. Jer 40:8; 42:1
Jezer. Gen 46:24; Num 26:49; 1 Chr 7:13
Jeziah. Ezra 10:25
Jeziel. 1 Chr 12:3
Jezliah. 1 Chr 8:18
Jezoar. 1 Chr 4:7
Jezrahiah. Neh 12:42
Jibsam. 1 Chr 7:2
Jidlaph. Gen 22:22
Jimnah. Gen 46:17; Num 26:44
Jiphtah. Josh 15:43
Jiphthahel. Josh 19:14, 27
Joahaz. 2 Chr 34:8
Joatham. Mat 1:9
Jobab. (1) Gen 10:29; 1 Chr 1:23. (2) Gen 36:33, 34; 1 Chr 1:44, 45. (3) Josh 11:1. (4) 1 Chr 8:9. (5) 1 Chr 8:18
Jochebed. Ex 6:20; Num 26:59
Joed. Neh 11:7
Joelah. 1 Chr 12:7
Joezer. 1 Chr 12:6
Jogbehah. Num 32:35; Judg 8:11
Jogli. Num 34:22
Joha. (1) 1 Chr 8:16. (2) 1 Chr 11:45
Joiada. Neh 12:10, 11, 22; 13:28
Joiakim. Neh 12:10, 12, 26
Joiarib. (1) Ezra 8:16. (2) Neh 11:5. (3) Neh 11:10; 12:6, 19
Jokdeam. Josh 15:56
Jokim. 1 Chr 4:22
Jokmeam. 1 Chr 6:68
Jokneam. (1) Josh 12:22; 19:11; 21:34. (2) 1 Ki 4:12
Jokshan. Gen 25:2, 3; 1 Chr 1:32
Joktan. Gen 10:25, 26, 29; 1 Chr 1:19, 20, 23
Joktheel. (1) Josh 15:38. (2) 2 Ki 14:7
Jonan. Luke 3:30
Jonath-elem-rechokim. Ps 56 title
Jorah. Ezra 2:18
Jorai. 1 Chr 5:13
Jorkoam. 1 Chr 2:44
Josaphat. Mat 1:8
Joshah. 1 Chr 4:34
Joshaphat. 1 Chr 11:43
Joshaviah. 1 Chr 11:46
Joshbekashah. 1 Chr 25:4, 24
Josibiah. 1 Chr 4:35
Josiphiah. Ezra 8:10
Jotbah. 2 Ki 21:19
Jotbathah. Num 33:33, 34; Deut 10:7
Jozabad. (1) 1 Chr 12:4. (2) 1 Chr 12:20. (3) 2 Chr 31:13. (4) 2 Chr 35:9. (5) Ezra 8:33. (6) Ezra 10:22. (7) Ezra 10:23. (8) Neh 8:7. (9) Neh 11:16
Jozachar. 2 Ki 12:21
Jozadak. Ezra 3:2, 8; 5:2; 10:18; Neh 12:26
Jubal. Gen 4:21
Jucal. Jer 38:1
Judith. Gen 26:34
Julia, Rom 16:15
Julius Acts 27:1, 3
Junia. Rom 16:7
Jushab-hesed. 1 Chr 3:20

KABZEEL. Josh 15:21; 2 Sam 23:20; 1 Chr 11:22
Kadmiel. (1) Ezra 2:40; Neh 7:43. (2) Ezra 3:9. (3) Neh 9:4, 5; 10:9; 12:8, 24
Kallai. Neh 12:20
Kanah. (1) Josh 16:8; 17:9. (2) Josh 19:28
Karkaa. Josh 15:3
Karkor. Judg 8:10
Kartah. Josh 21:34
Kartan. Josh 21:32
Kattath. Josh 19:15
Kedemah. Gen 25:15; 1 Chr 1:31,
Kedemoth. (1) Deut 2:26. (2) Josh 13:18; 21:37; 1 Chr 6:79
Kedesh. (1) Josh 12:22; 19:37. (2) Josh 20:7; 21:32; Judg 4:6; 9:10, 11; 2 Ki 15:29; 1 Chr 6:76. (3) 1 Chr 6:72. (4) Josh 15:23
Kehelathah. Num 33:22, 23
Kelaiah. Ezra 10:23
Kelita. (1) Ezra 10:23. (2) Neh 8:7. (3) Neh 10:10
Kemuel. (1) Gen 22:21. (2) Num 34:24. (3) 1 Chr 27:17
Kenan. 1 Chr 1:2
Kenath. Num 32:42; 1 Chr 2:23
Keren-happuch. Job 42:14
Keros. Ezra 2:44; Neh 7:47
Kezia. Job 42:14
Keziz. Josh 18:21
Kibroth-hattaavah. Num 11:34, 35; 33:16, 17; Deut 9:22
Kibzaim. Josh 21:22
Kinah. Josh 15:22
Kirjath. Josh 18:28
Kirjath-arim. Ezra 2:25
Kirjath-baal. Josh 15:60; 18:14
Kirjath-huzoth. Num 22:39
Kirjath-sannah. Josh 15:49
Kirjath-sepher. Josh 15:15, 16; Judg 1:11, 12
Kishi. 1 Chr 6:44
Kishion. Josh 19:20; 21:28
Kishon. Judg 4:7, 13; 5:21; 1 Ki 18:40; Ps 83:9
Kithlish. Josh 15:40
Kitron. Judg 1:30
Koa. Ezek 23:23
Kolaiah. (1) Neh 11:7. (2) Jer 29:21
Kore. (1) 1 Chr 9:19; 26:1, 19. (2) 2 Chr 31:14
Koz. Ezra 2:61; Neh 7:63
Kushaiah. 1 Chr 15:17

LAADAH. *1 Chr* 4:21
Laadan. (1) *1 Chr* 7:26. (2) *1 Chr* 23:7, 8, 9; 26:21
Lael. *Num* 3:24
Lahad. *1 Chr* 4:2
Lahairoi. *Gen* 24:62; 25:11
Lahmam. *Josh* 15:40
Lahmi. *1 Chr* 20:5
Lakum. *Josh* 19:33
Lapidoth. *Judg* 4:4
Lasea. *Acts* 27:8
Lasha. *Gen* 10:19
Lasharon. *Josh* 12:18
Lebanah. *Ezra* 2:45; *Neh* 7:48
Lebaoth. *Josh* 15:32
Lebonah. *Judg* 21:19
Lecah. *1 Chr* 4:21
Lehabim. *Gen* 10:13; *1 Chr* 1:11
Lehi. *Judg* 15:9, 14, 19
Leshem. *Josh* 19:47
Letushim. *Gen* 25:3
Leummim. *Gen* 25:3
Libni. (1) *Ex* 6:17; *Num* 3:18; *1 Chr* 6:17, 20. (2) *1 Chr* 6:29.
Likhi. *1 Chr* 7:19
Linus. *2 Tim* 4:21
Lod. *1 Chr* 8:12; *Ezra* 2:33; *Neh* 7:37; 11:35
Lodebar. *2 Sam* 9:4, 5; 17:27
Lotan. *Gen* 36:20, 22, 29; *1 Chr* 1:38, 39
Lubims. *2 Chr* 12:3; 16:8; *Nah* 3:9
Lud. (1) *Gen* 10:22; *1 Chr* 1:17. (2) *Isa* 66:19; *Ezek* 27:10
Ludim. *Gen* 10:13; *1 Chr* 1:11
Luhith. *Isa* 15:5; *Jer* 48:5
Lycia. *Acts* 27:5

MAADAI. *Ezra* 10:34
Maadiah. *Neh* 12:5
Maai. *Neh* 12:36
Maaleh-acrabbim. *Josh* 15:3
Maarath. *Josh* 15:59
Maasiai. *1 Chr* 9:12
Maaz. *1 Chr* 2:27
Maaziah. (1) *1 Chr* 24:18. (2) *Neh* 10:8
Machbanai. *1 Chr* 12:13
Machbenah. *1 Chr* 2:49
Machi. *Num* 13:15
Machnadebai. *Ezra* 10:40
Madai. *Gen* 10:2; *1 Chr* 1:5
Madmannah. (1) *Josh* 15:31. (2) *1 Chr* 2:49
Madmenah. *Isa* 10:31
Madon. *Josh* 11:1; 12:19
Magbish. *Ezra* 2:30
Magdalene. *Mat* 27:56, 61; 28:1; *Mark* 15:40, 47; 16:1, 9; *Luke* 8:2; 24:10; *John* 19:25; 20:1, 18
Magdiel. *Gen* 36:43; *1 Chr* 1:54
Magor-missabib. *Jer* 20:3
Magpiash. *Neh* 10:20
Mahalah. *1 Chr* 7:18
Mahalath. (1) *Gen* 28:9. (2) *2 Chr* 11:8. (3) *Ps* 53 title; *Ps* 88 title
Mahanehdan. *Judg* 18:12
Maharai. *2 Sam* 23:28; *1 Chr* 11:30; 27:13
Mahath. (1) *1 Chr* 6:35; *2 Chr* 29:12. (2) *2 Chr* 31:13
Mahazioth. *1 Chr* 25:4, 30
Mahlah. *Num* 26:33; 27:1; 36:11; *Josh* 17:3
Mahli. (1) *Ex* 6:19; *Num* 3:20; *1 Chr* 6:19, 29; 23:21; 24:26, 28; *Ezra* 8:18. (2) *1 Chr* 6:47; 23:23; 24:30
Mahol. *1 Ki* 4:31
Makaz. *1 Ki* 4:9
Makheloth. *Num* 33:25, 26
Makkedah. *Josh* 10:10, 16, 17, 21, 28, 29; 12:16; 15:41
Maktesh. *Zeph* 1:11
Malachi. *Mal* 1:1
Malchiah. (1) *1 Chr* 6:40. (2) *1 Chr* 9:12; *Neh* 11:12. (3) *1 Chr* 24:9. (4) *Ezra* 10:25. (5) *Ezra* 10:25. (6) *Ezra* 10:31. (7) *Neh* 3:11. (8) *Neh* 3:14. (9) *Neh* 3:31. (10) *Neh* 8:4. (11) *Neh* 10:3; 12:42. (12) *Jer* 21:1; 38:1
Malchiel. *Gen* 46:17; *Num* 26:45; *1 Chr* 7:31
Malchiram. *1 Chr* 3:18
Maleleel. *Luke* 3:37
Malothi. *1 Chr* 25:4, 26
Malluch. (1) *1 Chr* 6:44. (2) *Ezra* 10:29. (3) *Ezra* 10:32. (4) *Neh* 10:4; 12:2. (5) *Neh* 10:27
Manahath. (1) *Gen* 36:23; *1 Chr* 1:40. (2) *1 Chr* 8:6
Maoch. *1 Sam* 27:2
Maon. (1) *Josh* 15:55; *1 Sam* 25:2. (2) *1 Chr* 2:45
Maralah. *Josh* 19:11
Mareshah. (1) *Josh* 15:44; *2 Chr* 11:8; 14:9, 10; 20:37; *Mi* 1:15. (2) *1 Chr* 2:42. (3) *1 Chr* 4:21
Maroth. *Mi* 1:12
Marsena. *Esth* 1:14
Maschil. *Ps* 32 title, and 42, 44, 45, 52, 53, 54, 55, 74, 78, 88, 89, 142
Mash. *Gen* 10:23
Mashal. *1 Chr* 6:74
Masrekah. *Gen* 36:36; *1 Chr* 1:47
Massa. *Gen* 25:14; *1 Chr* 1:30
Matred. *Gen* 36:39; *1 Chr* 1:50
Matri. *1 Sam* 10:21
Mattanah. *Num* 21:18, 19
Mattaniah. (1) *2 Ki* 24:17. (2) *1 Chr* 9:15; *2 Chr* 20:14; *Neh* 11:17, 22; 12:8, 25, 35. (3) *1 Chr* 25:4, 16. (4) *2 Chr* 29:13. (5) *Ezra* 10:26. (6) *Ezra* 10:27. (7) *Ezra* 10:30. (8) *Ezra* 10:37. (9) *Neh* 13:13
Mattatha. *Luke* 3:31
Mattathah. *Ezra* 10:33
Mattenai. (1) *Ezra* 10:33. (2) *Ezra* 10:37. (3) *Neh* 12:19
Matthan. *Mat* 1:15.
Matthat. (1) *Luke* 3:24. (2) *Luke* 3:29
Mattithiah. (1) *1 Chr* 9:31. (2) *1 Chr* 15:18, 21; 16:5. (3) *1 Chr* 25:3, 21. (4) *Ezra* 10:43. (5) *Neh* 8:4
Meah. *Neh* 3:1; 12:39
Mearah. *Josh* 13:4
Mebunnai. *2 Sam* 23:27
Medan. *Gen* 25:2; *1 Chr* 1:32
Medeba. *Num* 21:30; *Josh* 13:9, 16; *1 Chr* 19:7; *Isa* 15:2
Mehetabel. (1) *Gen* 36:39; *1 Chr* 1:50. (2) *Neh* 6:10
Mehida. *Ezra* 2:52; *Neh* 7:54
Mehir. *1 Chr* 4:11
Mehujael. *Gen* 4:18
Mehuman. *Esth* 1:10
Mehunim. *Ezra* 2:50; *Neh* 7:52
Mejarkon. *Josh* 19:46
Mekonah. *Neh* 11:28
Melatiah. *Neh* 3:7
Melchishua. *1 Sam* 14:49; 31:2; *1 Chr* 8:33; 9:39; 10:2
Melea. *Luke* 3:31
Melech. *1 Chr* 8:35; 9:41
Melicu. *Neh* 12:14
Melita. *Acts* 28:1
Melzar. *Dan* 1:11, 16
Menan. *Luke* 3:31
Meonenim. *Judg* 9:37
Meonothai. *1 Chr* 4:14
Mephaath. *Josh* 13:18; 21:37; *1 Chr* 6:79; *Jer* 48:21
Meraiah. *Neh* 12:12
Meraioth. (1) *1 Chr* 6:6, 7, 52; *Ezra* 7:3. (2) *1 Chr* 9:11; *Neh* 11:11. (3) *Neh* 12:15
Merathaim. *Jer* 50:21
Mered. *1 Chr* 4:17, 18
Meremoth. (1) *Ezra* 8:33; *Neh* 3:4, 21. (2) *Ezra* 10:36. (3) *Neh* 10:5; 12:3
Meres. *Esth* 1:14
Meribbaal. *1 Chr* 8:34; 9:40
Merodath-baladan. *2 Ki* 20:12; *Isa* 39:1
Mesha. (1) *Gen* 10:30. (2) *2 Ki* 3:4. (3) *1 Chr* 2:42. (4) *1 Chr* 8:9
Meshelemiah. *1 Chr* 9:21; 26:1, 2, 9
Meshezabeel. (1) *Neh* 3:4. (2) *Neh* 10:21; 11:24
Meshillemith. *1 Chr* 9:12
Meshillemoth. (1) *2 Chr* 28:12. (2) *Neh* 11:13
Meshobab. *1 Chr* 4:34
Meshullam. (1) *2 Ki* 22:3. (2) *1 Chr* 3:19. (3) *1 Chr* 5:13. (4) *1 Chr* 8:17. (5) *1 Chr* 9:7. (6) *1 Chr* 9:8. (7) *1 Chr* 9:11; *Neh* 11:11. (8) *1 Chr* 9:12. (9) *2 Chr* 34:12. (10) *Ezra* 8:16. (11) *Ezra* 10:15. (12) *Ezra* 10:29. (13) *Neh* 3:4, 30; 6:18. (14) *Neh* 3:6. (15) *Neh* 8:4. (16) *Neh* 10:7. (17) *Neh* 10:20. (18) *Neh* 11:7. (19) *Neh* 12:13, 33. (20) *Neh* 12:16. (21) *Neh* 12:25
Meshullemeth. *2 Ki* 21:19
Mezahab. *Gen* 36:39; *1 Chr* 1:50
Miamin. (1) *Ezra* 10:25. (2) *Neh* 12:5
Mibhar. *1 Chr* 11:38
Mibsam. (1) *Gen* 25:13; *1 Chr* 1:29. (2) *1 Chr* 4:25
Mibzar. *Gen* 36:42; *1 Chr* 1:53
Micha. (1) *2 Sam* 9:12. (2) *Neh* 10:11. (3) *Neh* 11:17, 22
Michmas. *Ezra* 2:27; *Neh* 7:31
Michmash. *1 Sam* 13:2, 5, 11, 16, 23; 14:5, 31; *Neh* 11:31; *Isa* 10:28
Michmethah. *Josh* 16:6; 17:7
Michri. *1 Chr* 9:8
Michtam. *Ps* 16 title, and 56, 57, 58, 59, 60
Middin. *Josh* 15:61
Migdalel. *Josh* 19:38
Migdalgad. *Josh* 15:37
Migdol. (1) *Ex* 14:2; *Num* 33:7. (2) *Jer* 44:1; 46:14
Migron. *1 Sam* 14:2; *Isa* 10:28
Mijamin. (1) *1 Chr* 24:9. (2) *Neh* 10:7
Mikloth. (1) *1 Chr* 8:32; 9:37, 38. (2) *1 Chr* 27:4
Mikneiah. *1 Chr* 15:18, 21
Milalai. *Neh* 12:36
Miniamin. (1) *2 Chr* 31:15. (2) *Neh* 12:17, 41
Minni. *Jer* 51:27
Minnith. *Judg* 11:33; *Ezek* 27:17
Miphkad. *Neh* 3:31
Mirma. *1 Chr* 8:10
Misgab. *Jer* 48:1
Misham. *1 Chr* 8:12
Misheal. *Josh* 19:26; 21:30
Mishma. *Gen* 25:14; *1 Chr* 1:30; 4:25, 26
Mishmannah. *1 Chr* 12:10
Mispereth. *Neh* 7:7
Misrephothmaim. *Josh* 11:8; 13:6
Mithcah. *Num* 33:28, 29
Mithredath. (1) *Ezra* 1:8. (2) *Ezra* 4:7
Mitylene. *Acts* 20:14
Mizpar. *Ezra* 2:2
Mizraim. *Gen* 10:6, 13; *1 Chr* 1:8, 11
Mizzah. *Gen* 36:13, 17; *1 Chr* 1:37
Moadiah. *Neh* 12:17
Moladah. *Josh* 15:26; 19:2; *1 Chr* 4:28; *Neh* 11:26
Molid. *1 Chr* 2:29
Moreh. (1) *Gen* 12:6; *Deut* 11:30. (2) *Judg* 7:1
Moreshethgath. *Mi* 1:14
Mosera. *Deut* 10:6
Moseroth. *Num* 33:30, 31
Moza. (1) *1 Chr* 2:46. (2) *1 Chr* 8:36, 37; 9:42, 43
Mozah. *Josh* 18:26
Muppim. *Gen* 46:21
Mushi. *Ex* 6:19; *Num* 3:20; *1 Chr* 6:19, 47; 23:21, 23; 24:26, 30
Muthlabben. *Ps* 9 title

NAAM. *1 Chr* 4:15
Naamah. (1) *Gen* 4:22. (2) *1 Ki* 14:21, 31; *2 Chr* 12:13. (3) *Josh* 15:41
Naarah. *1 Chr* 4:5, 6
Naarai. *1 Chr* 11:37
Naaran. *1 Chr* 7:28
Naarath. *Josh* 16:7
Nachon. *2 Sam* 6:6
Nachor. *Luke* 3:34
Nahaliel. *Num* 21:19
Nahallal. *Josh* 19:15; 21:35; *Judg* 1:30

Naham. 1 Chr 4:19
Nahamani. Neh 7:7
Naharai. 2 Sam 23:37; 1 Chr 11:39
Nahath. (1) Gen 36:13, 17; 1 Chr 1:37. (2) 1 Chr 6:26. (3) 2 Chr 31:13
Nahbi. Num 13:14
Nahshon, see Naashon, p. 447
Nahum. Nah 1:1
Naphish. (1) Gen 25:15; 1 Chr 1:31. (2) 1 Chr 5:19
Naphtuhim. Gen 10:13; 1 Chr 1:11
Narcissus. Rom 16:11
Nathan-melech. 2 Ki 23:11
Neah. Josh 19:13
Neariah. (1) 1 Chr 3:22, 23. (2) 1 Chr 4:42
Nebajoth. (1) Gen 25:13; 28:9; 36:3; 1 Chr 1:29. (2) Isa 60:7
Neballat. Neh 11:34
Nebushasban. Jer 39:13
Necho. 2 Chr 35:20, 22; 36:4
Nedabiah. 1 Chr 3:18
Neginah. Ps 4 title
Nehiloth. Ps 5 title
Nehum. Neh 7:7
Nehushta. 2 Ki 24:8
Neiel. Josh 19:27
Nekeb. Josh 19:33
Nekoda. (1) Ezra 2:48; Neh 7:50. (2) Ezra 2:60; Neh 7:62
Nemuel. (1) Num 26:9. (2) Num 26:12; 1 Chr 4:24
Nepheg. (1) Ex 6:21. (2) 2 Sam 5:15; 1 Chr 3:7; 14:6
Nephishesim. Neh 7:52
Nephthalim. Mat 4:13, 15; Rev 7:6
Nephtoah. Josh 15:9; 18:15
Nephusim. Ezra 2:50
Nergal-sharezer. Jer 39:3, 13
Neri. Luke 3:27
Netophah. Ezra 2:22; Neh 7:26
Netophathi. Neh 12:28
Neziah. Ezra 2:54; Neh 7:56
Nezib. Josh 15:43
Nibhaz. 2 Ki 17:31
Nibshan. Josh 15:62
Nicolas. Acts 6:5
Nimrah. Num 32:3
Nimrim. Isa 15:6; Jer 48:34
Nobah. (1) Num 32:42. (2. Name of place) Num 32:42; Judg 8:1
Nod. Gen 4:16
Nodab. 1 Chr 5:19
Nogah. 1 Chr 3:7; 14:6
Nohah. 1 Chr 8:2
Non. 1 Chr 7:27
Nophah. Num 21:30

OBAL. Gen 10:28
Oboth. Num 21:10, 11; 33:43, 44
Ohad. Gen 46:10; Ex 6:15
Ohel. 1 Chr 3:20
Omar. Gen 36:11, 15; 1 Chr 1:36
Omega. Rev 1:8, 11; 21:6; 22:13
Omer. Ex 16:16, 18, 22, 32, 33, 36
Onam. (1) Gen 36:23; 1 Chr 1:40. (2) 1 Chr 2:26, 28
Ono. (1) 1 Chr 8:12; Ezra 2:33; Neh 7:37; 11:35. (2) Neh 6:2
Ophni. Josh 18:24
Ophrah. (1) Josh 18:23; 1 Sam 13:17. (2) Judg 6:11, 24; 8:27, 32; 9:5. (3) 1 Chr 4:14
Oren. 1 Chr 2:25
Osee (Hosea). Rom 9:25
Othni. 1 Chr 26:7
Ozni. Num 26:16

PADAN. Gen 48:7
Padon. Ezra 2:44; Neh 7:47
Pahath-moab. (1) Ezra 2:6; 10:30; Neh 3:11; 7:11. (2) Ezra 8:4. (3) Neh 10:14
Pai. 1 Chr 1:50
Palal. Neh 3:25
Pallu. Gen 46:9; Ex 6:14; Num 26:5, 8; 1 Chr 5:3
Palti. Num 13:9
Paltiel. (1) Num 34:26; (2) 2 Sam 3:15
Parah. Josh 18:23
Parmashta. Esth 9:9
Parnach. Num 34:25
Parosh. (1) Ezra 2:3; Neh 7:8. (2) Ezra 8:3. (3) Ezra 10:25. (4) Neh 3:25. (5) Neh 10:14
Parshandatha. Esth 9:7
Paruah. 1 Ki 4:17
Parvaim. 2 Chr 3:6
Pasach. 1 Chr 7:33
Pasdammim. 1 Chr 11:13
Paseah. (1) 1 Chr 4:12. (2) Ezra 2:49; Neh 7:51. (3) Neh 3:6
Pathrusim. Gen 10:14; 1 Chr 1:12
Patrobas. Rom 16:14
Pedahel. Num 34:28
Pedahzur. Num 1:10; 2:20; 7:54, 59; 10:23
Pedaiah. (1) 2 Ki 23:36. (2) 1 Chr 3:18, 19. (3) 1 Chr 27:20. (4) Neh 3:25. (5) Neh 8:4; 13:13. (6) Neh 11:7
Pekod. Jer 50:21; Ezek 23:23
Pelaiah. (1) 1 Chr 3:24. (2) Neh 8:7. (3) Neh 10:10
Pelaliah. Neh 11:12
Peleg. Gen 10:25; 11:16, 17, 18, 19; 1 Chr 1:19, 25
Pelet. (1) 1 Chr 2:47. (2) 1 Chr 12:3
Peleth. (1) Num 16:1. (2) 1 Chr 2:33
Peninnah. 1 Sam 1:2, 4
Peresh. 1 Chr 7:16
Perezuzzah. 2 Sam 6:8; 1 Chr 13:11
Perida. Neh 7:57
Peruda. Ezra 2:55
Pethahiah. (1) 1 Chr 24:16. (2) Ezra 10:23. (3) Neh 9:5. (4) Neh 11:24
Pethor. Num 22:5; Deut 23:4
Pethuel. Joel 1:1
Peulthai. 1 Chr 26:5
Phalti. 1 Sam 25:44
Phanuel. Luke 2:36
Phibeseth. Ezek 30:17
Phichol. Gen 21:22, 32; 26:26
Philemon. Philem 1
Phut. (1) Gen 10:6; 1 Chr 1:8. (2) Ezek 27:10. (3) Nah 3:9
Phuvah. (1) Gen 46:13; Num 26:23; 1 Chr 7:1. (2) Judg 10:1
Pildash. Gen 22:22
Pileha. Neh 10:24
Piltai. Neh 12:17
Pinon. Gen 36:41; 1 Chr 1:52
Piram. Josh 10:3
Pirathon. Judg 12:15
Pison. Gen 2:11
Pithom. Ex 1:11
Pithon. 1 Chr 8:35; 9:41
Pochereth. Ezra 2:57; Neh 7:59
Poratha. Esth 9:8
Prisca. See Priscilla
Prochorus. Acts 6:5
Ptolemais. Acts 21:7
Punon. Num 33:42, 43
Putiel. Ex 6:25

RAAMAH. (1) Gen 10:7; 1 Chr 1:9. (2) Ezek 27:22
Raamiah. Neh 7:7
Raamses. Ex 1:11
Rabbith. Josh 19:20
Rabmag. Jer 39:3, 13
Rabsaris. (1) Jer 39:3, 13. (2) 2 Ki 18:17
Rachal. 1 Sam 30:29
Raddai. 1 Chr 2:14
Raguel. Num 10:29
Raham. 1 Chr 2:44
Rakem. 1 Chr 7:16
Rakkath. Josh 19:35
Rakkon. Josh 19:46
Ramath. Josh 19:8
Ramathaim-zophim. 1 Sam 1:1
Ramathlehi. Judg 15:17
Ramathmizpeh. Josh 13:26
Rameses. Gen 47:11; Ex 12:37; Num 33:3, 5
Ramiah. Ezra 10:25
Reaiah. (1) 1 Chr 4:2. (2) 1 Chr 5:5. (3) Ezra 2:47; Neh 7:50
Reba. Num 31:8; Josh 13:21
Rechah. 1 Chr 4:12
Reelaiah. Ezra 2:2
Regem. 1 Chr 2:47
Regemmelech. Zech 7:2
Rehabiah. 1 Chr 23:17; 24:21; 26:25
Rehob. (1) Num 13:21; Josh 19:28, 30; 21:31; Judg 1:31; 2 Sam 10:8; 1 Chr 6:75. (2) 2 Sam 8:3, 12. (3) Neh 10:11
Rei. 1 Ki 1:8
Rekem. (1) Num 31:8; Josh 13:21 (2) 1 Chr 2:43, 44. (3) Josh 18:27
Remeth. Josh 19:21
Remmon. Josh 19:7
Remmon-methoar. Josh 19:13
Rephael. 1 Chr 26:7
Rephah. 1 Chr 7:25
Rephaiah. (1) 1 Chr 3:21. (2) 1 Chr 4:42. (3) 1 Chr 7:2. (4) 1 Chr 9:43. (5) Neh 3:9
Resen. Gen 10:12
Resheph. 1 Chr 7:25
Reu. Gen 11:18, 19, 20, 21; 1 Chr 1:25
Reuel. (1) Gen 36:4, 10, 13, 17; 1 Chr 1:35, 37. (2) Ex 2:18. (3) Num 2:14. (4) 1 Chr 9:8
Reumah. Gen 22:24
Rezeph. 2 Ki 19:12; Isa 37:12
Rezia. 1 Chr 7:39
Rezon. 1 Ki 11:23
Ribai. 2 Sam 23:29; 1 Chr 11:31
Riblah. Num 34:11; 2 Ki 23:33; 25:6, 21; Jer 39:5, 6; 52:9, 10, 26, 27
Rimmon-parez. Num 33:19, 20
Rinnah. 1 Chr 4:20
Riphath. Gen 10:3; 1 Chr 1:6
Rissah. Num 33:21, 22
Rithmah. Num 33:18, 19
Rogelim. 2 Sam 17:27; 19:31
Rohgah. 1 Chr 7:34
Romanti-ezer. 1 Chr 25:4, 31
Rumah. 2 Ki 23:36

SABTAH. Gen 10:7; 1 Chr 1:9
Sabtecha. Gen 10:7; 1 Chr 1:9
Sacar. (1) 1 Chr 11:35. (2) 1 Chr 26:4
Sadoc. Mat 1:14
Sala, Salah. Gen 10:24; 11:12, 13, 14, 15; Luke 3:35
Salamis. Acts 13:5
Salchah. Deut 3:10; Josh 12:5; 13:11; 1 Chr 5:11
Salim. Josh 3:23
Sallai. (1) Neh 11:8. (2) Neh 12:20
Sallu. (1) Neh 12:7. (2) 1 Chr 9:7; Neh 11:7
Salma. 1 Chr 2:51, 54
Samgar-nebo. Jer 39:3
Samlah. Gen 36:36, 37; 1 Chr 1:47, 48
Samos. Acts 20:15
Samothracia. Acts 16:11
Sansannah. Josh 15:31
Saph. 2 Sam 21:8
Saraph. 1 Chr 4:22
Sargon. Isa 20:1
Sarid. Josh 19:10, 12
Sarsechim. Jer 39:3
Sebat. Zech 1:7
Secacah. Josh 15:61
Sechu. 1 Sam 19:22
Secundus. Acts 20:4
Segub. (1) 1 Ki 16:34. (2) 1 Chr 2:21, 22
Seirath. Judg 3:26
Sela. 2 Ki 14:7; Isa 16:1
Sela-hammahlekoth. 1 Sam 23:28
Seled. 1 Chr 2:30
Sem. Luke 3:36
Semachiah. 1 Chr 26:7
Senaah. Ezra 2:35; Neh 7:38
Seneh. 1 Sam 14:4
Senir. 1 Chr 5:23; Ezek 27:5
Senuah. Neh 11:9
Seorim. 1 Chr 24:8
Sephar. Gen 10:30
Sepharad. Ob 20
Serah (Sarah). Gen 46:17; Num 26:46; 1 Chr 7:30
Sered. Gen 46:14; Num 26:26